SURGICAL PHARMACOLOGY OF THE EYE

Surgical Pharmacology of the Eye

Editors

Marvin L. Sears, M.D.
Professor and Chairman
Department of Ophthalmology
and Visual Science
Yale University School of Medicine
New Haven, Connecticut

Ahti Tarkkanen, M.D.
Associate Professor
Department of Ophthalmology
Eye Clinic
University Hospital of Helsinki
Helsinki, Finland

Raven Press ■ New York

Raven Press, 1140 Avenue of the Americas, New York, New York 10036

Made in the United States of America

Library of Congress Cataloging in Publication Data
Main entry under title:

Surgical pharmacology of the eye.

Based on a symposium organized at the Haikko
Estates in Porvoo, Finland in May 1984.
Includes bibliographies and index.
1. Eye—Surgery—Congresses. 2 Ocular pharmacology—Congresses. I. Sears, Marvin L., 1928–
II. Tarkkanen, Ahti. [DNLM: 1. Eye—surgery—
congresses. 2. Eye Diseases—therapy—congresses.
WW 168 S961 1984]
RE80.S85 1985   617.7'1   84-24974
ISBN 0-88167-047-2

The material contained in this volume was submitted as previously unpublished material, except in the instances in which credit has been given to the source from which some of the illustrative material was derived.

Great care has been taken to maintain the accuracy of the information contained in the volume. However, Raven Press cannot be held responsible for errors or for any consequences arising from the use of the information contained herein.

Second Printing, January 1986

Preface

Accessibility to important new biomedical and technical knowledge has had more than considerable impact on the ophthalmic surgeon. At the forefront of this information is the excitement and drama of extracapsular cataract surgery with implantation of a posterior chamber lens. Technical advances in surgery of the retina and vitreous as well as new ways of handling other ocular tissues are also being rapidly established. Still newer ones begin to appear. The ophthalmic arsenal of technology includes high quality optics that provide stereoscopic surgery, appropriate magnification, flexible systems of illumination that offer either coupled or separate light sources, the opportunity to observe structures deep within the eye, as well as the well known aspiration, cutting, and infusion devices. The development of such powerful instrumentation for surgery of the eye carries with it an invasiveness that threatens eye tissue. Even in "non-invasive" laser surgery protection of the treated tissues is essential.

Surgeons recognize that technical or bioengineering advances have been accompanied by striking progress in the development and application of old and new drugs that can be used to protect ocular tissues from trauma. The contributors to this volume wish to convey and consolidate this new knowledge for the ophthalmic surgeon. New information about the relationship of anesthesia, analgesia, antibiotics, and anti-inflammatory drugs to the eye patient as well as to the operating specifics of irrigating solutions, gases, and other useful drugs have been organized and are presented here in an effort to prevent, ameliorate, and treat damage done to the eye in the course of surgery. The receptor on the surface of ocular cells has been the conference room of the pharmacologist and the chemist, but, now, with information obtained from the basic scientist, the surgeon can deal more effectively with diseases of the eye with a newly acquired knowledge of the cellular basis of surgical trauma. Lessons from enzyme chemistry, especially the significance of enzyme inhibition as the basis of drug action, lessons from toxicology, and, from drug-receptor interaction, have been useful in the development and application of new compounds for clinical use. Several old and new substances and their methods of administration are important in the management of surgical patients.

The authors expect that *Surgical Pharmacology of the Eye* will produce improved understanding and treatment that will enhance still further the technical refinements of eye surgery.

Marvin L. Sears
Ahti Tarkkanen

Acknowledgments

A symposium organized at the Haikko Estates in Porvoo, Finland provided the forum for the discussion and development of the volume. The meeting was planned, organized, and implemented by Mr. George C. Andreassi and Mr. George Jamieson of Merck Sharp and Dohme and hosted by Merck Sharp Dohme Chibret. To these corporate people all of us owe our thanks and the editors are grateful for their collegiality and expertise.

Contents

Pharmacology of Specific Procedures

CONTENTS

Contributors

Thomas M. Aaberg, M.D.
Professor
Department of Ophthalmology
Director of Vitreal Retinal Service
Medical College of Wisconsin
8700 W. Wisconsin Avenue
Milwaukee, Wisconsin 53226

Daniel M. Albert, M.D.
Professor
Department of Ophthalmology
Director, Eye Pathology Laboratory
Harvard Medical School
Massachusetts Eye and Ear Infirmary
243 Charles Street
Boston, Massachusetts 02114

Joaquín Barraquer, M.D.
Professor
Instituto Barraquer
Laforja 88
Barcelona 21, Spain

Rafael I. Barraquer, M.D.
Instituto Barraquer
Laforja 88
Barcelona 21, Spain

Joseph Caprioli, M.D.
Assistant Professor
Department of Ophthalmology and
*   Visual Science*
Yale University School of Medicine
310 Cedar Street, P.O. Box 3333
New Haven, Connecticut 06510

Devron H. Char, M.D.
Ocular Oncology Unit
Department of Ophthalmology
University of California
San Francisco, California 94143

Manuel Datiles, M.D.
The Wilmer Institute
The Johns Hopkins Hospital
600 North Wolfe Street
Baltimore, Maryland 21205

Isabel DeLeon, M.D.
The Wilmer Institute
The Johns Hopkins Hospital
600 North Wolfe Street
Baltimore, Maryland 21205

David Denlinger, M.D.
The Wilmer Institute
The Johns Hopkins Hospital
600 North Wolfe Street
Baltimore, Maryland 21205

Henry F. Edelhauser, Ph.D.
Professor
Department of Physiology and
*   Ophthalmology*
Medical College of Wisconsin
8701 Watertown Plante Road
Milwaukee, Wisconsin 53226

Richard K. Forster, M.D.
Professor of Ophthalmology
Bascom Palmer Eye Institute
University of Miami School of Medicine
P.O. Box 016880
Miami, Florida 33101

Edmund Gerke, M.D.
University Eye Hospital
Hufelandstrasse 55
D 4300 Essen 1, Federal Republic of
*   Germany*

Nicholas M. Greene, M.D.
Professor
Department of Anesthesiology
Yale University School of Medicine
333 Cedar Street
New Haven, Connecticut 06510

F. Hoffmann, M.D.
Department of Ophthalmology
Klinikum Steglitz
Free University of Berlin
Hindenburgdamm 30
D 1000 Berlin 45, Federal Republic of
Germany

Lee M. Jampol, M.D.
Professor and Chairman
Department of Ophthalmology
Northwestern University School of
Medicine
303 E. Chicago Avenue
Chicago, Illinois 60611

Arthur Jampolsky, M.D.
Director
Smith-Kettlewell Institute of Visual
Sciences
2232 Webster Street
San Francisco, California 94115

Ali A. Khodadoust, M.D.
Professor
Department of Ophthalmology and
Visual Science
Yale University School of Medicine
310 Cedar Street, P.O. Box 3333
New Haven, Connecticut 06510

G. K. Krieglstein, M.D.
University Eye Hospital Würzburg
Kopfklinikum
Josef-Schneider-Strasse 11
D-8700 Würzburg, Federal Republic of
Germany

Leila Laatikainen, M.D.
Department of Ophthalmology
Helsinki University Central Hospital
Helsinki, 00290 Finland

Irving H. Leopold, M.D., D.Sc.
Professor Emeritus
Department of Ophthalmology
University of California, Irvine
College of Medicine
Irvine, California 92717

W. Leydhecker, M.D.
Director
University Eye Hospital Würzburg
Kopfklinikum
Josef-Schneider-Strasse 11
D-8700 Würzburg, Federal Republic of
Germany

Kanjiro Masuda, M.D.
Associate Professor
Department of Ophthalmology
University of Tokyo
School of Medicine
7-3-1 Hongo, Bunkyo-ku
Tokyo, Japan

Scott M. Mac Rae, M.D.
Assistant Professor
Department of Ophthalmology
University of Oregon
3181 S. W. Sam Jackson Park Road
Portland, Oregon 97201

Gerhard Meyer-Schwickerath, M.D.
Professor
University Eye Hospital
Hufelandstrasse 55
D-4300 Essen 1, Federal Republic of
Germany

Edward D. Miller, Jr., M.D.
Professor
Department of Anesthesiology
University of Virginia School of
Medicine
Box 238
Charlottesville, Virginia 22908

James E. Puklin, M.D.
Associate Professor
The Retina Study Center
Department of Ophthalmology and
Visual Science
Yale University School of Medicine
310 Cedar Street, P.O. Box 3333
New Haven, Connecticut 06510

Marvin L. Sears, M.D.
Professor and Chairman
Department of Ophthalmology and
*   Visual Science*
Yale University School of Medicine
310 Cedar Street, P.O. Box 3333
New Haven, Connecticut 06510

Walter J. Stark, M.D.
The Wilmer Ophthalmological Institute
The Johns Hopkins Hospital
600 North Wolfe Street
Baltimore, Maryland 21205

Johan Stjernschantz, M.D.
Star Pharmaceuticals
Niittyhaankatu 20
PL 33
33721 Tampere 72, Finland

Ahti Tarkkanen, M.D.
Associate Professor
Department of Ophthalmology
Eye Clinic
University Hospital of Helsinki
Haartmaninkatu 4 C
00290 Helsinki 29
Finland

Arlo C. Terry, M.D.
The Wilmer Ophthalmological Institute
The Johns Hopkins Hospital
600 North Wolfe Street
Baltimore, Maryland 21205

W. Frits Treffers, M.D.
Department of Ophthalmology
St. Radboud Hospital
15 Philips van Leydenlaan
Nijmegen, The Netherlands

Mark O. M. Tso, M.D.
Professor
Georgiana Theobald Ophthalmic
*   Pathology Laboratory*
University of Illinois
Eye and Ear Infirmary
1855 West Taylor Street
Chicago, Illinois 60612

Achim Wessing, M.D.
University Eye Hospital
Hufelandstrasse 55
D-4300 Essen 1, Federal Republic of
*   Germany*

M. Wiederholt, M.D.
Department of Clinical Physiology
Klinikum Steglitz
Free University of Berlin
Hindenburgdamm 30
D 1000 Berlin 45, Federal Republic of
*   Germany*

George A. Williams, M.D.
Department of Ophthalmology
Medical College of Wisconsin
8700 W. Wisconsin Avenue
Milwaukee, Wisconsin 53226

John J. Woog, M.D.
Department of Ophthalmology
Harvard Medical School
Massachusetts Eye and Ear Infirmary
243 Charles Street
Boston, Massachusetts 02114

SURGICAL PHARMACOLOGY OF THE EYE

Commentary

Anesthesia and Analgesia

Contemporary microsurgery has been accompanied by increased use of general anesthesia in adult as well as pediatric ophthalmic surgery. Surgeons frequently desire general anesthesia for their patients. For sedation and premedication there are hypnotics, pentobarbital, secobarbital or triclofos (Triclos®), tranquilizers, analgesics including morphine sulfate and fentanyl, and the anticholinergics. The latter are not used with modern anesthetic agents. Among the useful tranquilizers are diazepam, hydroxyzine, and droperidol. In children fear of separation from the parent is often great and may require a hypnotic dosage of one of the tranquilizing agents. The use of large doses results in prolonged sleep and requires careful postoperative care. If ketamine is to be used, glycopyrrolate may be an advantageous agent to dry secretions with less tachycardia. Unlike atropine or scopolamine glycopyrrolate does not cross the blood-brain barrier and produce central sedation. Sometimes premedication may be omitted if the parents can be allowed to come to the induction area.

Dr. Miller also addresses specific problems: the full stomach and open eye, the oculocardiac reflex, malignant hyperthermia, coughing and emesis, and intravitreal gas. In patients who may have recently had a meal, to prevent increase of intraocular pressure and/or aspiration of gastric contents the patient is given a nondepolarizing muscle relaxant and 45 sec later a large dose of thiobarbiturate is followed by intubation. This elegant method will certainly work in the hands of the expert but inducing neuromuscular blockade before anesthetic may be very hazardous in the hands of the occasional ophthalmic anesthesiologist. (Another way of handling this situation has been outlined in the chapter of J. E. Puklin. This includes the use of an antiemetic, such as droperidol intramuscularly, premedication, and intravenous lidocaine just prior to the intubation.) Neuromuscular blockade can be accomplished by one of the non-depolarizing agents that does not raise the intraocular pressure. Emesis after intraocular surgery may be annoying; Dr. Miller states that even small doses of droperidol (0.075 mg/kg) may be somewhat effective in preventing emesis. In a double-masked study it was recently shown that even 0.036 mg/kg may be effective in preventing vomiting (1). Intraocular pressure can be lowered during lens delivery or intraocular lens implantation by controlling (lowering) the $PaCO_2$ of the blood under general anesthesia. Neurosurgical anesthesiologists have long been aware of the value of hyperventilation. Respiratory alkalosis can shrink vascular components of the intracerebral volume. Hyperventilation results also decrease the intraocular pressure by reducing the choroidal volume. This procedure adds no further risks in experienced hands but is very helpful to the surgeon (2).

Without question success in ophthalmic surgery calls for close cooperation between ophthalmic surgeon and ophthalmic anesthesiologist.

The Editors

REFERENCES

1. Karhunen, U., and Orku, R. (1981): *Ophthalmic Surg.,* 12:810–822.
2. Smith, B. G. (1983): *Ophthalmic Anesthesia.* Edward Arnold, London.

Surgical Pharmacology of the Eye,
edited by M. Sears and A. Tarkkanen.
Raven Press, New York © 1985.

Anesthesia and Analgesia

Edward D. Miller, Jr.

*Department of Anesthesiology, University of Virginia School of Medicine,
Charlottesville, Virginia 22908*

SUMMARY: The primary aim of sedation should be to render the patient relaxed, ie., calm, but not unconscious. To produce this relaxed state, a primary element is the preoperative visit by the anesthesiologist. In children, few surgical operations can be done under local anesthesia. The routine use of premedication is questionable and, therefore, the need for an injection can be eliminated. If the child is uncooperative then oral premedication with triclofos (70 mg/kg), 2 hr prior to surgery, will result in an extremely sleepy child in whom a mask induction can then be performed. In adults, excellent analgesia of the eye and related structures can be obtained with local anesthetics. Therefore, many operations can be done without general anesthesia. For patients under local anesthesia either reassurance or a small amount of diazepam orally may be adequate. The older patient requires less preoperative medication. The more premedicants used, the greater the possibility of prolonged or delayed recovery.

General anesthesia for children or adults can be accomplished with a barbiturate induction and then maintained with a potent inhalational agent (e.g. halothane, enflurane, isoflurane). If an endotracheal tube is necessary, then the use of a muscle relaxant is often necessary. Succinylcholine transiently increases intraocular pressure and is not indicated in a patient with an open eye. The nondepolarizing muscle relaxants (e.g. curare, pancuronium) do not increase intraocular pressure. Intraocular pressure can be increased if certain gases are introduced into the eye while nitrous oxide is being administered. Other major concerns include recognition of malignant hyperthermia, prevention of coughing or vomiting, and prevention and treatment of oculocardiac reflexes.

Anesthetic agents and techniques are now available that provide excellent conditions for surgery of the eye. Communication between the surgeon and anesthesiologist will determine the best choice for each patient.

The ophthalmologist often requires the use of anesthetics to perform either examinations of the eye or surgical procedures on or about the eye. The needs of the surgeon may be met by either local or general anesthetics. The choice of which to use is a decision best arrived at by a discussion between the anesthesiologist and the surgeon. Several factors are important in that choice, including the pharmacologic properties of the agents available. The purpose of this chapter is to review the pharmacology of general anesthetics used in such a manner as to provide optimal operating conditions with the least risk to the patient. Since space prevents full discussion of all aspects of general anesthetics used for all types of ophthalmologic operations, emphasis is focused on the more common surgical procedures. Because of the great differences in dose, techniques, and types of procedures, the pediatric patient and the adult patient are discussed separately.

SEDATION AND PREMEDICATION

Pediatric

Most anesthesiologists agree that a satisfactory preoperative visit to the pediatric patient is more helpful in allaying anxiety than most of the drugs that are available. The young child who is able to identify with the anesthesiologist and surgeon prior to the surgical procedure does not view the experience as one of impending danger. Unfortunately, many circumstances, including the maturity of the child, may prevent a satisfactory preoperative visit. Furthermore, with some anesthetic techniques, the need to minimize secretions is necessary. The anesthesiologist must then choose between several types of premedicants that may sedate the child adequately. The aim of preoperative medication should be to diminish anxiety and to reduce secretions as necessary. Since there is not universal agreement on the best medication for children, any medication will, by necessity, be an individual matter. However, it should be stressed that preoperative medication that renders a child unconscious may be dangerous even if adequately monitored. Adequate surgical anesthesia should not be the goal of preoperative medication; rather, the goal is one of a calm, sleepy child.

Agents available for sedation in the child include hypnotics, tranquilizers, analgesics, and anticholinergics. Since any of these agents may alter the state of consciousness, attention should be given to when the last solids and liquids were ingested. Recommendations vary, but many feel that, in children, no solids or milk should be ingested 8 hr prior to induction of anesthesia. Clear liquids should be withheld 6 hr prior to induction in children over 1 year old. Children under 1 year of age are allowed clear liquids up until 4 hr prior to induction. These are conservative guidelines and err on the side of safety.

The timing of premedication is extremely important. At least 1 hr needs to elapse between the time of the premedication and the arrival of the child in the operating room suite. Hypnotics, e.g., secobarbital and pentobarbital, in 2- to 4-mg/kg dosage may be given orally or intramuscularly. Both have relatively long half-lives, and their effects may persist for several hours postoperatively (9). Secobarbital has a slightly shorter half-life than pentobarbital, but as a premedicant, this difference is not clinically significant. Hypnotics provide no analgesia and may even have antianalgesic properties. The disadvantage of long sleeping times and the necessity of intramuscular injection for adequate uptake may make hypnotics less than optimal. Triclofos sodium

(Triclos®, 50 to 70 mg/kg), a derivative of chloral hydrate, is an effective premedicant in children when given orally. However, in large quantities, triclofos has a variable absorption from the GI tract and may induce vomiting shortly after ingestion. Whether vomiting results from the drug or the carrier is unclear, but oral premedication may result in vomiting because of the irritant effects when given on an empty stomach. Once the premedication has been vomited, repeating of the dose is not indicated.

Tranquilizers have been used to circumvent some of the problems associated with hypnotics. The most commonly used parenteral agents are diazepam (Valium®) 0.2 mg/kg, hydroxyzine (Vistaril®) 0.5 to 1 mg/kg, and droperidol (Inapsine®) 0.1 mg/kg. Each of these agents has been used with some degree of success in children. However, the fear of separation from parent is great and is not diminished unless hypnotic doses of the agents are used. The use of the large doses results in prolonged sleeping times.

Parenteral analgesics, e.g., morphine sulfate (0.1 to 0.2 mg/kg) and meperidine (Demerol®) hydrochloride (1 to 2 mg/kg), produce the most reliable degree of sedation. This is due to the consistent absorption of the drug when given intramuscularly. Although the advantages of narcotics are obvious, the nausea and vomiting that are commonly seen with narcotics often make them undesirable in the preoperative and postoperative periods. A child with a potential open-eye injury could suffer severe eye damage if vomiting occurred prior to the induction of anesthesia. Furthermore, an intramuscular injection is often so upsetting to a child that the injection itself may defeat the purpose of giving this type of premedication.

Anticholinergics are often given as a routine medication prior to any general anesthetic, especially in children. This stems partly from the older types of anesthetics that cause copious secretions. Currently used general anesthetics do not have this unfavorable side effect. However, ketamine, an injectable anesthetic to be discussed later, does produce secretions. If ketamine is to be used, an anticholinergic must be given either orally or intramuscularly. Atropine (0.02 mg/kg, p.o.) is most frequently used, but glycopyrrolate (0.02 mg/kg, p.o.) may be advantageous in causing more intense drying with less tachycardia (16). Scopolamine hydrobromide, in contrast to the other agents, crosses the blood-brain barrier and produces central sedation. The resulting long-term sedation from this agent often makes it less desirable. All of the anticholinergic agents help prevent the bradycardia seen with halothane anesthesia or when succinylcholine is administered. It is also helpful in preventing the oculocardiac reflex. Some authorities believe that prevention of bradycardia is crucial in children to maintain normal cardiac output.

Each premedicant has disadvantages. With short surgical procedures, the somnolence in the postoperative period resulting from preoperative medication may prevent early discharge from the recovery room or from the hospital. With increasing familiarity with modern anesthetic techniques and the use of ambulatory surgical facilities, more emphasis is placed on the personal approach for sedation, rather than on one that uses drugs exclusively. Because of the need to employ less premedication, several institutions are recognizing the value of allowing parents to accompany the child to the operative suite. Anesthetic induction may then be accomplished without the need for premedication, since separation of child from parent does not occur.

Adults

Preoperative preparation of adults also relies on establishing good rapport with the patient. More and more patients are now requesting no preoperative medication prior to general anesthesia, whereas others demand a premedicant. As in the pediatric patient, the same types of medications are possible. However, since the majority of adult operations on the eye involve patients over 60 years of age, special problems need to be considered.

Many adult patients routinely rely on hypnotics to aid sleeping. When these patients receive a standard dose of 100 mg secobarbital or pentobarbital, little sedation may result. That this is due to tolerance to the drug seems likely, but definitive proof is not available to substantiate this. One of the advantages of hypnotics is the absence of significant cardiovascular effects. Blood pressure and heart rate are minimally depressed and approach patterns normally seen during sleep. The barbiturates minimally depress respiration in the normal doses employed and protective reflexes are maintained. Barbiturates have been proved to be reliable premedicants in adults. Unfortunately, drowsiness may persist for some time, and patients often complain of headache or, more commonly, a "hangover." Indeed, standard doses of barbiturates result in subtle but important disturbances in mood, judgment, and fine motor skills for as long as 24 hr. Also, sedation does not always result when barbiturates are used. Paradoxical excitement and antianalgesic effects may result and make preoperative or postoperative management difficult.

Tranquilizers are frequently used as premedicants in adults, especially the benzodiazepines. More than 2,000 benzodiazepines have been synthesized and more than 100 of these tested. The major advantage of benzodiazepines is their ability to produce sedation, decrease anxiety, and produce muscle relaxation. Oral diazepam (Valium®, 5 to 10 mg) is effective. The intramuscular route can be used but produces less predictable blood levels and is painful. Some patients may remain somnolent preoperatively for relatively long periods, but this effect can be reversed by small (1-mg) doses of physostigmine. Physostigmine is an anticholinesterase agent that crosses the blood-brain barrier and results in central stimulation. If given in large doses, physostigmine increases the incidence of nausea and vomiting (4). Lorazepam (Ativan®) has also been used, but long periods of sedation occur more frequently. Droperidol (2.5 to 5.0 mg, intramuscularly) produces 6 to 12 hr of sedation but may also produce restlessness and extrapyramidal dyskinesia (17). Droperidol, however, decreases nausea and vomiting and therefore may be useful prophylactically when postoperative vomiting would be injurious to the eye.

Narcotics should not be frequently used as a premedicant for eye surgery. The use of local anesthetics in and around the eye allows postoperative pain to be kept to a minimum. Morphine has a long half-life (4 to 6 hr), causes respiratory depression, and may induce nausea and vomiting. Meperidine (Demerol®, 50 to 100 mg) and other narcotics have disadvantages similar to those of morphine.

Anticholinergics are also frequently given to adult surgical patients. Not only are secretions decreased but patients with a tendency for bronchospasm may be aided by the bronchodilating properties of anticholinergics (7). However, in patients with undiagnosed angle-closure glaucoma, anticholinergics may precipitate an increase in intraocular pressure with some of these agents. Atropine is safe in patients with open-angle glaucoma and in patients with acute closure glaucoma who are in remission (19). However, scopolamine produces a greater degree of mydriasis than atropine and therefore increases risk of acute glaucoma. The greater anticholinergic potency of scopolamine may reflect the relative pharmacologic inactivity of the *d*-hyoscyamine that is found in atropine (*dl*-hyoscyamine) (8). If inhibition of secretion is necessary, atropine or glycopyrrolate is preferred to scopolamine.

GENERAL ANESTHESIA

General anesthesia is almost mandatory for the pediatric patient. Attempts to use larger amounts of sedatives instead of general anesthesia often result in sudden, unexpected movements that could be disastrous. Similarly, the adult patient who suddenly awakens during an eye procedure or who coughs can do irreparable eye damage.

The choice of anesthetic agents depends on the type of surgery required, the length of the procedure, and the age and physical status of the patient. For the young child scheduled for an examination of the eye, inhalation anesthesia using nitrous oxide and a potent agent such as halothane with an anesthesia mask is often sufficient for a good eye examination. At the end of the procedure, anesthetic agents are rapidly eliminated, and the patient, who recovers equally rapidly, may be discharged within a short time if cared for in an outpatient setting. The fewer the agents needed for sedation and for induction and maintenance of general anesthesia, the more rapidly a child awakens. For the adult patient, with a larger lung capacity, a mask induction would be unpleasant and may result in undue cardiovascular depression. Intravenous agents that produce unconsciousness are preferred by most adults for the induction of general anesthesia. This requires the establishment of an intravenous route, since most of these agents cause local tissue damage if not injected intravenously.

The most commonly used induction agents are the barbiturates. In the smaller child (less than 4 years old), where an intravenous route may not be readily available, rectal methohexital sodium (Brevital Sodium®, 30 mg/kg) produces unconsciousness in 5 to 10 min in 95% of patients. For the child in whom an intravenous route is available, and for most adults, sodium thiopental (3 mg/kg) intravenously is particularly popular. Thiopental, however, lowers intraocular pressure, as well as producing some degree of cardiovascular and respiratory depression (5). Thiopental and other thiobarbiturates produce rapid loss of consciousness because of the rapid equilibration of the drug within the brain. Use of these agents to maintain a state of drowsiness, however, is fraught with danger (e.g., prolonged central nervous system, cardiovascular, and respiratory depression). Barbiturates are known to cause acute tolerance. After a single dose of barbiturate, the plasma concentration on awakening may be higher than when sleep ensued. After a second dose, a higher level is required to reestablish sleep than with the first dose. Therefore, when using a thiobarbiturate as a sedative, instead of as a hypnotic, large quantities of the drug may be given for greatly prolonged degrees of sedation.

Etomidate is a recently released hypnotic with less cardiovascular and respiratory depression than thiopental. Though it can cause pain on injection, as well as myoclonic movements, newer formulations have diminished, but not eliminated, the incidence of these side effects. Awakening times are similar to those seen with thiopental (6).

Ketamine has often been used for induction of anesthesia in children, in part because it is effective either intravenously or intramuscularly. A struggling child, given 5 to 7 mg/kg of ketamine in the deltoid muscle, can be taken to the operating room rapidly and general anesthesia begun. However, ketamine causes copious secretions, and unless an anticholinergic has been given, coughing and laryngospasm may present real hazards to the patient. Initial reports that ketamine caused an increase in intraocular pressure have not been substantiated (3). However, ketamine, because it may cause nystagmus and blepharospasm may therefore not be a suitable agent for many ophthalmologic procedures.

For the older patient with compromised cardiovascular function, induction with diazepam may be indicated. Since diazepam causes less cardiovascular depression than thiopental, selected patients may benefit from this type of induction (18). The long half-life of the drug makes early recovery sometimes difficult if large doses have been used.

Once induction has been accomplished, maintenance of stable general anesthesia for the best surgical field is required. Except for brief eye examinations, general anesthesia requires the use of an endotracheal tube. This is required to give adequate surgical exposure, with the anesthesiologist removed from the surgical field. It also assures a clear airway for adequate artificial ventilation when needed during anesthesia and surgery. If ductal irrigation is part of the surgical procedure, tracheal intubation means that the irrigating solution can be removed from the posterior pharynx without the risk of laryngospasm or aspiration.

For the young child, the placement of an endotracheal tube can be done with the use of potent anesthetic agents alone. With older children or adults and patients with a potentially open eye, muscle relaxants are necessary for placement of an endotracheal tube without coughing or straining. Much has been written about the use of muscle relaxants in eye surgery. Most studies show that succinylcholine increases intraocular pressure because of sustained contraction of the extraocular muscles. Extrusion of vitreous after the use of succinylcholine in patients with open-eye injuries has been reported (10). The increase in intraocular pressure (approximately 8 mm Hg) occurs 1 to 4 min after injection of succinylcholine and returns to normal control levels within 7 min of injection. Attempts to block this effect of succinylcholine have included small doses of nondepolarizing muscle relaxants before injection of succinylcholine, but results have been varied (13). Other studies have examined the use of "self-taming" doses of succinylcholine (one-fifth the total dose) prior to the full paralyzing dose of succinylcholine. Although this method may be effective in many cases, small increases in intraocular pressure still may result (24). It should be remembered that echothiophate iodide is an anticholinesterase agent, and its prolonged use in patients results in an inhibition of the enzyme responsible for the hydrolysis of succinylcholine. Prolonged paralysis of patients treated with echothiophate who then receive succinylcholine has been reported.

Nondepolarizing muscle relaxants decrease intraocular pressure, but the onset of action is slower than the onset of action of succinylcholine. When large doses of nondepolarizing relaxants are used for tracheal intubation e.g., 0.1 mg/kg pancuronium (Pavulon®), intraocular pressure decreases as long as hypoxia and hypercarbia do not occur (11).

The patient who has recently eaten and has sustained an open-eye injury presents a particular challenge to the anesthesiologist. He must not only protect the patient from aspiration of gastric contents but must also prevent increases in intraocular pressure. One technique for prevention of these complications includes preoxygenation of the patient followed by a large dose of a nondepolarizing muscle relaxant. Forty-five seconds later a large dose of thiobarbiturate is given and intubation is performed. This sequence provides maximum relaxation of an unguarded airway with minimal time, while preventing increases in intraocular pressure. Another technique advocated by some is a smaller dose of a nondepolarizing muscle relaxant, followed by thiopental, succinylcholine, and intubation. Although in many cases this technique does not result in an increase in intraocular pressure, such rises in pressure are not assured. One of the consequences of this so-called rapid-sequence technique (sodium thiopental, succinylcholine) is the tachycardia and hypertension that often result (23). In the elderly patient or in the patient with significant hypertension, these changes may significantly increase myocardial work. If underlying coronary artery disease is present, myocardial oxygen demands may not be met, and myocardial ischemia or infarction could occur. A variety of techniques are available that can minimize the cardiovascular effects of intubation, including the use of intravenous lidocaine, sodium nitroprusside, propranolol, or fentanyl (22).

Once intubated, a variety of anesthetic agents and techniques may be used for maintenance of anesthesia. A technique using nitrous oxide, relaxant, and small doses of narcotics has often been used, because the patient rapidly awakens with the termination of the anesthetic. Close monitoring of the neuromuscular blockade is essential with this technique to assure that sudden movement intraoperatively does not occur. A disadvantage of this technique is the incidence of postoperative vomiting caused by the narcotic.

Potent inhalational anesthetics may be attractive because all decrease intraocular pressure (2). However, halothane also decreases blood pressure and heart rate by depressing myocardial contractility. Enflurane and isoflurane, on the other hand, decrease blood pressure by decreasing peripheral resistance rather than by decreasing myocardial contractility and cardiac output. For the elderly patient with significant cerebrovascular disease, large changes in blood pressure may be especially hazardous; a technique using muscle relaxants (nondepolarizing) and a low-dose, potent agent may be required. Since halothane causes sensitization of the myocardium to exogenous catecholamines, the use of halothane when large amounts of epinephrine are to be injected is contraindicated. However, the use of sympathomimetics in the anterior chamber of the eye during halothane anesthesia does not cause an increase in ventricular arrhythmias (20).

Since many ophthalmologists introduce an air bubble at the end of the surgical procedure, plans to prevent unacceptable increases in intraocular pressure should be considered. If used in the presence of nitrous oxide, the injected bubble can cause an increase in intraocular pressure because of the diffusion of nitrous oxide into the bubble. If sulfur herafluoxide gas is injected instead of air, the expansion is greater than that seen with air. It has been recommended that nitrous oxide be discontinued 15 min before the injection of the bubble and that the patient be maintained with 100% oxygen and low concentrations of potent anesthetic agents (21).

Intraoperative concerns of the anesthesiologist for patients having surgery on the eye are related to the type and length of surgery. A major cardiovascular problem is the oculocardiac reflex that is elicited by pressure on the globe or by traction on the conjunction, orbital structures, or extraocular muscles, especially the medial rectus. The afferent limb for this reflex is the trigeminal nerve, and the efferent limb is the vagus. Bradycardia is the most common rhythm disturbance, but other arrhythmias, including cardiac standstill, have been reported. Treatment is first directed at stopping the offending maneuver and then treating with an intravenous anticholinergic. Although there are several proponents of "treatment only when necessary," others believe that the condition is so common that all patients should have prophylactic intravenous anticholinergic therapy prior to surgery (14).

A second intraoperative concern is malignant hyperthermia. Although this condition is rare (1/15,000 anesthetics), it is more commonly seen in patients with ptosis and strabismus. Although the etiology, pathophysiology, and treatment cannot be discussed in detail here, the most important factor in patient survival is diagnosis of the disease. Untreated, malignant hyperthermia has a mortality rate of 50% to 80%. Increasing heart rate, temperature, and abnormal response to muscle relaxants should alert all in the operating room that the patient is at risk for malignant hyperthermia. This acute, fulminant, hypermetabolic state triggered by anesthetic agents can now be successfully treated if properly recognized (12). Treatment consists of discontinuation of all anesthetic agents, rapid ventilation with 100% oxygen, treatment of metabolic acidosis with sodium bicarbonate, and the use of dantrolene sodium (up to 10 mg/kg or until temperature decreases). Ventricular arrhythmias are treated with procainamide (maximum dose, 7 mg/kg); and hyperkalemia, with intravenous insulin. Cooling should be done simultaneously, using iced lavage of body cavities, cooling blankets, or immersion of the patient in an iced bathtub made through the use of plastic sheets. Mannitol (0.5 mg/kg), furosemide (2 mg/kg), and cold intravenous fluids should be administered to prevent renal failure. Later, problems with a consumption coagulopathy or central nervous system damage should be appropriately treated.

Because of the increasing complexity of intraocular operations, surgical procedures may prove lengthy. Hypothermia and bladder distention may occur during these procedures and may limit the length of operating time. In adults, ambient room temperature appears to be the determinant of body temperature. Since the anesthetic agents alter the patient's ability to regulate body temperature, the patient starts to lose heat to his environment. The wrapping of the patient, heating of fluids, and inspired gases all contribute to maintenance of normal body temperature, but if room temperature is too low, compensation cannot occur. This may result in temperatures near the ventricular fibrillation threshold (approximately 32°C). Monitoring of body temperature is crucial. Children are even more susceptible to heat loss, and all efforts must be directed to preserving heat. While heating blankets in adults are often of little avail, children whose body surface is less than 0.5 m^2 may benefit from such devices.

If long surgical procedures are planned and osmotic diuretics are needed, a urinary catheter should be inserted. Severe intraoperative hypertension and postoperative urinary retention have resulted from over-distended bladders.

At the end of the surgical procedure, the major concerns after intraocular surgery are coughing and emesis. Although no technique is totally reliable, the use of intravenous lidocaine (100 mg/70 kg) can decrease coughing and result in a smoother emergence. All types of surgical procedures cause some degree of nausea and vomiting, but the frequency of emesis is particularly high after ocular surgery (15). No one method is able to abolish this completely, but droperidol (0.1 mg/kg, i.v.) can markedly reduce its incidence, though often at the cost of prolonged postoperative sedation. Smaller doses (0.075 mg/kg) are somewhat effective in prevention of vomiting, whereas doses less than 0.05 mg/kg are ineffective. The prophylactic administration of droperidol at the end of surgery should be considered (1).

In summary, optimal conditions for surgery on the eye can be achieved through the use of proper premedicants, induction agents, and anesthetic agents. Most of the drugs used in anesthesia, however, have properties that may be undesirable for certain ophthalmologic procedures. The ophthalmologic patient presents special challenges for the anesthesiologist that can be met with the proper application of the known pharmacologic properties of the agents he uses.

REFERENCES

1. Abramowitz, M. D., Epstein, B. S., Friendly, D. S., Oh, T., and Greenwald, M. (1981): The effect of droperidol in reducing vomiting in pediatric strabismic outpatient surgery. *Anesthesiology*, 55:A329.
2. Ausinsch, B., Graves, S. A., Munson, E. S., and Levy, M. S. (1975): Intraocular pressures in children during isoflurane and halothane anesthesia. *Anesthesiology*, 42:167–172.
3. Ausinsch, B., Rayburn, R. L., Munson, E. S., and Levy, N. S. (1976): Ketamine and intraocular pressure in children. *Anesth. Analg.*, 55:773–775.
4. Bidwai, A. V., Stanley, T. H., Rogers, C., and Riet, E. K. (1979): Reversal of diazepam-induced postanesthetic somnolence with physostigmine. *Anesthesiology*, 51:256–259.
5. Conway, C. M., and Ellis, D. B. (1969): The hemodynamic effects of short acting barbiturates. *Anesthesiology*, 12:308–314.
6. Fragen, R. J., and Caldwell, N. (1979): Comparison of a new formulation of etomidate with thiopental—side effects and awakening times. *Anesthesiology*, 50:242–244.
7. Gal, T. J., and Surratt, P. M. (1981): Atropine and glycopyrrolate—effects on lung mechanics in normal man. *Anesth. Analg.*, 60:85–90.
8. Garde, J. F., Aston, R., Endler, G. C., and Sison, O. S. (1978): Racial mydriatic response to belladonna premedication. *Anesth. Analg.*, 57:572–576.
9. Kales, A., Bixler, E. O., Kales, J. D., and Scharf, M. B. (1977): Comparative effectiveness of nine hypnotic drugs: Sleep laboratory studies. *J. Clin. Pharmacol.*, 17:207–213.
10. Lincoff, H. A., Ellis, C. H., and DeVoe, A. G. (1955): The effect of succinylcholine on intraocular pressure. *Am. J. Ophthalmol.*, 40:501–505.
11. Litwiller, R. W., DiFazio, C. A., and Rushia, E. L. (1975): Pancuronium and intraocular pressure. *Anesthesiology*, 42:750–752.
12. McGoldrich, K. E. (1980): Malignant hyperthermia: A review. *J. Am. Med. Wom. Assoc.*, 35:95–98.
13. Meyers, E. F., Krupin, T., Johnson, M., and Zink, H. (1978): Failure of nondepolarizing neuromuscular blockers to inhibit succinylcholine-induced increased intraocular pressure, a controlled study. *Anesthesiology*, 48:149–151.
14. Meyers, E. F., and Tomeldan, S. A. (1979): Glycopyrrolate compared with atropine in prevention of the oculocardiac reflex during eye-muscle surgery. *Anesthesiology*, 51:350–354.
15. Nikki, P., and Pohjola, S. (1972): Nausea and vomiting after ocular surgery. *Acta Ophthalmol. (Copenh.)*, 50:525–531.
16. Oduro, K. A. (1975): Glycopyrrolate methobromide. II. Comparison with atropine sulfate in anaesthesia. *Can. Anaesth. Soc. J.*, 22:466–473.
17. Patton, C. M. (1975): Rapid induction of acute dyskinesia by droperidol. *Anesthesiology*, 43:126–131.
18. Reves, J. B., Corssen, G., and Holcomb, C. (1978): Comparison of two benzodiazepines for anesthetic induction: Midazolam and diazepam. *Can. Anaesth. Soc. J.*, 25:211–217.
19. Rosen, D. A. (1962): Anaesthesia in ophthalmology. *Can. Anaesth. Soc. J.*, 9:545–549.
20. Smith, R. B., Douglas, H., Petruscak, J., and Breslin, P. (1972): Safety of intraocular adrenaline with halothane anaesthesia. *Br. J. Anaesth.*, 44:1314–1317.
21. Stinson, T. W., and Donlon, J. V. (1979): Interaction of SF_6 and air with nitrous oxide. *Anesthesiology*, 51:S16.
22. Stoelting, R. K. (1979): Attenuation of blood pressure response to laryngoscope and tracheal intubation with sodium nitroprusside. *Anesth. Analg.*, 58:116–119.
23. Stoelting, R. K., and Peterson, C. (1976): Circulatory changes during anesthetic induction: Impact of d-tubocurarine pretreatment, thiamylal, succinylcholine, laryngoscopy and tracheal lidocaine. *Anesth. Analg.*, 55:77–84.
24. Verma, R. S. (1979): "Self-taming" of succinylcholine-induced fasciculations and intraocular pressure. *Anesthesiology*, 50:245–247.

Commentary

Clinical Pharmacology of Local Anesthetics
in Ophthalmologic Surgery

For local anesthesia the ophthalmic surgeon is concerned with the technique of administration and its duration of action. Greene offers an excellent, masterful review of the clinical pharmacology of agents used for topical and infiltrative anesthesia. The author points out that the longer a local anesthetic acts, the longer it takes to act. This is why mixtures of two local anesthetics, e.g. short acting 2% lidocaine with long-acting 0.75% bupivacaine are commonly used. However, mixing two solutions each with a different pH, may result in a pH that significantly alters the anesthetic action of either or both of the constituents. Furthermore, competition for the same binding sites may alter the predictability of the action of either or both drugs. The mixtures may not live up to their theoretical expectations. Adding hyaluronidase to the anesthetic will increase diffusion but it will also increase vascular absorption and, by so doing, decrease duration and increase systemic toxicity. Adding epinephrine 1:200,000 will double the duration of short-acting anesthetics while it only slightly increases the duration of long acting agents. On the other hand, this potent vasoconstrictor may increase the incidence of systemic and local side effects.

Systemic toxicity is determined by total plasma level of an agent. It will interest ophthalmologists to know that topical anesthetics applied to the eye may reach high plasma levels because the anesthetics may drain through the nasolacrimal duct and reach a large, absorptive area of the nasal mucosa.

Every ophthalmic surgeon should be alert to possible central nervous system side effects of local anesthetics. Prevention of high plasma levels is the key to their avoidance. Diazepam increases the threshold for toxic reactions. Yet it is valuable to know that treatment consists of further intravenous diazepam and oxygen. Although thiopental is useful, diazepam may be a safer agent in ophthalmology.

Finally, the success of local infiltration anesthesia lies in neuroanatomic precision of administration. Meticulous technique for retrobulbar injection avoids the local complications like intravascular insertion, rupture of a vessel, or injury to the optic nerve. Optic atrophy as a complication of cataract surgery and/or retrobulbar injection is still a puzzle. Direct needle trauma, the inclusion of epinephrine in the injection, arterial injury, and travel of anesthesia up the nerve sheath are all possible causes. The performance of retrobulbar injection with a blunt retrobulbar needle, avoiding aspiration of vascular tissue into the lumen of the needle, and keeping positive pressure on the plunger of the syringe as the injection proceeds are useful in diminishing the number of complications.

The Editors

Surgical Pharmacology of the Eye,
edited by M. Sears and A. Tarkkanen.
Raven Press, New York © 1985.

Clinical Pharmacology of Local Anesthetics in Ophthalmologic Surgery

Nicholas M. Greene

*Department of Anesthesiology, Yale University School of Medicine,
New Haven, Connecticut 06510*

SUMMARY: The best clinical results associated with use of local anesthetics in ophthalmic surgery depend on recognition of pharmacologic principles involved in determining their anesthetic action and toxicity.

This chapter emphasizes the factors governing the potency of local anesthetics, the rapidity of their onset of action, their duration of action, and the types of nerve fibers blocked. These factors in turn depend on the pKa, or dissociation constant, of the local anesthetics, the pH of the site at which they are applied, the concentrations of local anesthetic solution employed, the lipid solubility of the anesthetics, and the size and type of nerve fibers to which the local anesthetics are applied.

Toxicity of local anesthetics can be local or systemic. Local toxicity includes neuro- and myotoxicity, together with impairment of wound healing and hemostasis, as well as susceptibility to infection.

Systemic toxicity depends solely on plasma levels of local anesthetics. Allergy is rarely, if ever, involved. Plasma levels in turn depend on the rate of vascular absorption (amount of anesthetic used, vascular supply at the site of application, the time over which the anesthetic is administered, and the area of distribution) and the rate of elimination from the vascular system (by redistribution and metabolism). Central nervous system toxicity is characterized by hyperexcitability, including convulsions. Cardiovascular toxicity is characterized by hypotension or even cardiac arrest. Since anesthetic potency and systemic toxicity are directly related, the therapeutic ratios for all local anesthetics are essentially the same. The cardiovascular system is less sensitive to the toxic effects of local anesthetics than is the central nervous system.

The clinical pharmacology of local anesthetics determines efficacy and safety. This chapter considers the clinical pharmacology of local anesthetics in ophthalmologic surgery.

NEURONAL RESPONSES

Local anesthetics in ophthalmologic surgery are used by topical application to the conjunctiva and/or the cornea and by injection. Injection includes infiltration into tissues with little or no regard to the neuroanatomy involved. It also includes injection into neuroanatomically determined sites to block specific nerves. Though semantically inaccurate, both forms of injection local anesthesia will, for convenience, be termed infiltration anesthesia.

Topical Anesthetics

Topical anesthetics inhibit excitation of sensory receptors and thus prevent generation of afferent sensory impulses. The concentration of local anesthetic required to block neuronal excitation is about one-half that required to block axonal transmission. Effective topical anesthesia requires, nevertheless, concentrations of local anesthetic solutions substantially greater than those required to block axonal transmission during injection anesthesia. This is because local anesthetics applied to epithelial surfaces are extensively diluted as they diffuse through tissue barriers to their effector sites.

The rate at which local anesthetics applied topically to epithelial surfaces penetrate beneath the surface varies greatly. Penetrance of some local anesthetics, e.g., procaine (Novocain®) and bupivacaine (Marcaine®), is so slight that they are ineffective topical anesthetics. Penetrance of local anesthetics such as tetracaine (amethocaine; Pontocaine®) and lidocaine (lignocaine; Xylocaine®) is so great that onset of topical anesthesia occurs within minutes. Why penetrance is greater with some local anesthetics than with others remains unclear. There is no discernible relation to chemical structure, lipid solubility, or molecular weight. Nor is penetrance a function of the degree of ionization. Penetrance of topical anesthetics is, however, inversely related to the thickness of the tissue barriers to which they are applied. This, together perhaps with the unique chemical composition of skin, explains why most local anesthetics are ineffective when applied to intact cutaneous surfaces.

Duration of action of topical anesthetics is determined by the rate at which they undergo vascular absorption. Evanescent in highly perfused tissues, topical anesthesia is prolonged in poorly perfused tissues. Addition of epinephrine to topical anesthetic solutions fails to prolong duration of anesthesia. The penetrance of topical epinephrine is so low that vasoconstriction and a decrease in vascular absorption of local anesthetic in areas beneath the site of application do not occur. Vasoconstrictors such as phenylephrine (Neo-Synephrine®), on the other hand, are effective topical vasoconstrictors.

Duration of topical anesthesia is also a function of lipid solubility of local anesthetics. Local anesthetics highly soluble in lipids (e.g., tetracaine) are less susceptible to removal from effector sites by vascular absorption than are local anesthetics less soluble in lipids (e.g., lidocaine). They thus produce anesthesia that lasts longer.

There are no clinically significant differences in the sensitivity of different types of sensory receptors (pain, touch, heat, etc.) to the effects of topical local anesthetics. This stands in contrast to the differential blockade of nerve conduction produced by infiltration anesthetics.

Infiltration Anesthetics

Infiltration anesthetics block transmission of nerve impulses. The speed with which local anesthetics produce their effects (that is, latency) varies with different local anesthetics depending principally on pKa. The pKa of a local anesthetic is the pH at which 50% of the anesthetic exists in a cationic or ionized state, and 50% exists in the un-ionized state. Ionized molecules produce anesthesia. They do so by acting intracellularly to block sodium channels in nerve membranes and, by thus preventing nerve membrane depolarization, inhibit propagation of action potentials (27). Nerve membranes are, however, impermeable to charged forms of local anesthetics. It is in the uncharged, nonionized form that local anesthetics pass through nerve membranes. Once intracellular, part of the nonionized molecules dissociate into ionized molecules, which then exert their pharmacologic action. The pKa of tetracaine is 8.5. At a physiologically normal pH of 7.40, only 10% of tetracaine molecules are not ionized and thus capable of diffusing across nerve membranes. The pKa of lidocaine is 7.7. At a pH of 7.40, 30% of lidocaine molecules are un-ionized. Lidocaine, therefore, enters nerve cells more rapidly than tetracaine. Onset of anesthesia is accordingly more rapid with lidocaine than with tetracaine.

An increase in pH above 7.40 increases the percentage of local anesthetics in the nondissociated form. Onset of anesthesia is thus more rapid in the presence of alkalosis. In the presence of acidosis, as in infected or inflamed tissues, the availability of un-ionized local anesthetic molecules is so low that onset of anesthesia is prolonged, or indeed anesthesia may be difficult, if not impossible, to establish.

Rate of onset of action of infiltration anesthetics also depends, of course, on the accuracy with which the local anesthetic is deposited about nerves that are to be blocked. Differences in latency of local anesthetics have been ascribed to differences in the rates at which they diffuse down a concentration gradient from the site of injection to the site of action. *In vivo* differences in tissue diffusivity of local anesthetics in the presence of equal tissue concentration gradients have not, however, been pharmacokinetically quantitated. Most of the apparent differences in latency of local anesthetics can be ascribed to differences in concentration of local anesthetic in the solution injected and to differences in the rate at which anesthetics penetrate nerve membranes, i.e., pKa. Hyaluronidase increases diffusion of local anesthetics in tissue but is a weak substitute for neuroanatomic precision in injection of local anesthetics. Because hyaluronidase increases diffusion and so increases vascular absorption, it both decreases duration of anesthesia and increases the risk of systemic toxicity.

Potency of infiltration local anesthetics is defined as the number of anesthetic molecules required to block sodium channels. Potency also depends on pKa and thus on pH at the site of injection. The minimum effective blocking concentration of lidocaine is 100 times greater at pH 5.0 than at pH 7.0.

Lipid solubility also determines potency. The more lipophilic an anesthetic is, the lower the minimum effective blocking concentration. The solubilities of tetracaine and bupivacaine in lipids are so great that injection of concentrations of 0.15% and 0.5% effectively block neural transmission. Lidocaine, being less soluble in lipids, requires use of a 2% solution.

Potency of local anesthetics varies not only with lipid solubility and pKa, it also depends on nerve fiber size (12,13,24) and frequency of impulse transmission in nerves (7,26). Smaller nerve fibers are more sensitive than larger nerve fibers to the effects of local anesthetics. Autonomic nerve fibers, being smaller than somatic sensory fibers, are blocked before sensory fibers. Somatic sensory fibers, in turn being smaller than somatic motor fibers, are blocked before motor fibers. Also, the higher the frequency of transmission, the greater the sensitivity to local anesthetics. Differential nerve block thus often occurs during injection anesthesia. To the ophthalmologic surgeon differential nerve block means that evidence of autonomic blockade (change in pupillary size, conjunctival hyperemia) following injection of local anesthetic may not always be taken as evidence of sensory anesthesia. It also means that sensory anesthesia may not always be associated with akinesia of extraocular skeletal muscles. Apparent paradoxes in responses to injection of local anesthetics in the operating room are often the consequence of differential sensitivity of nerves to the effects of local anesthetics.

Duration of action of injected local anesthetics depends on the volume injected and the rate at which local anesthetics are removed from the site of injection. Concentration is more important than the amount injected. Anesthesia lasts longer when 500 mg is injected as 25 ml of a 2% solution than when 50 ml of a 1% solution is used, though the extent of anesthesia will be less with the former.

Removal of local anesthetic from the site of injection is by vascular absorption. *In situ* biotransformation does not occur. The greater the blood flow, the shorter the duration. Since tissue blood flow differs at different anatomic sites, the site of injection influences duration of local anesthesia. So too does age. Duration of action is greater in elderly patients because peripheral blood flow is decreased.

Duration of anesthesia may be pharmacologically prolonged by adding vasoconstrictors to the anesthetic solution to decrease the rate of vascular absorption. The best (and safest) vasoconstrictor is epinephrine. The effect of epinephrine on duration is concentration dependent up to a concentration of 1:200,000. Epinephrine 1:200,000 doubles duration of action of short-acting local anesthetics (e.g., lidocaine) but increases duration of action of long-acting anesthetics (e.g., bupivacaine) only about 50%. Concentrations of epinephrine in excess of 1:200,000 produce no further increase in duration of anesthesia. They are, however, associated with an increased incidence of potentially dangerous side effects.

Rate of vascular absorption of local anesthetics from the site of injection, and thus duration of action, is also governed by lipid solubility. The lipid solubility of tetracaine (80) is one of the reasons why tetracaine lasts longer than lidocaine (lipid solubility 2.9). The ratio between lipid solubility and duration is, however, not linear. Tetracaine is 27 times more soluble in lipids than lidocaine but lasts only about 5 times longer. Similarly, even though the affinity of tetracaine for lipids is 3 times greater than that of bupivacaine, the durations of action of tetracaine and bupivacaine are similar. Though duration of action of highly lipid soluble local anesthetics is prolonged by epinephrine, the prolongation is not as great as it is with local anesthetics with shorter durations of action and lesser solubilities in lipids.

The longer a local anesthetic acts, the longer it takes to act. This has led to clinical use of mixtures of two local anesthetics, one with rapid onset but short duration, the other with slow onset but long duration. The efficacy of such combinations remains, however, uncertain. Combining lidocaine with bupivacaine (8,22,33) or combining lidocaine, chloroprocaine (Nesacaine®), or mepivacaine (Carbocaine®) with tetracaine (23) has been reported to have no effect on either latency of the short-acting anesthetic or duration of action of the long-acting anesthetic. On the other hand, other studies have reported that combining local anesthetics with rapid onset of action, such as lidocaine (4,30) or chloroprocaine (6,18) with local anesthetics of long duration of action such as bupivacaine, although having no effect on latency of the shorter-acting anesthetic significantly decreases the duration of action of bupivacaine. In fact, duration of anesthesia with the combination of chloroprocaine and bupivacaine is the same as the duration of action of chloroprocaine alone. Mixtures of local anesthetics may not live up to theoretical expectations because the pHs of solutions of different local anesthetics as commercially supplied vary considerably. Since the action of local anesthetics is pH dependent, mixing two solutions, each with a different though appropriate pH for each of the two anesthetics, may result in a pH that significantly alters the anesthetic action of either or both of the constituent anesthetics. Combinations of local anesthetics may also be unpredictable because of competitive binding to nonspecific receptor sites.

LOCAL SIDE EFFECTS AND TOXICITY

Local anesthetics have the potential for producing histologic and functional changes at the site of injection.

Histologic Side Effects

Local anesthetics in current use are devoid of neurotoxicity. The only possible exception may be chloroprocaine. Chloroprocaine, unlike other local anesthetics, produces changes *in vivo* in nerves of experimental animals (2). The significance of this remains uncertain during infiltration anesthesia in clinical practice. The neurotoxic potential of local anesthetics is, however, revealed when greater than recommended concentrations are used. High concentrations of local anesthetics produce concentration-dependent nerve damage characterized chiefly by neurolysis. Though preexisting neurologic changes have been hypothesized as increasing the neurotoxicity of local anesthetics, there are no data either to substantiate or to refute such a possibility. However, many neurologic diseases are characterized by inexorable progression. Prudence dictates that local anesthetics are often best avoided in the presence of preexisting neurologic disease lest subsequent progression of the disease be ascribed, however erroneously, to the local anesthetic.

Though recommended concentrations of commonly used local anesthetics are devoid of neurotoxicity, nerve damage may be produced by the needle through which they are injected. Trauma to nerves during infiltration anesthesia is the most common cause of neurologic symptoms following regional anesthesia. This complication is most likely to occur when placement of the needle or injection of the anesthetic solution is accompanied by paresthesias (29). Vasoconstrictors injected with local anesthetic solutions to prolong duration of anesthesia do not increase the neurotoxicity of local anesthetics.

Though free of neurotoxicity, commonly used local anesthetics are associated with myotoxicity characterized by reversible breakdown of muscle fibers (11), a response accentuated by addition of epinephrine to the local anesthetic solution (35). Ophthalmologic surgeons should be aware that the intraorbital injection of local anesthetics may be followed by impairment of function of extraocular muscles for 2 to 3 weeks.

Functional Side Effects

Wound healing is adversely affected by local anesthetics, especially if used with epinephrine (3). This may be due to inhibition of cell replication (16,17) and/or inhibition of cell metabolism (10). Impairment by topical local anesthetics of healing of corneal wounds (31) is of particular importance in ophthalmology.

Operative hemostasis may also be adversely affected by local anesthetics. Though plasma levels of local anesthetics during infiltration anesthesia are insufficient to affect components of the clotting cascade, local anesthetics achieve concentrations at the site of injection sufficient to impair platelet aggregation (15). Local anesthetics also increase capillary permeability. The result may be an increase in frequency and size of hematomas at the site of surgery performed under infiltration or topical anesthesia. Such a possibility may be offset by the vasoconstrictor action of local anesthetics such as bupivacaine even in the absence of added epinephrine.

Local anesthetics have antibacterial and antifungal effects (9,28) that may decrease the frequency and severity of postoperative infections secondary to intraoperative contamination of the operative site. However, preservatives in commercial preparations of local anesthetics, especially chlorobutanol, inhibit the antimicrobial effects of local anesthetics. Also, local anesthetics impair leukocyte adherence (14). Neither incidence, type, nor magnitude of postoperative wound infections have, however, been shown to be affected by either infiltration or topical local anesthetics in ophthalmologic surgery.

SYSTEMIC SIDE EFFECTS AND TOXICITY

Local anesthetics appear in the systemic circulation as they are absorbed from the site of administration. Whether or not side effects (relatively minor systemic responses) or toxic effects (severe, even life-threatening systemic responses) occur depends principally on the plasma levels of local anesthetics achieved. Total plasma levels determine systemic toxicity, not the ratio between free and plasma protein anesthetic. Highly protein bound local anesthetics (e.g., etidocaine, bupivacaine) are as toxic at equal plasma levels as are less protein bound local anesthetics (e.g., lidocaine).

Plasma levels of local anesthetics are the product of no less than five simultaneously operative factors. First, the greater the amount of local anesthetic administered, the higher the plasma levels will be, if all other factors remain constant.

Second, plasma levels of local anesthetics are a function of vascular perfusion of the site at which they are applied. Topical application to or injection into highly vascular areas is associated with the rapid appearance of high concentrations of local anesthetics in the systemic circulation. Application to or injection into poorly perfused areas results in delayed appearance of low concentrations. Plasma levels of local anesthetics are greatest and are reached most rapidly if the local anesthetic solution is unintentionally injected intravascularly. Especially dangerous is inadvertent injection into an artery supplying the brain. Such injections, though not appreciably increasing systemic plasma concentrations of local anesthetic, cause delivery of a small volume of highly concentrated local anesthetic to the brain, with the immediate onset of severe central nervous system (CNS) toxic reactions, including transient blindness. The same danger exists when injection is made into an artery that, although it does not directly supply the brain, is accompanied by a proximal (upstream) artery that does supply the brain. Rapid injection into such an artery can produce retrograde flow of anesthetic to the branch of that artery supplying the brain, with consequent delivery of a toxic amount of anesthetic. The danger of acute, severe CNS toxicity from intra-arterial injection is greatest in ophthalmologic surgery during retrobulbar blocks.

Drugs such as epinephrine, used to prolong duration of local anesthesia, produce local vasoconstriction and so decrease the rate of vascular absorption of local anesthetics. By decreasing vascular absorption, they decrease blood levels and systemic toxicity of local anesthetics and thereby increase the amounts that may be safely administered.

Third, the greater the area over which a local anesthetic is distributed, the higher the plasma level and the more rapidly it is achieved. Blood levels after injection of a large volume of dilute local anesthetic solution may be higher than those following injection of a smaller volume of a more concentrated local anesthetic solution, because the former are exposed to a larger vascular absorptive surface area. The role of surface area is particularly important with topical anesthetics. Topical anesthetics are usually spread over a relatively large area, and vascular absorption may be correspondingly rapid. This is especially evident when topical anesthetics are used in the eye, the oral cavity, or the respiratory tract. In these areas blood levels approximate those observed when the same amount of local anesthetic is injected intravenously (1). Topical anesthetics applied to the eye may achieve unexpectedly high plasma concentrations because they may drain through the nasolacrymal duct and so become exposed to the greatly increased absorptive surface area represented by the nasal mucosa.

Fourth, blood levels of local anesthetics are inversely related to the time over which they are given. Blood levels are substantially greater when a given amount of local anesthetic is injected or applied topically all at once than when the same amount is administered over 10 min. Deliberate prolongation of administration of a local anesthetic is one of the most effective ways to avoid high blood levels and systemic reactions.

And, fifth, blood levels of local anesthetics are determined by the rate at which they are eliminated from the circulation. Tissue redistribution accounts for some of the elimination of local anesthetics from blood, but biotransformation is even more important. Ester-type local anesthetics (procaine, chloroprocaine, tetracaine) are metabolized by plasma pseudocholinesterase. Patients with either atypical forms of pseudocholinesterase (about 1 in 1,500 patients) or, due to liver disease, abnormally low plasma levels of pseudocholinesterase are especially liable to develop toxic reactions to ester-type local anesthetics. The systemic toxicity of chloroprocaine is the lowest of all local anesthetics because it is rapidly metabolized by pseudocholinesterase and because it is immediately exposed to pseudocholinesterase as soon as it enters the vascular system. Amide-type local anesthetics (lidocaine, bupivacaine) are metabolized by hepatic microsomal enzymes. Blood levels (and toxicity) of amide local anesthetics are thus increased by hepatic disease, decreases in hepatic blood flow associated with hypotension, congestive heart failure, etc., or the presence of drugs that inhibit microsomal enzymes (e.g., cimetidine).

Dosage of local anesthetics is but one of the factors that determine blood levels and systemic toxicity of local anesthetics. Safety based solely on calculations of the amounts of local anesthetics administered is both unreliable and a potentially dangerous oversimplification of a complex pharmacokinetic problem, even when calculated on a mg/kg basis. Calculation of "safe" doses of local anesthetics must be based on appreciation of all the pharmacokinetic determinants of blood levels of local anesthetics if systemic toxic reactions are to be avoided.

Allergic responses to local anesthetics, though often invoked to explain toxic reactions, are extremely rare (32). Only one immunologically proven case of allergy to a local anesthetic (lidocaine) has been reported (5). Allergy to preservatives present in commercial preparation of local anesthetic solutions may be more frequent than allergy to local anesthetics. The vast majority of adverse responses to local anesthetics are due to absolute or relative overdose. Relative overdose occurs because plasma concentrations of local anesthetics required to produce systemic toxicity in a large population of subjects form a Gaussian distribution curve. At one extreme are a few subjects who exhibit toxic reactions only with plasma concentrations substantially greater than those that elicit toxic responses in the majority of patients. At the other extreme are a few subjects who experience systemic toxicity only with plasma concentrations substantially less than the median toxic plasma level. The latter patients are hypersensitive, not allergic, to local anesthetics. In these patients, relative overdose can occur. Where an individual patient may fall on the Gaussian curve cannot be determined in advance.

Age influences sensitivity to local anesthetics in different ways with different local anesthetics, at least in experimental animals. Old mice are less sensitive to etidocaine (Duranest®) and bupivacaine than are immature mice, but there is no age-dependent difference in systemic toxicity of lidocaine and chloropro-caine (19). Whether these data can be extrapolated to humans is uncertain. If they can be, it would be despite the fact that the plasma half-life of lidocaine is significantly longer in older than in younger humans (25), a finding that suggests that the risk of systemic toxicity associated with a given dose of local anesthetic may be greater in older than in younger patients.

The systemic toxicity of local anesthetics is restricted to the CNS and the cardiovascular system. Aside from the production of methemoglobinemia by prilocaine (Citanest®) (21), other organ systems are not involved.

CNS Toxicity

Local anesthetics cross the blood-brain barrier rapidly. CNS concentrations of local anesthetics are thus immediately and directly determined by the plasma concentrations. When CNS concentrations reach a certain threshold, signs and symptoms due to blockade of cortical inhibitory synapses (34) start to appear. With low plasma levels, patients experience vertigo, tinnitus, lightheadedness, apprehension, and confusion. As plasma levels increase, tremors of the extremities and face occur, followed by convulsions and unconsciousness that may progress to respiratory arrest. The time course over which CNS reactions to local anesthetics develop depends on the plasma concentrations of local anesthetic achieved and the rate at which they are reached. With low plasma concentrations, CNS toxicity develops slowly and may never pass beyond the stage of vertigo and apprehension. With rapidly achieved high plasma concentrations, the onset of frank seizures, often within minutes, may be the first evidence of a toxic reaction.

The CNS toxicity of commonly used local anesthetics, as determined by intravenous administration in unanesthetized dogs, increases as a function of local anesthetic potency (20). Ratios of local anesthetic potencies (in man) of lidocaine, etidocaine, bupivacaine, and tetracaine are 1:2:4:4. Ratios of CNS toxicities are 1:3:5:6. The clinical safety is thus essentially the same for all commonly used local anesthetics. Those that have the least CNS toxicity require greater doses to provide anesthesia. Those that have the greatest CNS toxicity require the least doses to provide anesthesia.

Prevention of high plasma levels of local anesthetics is the key to avoidance of CNS toxicity. Also useful is the preoperative administration of diazepam (Valium®). Diazepam not only produces a relaxed, calm mental state, it also increases the CNS threshold for toxic reactions to local anesthetics.

Treatment of CNS reactions to local anesthetics consists of intravenous diazepam (5 to 20 mg in divided doses) and oxygen. Intravenous succinylcholine terminates convulsions but has no effect on CNS seizure activity and associated increases in CNS metabolism. Increases in CNS oxygen consumption associated with convulsions may result in cerebral hypoxia even though peripheral manifestations of CNS seizures have been eliminated by succinylcholine. Succinylcholine is rarely indicated in the management of convulsions induced by local anesthetics. If used, succinylcholine must be given only by those skilled and experienced in management of the respiratory arrest that succinylcholine produces.

Cardiovascular Toxicity

The cardiovascular system is less susceptible to local anesthetic toxicity than is the CNS. Ratios between toxic cardiovascular and CNS doses vary from 3.5 for lidocaine to 6.7 with tetracaine, with intermediate ratios for bupivacaine (4.1) and etidocaine (5.1) (20). It is thus possible for a patient to exhibit signs of CNS toxicity without cardiovascular toxicity. The reverse is less frequently encountered.

Cardiovascular toxicity, when it occurs, is the result of several actions of local anesthetics. First, local anesthetics, in common with general anesthetics, exert negative inotropic effects. They decrease the force of ventricular contraction and so decrease cardiac output. Local anesthetics also produce peripheral vasodilation both by direct action on vascular smooth muscle and by impairment of axonal and synaptic transmission in the sympathetic nervous system. Local anesthetics also have negative chronotropic and negative dromotropic actions. By decreasing heart rate, they further decrease cardiac output. Cardiovascular toxicity to local anesthetics is therefore characterized by arterial hypotension and bradycardia that, if untreated, may result in cardiac arrest. As with CNS toxicity, cardiovascular toxicity of local anesthetics is directly proportional to local anesthetic potency. Again, therefore, the more potent a local anesthetic is, the less need be used but the greater the potential for development of cardiotoxicity, and vice versa for less potent local anesthetics. As with CNS toxicity, the magnitude of cardiovascular responses to local anesthetics depends on the plasma concentrations of local anesthetics. Cardiovascular depression is greatest and most rapid in onset if the local anesthetic is inadvertently injected intravascularly. Cardiovascular responses may be relatively mild and slow in onset, with lower plasma concentrations, following vascular absorption from the site of injection.

Treatment of cardiovascular responses to local anesthetics consists of rapid placement of the patient in the head-down position to assure adequate venous return to the heart, the administration of oxygen, the rapid intravenous administration of a large volume of crystalloid solution (1,000 ml lactated Ringer's solution per 70 kg in 5 to 7 min), and the intravenous injection of a vasopressor. The best vasopressors are those with rapid onset and long duration of action and with positive inotropic and chronotropic effects but without arrhythmogenic potential. α-Adrenergic vasopressors such as methoxamine (Vasoxyl®) or phenylephrine (Neo-Synephrine®) are best avoided. By increasing peripheral vascular resistance they may, in the presence of left ventricular depression, further decrease cardiac output. Preferable are intravenous ephedrine or mephentermine (Wyamine®) (12 to 25 mg and 7.5 to 15 mg, respectively, in divided doses). Epinephrine is not as satisfactory. The difference between therapeutic and toxic doses of epinephrine is so small with intravenous bolus injections that safe yet effective doses may be difficult to give. The duration of action of epinephrine is also too brief. Intravenous infusions of dilute epinephrine solutions are useful in management of prolonged periods of cardiovascular depression, but their preparation wastes valuable time in an emergency and should not be relied on as the first step in treatment of cardiovascular toxic reaction to local anesthetics.

Epinephrine used to prolong the duration of local anesthetics may also be absorbed from the site of administration in amounts sufficient to produce cardiovascular responses that superficially resemble those observed during cardiovascular toxic responses caused by local anesthetics. The differential diagnosis is important, since therapy differs so greatly. High blood levels of epinephrine may be associated with apprehension similar to that seen in the early stages of CNS toxic reactions to local anesthetics, but apprehension due to epinephrine is not progressive, nor is it associated with tremors. Palpitations occur early with high blood levels of epinephrine. They do not occur with high blood levels of local anesthetics. Toxic responses to epinephrine are also characterized by hypertension, tachycardia, and ventricular arrhythmias, the latter especially frequent in elderly patients or those with coronary artery disease. Toxic reactions to local anesthetics, on the other hand, are characterized by hypotension and bradycardia. Treatment of reactions to epinephrine consists of the intravenous administration of propranolol (Inderal®, 1 to 2 mg, slowly in divided doses) or comparable β-adrenergic antagonists. Hypertensive crises may also be precipitated by topical application of phenylephrine to the conjunctiva. Especially frequent in young children, they are associated with pronounced bradycardia. Treatment consists of the intravenous injection of the α-adrenergic antagonist phentolamine (Regitine®, 5 mg in adults, 1 mg in children).

A final word about toxicity of local anesthetics: The ophthalmologic surgeon should not be so distressed by the preceding litany of local and systemic toxic responses to local anesthetics that the use of local anesthetics is abandoned in favor of general anesthetics. All anesthetics are associated with undesirable side effects and toxicity. All are associated with risk. The risk of general anesthesia may be just as great or greater than the risk of local anesthesia. The risk of local anesthesia can, however, be reduced by appreciation of pharmacologic and pharmacokinetic factors involved in determination of this risk, most particularly recognition of the determinants of plasma concentrations of local anesthetics and their potential for initiation of toxic responses.

REFERENCES

1. Adriani, J., and Campbell, D. (1956): Fatalities following topical application of local anesthetics to mucous membranes. *J.A.M.A.,* 162:1527–1530.
2. Barsa, J., Batra, M., Fink, B. R., and Sumi, S. M. (1982): A comparative in vivo study of local neurotoxicity of lidocaine, bupivacaine, 2-chloroprocaine, and a mixture of 2-chloroprocaine and bupivacaine. *Anesth. Analg.,* 61:961–967.
3. Bodvall, B., and Rais, O. (1962): Effects of infiltration anaesthesia on healing of incisions in traumatized and non-traumatized tissues. *Acta Chir. Scand.,* 123:83–91.
4. Bromage, P. R., and Gertel, M. (1972): Improved brachial plexus block with bupivacaine and carbonated lidocaine. *Anesthesiology,* 36:479–487.
5. Brown, D. T., Beamish, D., and Wildsmith, J. A. W. (1981): Allergic reaction to an amide local anaesthetic. *Br. J. Anaesth.,* 53:435–437.
6. Cohen, S. E., and Thurlow, A. (1979): Comparison of chloroprocaine-bupivacaine mixture with chloroprocaine and bupivacaine used individually for obstetric analgesia. *Anesthesiology,* 51:288–292.
7. Courtney, K. R., Kendig, J. J., and Cohen, E. N. (1978): Frequency-dependent conduction nerve block: The role of nerve impulse pattern in local anesthetic potency. *Anesthesiology,* 48:111–117.
8. Cunningham, N. L., and Kaplan, J. A. (1974): A rapid onset, long-acting regional anesthetic technique. *Anesthesiology,* 41:509–511.
9. Erlich, H. (1961): Bacteriologic studies and effects of anesthetic solutions on bronchial secretions during bronchoscopy. *Am. Rev. Respir. Dis.,* 84:414–421.
10. Fink, B. R., Kenny, G. E., and Simpson, W. E., III. (1969): Depression of oxygen uptake in cell culture by volatile, barbiturate, and local anesthetics. *Anesthesiology,* 30:150–155.
11. Foster, A. H., and Carlson, B. M. (1980): Myotoxicity of local anesthetics and regeneration of the damaged muscle fibers. *Anesth. Analg.,* 59:727–736.
12. Franz, D. N., and Perry, R. S. (1974): Mechanisms for differential block among single myelinated and non-myelinated axons by procaine. *J. Physiol. (Lond.),* 236:193–210.
13. Gasser, H. S., and Erlanger, J. (1929): The role of fiber size in the establishment of a nerve block by pressure or cocaine. *Am. J. Physiol.,* 88:581–591.
14. Giddon, D. B., and Lindhe, J. (1972): In vivo quantification of local anesthetic suppression of leukocyte adherence. *Am. J. Pathol.,* 68:327–338.

15. Gotta, A. W., and Sullivan, C. A. (1983): The effect of local anesthetics on platelet aggregation. *Regional Anesthesia,* 8:65–68.
16. Jackson, S. H. (1971): The metabolic effects of nonvolatile anesthetics on mammalian hepatoma cells in vitro. II. Inhibition of macromolecular precursor incorporation. *Anesthesiology,* 35:268–273.
17. Jackson, S. H., and Epstein, R. A. (1971): The metabolic effects of nonvolatile anesthetics on mammalian hepatoma cells in vitro. I. Inhibition of cell replication. *Anesthesiology,* 34:409–414.
18. Kim, J. M., Goto, H., and Arakawa, K. (1979): Duration of bupivacaine intradermal anesthesia when bupivacaine is mixed with chloroprocaine. *Anesth. Analg.,* 58:364–366.
19. Liu, P. L., Covino, B. M., and Feldman, H. S. (1983): Effect of age on local anesthetic central nervous system toxicity in mice. *Regional Anesthesia,* 8:57–60.
20. Liu, P. L., Feldman, H. S., Giasi, R., Patterson, M. K., and Covino, B. G. (1983): Comparative CNS toxicity of lidocaine, etidocaine, bupivacaine and tetracaine in awake dogs following rapid intravenous administration. *Anesth. Analg.,* 62:375–379.
21. Lund, P. C., and Cwik, J. C. (1965): Propitocaine (Citanest) and methemoglobinemia. *Anesthesiology,* 26:569–571.
22. Magee, D. A., Sweet, P. T., and Holland, A. J. C. (1983): Epidural anaesthesia with mixtures of bupivacaine and lidocaine. *Can. Anaesth. Soc. J.,* 30:174–178.
23. Moore, D. C., Bridenbaugh, L. D., Bridenbaugh, P. O., Thompson, G. E., and Tucker, G. T. (1972): Does compounding of local anesthetic agents increase their toxicity in humans? *Anesth. Analg.,* 51:579–585.
24. Nathan, P. W., and Sears, T. A. (1961): Some factors concerned in differential nerve block by local anaesthetics. *J. Physiol. (Lond.),* 157:565–580.
25. Nation, R. L., and Triggs, E. J. (1977): Lignocaine kinetics in cardiac and aged subjects. *Br. J. Pharmacol.,* 4:439–448.
26. Palmer, S. K., Bosnjak, Z. J., Hopp, F. A., von Colditz, J. H., and Kampine, J. P. (1983): Lidocaine and bupivacaine differential blockade of isolated canine nerves. *Anesth. Analg.,* 62:754–757.
27. Ritchie, J. M. (1975): Mechanism of action of local anaesthetic agents and biotoxins. *Br. J. Anaesth.,* 74:191–198.
28. Schmidt, R. M., and Rosenkrantz, H. S. (1970): Antimicrobial activity of local anesthetics: Lidocaine and procaine. *J. Infect. Dis.,* 121:597–607.
29. Selander, D., Brattsand, G., Lundborg, G., Nordborg, C., and Olsson, Y. (1979): Local anesthetics: Importance of mode of application, concentration and adrenaline for the appearance of nerve lesions. *Acta Anaesthesiol. Scand.,* 23:127–136.
30. Seow, L. T., Lips, F. J., Cousins, M. J., and Mather, L. E. (1982): Lidocaine and bupivacaine mixtures for epidural blockade. *Anesthesiology,* 56:177–183.
31. Smelser, G. K., and Ozanics, V. (1945): Effect of local anesthetics on cell division and migration following thermal burns of the eye. *Arch. Ophthalmol.,* 34:271–277.
32. Stoelting, R. K. (1983): Allergic reactions during anesthesia. *Anesth. Analg.,* 62:341–356.
33. Sweet, P. T., Magee, D. A., and Holland, A. J. C. (1982): Duration of intradermal anaesthesia with mixtures of bupivacaine and lidocaine. *Can. Anaesth. Soc. J.,* 29:481–483.
34. Tanaka, K., and Yamaski, M. (1966): Blocking of cortical inhibitory synapses by intravenous lidocaine. *Nature,* 209:207–208.
35. Yagiela, J. A., Benoit, P. W., Buon-Cristiani, R. D., Peters, M. P., and Fort, N. F. (1981): Comparison of myotoxic effects of lidocaine with epinephrine in rats and humans. *Anesth. Analg.,* 60:471–480.

Commentary

A Consideration of Selected Systemic Diseases Relating to the Surgical Pharmacology of the Eye

Many patients scheduled for ocular surgery are elderly and may be variously medicated. Preoperative medical consultations are often obtained. The ophthalmic surgeon is, obviously, a responsible participant. In this chapter Dr. Puklin reviews selected systemic conditions and indicates how they may interact with medications given during ocular surgery.

The most common cardiac lesions encountered are coronary artery disease and congestive heart failure. Unstable angina pectoris is a definite contraindication for any elective surgery. These patients should first have proper medical management, and, some may even require coronary artery bypass surgery. In evaluating the patients with congestive heart failure the simple "climb-test" may be helpful. If the patient is able to climb two or three flights of stairs without symptoms he or she may have an adequate cardiac reserve.

Surgical monitoring of the heart can be improved by use of a modified EKG utilizing an additional apical lead rather than lead 2. Mannitol or oral glycerin should not be used in patients with renal failure or in patients with congestive heart failure. Preoperative intraocular pressure should be lowered by local methods such as Vorosmarthy's pressure balloon, Honan manometer, and so on.

The chronic use of diuretics may lead to hypokalemia. The operation should be delayed when the serum potassium is 3 mEq/liter or less. The potassium deficit from diuretics may well be chronic and therefore cannot be corrected overnight. The preferred method of replacement is oral use of potassium chloride and deferral of surgery.

Insulin-dependent diabetics are common among our patients. Dr. Puklin gives a very clear regimen for their operative management. Similarly, asthmatic patients may require special management. The author has given valuable guidelines. If the patient requires preoperative corticosteroids it has been good practice to initiate them in moderate amounts at least 10 days prior to surgery. Anxiety may increase the secretion of catecholamines and cause an increase in heart rate and blood pressure and in myocardial oxygen consumption. "A quiet sit-down" with the patient providing him or her with relevant information combined with the appropriate premedication will reduce the level of anxiety.

The ophthalmologist in collaboration with the patient's physicians and anesthesiologist must reach the decision regarding the risks and benefits of delaying surgery. While the opinions of other physicians must be appreciated and enjoined, the ophthalmologist is the surgeon ultimately responsible for his patient.

The Editors

Surgical Pharmacology of the Eye,
edited by M. Sears and A. Tarkkanen.
Raven Press, New York © 1985.

A Consideration of Selected Systemic Diseases Relating to the Surgical Pharmacology of the Eye

James E. Puklin

*The Retina Study Center, Department of Ophthalmology and Visual Science,
Yale University School of Medicine, New Haven, Connecticut 06510*

The preparation of patients for ocular surgery, their management during the operation, and postoperative care are subjects ocular surgeons often take for granted. Much ocular surgery is of short duration and performed under local anesthesia. Nevertheless, most of our patients are elderly, and many are on a variety of medications that achieve varying levels of control for a variety of systemic problems. It is appropriate to consider a select number of frequently encountered or important systemic problems and how they and the medications used to control them may pharmacologically interact during ocular surgery. This chapter focuses on a number of these conditions.

CARDIOVASCULAR DISEASE

Coronary Artery Disease

The most common cardiac lesion encountered before elective noncardiac surgery is coronary artery disease (CAD). The patient's history as it relates to severity, progression, and functional limitations is important. Patients with borderline congestive heart failure (CHF) can be thrown into overt CHF during surgery by sedation, anesthesia, and intravenous fluids. Specific attention should focus on a patient's exercise tolerance represented by dyspnea, angina, orthopnea, recumbent cough, insomnia, unexplained fatigue, and complaints centering around excessive sympathetic nervous system activity such as palpitations and diaphoresis. A patient able to climb two or three flights of stairs without symptoms is likely to have an adequate cardiac reserve.

Angina is divided roughly into three forms: classical, unstable, and Prinzmetal's variant. Classical angina is the result of coronary arteries compromised by atherosclerosis. Increased demands for cardiac oxygenation during stress or exercise produce the symptoms. Angina is considered stable when there has been no recent change in precipitating factors, frequency, and duration. Unstable angina occurs with less than normal activity and may last for prolonged periods. It may also occur at rest. These symptoms may signal an impending myocardial infarction. Such patients can often be controlled by intensive medical management, with subsequent consideration given to coronary artery bypass surgery. Prinzmetal's angina variant is characterized by angina at rest and may be due to coronary artery spasms, in addition to atheromatous disease.

For a patient with CAD facing prospective, elective surgery the history of a previous myocardial infarction is extremely important because the incidence of myocardial reinfarction in the operative and postoperative period is related to the time elapsed from previous infarction (1). If surgery is undertaken within 3 months of the original infarct, the reinfarction rate is 27% to 37%; within 3 to 6 months of the infarction, 11% to 15%; and after 6 months, 6% to 7%. After 6 months the reinfarction rate stabilizes, but at a rate of 6% to 7% it is still about 50 times higher than the risk rate (0.1% to 1.5%) in patients undergoing similar operations but without a history of prior myocardial infarction.

Patients with CAD are usually receiving drugs that fall into three classes: nitrates, β-adrenergic blockers, and calcium channel blockers. The nitrates, which are taken sublingually, orally, or by preparations applied to the skin, are effective because of vasodilatation. A tachyphylaxis to this effect may occur with time. β-Blockers reduce the heart rate, myocardial contractility, and blood pressure. Propanolol is both a β_1- and a β_2-receptor blocker and is therefore contraindicated in patients with asthma and/or chronic obstructive pulmonary disease. Metoprolol is a relatively selective β_1-blocker and is preferred in these patients. These drugs are contraindicated in patients with CHF because they decrease myocardial contractility. Calcium channel blockers relieve coronary spasm and increase coronary blood flow. All three categories of medications should be continued during ocular surgery.

Additional preoperative evaluation should be directed to the role of digitalis and diuretics. Because of the chronic use of diuretics, patients may be hypokalemic and volume-depleted. The hypokalemia will potentiate a toxicity of certain drugs, such as digitalis. The electrocardiographic changes of hypokalemia include premature ventricular contractions and atrioventricular block. Both medications should be continued and elective surgery delayed when the serum potassium is below 3 mEq/liter. It is important to remember that a potassium deficit from diuretics is chronic and cannot be corrected the night before surgery (see section below on potassium). The ocular surgeon should anticipate hypokalemia in all patients who are on diuretics and begin potassium replacement therapy well in advance of surgery. The diuretics and digitalis should also be continued during surgery.

The best operative course will occur if patients arrive in the operating theater well informed and free of anxiety. The primary goal of the preanesthetic medications should be to reduce the anxiety level. Anxiety will cause an increase in catecholamine secretion manifested by increases in heart rate, blood pressure, and myocardial oxygen consumption. A well-informed patient and pharmacologic sedation (see E. Miller, *this volume*) that achieves maximum sedation without undesirable degrees of circulatory and respiratory depression is the goal. In our institution this can usually be accomplished by oral or intravenous diazepam.

During surgery the goal is to prevent myocardial ischemia. If general anesthesia is used, this is the responsibility of the anesthesiologist. Under local anesthesia any untoward event that produces tachycardia, systolic or diastolic hypertension, sympathetic nervous stimulation, or hypoxemia should be avoided. Patients should be attached to an electrocardiographic monitor. The detection of intraoperative myocardial ischemia depends entirely on monitoring the electrocardiogram for ST-segment changes.

Early postoperative mobilization is of great importance in this patient group because of the increased risk of peripheral thromboembolic phenomena with consequent pulmonary emboli. Routine medications should be resumed as quickly as possible. Pain should be controlled with suitable medications. We find that acetaminophen, 650 mg orally every 4 hr p.r.n., is usually sufficient for the postoperative pain following most ocular procedures. If pain is not relieved by acetaminophen, we use a narcotic analgesic such as meperidine hydrochloride and an antiemetic such as trimethabenzamide hydrochloride.

Valvular Heart Disease

Patients with valvular heart disease approaching eye surgery should be managed in accordance with the basic principles of their underlying valvular problem(s) (1) in cooperation with the cardiologist. Because of the added risks of bacterial endocarditis it is essential to administer appropriate systemic antibiotic coverage before, during, and after the surgery. General guidelines state that antimicrobial prophylaxis be started 30 min to 1 hr prior to the predictable bacteremia, rather than 24 hr in advance, so as to reach maximum therapeutic levels but not to obtain superinfection with unusual pathogens (2). When the possibility of an infection exists, or if the surgery itself was undertaken for an infective problem such as endophthalmitis, serial blood cultures should be performed to be certain that the antibiotic being administered is fully effective. The antibiotic chosen should be aimed at the statistically most common pathogen.

Hypertension

Patients with hypertension should be fully controlled and stable prior to ocular surgery. Patients coming to ocular surgery with hypertension that has not been treated should be referred for proper evaluation and the institution of a suitable treatment regimen. When the blood pressure is stable, elective ocular surgery can be undertaken.

Patients with hypertension are likely to be on a wide range of systemic medications. These medications are divided into three groups: diuretics, adrenergic inhibitors (sympatholytics), and vasodilators. Among the diuretics there are the thiazides and their derivatives, the loop diuretics, and potassium-sparing diuretics. The thiazide diuretics are the most commonly used, and their major effect is through diuresis that decreases the intravascular volume. Dietary supplements will prevent hypokalemia, but once it is established they will not correct it. Potassium supplements or potassium-sparing diuretics will be needed. The potassium-sparing diuretics are spironolactone, triamterene, and amiloride. They are weak diuretics and are used mainly as adjuncts to thiazide therapy to prevent hypokalemia. The loop diuretics are furosemide and ethacrynic acid. These are used mainly for hypertensive emergencies.

The adrenergic inhibitors include (a) the β_1- and β_2-receptor blockers (propanolol, timolol, nadolol, and pindolol); (b) the β_1-receptor blockers (antenolol and metoprolol); (c) methyldopa and clonidine, central nervous system agonists inhibiting central sympathetic outflow; (d) guanethidine, a peripheral sympathetic nerve blocker; and (e) reserpine, a catecholamine store depleter. Other adrenergic-inhibiting agents include phentolamine and trimethaphan, which are used intravenously for the rapid lowering of blood pressure in emergency situations.

The vasodilators include (a) hydralazine, an arteriole dilator; (b) prazosin, a postsynaptic α-adrenergic blocker; and (c) minoxidil, a direct relaxer of arteriolar smooth muscle. Other vasodilators, such as diazoxide and nitroprusside, are used intravenously and only for hypertensive emergencies.

The medications that a patient requires for the control of blood pressure should be continued up to and including the day of the operation. On the day of surgery the usual medications should be given by the usual route with sips of water. This does not seriously violate the NPO policy and prevents a serious rebound effect caused by interrupting the antihypertensive medications.

Regardless of the anesthetic choice the patient should be pain- and anxiety-free to prevent a catecholamine response. In local cases the addition of epinephrine hydrochloride to the retrobulbar anesthesia should be avoided. Additionally, the use of dilating drops such as 10% phenylephrine during the surgical procedure to prolong mydriasis should be avoided. Systemic absorption occurs and can raise the blood pressure significantly. Electrocardiographic monitoring should be employed. Cardiac-depressant drugs and excessive sedation should be avoided.

In patients who fear local anesthesia it is appropriate to use general anesthesia for greater patient comfort. Often, in the very ill hypertensive patient better control of the patient, the airway, the circulation, and the depth of anesthesia can be achieved by general anesthesia.

The postoperative care of the hypertensive patient involves adequate pain control and sedation. If the surgery has lasted several hours, as in complex retinal detachment or vitrectomy procedures, it is possible that a dose of the antihypertensive medication has been missed. This factor must be considered in the differential diagnosis of a rise in the blood pressure in the immediate postsurgical period. Suitable medications must be used to control the blood pressure during this time until the normal therapeutic regimen can be resumed.

Pacemakers

Patients with pacemakers are becoming more common. More than half of patients with pacemakers are over 70 years of age. It is important for the ocular surgeon to understand several aspects regarding patients who have pacemakers.

Permanent artificial pacemakers are used when patients have defects in impulse formation or impulse conduction resulting in a heart rate and cardiac output that does not provide adequate cerebral and coronary perfusion. The preoperative evaluation should include understanding the reason for pacemaker implantation and should insure that symptoms are stable and that medical therapy is adequate. It is probably advisable to institute prophylactic therapy for bacterial endocarditis in a manner similar to the procedure outlined for valvular heart disease.

General anesthetic techniques have been previously addressed. Under local anesthesia, cardiac and blood pressure monitoring is essential. The most important intraoperative concern is the potentially dangerous effect of electromagnetic fields on the pacemaker. The bone saws and electrical cautery used for dacryocystorhinostomies and extensive orbital procedures may produce interference. For *fixed-rate* (asynchronous) pacemakers, currently rarely used, the problem is minor, because these are relatively insensitive to electrical interference. *Demand* pacemakers (synchronous) may sense an electrical pulse generated from a source other than the heart (they sense and are suppressed by spontaneous P or R wave formation). Thus, the external electrical activity may suppress a demand pacemaker and the patient will revert to the rhythm for which the pacemaker therapy was instituted, and cardiac standstill may ensue.

For electrocautery, the indifferent plate of the cautery unit should be as far away from the pulse generator as possible. Pulse palpation or auscultation with a stethoscope will be needed, as the electrocardiogram will be useless owing to the electrical surges. The use of electrocautery should be avoided in all patients with pacemakers. The battery-powered disposable cauteries do not cause problems. An electromagnet of 10,000 gauss, such as used for removal of intraocular foreign bodies, will produce interference on the electrocardiogram monitor and will temporarily convert a demand pacemaker to a fixed-rate pacemaker. The pacemaker will revert back to its demand mode when the magnet is turned off.

ENDOCRINE DISEASE

Diabetes Mellitus

Diabetes mellitus is the most common endocrine disorder in clinical medicine and affects approximately 2% to 4% of the Western population. It is a chronic metabolic disorder of carbohydrate metabolism resulting in inappropriately high blood glucose levels. Many patients coming to eye surgery have diabetes because of the association of diabetes with an increased incidence of cataracts and because of the complications of diabetic retinopathy. As a group they often represent some of the most severely ill patients requiring surgery, particularly those who need vitrectomy surgery for end-stage diabetic retinopathy.

Diabetes mellitus is commonly divided into two groups (3). Type I diabetes is generally associated with an abrupt onset of symptoms, a dependence on injected insulin to sustain life, and a proneness to ketosis. The causes of type I diabetes include an association with certain genetically determined cell surface antigens of lymphocytes (HLA haplotypes), the association with certain viral infections (coxsackievirus [group B], mumps, rubella, and cytomegalovirus) preceding the onset of diabetes, immunologic mechanisms associated with humoral and cell-mediated B-cell destruction, and possible environmental chemical injury to the B-cells (4).

Type II diabetes is generally non-insulin dependent (although some patients may require insulin for optimal control) and is not prone to ketosis nor dependent on insulin to prevent ketonuria. The causes of type II diabetes are less well established but probably also comprise several subsets. There tends to be family aggregation of this type of diabetes and a high association with obesity (60% to 90% of patients), but HLA haplotypes and autoimmune responses do not play a role.

Diabetics who are under loose control are characterized by a body-fuel metabolism represented by (in addition to an elevated blood glucose level) hyperaminoacidemia, hyperlipidemia, excessive urinary calcium and phosphate loss, and elevated plasma levels of catecholamines, growth hormone, and glucagon. Improvement in metabolic control can return these abnormalities to near-normal levels, but there is currently little evidence to support the premise that tight metabolic control influences the microvascular complications that diabetic patients develop (5). The abnormal metabolic events are eventually accompanied by atherosclerotic and microangiopathic cardiovascular disease, neuropathies, nephropathies, arthropathies, dermopathies, cataracts, retinopathy, and neovascular glaucoma.

A patient with diabetes who is to undergo elective ocular surgery should be in the best medical condition possible. The development of large- and small-blood-vessel disease in these patients requires that they be considered older than their chronological age. Diabetic patients are about 5 to 10 times more likely to have a myocardial infarct in the intraoperative period than their cohorts in the general population. Careful attention should be given to the presence of hypertension, angina, heart failure, and myocardial infarction. Potassium metabolism may be abnormal because potassium may be depleted due to osmotic diuresis and moved intracellularly by more insulin. Patients on digitalis may develop arrythmias if they are hypokalemic.

For patients with type II diabetes treated with oral hypoglycemic agents and undergoing elective ocular surgery under local anesthesia it is not necessary to modify their drug regimen. For type II diabetic patients on insulin management, one-half to three-quarters of the regular morning insulin dose is given, and an intravenous infusion of 5% glucose is begun at the rate of about 50 cc/hr. Type I diabetic patients undergoing elective ocular surgery under local anesthesia may also be managed without a change in their regimen. Our usual practice, however, is to give such patients one-half to three-quarters of their normal morning insulin dose and to begin an intravenous drip of 5% glucose at the rate of about 50 cc/hr. About 1,000 cc of a 5% glucose solution is infused over each 8-hr period. Subsequent to surgery, the remaining dose of insulin for that day is administered and, when food intake is resumed, the intravenous drip is discontinued.

Patients undergoing general anesthesia require greater modification of their diabetic management. The goals of such management are to prevent acidosis and to prevent severe fluid loss and hypoglycemia. A number of regimens have been advocated.

Patients who are taking oral hypoglycemic agents should stop their medications as follows: Those taking tolbutamide (half-life, 5 hr; duration of action, 10 hr) and acetohexamide (half-life, 6 hr; duration of action, 12 to 24 hr) should not take their pills on the day of surgery. Chlorpropamide (half-life, 35 hr; duration of action, 60 hr) should be discontinued 2 days prior to surgery. These patients should then be managed with insulin during the operation and the immediate postoperative period.

For patients on insulin our procedure is to give the patient one-half the normal morning insulin dose and begin an intravenous infusion of 5% glucose and one-half normal saline at the rate of about 50 cc/hr. For surgical procedures more than 2 hr in length we obtain a blood glucose level in the operating room. Postoperatively, all patients have blood glucose determinations in the recovery room. Repeat blood glucose assessments may be obtained at 6-hr intervals. Regular insulin is used to manage the patient for the rest of that day. For blood glucose levels of less than 120 mg/dl the rate of glucose infusion is increased or changed to a solution of 10% glucose. For glucose levels between 120 and 200 mg/dl no additional insulin is given. When the blood glucose is between 200 and 300 mg/dl, we give about 4 U regular insulin; between 300 and 400 mg/dl, about 8 U; and between 400 and 500 mg/dl, about 12 U. Patients are encouraged to resume their normal oral caloric intake and regular insulin dosage as soon as possible, which is usually on or before the first postoperative day. It is important in the postoperative period to avoid hypoglycemia. Mild glycosuria and glycosemia are more desirable than glucose-free urine and euglycemia.

Additional Caveats About Drug Interactions During Surgery

In addition to hypokalemia and its potential effects on the cardiac status during surgery, several other pharmacologic interactions as they relate to the diabetic patient are important. Nonselective β-adrenergic blocking agents have gained wide acceptance. Propanolol, and now timolol, are used systemically for the treatment of hypertension, the prophylaxis of angina pectoris, and the control of certain types of cardiac arrythmias (see above). These drugs, taken systemically, augment the hypoglycemic action of insulin and mask the tachycardia that is an important sign of developing hypoglycemia. Patients susceptible to hypoglycemia must be alerted to the subtle signs of its development and respond appropriately. Surgeons operating on diabetic patients who also take oral β-adrenergic blocking agents must be aware that the usual signs of developing hypoglycemia may not occur. Timolol is widely used as eye drops for the control of glaucoma. Systemic absorption of the drug occurs and, in addition to other systemic responses, may mask the usual signs of developing hypoglycemia.

Thyroid

Patients who are hyperthyroid or hypothyroid present greater surgical and anesthetic risks than do patients who are euthyroid. Patients who are not euthyroid should be brought to the euthyroid state prior to surgery. For the hyperthyroid patient this can be accomplished preoperatively by therapeutic doses of radioactive iodine, antithyroid drugs, or a subtotal thyroidectomy. Usually, an antithyroid drug such as propylthiouracil or methimazole can be given for several weeks to achieve a euthyroid state. The usual daily dose of propylthiouracil is 400 to 600 mg in three or four divided doses. The equivalent dose of methimazole is about one-tenth that of propylthiouracil. Patients who have severe hyperthyroidism may require larger doses, up to 800 to 1,000 mg of propylthiouracil per day.

If emergency surgery is necessary before a hyperthyroid patient can be brought to the euthyroid state, the premedication must be modified. More sedation is indicated. Short-acting barbiturates have a moderate hypnotic effect and help to relieve apprehension. Narcotics in larger than usual doses decrease the metabolic rate and cause patients to be less concerned. Anticholinergic drugs in high doses will aggravate the tachycardia, but small doses of scopolamine will provide sedation as well as anticholinergic effect. The β-adrenergic blocker propranolol may also be used.

For the hypothyroid patient, treatment involves gradually increasing doses of thyroid replacement hormone. Adequate daily replacement is obtained with 0.1 to 0.2 mg of L-thyroxine (T_4) or an equivalent dose of pure T_3, or mixtures of T_3 and T_4. Once the euthyroid state is reached, the surgical risks are reduced and surgery may be undertaken with greater safety.

Hypoparathyroidism and Pseudohypoparathyroidism

Hypoparathyroidism, a disorder of mineral metabolism that occurs from the deficient secretion of parathyroid hormone (PTH), may be idiopathic but usually is the result of inadvertent removal of the parathyroid glands during thyroid surgery. Pseudohypoparathyroidism, a disorder of mineral metabolism in which the end organ is unresponsive to PTH, is rare and probably transmitted as a sex-linked dominant trait. The clinical manifestations of these two disorders include tetany and/or seizures, cataracts, and calcification of the basal ganglia. The treatment for both includes calcium and vitamin D. Occasionally, patients with cataracts associated with these two disorders come to surgery. If surgery is to be with local anesthesia, no special precautions are required. With general anesthesia, low ionized serum calcium increases the surgical risk because of cardiac and skeletal muscle irritability. The use of an intravenous solution of calcium gluconate will alleviate these problems. To prevent unwanted extraocular muscle fasciculations and contracture while the globe is open it may be inappropriate to use a retrobulbar block as well.

RENAL DISEASE

The development of hemodialysis and the widespread establishment of dialysis centers in the past two decades have resulted in a rapid increase in the number of patients surviving with chronic end-stage renal disease (6). The number of patients on maintenance hemodialysis is a rapidly emerging subgroup of society, and for reasons relating to the disease causing their end-stage renal failure and associated therapy, these patients will often be candidates for ocular surgery. Their problems range from cataracts associated with diabetes or the prolonged corticosteroid therapy for immunosuppression to corneal ulcers and perforation, epiretinal membrane formation, retinal detachment, and vitreous hemorrhage. It is necessary to manage these patients cooperatively with the nephrologist and the anesthesiologist and to have a basic understanding of the interrelated medical problems confronting them.

Preoperative Factors

Attention should be directed to the dialysis schedule and the current medications. Preoperative dialysis should be accomplished within 24 hr prior to surgery (7). Heparin is required for the extracorporeal circuit, and careful preoperative dialysis using the slow-infusion technique (rather than bolus or regional heparinization) will insure that patients are at no greater risk from bleeding complications than are normal patients (8).

Serum potassium levels should be as low as possible and should not exceed 5.5 mEq/liter. The hospital diet should strictly limit sodium and potassium intake, and salt substitutes should be avoided. Fluid intake must also be severely limited to insure optimal blood pressure and cardiac output. If possible, intravenous infusion should be avoided altogether. If intravenous infusions are necessary, small-bore tubing should be used, and intravenous solutions containing potassium, such as Ringer's lactate, should be avoided.

Most patients on chronic dialysis are receiving many medications. These should be maintained, and with the help of the nephrologist the potassium-digitalis interaction should be carefully watched to prevent digitalis toxicity (8). Uremic patients have a chronic normocytic-normochromic anemia resulting from (a) reduction of erythropoietin and erythrocyte production, (b) hemolysis, and (c) gastrointestinal bleeding. These patients are adjusted to their anemia. Rarely do they have a hemoglobin greater than 9 g/dl or a hematocrit greater than 27%. Higher levels are difficult to obtain and should not be a preoperative therapeutic goal. Circulatory overload can result from transfusion and the hematocrit will promptly return to its baseline level within a few days of the transfusion. If a transfusion is needed, washed, leukocyte-poor, packed red cells should be used to reduce the potassium load and to reduce the risk of rejection of a future renal transplant (9). The exact nature of the platelet dysfunction associated with renal failure is unknown but it appears to be an extrinsic defect because platelet function is restored to normal after dialysis. This defect will not be reflected in the platelet count, which will be normal.

The arteriovenous fistula is the hemodialysis patient's lifeline. Attention must be given to its preservation. No intravenous infusions or injections should be introduced into that extremity, and the extremity must be positioned to avoid an inadvertent closure of the fistula, which will require additional surgery.

Chronic renal failure patients exhibit suppressed cell-mediated immunity and altered skin and mucosal barriers (10). Hemodialysis creates granulocyte dysfunctions. Thus, lengthy operations may increase the risk of infections. There is no evidence to indicate that special precautions need to be taken for antibiotics administered topically or subconjunctivally. Most of these ophthalmic drugs are generally safe because small amounts of the drug reach the circulation and alternative excretory pathways exist. Parenteral antibiotics and other systemic medications will usually require dose modification to prevent toxicity, and these should be carefully monitored with the help of the nephrologist (11,12).

Mannitol and oral glycerin are not to be used. Both are commonly used preoperatively in order to shrink the vitreous and occasionally postoperatively to lower intraocular pressure rises. They are also used to treat narrow-angle glaucoma. These drugs increase the osmolarity of the intravascular compartment, and as they depend entirely on the kidney for elimination, they will circulate unchanged until the next dialysis. Small doses in the patient with renal failure will precipitate pulmonary edema, metabolic acidosis, hyponatremia, and hyperosmolar nonketotic coma (11).

Operative Factors

Local anesthesia is preferable in these patients because it will reduce the risks of complications. The intravenous use of diazepam or diphenhydramine is safe as a hypnotic agent. Local anesthetic agents such as lidocaine, mepivacaine, or bupivacaine should be selected on the basis of the anticipated length of the case. Adrenergic agonists such as epinephrine add excessive risks and little benefit to these patients and should be avoided.

If general anesthesia is indicated, most commonly used inhalation anesthetics can be used along with narcotics and skeletal muscle relaxants (10). The lightest anesthesia plane possible is preferred so as to avoid a depressed cardiac output.

Postoperative

The postoperative care of the patient with renal failure relies on principles previously mentioned. Hyperkalemia is the leading cause of postoperative morbidity (7). Thus, serum electrolytes should be obtained every 6 to 8 hr in the first postoperative day. Attention must also be given to the serial electrocardiograms for the hyperkalemic changes that they may reflect. Fevers should be vigorously investigated because infection is the leading cause of mortality in these patients. An elevated blood pressure usually represents fluid overload. Hypotension results from pericardial effusion, myocardial infarction, autonomic dysfunction, or medications. The first postoperative dialysis should be delayed to 48 to 72 hr after surgery to reduce bleeding complications.

PULMONARY DISEASE

Many elderly patients undergoing ocular surgery have chronic obstructive pulmonary disease (COPD). It is essential that these patients be in the best possible pulmonary condition prior to surgery so that the operative and postoperative periods pass as free of complicating events as possible. Demonstrable abnormalities of pulmonary function are usually associated with obesity and cigarette smoking, and these environmental or acquired abnormalities are often superimposed on the changes of lung function that constitute the normal aging process. Thus, a good preoperative history should include a careful inquiry about coughing, allergy or wheezing, and smoking. A drug history is important, because drugs such as reserpine, steroids, diuretics, and bronchodilators may alter the cardiorespiratory responsiveness during and after surgery. An excessive use of bronchodilators may cause a paradoxical increase in airway resistance.

Clinically, these patients may demonstrate many signs of pulmonary disease. These include a cough, general muscle mass wasting and weakness, cyanosis, digital clubbing, tracheal deviation, and the typical signs of respiratory acidosis, which are vasodilatation and bounding pulses. A general indicator of the severity of the obstructive pulmonary disease is the height of the jugular venous pulse, which is the result of an increased intrapleural pressure interfering with venous return.

Whether a patient has intrinsic chronic obstructive or restrictive lung disease or a major systemic disease with pulmonary sequelae, it is helpful and important to have an estimate of the mechanics of ventilation obtained by pulmonary function tests. Arterial blood gases will provide additional information about blood-gas exchange.

On the basis of history, physical examination, and laboratory data the level of pulmonary dysfunction can be ascertained. Prior to surgery a patient's pulmonary status must be put into the most stable state. The ophthalmologist, in collaboration with a patient's other physicians and an anesthesiologist, must often reach a decision early regarding the risks and benefits of delaying surgery. Improvement in respiratory function is often possible using techniques of respiratory therapy. Respiratory therapy often requires varying periods of time to stabilize a patient maximally, and this depends on the type and severity of the existing pulmonary problems.

There are many specific measures that can be employed. Patients who smoke should stop. A demonstrable improvement in airway clearing mechanisms will occur in 2 to 3 weeks time. If bronchospasm exists, bronchodilators may be used orally, intravenously, or by inhalation. Thick secretions will be loosened by adequate hydration. Intraluminal hydration with an ultrasonic nebulizer after pretreatment with a bronchodilator will prevent increased airway resistance and assist pulmonary drainage. Persistently thick secretions may respond to acetylcysteine or pancreatic dornase administered by a nebulizer, with proper pretreatment to prevent bronchospasm. Pulmonary physiotherapy should be employed, using chest vibration and percussion and stimulation of the cough mechanism. If corticosteroids have been used to treat pulmonary problems preceding surgery, they should be maintained prior to surgery, increased on the day of surgery and the day following surgery, and then tapered over the next few days to a maintenance level.

Eye surgery patients with pulmonary disease represent a difficult group of patients. This is because the patients must lie flat, and the surgical draping technique includes drapes that, to some extent, pass over the face and nose. As these patients are aware of their pulmonary problems, they frequently become anxious beneath the drapes, fearing a lack of oxygen or actually experiencing dyspnea. Coughing is also frequently difficult to control. The best technique for local anesthesia is to prepare the patient properly for the operating room experience by informing the patient of what is to happen. Then light sedation with good local and regional block and swift surgery will help to insure the best result. Nasal cannulas with air flowing through will give the patient a strong sense of confidence and security.

For the most severe pulmonary cases or for surgical procedures that will take a long time our anesthesia department prefers general anesthesia with periodic arterial blood gas monitoring. This affords the surgeon a quiet environment free of the unexpected surprises that patients with severe pulmonary disease frequently provide and also insures that the patient will be properly controlled.

The postoperative care of pulmonary patients centers around preserving an adequate exchange, with good hydration and pulmonary physiotherapy. The ocular surgeon can best insure excellent results by recognizing that the postoperative course will involve coughing and other pulmonary straining. Ocular wounds should be sewn tightly to guard against an undesirable wound dehiscence.

TRAUMA

Trauma may be generalized, or localized to several organs or organ systems. The eye and its adnexa may be the only organ system involved or may be part of a more widespread systemic trauma. Although trauma does not constitute a "systemic disease," it is appropriate to consider certain aspects of trauma relating to the eye. Trauma patients may, of course, have a variety of other systemic diseases and these must also be given attention.

The Traumatized Eye and Adnexa

The principles of evaluating ocular trauma have been extensively discussed (13,14). Those emergencies requiring urgent surgery include globe lacerations, intraocular foreign bodies, severe lid lacerations, some craniofacial fractures, and many endophthalmitis cases. Surgery for other ocular injuries may be delayed for a more optimal time. These traumas include total or blackball hyphema, many orbital fractures, lens dislocation, vitreous hemorrhage, and retinal detachment not associated with an open globe. In this latter group a patient's general medical condition can be properly evaluated and timely, safe surgery undertaken. Systemic conditions should be managed before, during, and subsequent to surgery, as in all previously discussed disease entities.

When urgent or emergent surgery is necessary, time must still be taken to obtain a comprehensive history and to perform a comprehensive examination. It is often not possible, however, to wait until the patient is in optimal medical condition for the surgery. The primary problems center around operating on patients with opened globes and/or a full stomach.

The patient with severe trauma who is in pain and has a full stomach deserves emphasis, because aspiration pneumonitis remains a major cause of anesthesia morbidity and mortality. Gastric motility is reduced or ceases under the stimulus of either somatic or visceral pain, and thus the stomach is not likely to empty normally even if the operative procedure is delayed. Patients sustaining severe eye injury within several hours of eating are still likely to have a full stomach up to 10 hr later unless they have actively vomited. Thus, the interval between the last meal and the time of the accident is more important than the interval between the last meal and the induction of anesthesia (15). In addition, such patients may have stimulation of the chemoreceptor trigger zone and the induction of vomiting when the commonly used synthetic opioid, fentanyl, is used for anesthetic induction. Fentanyl's role in the rapid anesthetic induction of patients with a full stomach is not yet well defined. Large doses may be contraindicated since they will suppress spontaneous respiration and may induce truncal rigidity (16).

Succinylcholine is a neuromuscular blocking agent that acts to depolarize membranes in a manner similar to acetylcholine. As succinylcholine persists in the neuromuscular junction longer than acetylcholine, the depolarization is longer lasting, resulting in transient muscular fasciculations followed by a paralytic effect lasting about 5 min. The rise in intraocular pressure averages about 8 mm Hg 2 to 3 min after injection (17,18). The pressure falls to normal levels in about 6 min. Maximum elevations have reached levels above 30 mm Hg. It is thought these pressure rises are due to the transient fasciculations of the extraocular muscles. Thus, the popular use of succinyl-choline is to be avoided when choosing a neuromuscular blocking agent for surgery of an open globe. Additionally, it should be avoided when "exploratory" surgery is carried out to ascertain the presence of a suspected ruptured globe. Other neuromuscular blocking agents, such as D-tubocurarine, metocurine, gallamine, and pancuronium are nondepolarizing agents. They act as competitive neuromuscular blockers and bind at the cholinergic receptor site in the postjunctional membrane, competitively blocking the transmitter action of acetylcholine. They directly paralyze the extraocular muscles without the depolarizing fasciculations associated with succinylcholine and do not, therefore, acutely raise the intraocular pressure.

Thus, patients with ocular trauma requiring urgent or emergent surgery should be assumed to have a full stomach. The choices of techniques and of pharmacology should prevent emesis and aspiration of gastric contents and prevent an increase in intraocular pressure. They may include using an antiemetic such as droperidol, intramuscularly, in the premedication and intravenous lidocaine just prior to the intubation to lessen sympathetic response. Preoxygenation may be accomplished with a mask while the ocular area is protected by a metal shield. Laryngoscopy and intubation should be done after achieving deep general anesthesia with an intravenous medication such as thiopental. Neuromuscular blockade should be accomplished first by one of the nondepolarizing competitive blockers. If succinylcholine is needed it may then be used without a rise in the intraocular pressure. A nasogastric or orogastric tube should be used to decompress the stomach. Patients should be extubated while awake after a smooth emergence and careful pharyngeal suctioning.

The Trauma Patient with Ocular Involvement

In cases involving severe explosions, chemical burns, or thermal burns one or both eyes may be badly damaged. The initial care is directed toward shock management and airway maintenance. Severe trauma, hemorrhage, and shock cause a reduction in oxygen transport to tissues, which will lead to cellular hypoxia and death if uncorrected. Factors influencing a patient's homeostatic mechanisms and ability to deal with hypovolemia include the preexisting physiologic status, presence or absence of major organ system pathology, presence of acute intoxication, current drug therapy, and condition of the stomach. For an organ system to survive shock and hemorrhage the microcirculation must be maintained. Little is known about the effect of this form of trauma on the microcirculation to the retina, choroid, optic nerve, and the rest of the visual pathway.

When the usual principles of managing the traumatized patient have been met and the patient is stable, the previously discussed factors affecting the potentially open globe should be met and timely surgery undertaken.

HEMOGLOBINOPATHIES

Hereditary diseases affecting the structure of hemoglobin are of particular interest to ophthalmologists and anesthesiologists alike. Patients with sickle cell disease and sickle cell trait may require anterior segment surgery. Proliferative sickle cell retinopathy can occur in patients with homozygous sickle cell disease (SS), sickle cell-C disease (SC), sickle cell thalassemia disease (S-thal), sickle cell O-Arab disease (S-O Arab), sickle cell trait (AS), and hemoglobin C trait (AC). Retinal detachment is generally related to vitreous traction, peripheral neovascularization, and retinal tears. It has been reported to occur in 4.3% of patients with SC disease and 1.4% of patients with SS disease (19,20).

Retinal detachment and vitrectomy surgery is often difficult owing to fibrovascular membranes and vitreous hemorrhage, which may obscure holes or tears. These cases often require lengthy operations involving broad, high buckles. Anterior segment ischemia, a syndrome consisting of conjunctival edema, corneal edema with folds in Descemet's membrane, iris bogginess followed by necrosis, loss of pupillary tone, rubeosis iridis, cataract formation, and hypotony has occurred in up to 60% of such cases undergoing ocular surgery (21). The cause is believed to be intraoperative intravascular sickling causing hypoxia to the anterior eye.

Current operative management of patients with sickling hemoglobinopathies involves exchange blood transfusions. Although the exact level of hemoglobin-A that will protect the eye from anterior segment ischemia is not known, a hemoglobin-A level of 50% or more is believed sufficient to protect the anterior segment from intraoperative sickling and subsequent hypoxia. Thus, achieving this level by partial exchange transfusions appears to make it possible to perform the extensive surgical techniques required for complex retinal detachment and vitrectomy procedures without modification of other aspects of the procedure or the development of anterior segment ischemia (22,23). Exchange transfusions also probably help to prevent intraoperative and postoperative systemic sickling that can result in thromboembolic complications.

Secondary glaucoma may develop as the result of anterior segment blood in patients with these hemoglobinopathies (24). The nonpliable sickled cells obstruct the trabecular meshwork and may lead to secondary glaucoma and corneal blood staining. Intraocular hemorrhages in the immediate postoperative period after vitrectomy and lensectomy will contain few cells with sickle hemoglobin after the partial exchange transfusion, thereby reducing the chances of this form of postvitrectomy glaucoma.

Anesthetic procedures should reduce the risk of hypoxia, acidosis, stasis, and cooling. Special attention should be given to the arterial oxygen tensions, which should be measured prior to surgery, intraoperatively, and postoperatively. Postoperatively, supplemental oxygen should be administered for up to 2 days, with periodic blood gas assessments and additional exchange transfusions as needed.

MUSCLE DISEASE

Malignant Hyperthermia

Malignant hyperthermia is a systemic metabolic disorder of muscle. Most cases are nonfamilial, but it can be genetically transmitted as an autosomal dominant disorder. Questions about its penetrance and expressivity are unresolved (25). The incidence of malignant hyperthermia is 1 in 15,000 cases of anesthetized children and 1 in 50,000 cases of anesthetized adults, and it is therefore fairly uncommon. It is, however, potentially fatal, with a mortality rate as high as 70%, and occurs with greater frequency in patients with known musculoskeletal abnormalities such as ptosis and strabismus. It is for these reasons that it is an important concern to the ophthalmic surgeon. Other systemic musculoskeletal abnormalities with which malignant hyperthermia is associated include hernias, kyphoscoliosis, clubfoot, joint hypermobility, and local muscle weakness.

The cause of malignant hyperthermia is unproved, but it is believed that abnormal calcium movements within muscle cells produce the clinical signs and symptoms. Calcium release and reuptake is regulated by muscle membrane depolarization, calcium intracellular concentrations, and adenosine triphosphate (ATP) concentrations.

The preoperative diagnosis of malignant hyperthermia cannot be made in the sporadic case, but it should be suspected during the anesthetic induction if there is a tachycardia or isolated masseter muscle spasm during the administration of succinylcholine (a paradoxical response). These signs (together or separate), not a rise in temperature, are the first signs of malignant hyperthermia, and elective surgical procedures should be terminated immediately (26). When there are reasons to believe that malignant hyperthermia exists, the screening methods used are nonspecific, and several tests must be used together to make a confident judgment. One-third of patients susceptible to malignant hyperthermia have normal creatine phosphokinase (CPK) levels; thus, CPK levels are not diagnostic. Assessing the isozymes of CPK may be more useful (27). Other predictive tests (28) include an abnormal platelet aggregation response to epinephrine hydrochloride, abnormal platelet ATP reduction, and muscle biopsies showing *in vitro* caffeine-induced or halothane-induced contraction responses. The triad of an elevated CPK level, a family history of susceptibility to malignant hyperthermia, and a musculoskeletal abnormality such as strabismus or ptosis is highly suggestive as an indicator of malignant hyperthermia susceptibility.

The classic signs of malignant hyperthermia include muscle rigidity, tachycardia, tachypnea, metabolic and respiratory acidosis, paradoxical reaction to succinylcholine, and hyperthermia. In general the higher the temperature, the higher the mortality rate. Several anesthetic agents may trigger malignant hyperthermia (see E. Miller, *this volume*). The treatment of malignant hyperthermia includes discontinuing the anesthesia, hyperventilation with 100% oxygen, aggressive cooling, the maintenance of adequate urine output, and other intensive monitoring measures (29). The intravenous use of dantrolene, a direct skeletal muscle relaxant, should be started.

It is wise to avoid elective surgery in patients who are known to be susceptible to malignant hyperthermia. Should surgery be necessary, it can be done with little risk if adequate precautions are taken. If possible, local anesthesia should be used. Tetracaine and procaine are safe. General anesthesia should be done with barbiturates, nitrous oxide, narcotics, and pancuronium. Prophylactic preoperative dantrolene may also be used. Ketamine and chlorpromazine should be avoided.

Myotonic Muscular Dystrophy

Myotonic muscular dystrophy is also known as Steinert's disease, Batten-Curschmann's disease, or myotonia atrophica. It is autosomal dominant and characterized by a myotonia, distal muscle wasting, testicular atrophy, cardiac conduction blocks, pulmonary hypoventilation, abnormal glucose tolerance, and cataracts. Its incidence is about 3 to 5 per 100,000, and it becomes symptomatic in adolescence or early adult life. A biological ocular hypotony exists in these patients presumably as a result of the elevated gonadotropin (follicle-stimulating hormone) stimulating the adenylcyclase-receptor complex, reducing net aqueous flow (30). The basic myotonic phenomenon is a contracture due to abnormal muscle membrane activity with electrical silence in the efferent motor nerves and at the myoneural junction. Thus, anticholinesterases generally make the myotonia worse, and total neuromuscular blockage with curare has no effect. Neuromuscular junction depolarizers such as succinylcholine lead to contracture. The treatment is with muscle-membrane-stabilizing drugs such as quinine, procainamide, and phenytoin.

Patients with myotonic muscular dystrophy occasionally come to cataract surgery and the achievement of muscle relaxation is one of the most difficult anesthetic problems. Surgery under local anesthesia presents the lowest risk, and the myotonia may be completely blocked by retrobulbar injection and local muscle infiltration with an agent such as lidocaine. General anesthesia poses many problems (31) regarding cardiac stability and myotonia of the thoracic and laryngeal musculature. Adequate airway maintenance and oxygen exchange may be difficult. Deep general anesthesia will depress respiration for a prolonged period. For open ocular surgery a quiet globe is best assured by adding a retrobulbar and infiltrative muscle block.

HEPATIC DISEASE

Although hepatic disease is a serious systemic problem, there are only a few aspects that relate directly to the care of the eye surgery patient. These center primarily on the chronic anemia, often associated with a leukopenia and thrombocytopenia, and the coagulation defects that occur. Patients with hepatic disease generally fall into two categories: (a) those with unsuspected liver disease and (b) those with known liver dysfunction due either to extrahepatic obstruction or to documented liver disease.

The ocular surgeon must be careful to detect the patient with unsuspected liver disease who is to undergo surgery. An example is the "secret" drinker who has nodular cirrhosis. A careful inquiry will elicit a history of prior hepatitis, jaundice, dark urine, or alcohol abuse. Physical signs include the typical spider nevi, palmar erythema, pruritus, nail clubbing, and an increase in cutaneous melanin pigment. The preoperative laboratory screening should include the usual tests of liver function such as bilirubin, transaminase, alkaline phosphatase, leucine aminopeptidase, and gamma-glutamyl transpeptidase. For patients with known liver disease, whether extrahepatic or intrahepatic, the diagnosis has been established and therapy previously instituted.

Preoperative coagulation defects present the major problems in patients with hepatic disease. Factors VII, IX, and X are produced by the liver and may be deficient. A thrombocytopenia secondary to hypersplenism, or in the alcoholic due to bone marrow depression, has important implications. Prothrombin production is usually reduced and the prothrombin time prolonged. This correlates with both the severity of the parenchymal liver disease and the vitamin K deficiency secondary to malabsorption. Parenteral vitamin K will restore prothrombin production in cases of biliary obstruction but may not be effective if hepatocellular disease is severe. To prevent excessive bleeding at surgery in these patients fresh blood should be transfused and fresh-frozen plasma and cryoprecipitates given as needed. Occasionally platelet transfusions may be needed to overcome the thrombocytopenia.

The hepatic microsomes play a key role in the detoxification and metabolism of many drugs. Thus, preoperative analgesics and sedatives must be given cautiously, and a good rule to follow is to administer about 25% of the normal amount given to a similar patient of comparable age and weight with normal hepatic function. If a hepatic encephalopathy is present, sedatives should not be given and analgesics should be administered with great caution. Most currently used intravenous and inhalation anesthetic agents do not appear to cause liver damage by direct toxic effects. Suspicion exists that the hepatitis, on rare occasions, follows halothane anesthesia and may be related to its hepatic metabolism. All anesthetic agents and techniques reduce hepatic blood flow by either a fall in blood pressure or by a reduction in splanchnic blood flow. Pseudocholinesterase is an enzyme, the production of which is impaired by hepatic disease, and a fourfold reduction is required before the depolarizing neuromuscular blockade of succinylcholine is prolonged. Drugs such as lidocaine, meperidine, and diazepam have prolonged plasma half-lives in severe chronic liver disease. Postoperatively, the usual catabolic state that follows surgery is accentuated in the already catabolic patient with liver disease. Efforts to improve anabolism should be made preoperatively and postoperatively. Cirrhotics are more prone to postoperative infections, and these infections must be diagnosed early and treated vigorously.

PREGNANCY

Teratogenicity for virtually all drug and anesthetic agents has been implicated under certain conditions. At present, however, there is no proof that any anesthetic drug, premedicant, intravenous induction agent, inhalation agent, or local anesthetic is teratogenic in humans. Nevertheless, it is probably safe to assume that some potential for teratogenicity does exist and postpone elective surgery until after pregnancy (32,33). The period of organogenesis is the first 12 weeks of gestation, and medication and surgery should be avoided during this period if at all possible. If surgery cannot be delayed unduly (such as in retinal detachment), the usual systemic preparations should be made and a local anesthetic used if possible. If a general anesthetic is needed, it should be accomplished without halogenated agents. In the last trimester of pregnancy the presence or absence of uterine contractions should be determined and fetal heart rates should be monitored. In the later parts of pregnancy special positioning on the operating table may be needed to avoid uterine compression of the large abdominal vessels during the surgery.

Another consideration that occurs less frequently is the timing of surgery and choice of drugs in the lactating mother. Most of the substances given to the mother will be excreted in the breast milk.

While fluorescein has not been shown to be teratogenic in humans, we do not perform fluorescein angiograms on patients known to be pregnant. Fluorescein angiography is, however, usually performed as needed on postpartum lactating mothers. We feel that the breast secretions with fluorescein will have no effect on the infant. Surgical procedures on the lactating mother are performed under local anesthesia if possible and under general anesthesia if needed. In the latter case infants are fed bottles for a day or two subsequent to surgery, and breast pumps are used to relieve the mother until normal feeding resumes. It is unlikely that isolated maternal exposure to these drugs will affect the breast-fed neonate (34).

INFECTIONS

Patients with ocular infections may often require systemic antibiotics for proper treatment of the infection. In the case of a severe endophthalmitis the ocular aspiration will probably be performed prior to initiating therapy. It may, however, be appropriate to do a vitrectomy and a scleral buckle before the therapeutic course of the antibiotics is over. Additionally, patients with various types of penetrating ocular trauma may be placed on broad-spectrum antibiotic coverage and subsequently, while still on the medication, require more surgery. It is therefore important to know that certain antibiotics may also cause a neuromuscular blockade.

Among the antibiotics frequently used in ophthalmology (35) there is no evidence for neuromuscular blockade with erythromycin, oleandomycin, and vancomycin. Neuromuscular blockade probably does not occur with penicillin, chloramphenicol, or bacitracin. The following antibiotics have been shown to enhance neuromuscular blockade from muscle relaxants (36): neomycin, streptomycin, gentamicin, kanamycin, polymyxin A and B, colistin, tetracycline, and lincomycin. There is disagreement regarding the mechanism by which these antibiotics affect the neuromuscular junction (37). It is not clear whether they may act as depolarizers or nondepolarizers. The mechanisms are probably different for each of the various antibiotics. Prolonged blockade may be reversed by neostigmine, up to 5 mg/kg, and by controlling the ventilation until the neuromuscular blockade terminates spontaneously (36).

POTASSIUM

Potassium is the predominant intracellular cation and diffuses readily through cell membranes. Sodium, the predominant extracellular cation, does not diffuse readily through cell membranes. The result is a resting transmembrane potential such that electrical charge on the interior of depolarizable cell membranes in nerve, heart, and muscle is 90 mV less than that on the outer side of cell membranes. The propagation of an action potential generated by membrane depolarization eliminates or reverses the transmembrane potential. The first step of depolarization is an increase in permeability of the cell membrane to sodium. Sodium ions enter the cell and reverse the potential from negative to positive. Membrane permeability to potassium increases, and potassium ions move out of the cell, returning the resting potential to normal. Intra- and extracellular potassium and sodium concentrations are restored as sodium is pumped out of the cell and potassium is pumped back in. Changes in extra- and intracellular potassium concentrations thus alter the ability of nerves, muscles, and cardiac conductive tissue to generate action potentials.

Although a decrease in extracellular potassium with normal total body potassium may occur in conditions such as acute alkalosis, insulin therapy, glucose infusion, and cortisol infusion, the most common situation is a decrease in total body potassium. By far the most common cause of this situation is the use of diuretics. Because of the increased risk of ventricular arrythmia intraoperatively when serum potassium levels are about 3 mEq/liter or less it is generally agreed that a serum potassium of about 3.2 mEq/liter is required preoperatively. A deficit of 1 mEq/liter in serum potassium level represents a 20% decrease in total body potassium. Thus, in a 70-kg man a fall in the serum potassium level from 4 to 3 mEq/liter represents a total body potassium deficit of about 700 mEq. Potassium can be replaced at a rate of about 240 mEq/day at a rate not faster than 20 mEq/hr for all but life-threatening situations. Thus, intravenous administration of potassium the night before surgery cannot adequately correct chronic hypokalemia represented by a serum potassium level of 3 mEq/liter.

For the potassium-deficient eye patient, the preferred method of replacement is oral, using potassium chloride. Therapy should be started well in advance of scheduled surgery to insure adequate replacement. For urgent or emergent cases potassium can be administered at a rate of 50 mEq/hr through a central venous catheter under electrocardiographic monitoring and hourly electrolyte determinations. When half of the estimated deficit has been administered, the infusion rate should be halved. There is a danger of phlebitis if potassium is infused at high rates through peripheral veins.

REFERENCES

1. Salem, D. N., Homans, D., McNally, J. W., and Banas, J. S. (1982): Cardiology. In: *Management of Medical Problems in Surgical Patients,* edited by M. Molitch, pp. 73–130. F. A. Davis, Philadelphia.

2. Committee on Prevention of Rheumatic Fever and Bacterial Endocarditis of the American Heart Association. (1977): Prevention of bacterial endocarditis. *Circulation,* 56:139a–143a.
3. National Diabetes Data Group. (1979): Classification and diagnosis of diabetes mellitus and other categories of glucose intolerance. *Diabetes,* 28:1039–1057.
4. Craighead, J. E. (1978): Current views on the etiology of insulin-dependent diabetes mellitus. *N. Engl. J. Med.,* 299:1439–1445.
5. Tamborlane, W. V., Puklin, J. E., Bergman, M., et al. (1982): Long-term improvement of metabolic control with the insulin pump does not reverse diabetic microangiopathy. *Diabetes Care,* 5(Suppl. 1):58–64.
6. Stuart, F. P., Simonian, S. J., and Hill, J. L. (1976): Special considerations in surgical management of patients on hemodialysis after successful kidney transplantation. *Surg. Clin. North Am.,* 56:15–19.
7. Wish, J. B., and Cohen, J. J. (1982): Renal disease and hypertension. In: *Management of Medical Problems in Surgical Patients,* edited by M. E. Molitch, p. 533. F. A. Davis, Philadelphia.
8. Brenowitz, J. B., Williams, C. B., and Edwards, W. S. (1977): Major surgery in patients with chronic renal failure. *Am. J. Surg.,* 134:765–769.
9. Blythe, W. (1979): The management of intercurrent medical and surgical problems in the patient with chronic renal failure. In: *Strauss & Welt's Diseases of the Kidney,* edited by L. Early and C. Gottschalk, p. 522. Little, Brown, Boston.
10. Goldblum, S. E., and Reed, W. P. (1980): Host defenses and immunologic alterations associated with chronic hemodialysis. *Ann. Intern. Med.,* 93:597–613.
11. Cheigh, J. S. (1977): Drug administration in renal failure. *Am. J. Med.,* 62:555–563.
12. Wish, J. B., and Cohen, J. J. (1982): Renal disease and hypertension. In: *Management of Medical Problems in Surgical Patients,* edited by M. E. Molitch, pp. 526–533. F. A. Davis, Philadelphia.
13. Payton, D., and Goldberg, M. F. (1976): *Management of Ocular Injuries.* W. B. Saunders, Philadelphia.
14. Freeman, H. F. (1979): *Ocular Trauma.* Appleton-Century-Crofts, New York.
15. Morris, R. E., and Miller, G. W. (1976): Pre-operative management of the patient with a full stomach. *Clin. Anesth.,* 11:25–29.
16. Crowley, R. A., and Trump, B. E. (1982): *Pathophysiology of Shock, Anoxia, and Ischemia.* Williams & Wilkins, Baltimore.
17. Lincoff, H. A., Ellis, C. H., DeVoe, A. G., et al. (1955): The effects of succinylcholine on intraocular pressure. *Am. J. Ophthalmol.,* 40:501–510.
18. Pandey, K., Badola, R. P., and Kumar, S. (1972): Time course of intraocular hypertension produced by suxamethonium. *Br. J. Anaesth.,* 44:191–196.
19. Condon, P. I., and Serjeant, G. R. (1972): Ocular findings in hemoglobin-SC disease in Jamaica. *Am. J. Ophthalmol.,* 74:921–931.
20. Condon, P. I., and Serjeant, G. R. (1972): Ocular findings in homozygous sickle cell anemia in Jamaica. *Am. J. Ophthalmol.,* 73:533–543.
21. Ryan, S. J., and Goldberg, M. F. (1971): Anterior segment ischemia following scleral buckling in sickle cell hemoglobinopathy. *Am. J. Ophthalmol.,* 72:35–50.
22. Jampol, L. M., Green, J. L., Jr., Goldberg, M. F., and Peyman, G. A. (1983): An update of vitrectomy surgery and retinal detachment repair in sickle cell disease. *Arch. Ophthalmol.,* 100:591–593.
23. Caprioli, J., and Puklin, J. E. Retinal detachment and vitrectomy surgery in patients with sickle hemoglobinopathy: The role of pre-operative exchange transfusions (*in preparation*)
24. Goldberg, M. F. (1979): The diagnosis and treatment of secondary glaucoma after hyphema in sickle cell patients. *Am. J. Ophthalmol.,* 87:43–49.
25. Gordon, R. A., Britt, B. A., and Kalow, W. (1973): *International Symposium on Malignant Hyperthermia.* Charles C. Thomas, Springfield, Illinois.
26. McGoldrick, K. E. (1982): Letter to the editor. *Arch. Ophthalmol.,* 100:842.
27. Meltzer, H. Y., Hassan, S. B., Russo, P., et al. (1976): Isoenzymes of creatinine phosphokinase in serum of families with malignant hyperpyrexia. *Anesth. Analg.,* 55:797–799.
28. Aldrete, J. A., and Britt, B. A. (1978): *Malignant Hyperthermia: Proceedings of the Second International Symposium.* Grune & Stratton, New York.

29. Miller, J., and Lee, C. (1981): Muscle diseases. In: *Anesthesia and Uncommon Diseases,* edited by J. Katz, J. Benumof, and L. B. Kadis, pp. 545–550. W. B. Saunders, Philadelphia.
30. Sears, M., and Mead, A. (1983): A major pathway for the regulation of intraocular pressure. *Int. Ophthalmol.,* 6:201–212.
31. Miller, J., and Lee, C. (1981): Muscle diseases. In: *Anesthesia and Uncommon Diseases,* edited by J. Katz, J. Benumof, and L. B. Kadis, pp. 530–537. W. B. Saunders, Philadelphia.
32. Pederson, H., and Finster, M. (1979): Anesthetic risk in the pregnant surgical patient. *Anesthesiology,* 51:439–451.
33. Levinson, G., and Shnider, S. M. (1979): Anesthesia for operations during pregnancy. In: *Anesthesia for Obstetrics,* edited by S. M. Shnider and G. Levinson, pp. 312–320. Williams & Wilkins, Baltimore.
34. Knowles, J. A. (1965): Excretion of drugs in milk—a review. *J. Pediatr.,* 66:1068–1082.
35. Miller, R. D. (1976): Antagonism of neuromuscular blockade. *Anesthesiology,* 44:318–329.
36. Miller, R. D., and Savarese, J. J. (1981): Pharmacology of muscle relaxants, their antagonists, and monitoring of neuromuscular function. In: *Anesthesia,* edited by R. D. Miller, pp. 523–524. Churchill Livingstone, New York.
37. Singh, Y. N., Marshall, I. G., and Harvey, A. L. (1979): Depression of transmitter release and post-junctional sensitivity during neuromuscular block produced by antibiotics. *Br. J. Anaesth.,* 51:1027–1033.

Commentary

Antibiotics and Asepsis

In an outstanding review Dr. Forster states that a careful pre-surgical examination is the most important prophylactic step in the prevention of endophthalmitis. In routine cultures *S aureus* is found in 21% of normal subjects at any given time. This figure agrees well with the 25% incidence of *S aureus* found in the nasopharyngeal area. The author does not recommend either routine preoperative cultures or topical antibiotics. Indeed, routine use of antibiotics could easily lead to the development of resistant organisms. But, patients with diabetes mellitus, allergy, blepharoconjunctivitis, contact lens wearers, and those with a prosthesis are a group deserving of preoperative cultures and treatment.

There may be a clinical difference between a highly selected private practice and a teaching hospital. In Helsinki (about 1,600 intraocular operations per year) preoperative smears and cultures have been obtained for the past 20 years. The value of these measures lies mainly in the preoperative discovery of unsuspected streptococci or gram-negative bacilli. The patients who harbor streptococci in the conjunctiva do so often also in their pharynx. Preoperative microbiological studies may serve as an additional safety measure. In terms of cost they add very little when compared to the price of viscous solutions and intraocular lens implants.

Preoperative polyvidon-iodide baths have been used successfully in vascular surgery in reducing the bacterial flora of the skin. Dr. Forster recommends polyvidon-iodide prep of the periocular skin and face and cleansing of the lid margins. A half strength povidone-iodine solution can be used as part of the preparation of the eye for surgery utilizing the solution as a conjunctival scrub. One of us has been using this preparation for two years with good success [see Apt, et al. (1984): *Arch. Ophth.,* 102:728–734].

A commentary on this excellent chapter may well be superfluous. In addition to the aforementioned, we should possess an awareness of irregularities that may occur in outpatient surgery, the occasional chemosis seen after the use of the aminoglycosides, and careful attention to the toxic levels of intraocular antibiotics, and, anticipation of the third generation of cephalosporins, which may prove to be extraordinarily useful in the prophylaxis of infection.

The Editors

Surgical Pharmacology of the Eye,
edited by M. Sears and A. Tarkkanen.
Raven Press, New York © 1985.

Antibiotics and Asepsis

Richard K. Forster

*Bascom Palmer Eye Institute, University of Miami School of Medicine,
Miami, Florida 33101*

SUMMARY: 1. Background and rationale for the selection of prophylactic antibiotics and asepsis are presented, and specific guidelines and recommendations for use of antibiotics and aseptic techniques are discussed.

2. A careful pre-surgical examination is probably the most important step in the prevention of postoperative infections.

3. Preoperative cultures are of little value in the selection of prophylaxis, but, if there is a suggestion of skin or adnexal infection, or if the patient wears an extended wear contact lens or prosthesis, then cultures should be performed to determine and quantify the organisms present, and to select appropriate antibiotics.

4. Choose one of two approaches to prophylactic preoperative topical antibiotics: (a) Routine use of gentamicin 3 mg/ml, tobramycin 3 mg/ml, or polymixin, gramacidin-neomycin, and augment with gentamicin ointment the night before surgery; or (b) selective use of the above antibiotics in patients with mild blepharitis, conjunctival hyperemia or contact lens wear.

5. If preoperative cultures are indicated, treat patient for 5–7 days prior to surgery; remove prosthetic shell, and treat nasolacrimal obstruction definitively.

6. Prophylactic subconjunctival treatment: gentamicin 20 mg and cefazolin 50 mg.

7. Aseptic surgical preparation should include a povidone-iodine solution preparation and draping with self-adherent plastic drape.

8. In ocular trauma, prophylaxis of infection should include: tetanus toxoid; cefazolin 500 mg every 6 hours, i.m. or i.v.; topical antibiotics; and subconjunctival gentamicin and cefazolin at surgery.

9. In retinal surgery, use topical antibiotics, intraoperative soaking of buckling elements and irrigation of the bed of buckle, subconjunctival gentamicin and cefazolin. After reoperations, the eye should be treated topically for 7–14 days because of problems with conjunctival closure.

The purpose of this chapter is to review and recommend the best prophylaxis and pharmacotherapy for the prevention of postoperative ocular infections. The specific aims are to provide

1. Background and rationale for the selection of prophylactic antibiotics and asepsis.
2. Specific guidelines and recommendations for use of antibiotics and aseptic techniques.

The rationale for selection of prophylactic management in ocular surgery should be based on recognized risk factors and the profile of reported infections. These factors include the exogenous source of microbial flora, the local pathologic status of the eye, the type of surgery to be employed, and the status of the host.

The types of ocular surgery to be considered include anterior segment procedures such as cataract extractions and glaucoma filtering surgery, retinovitreous surgery, and the management of ocular trauma. Guidelines and recommendations are directed primarily toward the prevention of endophthalmitis; in the case of retinal surgery, prevention of infected scleral buckles; and in trauma surgery, prevention of endophthalmitis and adnexal infections.

THE PROBLEM—BACKGROUND AND RATIONALE FOR THE SELECTION OF PROPHYLACTIC ANTIBIOTICS AND ASEPSIS

Incidence

Infectious endophthalmitis is one of the most catastrophic complications of intraocular surgery and penetrating injuries of the eye. The true incidence and cause is difficult to confirm because most cases are probably unreported. Until recently, the more frequently quoted studies often did not have confirmation of an infectious agent from intraocular cultures but instead attributed endophthalmitis to a microbial agent that might have been cultured from the conjunctiva and lids, and clinical studies are difficult to control for variables that may influence the incidence and the cause of postoperative infections. An apparent decrease in the incidence of infectious endophthalmitis, however, has been noted in the past two decades and has been attributed to improved sterile technique and asepsis, more delicate surgical instrumentation, manipulation, and wound closure, and the use of preoperative and intraoperative prophylactic antibiotics. Recognizing the limitations of study design, there are several reported series that attempt to clarify the incidence of postoperative endophthalmitis.

Christy and Lall (1), operating on a native population in Pakistan, have published the largest series of postoperative endophthalmitis. From a total of 77,093 cataract extractions they reported 382 cases of endophthalmitis, an incidence of approximately 0.5% (5 infections per 1,000 operations). They observed and cautioned that success in a few hundred cases does not insure success in a larger series, and this was borne out in their study by three groups of more than 1,000 consecutive operations without an apparent infection.

In another large clinical study, Allen and Mangiaracine (2,3) reported 22 infections in a series of 20,000 operations (0.11%) and only 9 infections in a second series of 16,000 consecutive operations (0.056%). Therefore, on the bases of these two large studies and others reporting a similar incidence of endophthalmitis, and recognizing that control of variables and culture-proved infections was often lacking, we can estimate that an overall incidence of postoperative endophthalmitis of 0.05% (1 in 2,000 cases) to 0.5% (1 in 200) might be expected. Since endophthalmitis represents such a catastrophic complication of surgery, we must carefully analyze those variables that can be effected to further reduce the incidence of infections following anterior segment intraocular procedures.

The incidence of infectious endophthalmitis following trauma is even more difficult to determine and affect. In a retrospective review of 82 consecutive eyes with penetrating trauma seen in 1974 and 1975 at the Bascom Palmer Eye Institute in Miami (4), only two infections were proved by culture (2.4%); 77 of the 82 cases were treated prophylactically with cephalosporins intravenously and with periocular gentamicin and topical antibiotics after surgical correction. Barr (5) reported on the prognostic factors in corneoscleral lacerations in 122 patients repaired during a 4-year period and documented culture-proved endophthalmitis in 4 (3.3%) of the traumatized eyes. Organisms that are rare as causes of postoperative endophthalmitis, such as bacilli and fungi, are more common in posttraumatic endophthalmitis (4).

The incidence of microbial-related extruded or infected episcleral exoplants is likewise difficult to determine because of the variable criteria for infection and accuracy of the culture technique. Seven studies published between 1970 and 1979 report an incidence of infected scleral exoplants of 1.3% to 24.4%. Russo and Ruiz (6) emphasize that early infections probably represent surgical contamination, whereas late infections develop secondary to mechanical erosion of the scleral exoplant with subsequent infection.

Microbiology

A number of repeating potential microbes must be considered in evaluating appropriate asepsis and selection of prophylactic antibiotics. Isolated cases or clustered outbreaks of postoperative endophthalmitis have been attributed to contaminated instruments, irrigating solutions, and intraocular lenses, and also to presumed airborne contamination from operating room personnel and contaminants on donor corneas or scleral exoplants. It is likely, however, that in most cases the infectious organism was present on the patient's skin and conjunctiva. The former causes should be well controlled by meticulous aseptic technique, whereas the majority of cases, which are presumably traced to the patient, are more difficult to prevent and require an understanding of the organisms isolated from culture-proved cases and appropriate preoperative prophylactic pharmacotherapy.

We have reported culture results in 140 eyes with endophthalmitis and identified positive cultures from anterior chamber and/or vitreous fluid in 78 eyes (56%) (7). Forty of the isolates were in patients with recent surgery and had isolation of gram-positive organisms in 24, gram-negative organisms in 14, and fungi in 2. Fifteen positive cultures in eyes developing endophthalmitis following trauma had gram-positive organisms in 10 (66%). In a more recent, subsequently published study (8) of 29 culture-positive isolates from 40 cases of suspected endophthalmitis following anterior segment surgery, gram-positive organisms were cultured from 26 eyes, gram-negative organisms from 2 eyes, and fungi from 1 eye. The increased recognition of *Staphylococcus epidermidis* as an etiologic agent in endophthalmitis, supported by the work of Valenton and co-workers (9), Puliafito (10), O'Day (11), and by our culture results (12), indicates that *S epidermidis* is probably the most frequently isolated organism from cases of endophthalmitis following recent surgery.

In endophthalmitis following trauma two-thirds of the infections are due to gram-positive organisms, but in contrast to anterior segment surgery bacilli predominate. In our review of 34 cases of traumatic endophthalmitis (13), positive cultures were obtained in 21 eyes (62%); specifically with gram-positive organisms isolated in 58%, gram negative organisms in 25%, and fungi in 17%. The 14 gram-positive isolates included bacilli, 5; streptococci, 4; *Staphylococcus epidermidis,* 4; and Clostridia, 1. The six gram-negative isolates included *Klebsiella pneumoniae,* 2; *Enterobacter* organisms, 2; *Pseudomonas stutzeri,* 1; and *Aeromonas hydrophilia,* 1. The four fungal isolates each represented a separate genus and species. Consistent with the nature of such injuries, there were three cases with multiple isolates.

The organisms associated with infected or extruded scleral exoplants have recently been examined in our facility in a retrospective chart review from 1977 through 1982 (14); 33% of the removed exoplants were culture-negative, 42% had isolation of a gram-positive organism, 24% had isolation of a gram-negative organism, and 1% had isolation of fungi. Of the gram-positive organisms cultured, *S epidermidis* (in 13 cases) and *S aureus* (in 10 cases) predominated; diphtheroids were isolated in the remaining 3 cases. Of the 15 gram-negative organisms isolated from removed exoplants there were *Proteus mirabilis,* 4; *Serratia marcescens,* 3; *Pseudomonas* organisms, 3; *Enterobacter* organisms, 2; *Escherichia coli,* 2; and *Neisseria catarrhalis,* 1. The one fungal isolate represented *Candida albicans.*

Preoperative Examination and the Role of Preoperative Cultures

A careful presurgical examination is probably the most important prophylactic step in the prevention of endophthalmitis. Attention should be directed to the skin, not only regarding dermatitis around the eyes but also on the body and limbs. Diabetics and patients with peripheral vascular disease should be specifically questioned and examined regarding infectious, gangrenous toes, and extremities. The lid margins should be carefully examined to avoid operating on patients with infectious blepharitis. The conjunctiva and lacrimal apparatus should likewise be examined, and if inflammation is evident, if the lacrimal sac is tender, or if mucopurulent material is expressed, then definitive therapy should be undertaken prior to surgery. It is advisable to perform preoperative conjunctival and lid cultures in patients with blepharitis, those with extended-wear contact lenses, and those with a contralateral ocular prosthesis, as there appears to be a higher incidence of asymptomatic colonization with gram-negative bacteria in these patients than in the general population.

Starr (15) has summarized and critically reviewed the literature on the value of performing preoperative cultures and the selection of prophylactic antibiotics. I would like to review some of these studies to arrive at a rationale for prophylactic cultures and the use of antibiotics.

Dunnington and Locatcher-Khorazo (16) reported the results of preoperative cultures from 2,508 eyes prior to cataract surgery. Postoperative endophthalmitis occurred in 11 eyes of 529 patients who had *S aureus* cultured from the lids preoperatively, whereas no eyes harboring more benign organisms, such as *S epidermidis* (1,706 eyes), developed postoperative endophthalmitis. They concluded that pathogenic staphylococci present preoperatively on the lids and conjunctiva increased the risk of postoperative infection. Unfortunately, they did not include a comparison of the preoperative cultures with cultures from the intraocular contents, so we do not know what microbes were responsible for the presumed infectious endophthalmitis in those cases.

In a challenge of the value and significance of obtaining routine preoperative cultures Allansmith et al. (17) cultured the lids and conjunctiva of normal subjects on a daily and weekly basis and found the presence of staphylococci to vary from day to day. The authors found a 21% chance that *S aureus* would be present at any given time on the lid margins, regardless of prior negative cultures. Variations in cultured organisms found preoperatively also were noted by Nolan (18) in 35% of 109 eyes cultured prior to cataract surgery. Such data renders routine positive or negative preoperative cultures of less value as an indicator of the type or quantity of bacteria present at the time of cataract surgery. Likewise, the method by which the cultures are obtained also raises questions as to reproducibility, reliability, and prognostic value for selection of antimicrobial therapy.

In contrast to the observations of Dunnington and Locatcher-Khorazo, in which no apparent eyes with *S epidermidis* on the lids or conjunctiva developed endophthalmitis, recent reports supporting the observation that *S epidermidis* is probably the most common cause of postoperative endophthalmitis raises even further questions as to which organisms to consider pathogenic. Therefore, if all eyes with organisms cultured from the lids or conjunctiva are to be treated prophylactically, then obtaining routine preoperative cultures becomes an unnecessary procedure. On the other hand, in clinical situations where there is inflammation of the lids, conjunctiva, or lacrimal apparatus or when an eye harboring a contact lens or prosthesis is cultured, if there is growth of specific organisms frequently related to clinical infection, or if one places value on the quantity rather than the specific genus and species, then an argument can perhaps be made for selective cultures. If the presence of any organism is of significance, perhaps all patients should receive preoperative treatment, thus eliminating the need for preoperative cultures. Although it is interesting to speculate about the importance of preoperative cultures, their routine use is probably not practical nor beneficial, and it certainly does not replace a careful preoperative examination. Likewise, the argument that knowledge of preoperative cultures might allow for more rational initial therapy if postoperative infection occurs gives a surgeon a false sense of security, since there are no data to compare preoperative cultures to specific etiologic microbial agents in postoperative endophthalmitis.

In our experience managing postoperative infections, there may, however, be a place for culturing the conjunctiva in patients with extruded or presumed infectious exoplants for the purpose of selecting antibiotic agents. This is borne out by the correlation of the conjunctival organism cultured prior to removal of the exoplant compared to the organism isolated from the exoplant after removal. In a study at our institution (14), the conjunctival cultures predicted the exoplant organism correctly in 3 of 4 cases in which there was no growth from the exoplant, in 12 of 22 cases in which gram-positive organisms were cultured (including 5 of 8 cases with *S aureus*), and in 8 of 9 cases in which gram-negative organisms were cultured. Whether more specific antimicrobial therapy would be beneficial and obviate the need for subsequent removal of an infected scleral implant is speculative, but the data is certainly in sharp contrast to the negative correlation of conjunctival and lid cultures compared to the organism isolated from intraocular cultures in our series of patients managed with postoperative endophthalmitis.

The Rationale for Prophylactic Antibiotics

Topical Antibiotics

The recommendation to use preoperative topical antibiotics as prophylactic therapy to prevent endophthalmitis requires a careful examination of *in vitro* sensitivity testing to organisms considered at risk and, more important, to the *in vivo* efficacy in studies utilizing topical antibiotics.

Locatcher-Khorazo (19) studied patients undergoing cataract surgery who received one of three antibiotic ointments applied to the conjunctiva and lids every 2 hr for five or six applications in the 24 hr prior to surgery. Quantitative cultures were taken before and after treatment, including preoperatively on the morning of surgery. Chloramphenicol 1% produced no decrease in post-treatment colony counts in 52 of 56 patients; terramycin 0.5% was ineffective in 37 of 56 patients; but a combination of penicillin-G 1,000 U and streptomycin sulfate 20 mg/g was effective in reducing the number of isolated organisms in 100% of 147 patients. Although this study did not randomly allocate patients to different treatment groups, nor were controls included, it did suggest the varying efficacy of different antibiotic ointments in reducing ocular flora and an apparent difference in the *in vitro* and *in vivo* antibiotic efficacy.

Burns and associates have reported several studies in which patients were randomly allocated to different treatment groups and masked for the therapeutic agents. In one study (20) controls were treated with a lubricating ointment, and treated patients received either neomycin sulfate ointment 0.5% or gentamicin ointment 0.3%. The antibiotics were administered postoperatively at the dressing change, and cultures were taken on the fifth postoperative day. Eleven percent of the controls (2 of 18) showed a decrease in the bacterial count, whereas the remaining control eyes showed an increase in the bacterial count. The eyes receiving neomycin or gentamicin ointment showed reduction in bacterial counts of 48% and 86%, respectively. This study indicated a significant superiority of both antibiotics over the control and the superiority of gentamicin compared to neomycin. In a subsequent study of similar design, Burns and Oden (21) demonstrated the superiority of gentamicin 0.3% over chloramphenicol 0.5%, both administered in drop form for 1 to 2 days preoperatively, four times a day, as well as postoperatively. Mean pretreatment bacterial counts of *S epidermidis* were greater in the gentamicin-treated patients, but mean posttreatment counts of this organism were dramatically reduced in the gentamicin group, whereas chloramphenicol drops demonstrated increased posttreatment counts. In a separate series of patients untreated with antibiotics, 92 of 114 various bacterial isolates showed postoperative increase after 2 to 3 days of patching, suggesting as did the first study, that an increase in the external eye temperature was associated with increased bacterial flora. A third study by Burns et al. (22) compared the effects of gentamicin 0.3% drops, gentamicin 0.3% ointment, sulfacetamide 30% drops, and neomycin-polymyxin-B-gramicidin drops. Gentamicin drops and ointment were comparable, with 100% of 67 patients treated with either formulation showing a decreased bacterial count postoperatively. Neomycin-polymyxin-B-gramicidin was somewhat less effective, with 25 of 33 eyes showing decreased counts, and sulfacetamide less so, with decreased counts in only 15 of 25 eyes. It should be noted, however, that the reference time for quantitating the cultures followed 2 to 3 days of patching, and if our understanding of the mechanism of infection is correct, the critical time when microbial flora must be reduced or eliminated is at the time of surgery, not 2 to 3 days later after patching.

Fahmy (23) assigned 60 cataract patients to one of six treatment groups, each received a different antibiotic five times a day before surgery, and cultures were obtained shortly before the surgical procedure. Gentamicin 0.3% drops were effective in eliminating bacteria from the eye prior to surgery in 9 of 10 eyes. The other groups showed positive bacterial growth after treatment in the majority of eyes following use of chloramphenicol 0.5% drops, oxytetracycline chloride 3%, polymyxin B sulfate 0.1% ointment, sulfamethizide 4% drops, bacitracin 1%–neomycin sulfate 0.5% drops, and ristocetin sulfate 0.5%–polymyxin B sulfate 0.25% drops.

The relative efficacy of topical antibiotics also was reported by Whitney et al. (24), comparing pre- and posttreatment counts of lid margin staphylococci after seven different prophylactic regimens in 153 preoperative patients and volunteers. All antibiotics tested produced a reduction in bacterial counts compared to untreated fellow eyes, but only gentamicin 1% (10 mg/ml) drops more significantly reduced microbial counts. Although the other antibiotics reduced the bacterial counts, the major difference was noted between gentamicin, which eradicated bacteria in 44% of the eyes treated when given every 10 min for 2 hr, compared to chloramphenicol drops, which failed to reduce bacterial counts.

These studies indicate that topical antibiotics administered for a brief preoperative regimen reduce the numbers of lid and conjunctival bacteria compared to untreated controls. They also point out that the degree to which the flora will be reduced depend on the choice of antibiotic and probably to its frequency and duration of administration. The bacteria must be susceptible to the antibiotics, suggesting that a broad spectrum of coverage is more efficacious than an antibiotic of limited spectrum.

Although we have suggested that there may be a lack of correlation between *in vitro* and *in vivo* bacterial sensitivity, in a study of 32 *S epidermidis* isolates from clinical endophthalmitis, we found six isolates in which there was *in vitro* resistance to gentamicin by the Kirby-Bauer technique; and after tube dilution sensitivities were performed, two still showed relative resistance (25). In examining *S epidermidis* isolates from ocular sources other than endophthalmitis in our laboratory, using the Kirby-Bauer disc sensitivity technique, approximately 85% showed sensitivity to gentamicin *in vitro,* compared to nearly 100% sensitivity for *S aureus.* The cephalosporins appear to be nearly 100% effective *in vitro* against both *S epidermidis* and *S aureus.* It is clear from the above studies that gentamicin is the most effective antibiotic of those tested to date to reduce the quantity of persistent bacterial flora on the lids and conjunctiva.

The effect of topical prophylactic antibiotics on the incidence of endophthalmitis is less clear because of the lack of controls and the frequent lack of microbiologic confirmation of an intraocular organism in endophthalmitis. Hughes and Owens (26) reported an incidence of endophthalmitis of 0.17% in 1,200 cataract operations in which preoperative penicillin drops or ointment were given 1 week or more before surgery. By comparison, an earlier series of 2,086 operations without prophylactic topical antibiotics had an incidence of endophthalmitis of 1.0%. Dunnington and Locatcher-Khorazo (16) reported no cases of postoperative infection in 663 patients treated with either topical penicillin or sodium sulfathiazole ointment. A subsequent study by Locatcher-Khorazo (27) of 7,095 cataract patients with various antibiotics administered five times on the day before surgery had six infections (0.08%).

The most impressive study showing efficacy of topical antibiotics in the prevention of endophthalmitis was reported in two parts by Allen and Mangiaricine (2,3). In the initial study there were 5 infections in 600 operations performed without use of preoperative antibiotics (0.75%), whereas among

19,340 patients prophylactically treated with various topical antibiotic regimens there were 17 postoperative infections (0.08%). The second series compared the efficacy of two combinations—neomycin 0.5% and chloramphenicol 0.4%—each used with polymyxin B sulfate 0.1% and erythromycin 0.5% ointment. Six infections occurred among 1,000 patients receiving the neomycin regimen, compared to three infections in 15,000 operations receiving the chloramphenicol regimen. In the total of 36,000 consecutive cataract operations, excluding 3 infections due to *Pseudomonas* organisms that were attributed to contaminated solutions, there were 6 infections in 26,307 cases in which chloramphenicol preparations were used and 22 infections in 9,693 cases in which chloramphenicol was not used.

Subconjunctival Antibiotics

Whereas administration of topical antibiotics is intended to reduce or eliminate the ocular flora prior to surgery, subconjunctival injections given usually at the completion of the operative procedure or occasionally before opening the eye are intended to inhibit inadvertent bacterial contamination that may occur during the operative procedure. Since there may be a significant number of organisms either on the wound margin or in the eye at the completion of surgery, the intent of the periocular injection of antibiotics is to produce bactericidal levels in the immediate postoperative period.

Burns (22) has shown that 20 mg gentamicin injected subconjunctivally at the time of cataract surgery is nearly as effective in lowering the conjunctival bacterial flora at 48 hr postoperatively as are gentamicin drops or ointment instilled daily at the time of dressing change. However, the effectiveness of reducing the incidence of endophthalmitis by use of prophylactic subconjunctival antibiotics is less well defined than by use of topical antibiotic prophylaxis. Pearlman (28) reported an incidence of 0.51% intraocular infections (9 in 1,773 cases) when no subconjunctival antibiotics were used, and he reduced this to no infections in 3,226 eyes by the administration of penicillin and streptomycin subconjunctivally at the completion of surgery. Aronstam (29) recognized eight infections over 20 months, four in patients receiving subconjunctival penicillin and streptomycin and four in patients not receiving subconjunctival prophylaxis. The interval between surgery and infection averaged 26.5 days in the treated group and 4.5 days in the untreated group, and the authors suggested that subconjunctival antibiotics may have only delayed the manifestations of postoperative infection. Unfortunately, neither Pearlman nor Aronstam confirmed the clinical diagnosis of endophthalmitis by intraocular cultures. Chalkley and Shoch (30) observed findings similar to those of Aronstam when they compared 571 patients receiving penicillin and streptomycin subconjunctivally, in whom two delayed infections occurred, with 281 patients who had not received treatment, in whom two immediate infections occurred postoperatively at 1 and 3 days.

Kolker et al. (31) conducted a prospective controlled series with alternative assignment of 974 patients undergoing intraocular surgery. No patients received pre- or postoperative topical or systemic antibiotics, and the study evaluated only subconjunctival prophylaxis versus no prophylactic antibiotics at all; 480 patients in the treatment group received subconjunctival penicillin G 100,000 U and streptomycin 66 mg, and 494 control patients received no antibiotics. Seven intraocular infections developed in the control group (1.42%), whereas only one infection occurred in the treated group (0.21%). Although this study would tend to substantiate the prophylactic value of subconjunctival antibiotics, it should be noted that this was a relatively small study in patient numbers, there was no prophylaxis for gram-negative organisms, and bacteriologic confirmation of the infectious agent in the cases of endophthalmitis was lacking. The authors were not able to substantiate the observation of delay in the manifestations of an infection, as had been suggested by Aronstam and by Chalkley and Shoch.

A more recent study by Christy and Lall (1) included the use of gentamicin, with better antibiotic coverage for staphylococci and *Pseudomonas* organisms than the previously mentioned streptomycin and penicillin subconjunctival regimens. Although the series is less well controlled and used concomitant topical antibiotics, the authors compared six treatment groups, including a control group of 3,798 patients who received topical antibiotics only; another group of 40,676 patients who also received chloramphenicol topically from day 1 preoperatively to postoperative day 3 or 5; and four other groups treated with subconjunctival antibiotic injection at the time of surgery who received either framycetin sulfate 100 mg, chloramphenicol succinate 100 mg, gentamicin sulfate 10 mg, or penicillin sodium 500,000 U. The authors did not recognize a significant reduction in postoperative infection with broader-spectrum antibiotics such as gentamicin. Furthermore, the overall incidence of infection in patients receiving subconjunctival antibiotics of any kind (0.521% in 9,787 patients) was higher than the incidence in patients who received no subconjunctival antibiotics (0.405% in 44,474 patients). The authors likewise did not note delay of infection during the first 12 postoperative days in patients who received subconjunctival antibiotics. This study is of interest in that it may suggest that if sufficient inoculum of microbial organisms enter the eye, no prophylactic antibiotic approach—either topical or subconjunctival—will halt the progression of infection.

Christy and Sommer (32) reported a subsequent series of 6,618 patients who underwent cataract surgery and were allocated to treatment or control groups in a masked fashion. The control group was treated with topical chloramphenicol and sulfadimadene as well as postoperative 5% sulfadimadene drops, and the treatment groups in addition received an injection of subconjunctival penicillin 500,000 U at the time of surgery. The infection rate in the control group was 0.45% and in the treatment group 0.15%. The authors concluded that combined prophylactic therapy was superior to topical antibiotics alone, and also noted that combined therapy in 21,829 patients was superior to subconjunctival penicillin alone in 2,071 cases. In this large series (1,32), granting that it was not well controlled and that the diagnosis of endophthalmitis was not proved by culture (it would be especially interesting to note which organisms are or are not successfully reduced), the authors concluded that combined therapy was superior to either topical or subconjunctival prophylaxis alone.

Systemic Antibiotics and Other Prophylactic Routes of Administration

Due to the lack of control studies and the recognized poor intraocular absorption of systemic antibiotics, the risk-benefit ratio of such use does not warrant consideration of systemic antibiotics in the prophylaxis of endophthalmitis.

Peyman et al. (33) compared the rate of postoperative infection among cataract patients operated on in southern India who had received both topical and oral chloramphenicol to a second group who received only intracameral gentamicin 50 μg at the conclusion of surgery without pre- or postoperative antibiotics administered by any other route. In the former group of 219 patients there were six presumed cases of endophthalmitis, an incidence of 2.9%, compared to the latter group of 1,626 patients, receiving only intracameral gentamicin, in which there were six infections, an incidence of 0.37%. Eleven of the eyes with presumed infections were culture-positive for one or more organisms that were sensitive to gentamicin, including those patients who had received intracameral gentamicin. This study further supports the observation that a large inoculum of organisms introduced into the eye at surgery may not be eliminated by prophylactic antibiotics regardless of the single or combined routes of prophylactic antibiotic delivery.

Surgical Asepsis

Leopold and Apt (34) concluded that "if antibiotic or chemotherapeutic agents had to be used prophylactically, they must be used as an adjunct to and not a substitute for an aseptic surgical technique or the reduction of regional bacterial flora by mechanical cleansing." Therefore, one must be aware of the potential sources of infection during ocular surgery and the importance of aseptic technique. Allan and Mangiaricine (2) have summarized the potential sources of infection during eye surgery, and although these will not be discussed individually, since we do not know the relative contributing role to infection for each of the individual sources, we should nevertheless be cognizant of the many potential sources that lead to intraocular infections (Table 1). Although total sterility of the operating field cannot be guaranteed, an attempt should be made to approach sterility as nearly as possible. Allan and Mangiaricine discuss the importance of technique; Theodore (35) considers

TABLE 1. *Potential sources of infection during eye surgery*

Airborne contaminants
   Respiratory origin
   Surface origin (e.g., skin, clothing)
   Air-conditioning system
Solutions and medications
   Saline for irrigation and other purposes
   Collyria
   Ointments
   Instrument disinfectants
   Skin antiseptics
   α-Chymotrypsin
Tissues
   Skin of hands
   Skin of operative field
   Lid margins and lashes
   Conjunctival sac
   Lacrimal sac
   Nasal mucosa
   Corneal grafts
   Vitreous implants
   Fellow eyes
Objects and materials
   Optical instruments
   Surgical instruments
   Tonometers
   Magnets
   Hypodermic needles, blood lancets
   Cotton balls, swabs, drapes, dressings, masks, gowns
   Rubber gloves, bulbs, droppers
   Glass syringes, bottles, irrigating tips
   Plastic tubing, sheeting, retractors
   Contact lenses
   Orbital implants
   Intraocular lenses
   Sutures

From ref. 2, with permission.

most of these factors; and Jaffe (36) discusses his personal experience with operating room technique.

Apt and Isenberg (37) surveyed 214 ophthalmologists worldwide to determine methods of preoperative chemical preparation of the eye and adnexa. Although a wide diversity of agents was reportedly used, povidone-iodine was the most popular agent applied to the skin, whereas the conjunctiva was either ignored or rinsed with a saline solution. Approximately one out of four used mild silver protein (Argyrol®) on the conjunctiva. Since this study had found that 42% of the respondents irrigated the conjunctival sac with dilutions that were not intended to be antimicrobial (such as normal saline), Isenberg et al. (38) investigated the effect on bacterial flora by use of conjunctival irrigation as part of chemical preparation of the eye before surgery. Forty consecutive patients had conjunctival irrigation with saline solution in a randomly selected eye. Aerobic and anaerobic conjunctival cultures were taken in a masked fashion before and after preparation. In nonirrigated eyes, colony counts before and after chemical preparation of the lids was virtually identical; in irrigated eyes the colony count increased 18% and the species count increased 46%. These findings suggest that irrigation with a saline solution does not reduce bacterial flora of the conjunctiva. In a second study, Isenberg et al. (39) evaluated the effectiveness of a mild silver protein solution. This was studied on 32 patients in a masked fashion, and the bacteriologic studies showed that a mild silver protein solution was no more effective in reducing the number of species and colonies in the treated eye than in the untreated eye. It did show staining of mucus and other debris on the eye, which might facilitate irrigation, but it did not demonstrate a significant bactericidal effect. A third study, by Apt et al. (40), evaluated the effectiveness of a diluted povidone-iodine conjunctival irrigation. In contrast to the conjunctival irrigation alone or the use of mild silver protein solutions, the povidone-iodine irrigation did reduce the colony counts and species isolated.

To reduce accidental or inadvertent contamination of the operative field and intraocular contents and to reduce the chance of heavy intraocular or wound contamination, the clinician must exercise alertness and respect for infection at all times in the operating room. Careful preoperative preparation of the skin and eye, the use of plastic occluding drapes with appropriate coverage of the lashes and lid margin, external irrigation prior to opening the globe, reduction in pooling of irrigating solutions in the conjunctiva, careful tissue manipulation and discreet use of intraocular solutions, and a minimum of conversation and traffic in the operating room will keep the potential bacterial contaminants to a minimum.

SPECIFIC GUIDELINES AND RECOMMENDATIONS FOR USE OF ANTIBIOTICS AND ASEPTIC TECHNIQUES

Guidelines and recommendations for use of antibiotics and asepsis will be directed primarily to elective anterior segment surgical procedures such as cataract extractions and glaucoma filtering surgery. Specific tailoring of recommendations for retinovitreous surgery and trauma surgery will include only variations in technique and specific antibiotic selection.

General—Anterior Segment Surgery

Preoperative Evaluation

At the time it is determined that a patient needs a surgical procedure, the examination should include a physical assessment of the patient's facial skin, ocular adnexa including the lids and lacrimal apparatus, and ocular surface. Inquiries should be made of the patient regarding generalized dermatologic conditions and whether there are any specific draining or presumed infectious processes. The use of an extended-wear contact lens in the fellow eye, the presence of a prosthesis, or a phthisical fellow eye should be noted, since there is a tendency for gram-negative organisms to inhabit the conjunctiva and the lids in patients under these circumstances.

Preoperative Cultures

I do not recommend *routine* preoperative cultures; however, if on the basis of examination there is a suggestion of a skin or adnexal infection or if the patient is wearing an extended-wear contact lens or a prosthesis on the fellow side, then lid and conjunctival cultures should be performed to determine the microbial organisms present, to quantitate the microbes, and to select appropriate preoperative prophylactic antibiotics. Such cultures should be obtained by moistening a cotton applicator with a nutrient liquid medium such as trypsinase soy broth, rubbing the conjunctiva and lid margins with the moistened applicator, and by inoculating a blood agar plate to be maintained at body temperature (37°C).

If there are symptoms of nasolacrimal obstruction and reflux of mucopurulent material through the punctum with pressure over the lacrimal sac, then that material should be cultured and definitive correction of the condition undertaken either by successful probing of the nasolacrimal system and systemic antibiotics or a dacryocystectomy or dacryocystorhinostomy.

Preoperative Prophylactic Topical Antibiotics

I do not recommend the *routine* use of preoperative prophylactic topical antibiotics prior to elective intraocular surgery. I recommend a careful preoperative examination, and if there is no evidence of periocular inflammatory disease I do not favor topical antibiotic prophylaxis. The clinical studies discussed in the first part of this chapter on the one hand demonstrate that short-term use of certain antibiotics, particularly chloramphenicol, do not uniformly reduce the lid and conjunctival microbial flora; on the other hand, granting the authors some leniency regarding study design and selection of treatment, Allan and Mangiaricine (2,3) in two studies have shown that prophylactic antibiotic preparations significantly reduced the likelihood of postoperative infection.

Therefore, I would recommend that the ophthalmologist choose one of two approaches. The *first* would be the routine use of topical prophylactic antibiotics, using either gentamicin sulfate 3 mg/ml, tobramycin 3 mg/ml, or combined polymyxin-B-gramicidin-neomycin drops at hourly intervals for five to six administrations the day prior to and the morning of intraocular surgery. The surgeon may wish to augment this with gentamicin 3 mg/g ointment at bedtime the night before surgery. It should be noted that topical administration of aminoglycoside antibiotics (gentamicin sulfate, tobramycin, or neomycin) may produce immediate hypersensitivity reactions characterized by tearing, lid edema, chemosis, and conjunctival hyperemia, as well as punctate corneal erosions. Despite the apparent efficacy shown with use of chloramphenicol by Allan and Mangiaricine (3) and its recommendation by Baum (41), the studies of Burns and associates (21,22) indicate that if one is to use prophylactic topical antibiotics, gentamicin drops or ointment have been shown to be superior to chloramphenicol in reducing the quantity as well as species of lid and conjunctival microbial organisms.

The *second* approach, which I favor, is the selective use of the above-recommended prophylactic antibiotics in patients who have mild blepharitis or conjunctival hyperemia or who have been wearing a contact lens in either eye. If, on the other hand, a blepharoconjunctivitis is noted or if the patient is wearing a prosthetic shell in the fellow eye, I obtain lid and conjunctival cultures from both eyes. If the problem appears to be primarily a blepharitis, I treat the patient for 5 to 7 days prior to surgery with bilateral use of gentamicin or tobramycin drops, as well as lid scrubs using gentamicin or tobramycin ointment. If the patient is wearing a prosthetic shell, I remove it and instruct the patient to leave it out until I advise resuming its wear in the postoperative period, and I apply the same antibiotic drops for 5 to 7 days, q.i.d., to both eyes until surgery. If the patient shows evidence of nasolacrimal obstruction, I treat that also with aminoglycoside topical antibiotic drops; if the obstruction is total, with regurgitation of mucopurulent material, I recommend deferring elective surgery if possible until definitive lacrimal surgery in the form of a dacryocystorhinostomy or dacryocystectomy is performed.

Although I do not use prophylactic topical antibiotics if the eye and adnexa appear normal and have no evidence of inflammation, I am personally aware of three instances in which both preoperative cultures and prophylactic topical antibiotic treatment certainly influenced the favorable outcome, which might have been disastrous if cultures and treatment had been overlooked. Although anecdotal, each of these cases emphasizes the need to be selective in obtaining preoperative cultures and in selecting treatment preoperatively.

The first was a woman scheduled to undergo a penetrating keratoplasty. The eyes looked essentially quiet and free of apparent infection the night before surgery, but on the morning of surgery the eye to be operated on had a marked conjunctival hyperemic response. Surgery was canceled, the patient's lids and conjunctiva were cultured, and she was started on topical gentamicin drops. Surgery was again tentatively scheduled for 48 hr later, but the culture report at 18 hr showed β-hemolytic streptococcus with poor sensitivity to aminoglycosides. Therefore, the patient was treated with polymyxin-B-neomycin-gramicidin drops and bacitracin ointment. She was discharged from the hospital and treated for 7 days, and then 1 week after completion of treatment the lids and conjunctiva were recultured, at which time there was no evidence of streptococci on culture. The patient was admitted for penetrating keratoplasty with the same selection of antibiotics that had rendered her culture-negative, and she underwent uneventful surgery and visual recovery.

A second case is that of a one-eyed patient who was noted to have mucopurulent discharge and obstruction of the nasolacrimal system in the fellow eye the night prior to elective cataract surgery. Cultures showed a heavy growth of *Pseudomonas aeruginosa* from both eyes but predominantly from the blind eye, and the patient underwent a dacryocystorhinostomy and subsequent uneventful cataract surgery.

The third case is a patient who was successfully treated for a *Proteus mirabilis* endophthalmitis by use of conventional and intraocular antibiotics and 3 years later presented for consideration of cataract surgery in the fellow eye. Cultures of the lids and conjunctiva of both eyes were positive for *P mirabilis,* apparently the same microbe that had been responsible for an endophthalmitis in the fellow eye 3 years before. The organism was sensitive to gentamicin sulfate, and the patient was treated for 1 week with both drops and ointment; treatment was then discontinued for 2 weeks, at the end of which time cultures were repeated and found to be negative. The patient was again treated for 5 days with topical gentamicin prior to successful cataract surgery.

I choose to share these three cases because they point out the need to examine carefully every patient preoperatively, and if the history or physical findings suggest an apparent increased likelihood of complicating factors that might result in the catastrophe of postoperative bacterial endophthalmitis, then definitive management should be undertaken prior to elective surgery. This should include (a) preoperative cultures, (b) an examination of the results as to both quantity and type of microbes isolated, (c) the obtaining of sensitivity data if either a virulent organism or heavy quantity of growth is noted, (d) cancellation of the surgery and institution of prophylactic antibiotics, (e) confirmation after termination of antibiotic therapy that the infection is indeed controlled, and then (f) reinstitution of prophylactic topical antibiotics prior to surgery.

Prophylactic Subconjunctival Antibiotic Treatment at Surgery

Although cultures of the anterior chamber fluid at the conclusion of cataract surgery are usually negative (42), there is little question that with the exception of postoperative infections due to poor wound closure and vitreous wick syndromes, most cases of endophthalmitis probably originate from contamination of the anterior chamber and/or vitreous with organisms of sufficient quantity to overcome protective effects of the anterior chamber and initiate infection. Therefore, the critical time to establish bactericidal levels of antibiotics is either during or at the completion of surgery. It is also well recognized that although topical antibiotics may reduce the conjunctival and lid flora, there may still be organisms that gain access to the wound or intraocular contents. The conflicting clinical data of Kolker and associates (31), who found a significant reduction in endophthalmitis by use of subconjunctival antibiotics; that of Christy and Lall (1), who demonstrated no apparent reduction in endophthalmitis in a population in Pakistan; and the work of Pearlman (28) or Chalkey and Shoch (30), who suggested that subconjunctival antibiotics delay the presentation of infection, nevertheless suggest that it would seem prudent to use subconjunctival prophylactic antibiotics at the completion of surgery. I would have no argument with such subconjunctival injection to be used at the beginning of surgery except that such an approach might result in conjunctival edema and retention of the injection, making surgery perhaps somewhat more difficult. I use and recommend the same subconjunctival prophylactic antibiotic injections favored by D. B. Jones, of gentamicin sulfate 20 mg and cefazolin sodium 50 mg when intraocular surgery is concluded (41). I do not use cefazolin if there is a history of significant penicillin allergy because there is a small but recognized cross-sensitivity of the cephalosporins with the penicillin-derived antibiotics. The rationale for two subconjunctival antibiotics is that although gentamicin has a broad spectrum with efficacy against most gram-positive and gram-negative microbes, it nevertheless has variable efficacy against streptococci and *S epidermidis,* two of the more frequently isolated organisms in cases of bacterial endophthalmitis. If one is concerned with the use of cefazolin or other cephalosporin antibiotics in patients with presumed penicillin allergy, the alternative would be to use gentamicin alone or to use vancomycin 25 mg instead of a cephalosporin. Although there is a question of whether therapeutic bactericidal levels of antibiotics can be achieved in the vitreous following subconjunctival delivery, adequate levels seem to be achievable within the anterior chamber.

Several years ago, Liesegang and I measured the gentamicin level in the anterior chamber at the beginning of cataract surgery after an injection of 20 mg gentamicin via one of three approaches—true subconjunctival (adjacent to the limbus in the bulbar conjunctiva), subconjunctivally in the cul-de-sac adjacent to the orbital rim, and infraorbitally via an injection with a ⅝-inch needle through the lower lid. The injections were given 20 min to 3 hr prior to surgery. Suffice it to say that negligible levels of gentamicin were found in the anterior chamber fluid by radioimmunoassay when administered either through the lid or in the cul-de-sac adjacent to the orbital rim, whereas therapeutic levels were achieved in most cases when the antibiotic was delivered via the bulbar subconjunctival approach. It was of interest that in five cases of aphakic corneal transplantation in which vitrectomy was utilized no recognizable vitreous levels of gentamicin were obtained by any route.

Although the cephalosporins rarely cause immediate or delayed hypersensitivity reaction, the aminoglycosides such as gentamicin, tobramycin, and neomycin not infrequently will result in typical features of a hypersensitivity response characterized by tearing, chemosis, and lid edema, usually evident the day following surgery. It is also important to modify the dose of antibiotics administered subconjunctivally to infants and young children, who may have an adverse reaction to aminoglycosides.

Postoperative Antibiotics

Although frequently used as a combination of topical corticosteroid and antibiotic, the administration of routine postoperative topical antibiotics

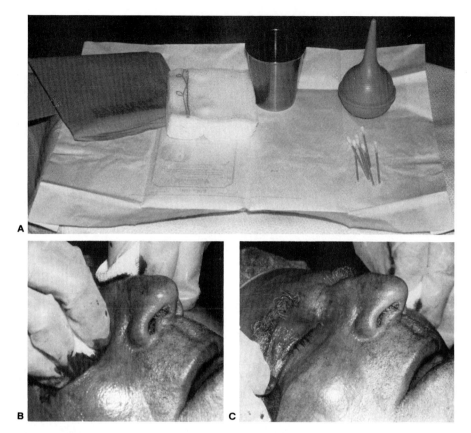

FIG. 1. Surgical prep. **A:** Materials for prep include sterile gloves, 4 × 4 cotton gauze pads, cotton applicators, povidone-iodine solution, irrigating bulb with saline, and sterile towel. **B & C:** Bilateral upper facial and lid prep with povidone-iodine solution and 4 × 4 cotton gauze pads.

probably has a rationale only in certain selected circumstances such as inadequate wound closure or wounds that are closed with exposed silk or absorbable sutures, with an increased risk for wound infections. The other case where postoperative prophylactic topical antibiotics might well be administered is either preceding or following suture cutting or removal. With the increased use of nonabsorbable nylon sutures such suture removal is perhaps less common. On the other hand, to effect and control astigmatism following cataract surgery and keratoplasty, sutures are not infrequently cut; in such circumstances I recommend the application of 1 or 2 drops of prophylactic topical antibiotic (preferably gentamicin or tobramycin).

Ocular Trauma

Patients who sustain penetrating ocular and adnexal trauma are more prone to become infected by microbes that are ubiquitous, such as bacilli and other

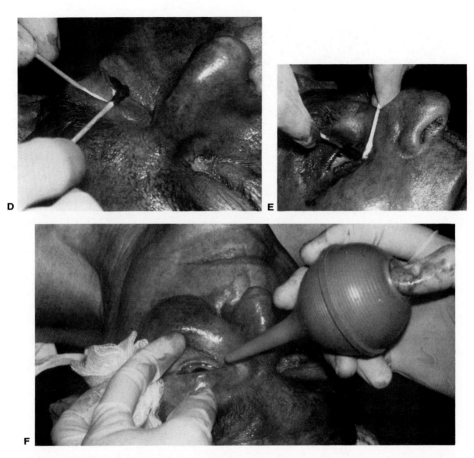

FIG. 1. Cont. D & E: Prep of the lid margins and lashes with povidone-iodine moistened cotton applicators. **F:** Irrigation of the ocular surface and conjunctiva with saline to remove debris and residual prep material.

soil contaminants, and anaerobic organisms associated with animal or human bites. Therefore, all patients who are admitted with ocular or periocular trauma and who are to undergo surgery should be treated prophylactically.

An updated history of the status of tetanus immunization should be obtained, and patients should be given a booster of tetanus toxoid. Unless there is a history of anaphylactoid penicillin antibiotic allergy, I recommend the use of cefazolin 500 mg, every 6 hr, intramuscularly or intravenously. This dosage is maintained for 3 to 5 days but modified according to clinical response. I also recommend the use of topical antibiotics prior to surgical repair of the traumatized eye with either gentamicin, tobramycin, or a combination of polymyxin-B, gramicidin, and neomycin for five to six doses. This application needs to be modified according to the severity of the injury, particularly if it is desired not to try to open the lids in extensive penetrating

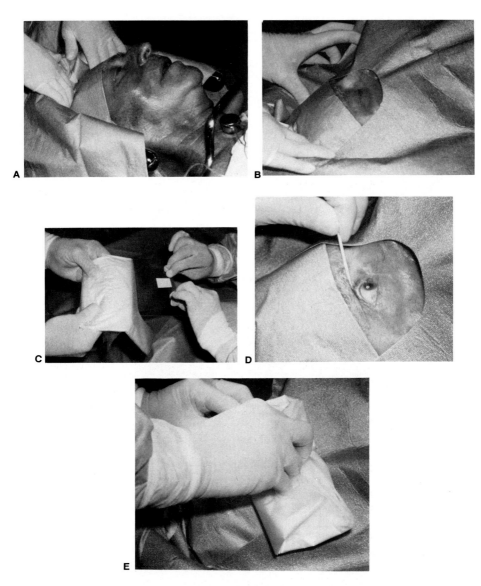

FIG. 2. Draping the surgical field. **A:** Placement of the forehead drape and positioning of wrist support. **B:** Placement of the split sheet with adherence to forehead drape. **C:** Removal of plastic cover from adhesive portion of plastic drape. **D:** Raising upper lid for application of sterile plastic drape. **E:** Adhesive surface of plastic drape applied directly to open eye.

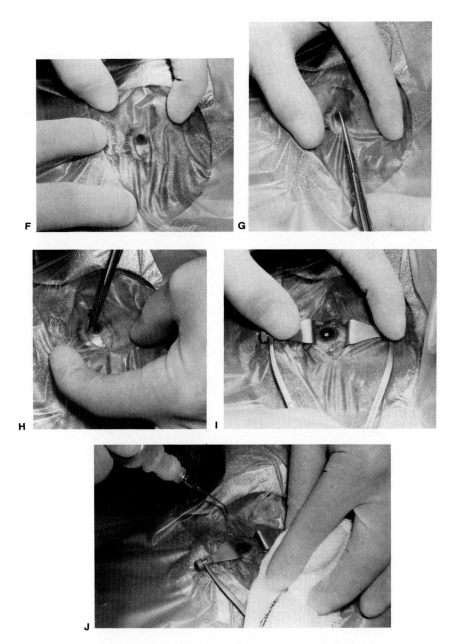

FIG. 2. Cont. F: Positioning of plastic drape with adhesion over the lids, lashes, and periorbital skin. **G:** Linear opening of drape over eye (note that the adhesive portion of drape does not adhere to the wet corneal and conjunctival surface). **H:** Vertical splitting of drape prior to application of lid speculum. **I:** Application of solid lid speculum with plastic drape material rolled around and under lid margin. **J:** Irrigation of cornea and conjunctival surface to remove any residual debris or prep solution prior to initiation of surgical procedure.

injuries. In such cases, application of either gentamicin or tobramycin ointment to the conjunctiva and lids should suffice and precludes frequent, repeated applications of drops. Following surgical repair, gentamicin 20 mg and cefazolin 50 mg should be injected subconjunctivally. Since gram-positive organisms tend to predominate, if the patient has an allergy to penicillin derivatives, then vancomycin may be substituted for the cephalosporins.

Not infrequently there may be a delay of more than 24 hr between injury and surgical correction, and in such cases if there is a high index of suspicion that an endophthalmitis has ensued, I recommend obtaining anterior chamber and/or vitreous cultures, and the injection of intracameral antibiotics consisting of gentamicin 0.1 mg in a volume of 0.1 ml and cefazolin 2.25 mg in a volume of 0.1 ml. In such cases of suspected early traumatic endophthalmitis, I recommend doubling the prophylactic subconjunctival antibiotic dosage to include gentamicin 40 mg and cefazolin 100 mg.

Retinal Surgery

Patients scheduled for primary retinal detachment repair with scleral buckling who have not had recent ocular surgery are usually managed with a selection of prophylactic antibiotics in a manner similar to elective primary anterior segment surgical procedures; that is, the patient may be treated the day before and morning of surgery with topical antibiotics or only on a selected basis, depending on the ocular history and examination. Intraoperatively, we suggest soaking the scleral buckling elements and irrigation of the bed of the buckle prior to conjunctival closure with diluted gentamicin (2 mg/ml), followed by subconjunctival injections of gentamicin 20 mg and cefazolin 50 mg.

In retinal detachment reoperations, I would recommend routine prophylactic antibiotic drops, and since conjunctival closure over the buckling element may be less than ideal, it is probably advisable to continue prophylactic drops postoperatively for at least 7 to 14 days, until the conjunctiva has adequately healed. This approach addresses the emphasis made by Russo and Ruiz (6) that early postretinal detachment infection probably represents surgical contamination, whereas the later infections tended to develop secondary to mechanical erosion of the scleral exoplant.

Aseptic Surgical Preparation

I recommend a povidone-iodine prep of the periocular skin and face and cleansing of the lid margins, preferably by the use of moistened cotton applicators (Fig. 1). Although there is no evidence that saline solution irrigation or mild silver-protein solution (Argyrol®) reduces the bacterial inhabitants on the conjunctiva, silver-protein solution does identify debris and mucus, and cleansing and removal of debris seems appropriate. For patients demonstrating allergy to iodine preparations, I recommend substitution of povidone-iodine with hexachlorophine (pHisoHex®).

Draping the patient and use of either disposable or laundered-sterilized head drape and split sheets should be individualized according to hospital policy. However, the use of self-adhering plastic drapes is recommended; they have the advantages of isolating the eye and conjunctiva from the surrounding facial skin, holding down the lashes to prevent their exposure to the operative field and, with proper application of a lid speculum, protecting the lid margin, thus occluding it from the operative field (Fig. 2).

All practical procedures, manipulations, and adjustments called for by common sense and surgical judgment need to be adhered to and combined in harmony to ensure the best prophylaxis and pharmacotherapy for the prevention of postoperative ocular infections.

REFERENCES

1. Christy, N. E., and Lall, P. (1973): Postoperative endophthalmitis following cataract surgery. *Arch. Ophthalmol.,* 90:361–366.
2. Allen, H. F., and Mangiaracine, A. B. (1964): Bacterial endophthalmitis after cataract extraction. *Arch. Ophthalmol.,* 72:454–462.
3. Allen, H. F., and Mangiaracine, A. B. (1974): Bacterial endophthalmitis after cataract extraction. II. Incidence in 36,000 consecutive operations with special reference to preoperative topical antibiotics. *Arch. Ophthalmol.,* 91:3–7.
4. Forster, R. K. (1982): Endophthalmitis. In: *Clinical Ophthalmology,* vol. 4, edited by T. D. Duane, chap. 24. Harper & Row, Hagerstown, MD.
5. Barr, C. C. (1983): Prognostic factors in corneoscleral lacerations. *Arch. Ophthalmol.,* 101:919–924.
6. Russo, C. E., and Ruiz, R. S. (1971): Silicone sponge rejection early and late complication in retinal detachment surgery. *Arch. Ophthalmol.,* 85:647–650.
7. Forster, R. K., Abbott, R. L., and Gelender, H. (1980): Management of infectious endophthalmitis. *Ophthalmology,* 87:313–318.
8. Olson, J. C., Flynn, H. W., Forster, R. K., and Culbertson, W. W. (1983): Results in the treatment of postoperative endophthalmitis. *Ophthalmology,* 90:692–697.
9. Valenton, M. J., Brubaker, R. F., and Allen, H. F. (1973): *Staphylococcus epidermidis* (albus) endophthalmitis. *Arch. Ophthalmol.,* 89:94–96.
10. Puliafito, C. A., Baker, A. S., Haaf, J., and Foster, C. S. (1982): Infectious endophthalmitis. Review of 36 cases. *Ophthalmology,* 89:921–928.
11. O'Day, D. M., Jones, D. B., Patrinely, J., et al. (1982): *Staphylococcus epidermidis* endophthalmitis. Visual outcome following noninvasive therapy. *Ophthalmology,* 89:354–360.
12. Forster, R. K. (1982): Discussion: Infectious endophthalmitis. Review of 36 cases (Puliafito et al.). *Ophthalmology,* 89:928–929.
13. Affeldt, J. C., Forster, R. K., and Mandelbaum, S. (1983): Traumatic endophthalmitis. *Invest. Ophthalmol. Vis. Sci.,* 24:173. (Abstract.)
14. Demartini, D., and Forster, R. K. (1983): The microbiology of extruded or infected episcleral exoplants. *Invest. Ophthalmol. Vis. Sci.,* 24:233. (Abstract.)
15. Starr, M. B. (1983): Prophylactic antibiotics for ophthalmic surgery. *Surv. Ophthalmol.,* 27:353–373.
16. Dunnington, J. H., and Locatcher-Khorazo, D. (1945): Value of cultures before operation for cataract. *Arch. Ophthalmol.,* 34:215–219.
17. Allansmith, M. R., Anderson, R. P., and Butterworth, A. (1969): The meaning of preoperative cultures in ophthalmology. *Trans. Am. Acad. Ophthalmol. Otolaryngol.,* 73:683–690.
18. Nolan, J. (1967): Evaluation of conjunctival and nasal bacterial culture before intraocular operations. *Br. J. Ophthalmol.,* 51:483–485.
19. Locatcher-Khorazo, D. (1953): The effect on the ocular bacterial flora of local treatment with chloromycetin (chloramphenicol), terramycin or penicillin-streptomycin ophthalmic ointments in preoperative cataract cases and miscellaneous infections. *Am. J. Ophthalmol.,* 36:475–479.
20. Burns, R. P., Hansen, T., Fraunfelder, F. T., Klass, A., and Allen, A. (1968): An experimental

model for evaluation of human conjunctivitis and topical antibiotic therapy: Comparison of gentamicin and neomycin. *Can. J. Ophthalmol.,* 3:132–137.

21. Burns, R. P., and Oden, M. (1972): Antibiotic prophylaxis in cataract surgery. *Trans. Am. Ophthalmol. Soc.,* 70:43–57.

22. Burns, R. P. (1972): Effectiveness study of antibiotics. *Symposium on Ocular Therapy,* 5:105–112.

23. Fahmy, J. A. (1980): Bacterial flora in relation to cataract extraction. V. Effects of topical antibiotics on the preoperative conjunctival flora. *Acta Ophthalmol. (Copenh),* 58:567–575.

24. Whitney, C. R., Anderson, R. P., and Allansmith, M. R. (1972): Preoperatively administered antibiotics. *Arch. Ophthalmol.,* 87:155–160.

25. Bode, D., Forster, R. K., and Rebell, G. (1982): Antibiotic sensitivities for *S. epidermidis* endophthalmitis. *Invest. Ophthalmol. Vis. Sci.,* 22:2. (Abstract.)

26. Hughes, W. F., and Owens, W. C. (1947): Postoperative complications of cataract extraction. *Arch. Ophthalmol.,* 38:577–595.

27. Locatcher-Khorazo, D., and Gutierrez, E. (1956): Eye infections following cataract extraction. *Am. J. Ophthalmol.,* 41:981–987.

28. Pearlman, M. D. (1956): Prophylactic subconjunctival penicillin and streptomycin after cataract extraction. *Arch. Ophthalmol.,* 55:516–518.

29. Aronstam, R. H. (1964): Pitfalls of prophylaxis. Alteration of postoperative infection by penicillin-streptomycin. *Am. J. Ophthalmol.,* 57:312–315.

30. Chalkey, T. H. F., and Shock, D. (1967): An evaluation of prophylactic subconjunctival antibiotic injection in cataract surgery. *Am. J. Ophthalmol.,* 64:1084–1087.

31. Kolker, A. E., Freeman, M. I., and Pettit, T. H. (1967): Prophylactic antibiotics and postoperative endophthalmitis. *Am. J. Ophthalmol.,* 63:434–439.

32. Christy, N. E., and Sommer, A. (1979): Antibiotic prophylaxis of postoperative endophthalmitis. *Ann. Ophthalmol.,* 11:1261–1265.

33. Peyman, G. A., Sathur, M. L., and May, D. R. (1977): Intraocular gentamicin as intraoperative prophylaxis in South India eye camps. *Br. J. Ophthalmol.,* 61:260–262.

34. Leopold, I. H., and Apt, L. (1960): Postoperative intraocular infections. *Am. J. Ophthalmol.,* 50:1225–1247.

35. Theodore, F. H. (1965): Prevention of infection following cataract surgery. *Int. Ophthalmol. Clin.,* 5:155–182.

36. Jaffe, N. S. (1981): Endophthalmitis. In: *Cataract Surgery and Its Complications,* 3d ed., edited by N. S. Jaffe, ch. 22. C. V. Mosby, St. Louis.

37. Apt, L., and Isenberg, S. (1982): Chemical preparation of skin and eye in ophthalmic surgery: An international survey. *Ophthalmic Surg.,* 13:1026–1029.

38. Isenberg, S., Apt, L., and Yoshimuri, R. (1983): Chemical preparation of the eye in ophthalmic surgery. I. Effect of conjunctival irrigation. *Arch. Ophthalmol.,* 101:761–763.

39. Isenberg, S., Apt, L., and Yoshimuri, R. (1983): Chemical preparation of the eye in ophthalmic surgery. II. Effectiveness of mild silver protein solution. *Arch. Ophthalmol.,* 101:764–765.

40. Apt, L., Isenberg, S. J., Paez, J. H., and Yoshimuri, R. (1984): Chemical preparation of the eye in ophthalmic surgery: III. Effect of povidone-iodine on the conjunctiva. *Arch. Ophthalmol.,* 102:728.

41. Baum, S., and Forster, R. K. (1983): Module 9: Infectious endophthalmitis. Focal points: Clinical modules for ophthalmologists. American Academy of Ophthalmology.

42. Constantaras, A. A., Metzger, W. I., and Frenkel, M. (1972): Sterility of the aqueous humor following cataract surgery. *Am. J. Ophthalmol.,* 74:49–51.

Commentary

Nonsteroidal and Steroidal Anti-Inflammatory Agents

Surgical trauma is direct mechanical trauma to cell membranes. There are several immediate consequences for the cell involved:

1. Membrane associated enzymes lose function. Thus the protein we call the Na-K pump (ATPase) is compromised, sodium enters the cell and potassium leaks out. A loss of the control of cell volume occurs. Entry of sodium and calcium increases cell water, and, as permeability is further enhanced, a continued loss of intracellular components occurs. The cell swells and may eventually rupture.

2. Direct membrane trauma also activates phospholipases to synthesize prostaglandins and/or leukotrienes, further increasing permeability and permitting further entry of ions with additional swelling.

3. As the intracellular organelles, such as the mitochondria, become involved, a reduction in ATP occurs. Loss of ATP begins to simulate an acute ischemic injury with a metabolic shift to anaerobic glycolysis, a consequent accumulation of lactate, and a decrease in cell pH leading to additional damage, such as effects on the cell chromatin and RNA synthesis. Changes in the permeability of the lysosomal membranes cause swelling lysis and release of hydrolases, lysosomal enzymes, degrading the cell constituents still further.

4. Conformational changes in the cell membrane also occur after injury. The microvilli of the membrane become elaborate and blebs form from the surface of the cell membrane. Separation of junctional complexes takes place. Conformational changes also take place in the endoplasmic reticulum and mitochondrial and lysosomal systems.

Mechanical injury activates certain enzymes called phospholipases, which free arachidonic acid from the phospholipids contained in the affected cell membranes. The arachidonic acid is converted to several products by one and/or two pathways, the cyclooxygenase and lipoxygenase: by the cyclooxygenase pathway to the prostaglandins, endoperoxides PGG_2 and PGH_2, which give rise to TXA_2 (thromboxane A_2) in platelets, and to prostacyclin PGI_2 in vessel walls, respectively, and to PGE_2, PGD_2, and $PGF_{2\alpha}$; by the lipoxygenase pathway to the HETES or hydroxyeicosatetranoic acids. The production of prostaglandins from the endoperoxides is accompanied by the formation of oxygen-derived free radicals.

Evidence of the relationship between prostaglandins and the pathogenesis of disease is frequently derived from the effects of cyclooxygenase inhibition, using acetylsalicylic acid or other newer nonsteroidal anti-inflammatory drugs.

The first demonstration of the endogenous involvement of the prostaglandins in ocular trauma (2,3) led to a host of subsequent studies (5). It should be remembered, however, that the lipoxygenase pathway (*not* directly affected by the nonsteroidals currently available), leads to the formation of the leukotrienes, one of which, LTB_4, is very effective as a cellular chemotactic agent, and promotes the important cellular component part of inflammation, cellular infiltration (1). Anti-inflammatory corticosteroids can enter into injury-response mechanisms. They can effectively block both arachidonic pathways by the nuclear induction of a molecule that inhibits the phospholipase A_2, which is responsible for arachidonic breakdown.

Translated into the arena of ophthalmic surgery, we can say the following: with instability of the blood aqueous barrier, or, with excessive surgical trauma to it, breakdown surely occurs as a result of vasodilation and plasma leakage, very likely by the action of the prostaglandins with increased hydrostatic pressure in the uveal stroma. Rupture of the junctions joining cells occurs. Lipoxygenase products are also activated to contribute the cellular part of the response to the trauma. Pretreatment of our patients with a cyclooxygenase inhibitor such as indomethacin, separately or together with corticosteroids, may well protect the eye (the blood-ocular barrier) (4).

Systemic administration of nonsteroidals should not be taken lightly by the prescribing physician because of adverse side effects (CNS and GI), but topical use is recommended. We await new inhibitors acting on the lipoxygenase pathway, as we continue for the moment to use prophylactic anti-inflammatory steroids and/or nonsteroidal agents, alone, or, in combination.

The Editors

REFERENCES

1. Kulkarni, P. S., and Srinivasan, D. (1985): Comparative *in vivo* inhibitory effects of nonsteroidal anti-inflammatory agents on prostaglandin synthesis in rabbit ocular tissues. *Arch. Ophthalmol.,* 103:103–106.
2. Neufeld, A. H., Chavis, R. M., and Sears, M. L. (1973): Degeneration release of norepinephrine causes transient ocular hyperemia mediated by prostaglandins. *Invest. Ophthalmol.,* 12:167–175.
3. Neufeld, A. H., Jampol, L., and Sears, M. (1972): Aspirin prevents the disruption of the blood aqueous barrier. *Nature,* 238:158–159.
4. Sanders, D. R. and Kraff, M. (1985): Steroids and nonsteroidal anti-inflammatory agents. *Arch. Ophthalmol.,* 102:1453–1457.
5. Sears, M. L., Neufeld, A. H., and Jampol, L. (1973): Prostaglandins. *Invest. Ophthalmol.,* 12:161–164.

Surgical Pharmacology of the Eye,
edited by M. Sears and A. Tarkkanen.
Raven Press, New York © 1985.

Nonsteroidal and Steroidal Anti-Inflammatory Agents

Irving H. Leopold

*Department of Ophthalmology, University of California at Irvine,
Irvine, California 92717*

Surgery on the eye is trauma. This trauma induces many alterations in the ocular tissues and fluids, including the release of prostanoids, eicosanoids, neurohormones, neuropeptides, histamines, bradykinin, and others, all of which may contribute to alterations in ocular appearance and function. Most of these may bring about heat, swelling, redness, and pain, which are the characteristics of inflammation. Surgeons for centuries have attempted to find agents that will reduce the severity of this reaction to surgical intervention in an effort to speed recovery, minimize discomfort, and allow rapid healing. Pharmacologic agents used to abet this desire include drugs acting through the autonomic system, steroids, and nonsteroidal anti-inflammatory agents.

SURGICAL INFLAMMATION

Inflammation is a term used to describe a series of responses of vascularized tissues of the body to injury. The clinical signs of this phenomenon can now be related to increased flow in local blood vessels, which produces the heat and redness, increased vascular permeability, and/or cellular infiltration, causing the swelling and pain and the release of a variety of materials at the site of inflammation. Loss of function was later considered an additional cardinal sign of inflammation. Mechanisms by which the function of a given tissue is impaired depend greatly on the nature of the tissue and on the detailed processes that contribute to the inflammatory reaction. There are varied and complex responses in different tissues and the same tissues at different times. Each operative trauma may result in a different mix of these responses. The inflammatory process is influenced also by the nutritional and hormonal status of the individual as well as by genetic factors.

Inflammation can be considered the beneficial reaction of tissue to injury. If there are deficiencies in this reaction, such as in the white blood cell response, this may produce defective inflammatory responses and insufficient protection against infection. The beneficial reaction of the inflammation is its ability to remove the inciting agent and repair the injured site. Although it produces discomfort and loss of function temporarily, in the end it is protective. A large number of surgical inflammatory situations, however, represent uncontrolled inflammatory action that if continued unchecked can produce permanent tissue destruction, or they may heal but only by inappropriate deposition of fibrous tissue or collagen and subsequent scar formation. This can be disastrous to vision.

The immune system also plays a part in the inflammatory action but is called into play after other elements of the inflammation have formed the picture and developed. The immune system may be looked on as a protective one. It adds specificity to the reaction. The antigen-stimulated lymphocytes provide a wealth of mediator functions themselves as well as modulating the immune response. All of the elements that play a part in inflammation, although complex and variable, tend to increase vessel permeability and induce emigration of inflammatory cells from the blood. Once they have reached the site of injury the emigrates are stimulated to phagocytize bacteria and debris and secrete many of their preformed and newly synthesized constituents. Molecules promoting these events may be called mediators. Reactions are controlled throughout by positive and negative feedback reactions, again involving mediators and inhibitors.

Hemodynamic changes may precede the inflammatory changes. They are of critical importance. Cohnheim's dictum, "without vessels—no inflammation," was later, however, rephrased by Metchnikoff as "there is no inflammation without phagocytes" (113). Nonetheless, vasodilatation, increased flow, and permeability are key early elements preceding inflammation. It may be presumed that their purpose is to allow maximum opportunity to recruit inflammatory cells and to bring plasma proteins to the site of injury. These plasma proteins can contribute to initiation or perpetuation of the response to the complement fragments involved or to the resolution of the response due to plasma protease inhibitors. The site of these reactions has not been definitely located. It may be in the postcapillary venules or in the capillaries (113).

It is obvious that neutrophils accumulate in these sites, as well as mononuclear phagocytes or macrophages. In order to bring about recovery, this influx of new cells must be halted, injurious oxygen radicals and proteases must be inactivated, fluids and proteins must be removed or reabsorbed, inflammatory cells and debris must be removed, and damaged cells must be replaced. In other circumstances, tissue fibroblasts may be similarly induced to divide and secrete connective tissue elements such as collagen. The mediators that induce all of this are beginning to receive specific attention (Table 1).

Definition of Mediators

An inflammatory mediator can be thought of as a chemical messenger that will act on blood vessels and nerve cells to contribute to the inflammatory

TABLE 1. *Examples of possible mediators contributing to surgical inflammation*

Mediator	Structure/chemistry	Probable origin	Most likely effects
Prostaglandin E_2		Arachidonic acid	Vasodilatation, potentiate permeability effect of histamine and bradykinin, increase permeability when acting with leukotactic agent, potentiate leukotriene effect
Thromboxane A_2		Arachidonic acid Thromboxane synthetase located in platelets	Vasoconstrictor platelet aggregator, decreased cyclic AMP
PGI_2		PGI_2 synthetase of vessel walls	Vasodilator; antiaggregator of platelets, stimulates adenylcyclase, potentiate leukotriene effects
Histamine	B-Imidazolylethelamine	Mast cells, basophils	Increase vascular permeability (venules), chemokinesis, mucus production, smooth muscle contraction
Serotonin	5-Hydroxytryptamine	Mast cells, platelets	Increase vascular permeability (venules), smooth muscle contraction
Bradykinin	Nonapeptide	Kininogen (by proteolytic cleavage)	Vasodilation, increase in vascular permeability, production of pain, smooth muscle contraction
Neutrophil chemotactic factor		Mast cells (?)	Chemotaxis of neutrophils
C3a	77-Amino-acid peptide	C3 complement protein	Degranulation of mast cells, smooth muscle contraction
C5 fragments C5a C5a desArg	74-Amino-acid peptide 73-Amino-acid peptide	C5 complement protein	Degranulation of mast cells, chemotaxis of inflammatory cells, oxygen radical production, neutrophil secretion, smooth muscle contraction
Vasoactive intestinal peptide	28-Amino-acid peptide	Mast cells, neutrophils, cutaneous nerves	Vasodilation, potentiate edema produced by bradykinin and C5
Substance P	Undecapeptide	Nerves	Vasodilatation, miosis, stimulation of smooth muscle

continued

TABLE 1. *Continued*

Mediator	Structure/chemistry	Probable origin	Most likely effects
Leukotriene B$_4$		Arachidonic acid (lipoxygenase pathway)	Chemotaxis of neutrophils, increase vascular permeability in the presence of PGE$_2$
Leukotriene D$_4$		Arachidonic acid (lipoxygenase pathway)	Smooth muscle contraction, increase vascular permeability
Platelet-activating factor		Basophils, neutrophils, monocytes, macrophages	Release of mediators from platelets, neutrophil aggregation, neutrophil secretion, superoxide production by neutrophils, increase vascular permeability, smooth muscle contraction
Interferon	Glycoprotein	T-lymphocytes	Activation of macrophages, modulation of immune reactions
Interleukin 1	Peptide	Macrophages	Fever, fibroblast proliferation, induction of collagenase and prostaglandin production

response. A mediator may be distinguished from a neurotransmitter on the one hand and a hormone on the other largely by the extent of its sphere of influence (neither at a nerve ending nor alternatively throughout the body). Douglas (44) introduced the term autacoids to refer to many of these substances that are considered mediators (128). He defined autacoids as substances of intense pharmacologic activity that are normally present in the body and cannot be conveniently classified as neurohormones or hormones.

Origin of Mediators

Chemical messengers or mediators may be exogenous, coming from outside the body, or endogenous, coming from within. Examples of exogenous mediators would be bacterial products and toxins (93,216). Endogenous mediators come from the plasma, blood cells, or tissues. Blood plasma contains three major mediator-producing systems, kinin, coagulation, and complement, which interact in defined manners to generate the flow of phlogistic compounds. Other mediators are cell derived, and within these cells of origin may be preformed or in storage granules, such as histamine in mast cells and cationic proteins in neutrophils, or they may be newly synthesized by the cells. The importance of these distinctions lies in part in the rapidity of release of the molecules and also in therapeutic approaches that may be taken to modify their effect.

Lipid mediators are generally synthesized within the cells when these cells are activated. Little is known as yet about the mechanism of secretion. Arachidonic acid is the precursor of a wide variety of molecules collectively termed prostanoids and eicosanoids. Arachidonic acid is derived from membrane phospholipids by the direct action of phospholipase A_2 or indirectly following the effect of phospholipase C. The arachidonic acid may then be converted into prostaglandins and thromboxanes by way of the cyclooxygenase and subsequent enzymes or into hydroperoxy and hydroxyeicosatetraenoic acids (HPETEs) and (HETEs) by the lipoxygenase enzymes. Leukotrienes C_4, D_4, and E_4, slow reacting substances, as well as B_4, a potent chemotactic agent, are derivatives of the lipoxygenase pathway. These metabolic events appear to be of great importance in the inflammatory action associated with surgical trauma (Figs. 1–3).

No convincing evidence has been obtained that the normal physiologic actions of prostanoids and eicosanoids are mediated by changes in plasma levels of the metabolite. Consequently, it is believed that both prostanoids and eicosanoids act as local modulators of biochemical activity in the tissues in which they are formed. Most are short-lived in the circulation because of chemical instability and/or rapid degradation.

FORMATION OF PROSTANOIDS AND EICOSANOIDS

Prostaglandin, the first arachidonic acid metabolite to be recognized, was so named because it was originally identified in seminal fluid and thought to be

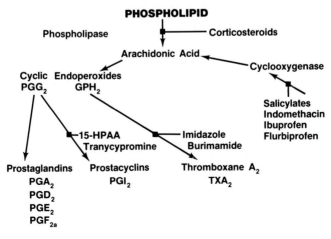

FIG. 1. Formation of prostanoids.

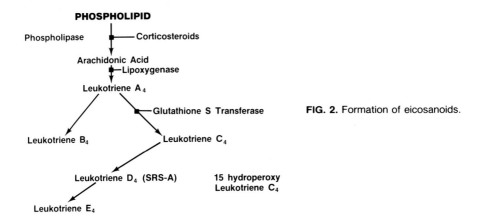

FIG. 2. Formation of eicosanoids.

secreted by the prostate (213). Other active metabolites were characterized subsequently and it was established they were formed by one of two synthetic pathways: a cyclooxygenase or the lipoxygenase system (4). These synthetic pathways and the structures of representative metabolites (Figs. 1–3), as well as prostaglandins and thromboxanes (69), the products of the cyclooxygenase pathways, are collectively termed prostanoids; the products of the lipoxygenase pathway are called eicosanoids.

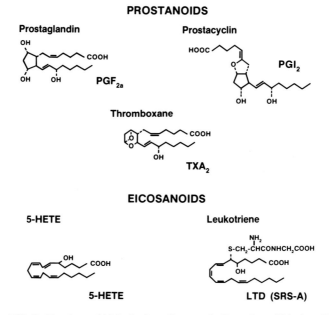

FIG. 3. Structure of biologically active metabolites of arachidonic acid.

The first step takes place in the plasma membranes themselves. Where arachidonic acid is cleaved from phospholipid, free arachidonic acid can then be metabolized by the cyclooxygenase or lipoxygenase pathway. The first product of the cyclooxygenase is the cyclic endoperoxide PGG_2, which is then converted to PGH_2. PGG_2 and PGH_2 are the key intermediates in the formation of the classical prostaglandins PGA_2, PGD_2, PGE_2 and $PGF_{2\alpha}$, prostacyclin (PGI_2) and thromboxane A_2 (TXA_2). The first product of the lipoxygenase pathway is hydro-peroxy-eicosatetraenoic acid (HPETE), which is an intermediate in the formation of 5-hydroxy-eicosate-traenoic acid (HETE) and the leukotrienes (LTA, LTB, LTC, LTD). There are fatty acids other than arachidonic that can be converted to metabolites closely related to the prostanoids and the eicosanoids.

All cells have the necessary substrates and enzymes to form some of the metabolites of arachidonic acid, but tissues differ widely in the amounts of the various enzymes and consequently in the amounts of the various products formed. Prostanoids and eicosanoids are synthesized according to immediate need and are not stored in significant amounts for later release (115).

The classical prostaglandins A_2, D_2, E_2, and $F_{2\alpha}$ are formed from the cyclic endoperoxide PGG_2 and PGH_2. Of these, PGE_2 and PGF_2 appear to be physiologically important. PGA_2, a degradation product of PGE_2, is supposed to have strong vasodepressor activity, but its physiologic relevance is uncertain. The two basic families of compounds involved are PGE and PGF. The 1, 2, and 3 subscripts refer to the number of double bonds, and the differences between the PGEs and the PGFs lie in the presence of 9-keto derivatives of the Es compared with the hydroxy derivation of the Fs.

Prostacyclin or PGI_2 can be synthesized in the vessel wall, not only from its own endogenous endoperoxides but also from those of platelets. At injury the initial response is platelet adherence to the vessel wall, which perhaps reflects this platelet/vessel wall interaction. Prostacyclin is the strongest inhibitor of platelet aggregation discovered to date and a potent vasodilator. In a number of *in vivo* animal experiments prostacyclin has inhibited thrombus formation when given locally or systemically. It stimulates adenylate cyclase, resulting in elevation of platelet cyclic adenosine monophosphate (AMP) levels and reduced platelet aggregation (210). Prostacyclin seems to have some potential for relief of ischemic diseases. In a study of patients with ischemic stroke, marked response was achieved in all 10 patients who received prosta-cyclin infusion, and at 6 months follow-up, 9 had maintained return of function.

Thromboxane Synthetase

Thromboxane synthetase catalyzes the incorporation of an oxygen atom into the ring of the endoperoxide PGH_2 to form the thromboxane TXA_2 synthesized by platelets and acts to enhance platelet aggregation.

The Effect of Drugs on the Synthesis of Prostanoids and Eicosanoids

Many drugs block the synthesis of prostanoids and eicosanoids by inhibiting one or more enzymes in the biosynthetic pathway. Glucocorticoids and several antimalarial drugs interfere with the cleavage of arachidonic acid from phospholipids (Fig. 2).

Cyclooxygenase, an enzyme in the pathway, is directly inhibited by non-steroidal anti-inflammatory drugs including the salicylates indomethacin, flurbiprofen, ibuprofen, and others. These same drugs also inhibit the peroxidase-mediated step that converts HPETE to HETE.

A multitude of newly created compounds have been developed to inhibit prostaglandin formation. Many of these differ little in their pharmacologic or clinical effect. All are successfully useful as analgesics in arthritis, particularly rheumatoid arthritis, but it would be wrong to consider them as nonspecific suppressors of inflammation, and it is perhaps unfortunate that the general term anti-inflammatory has been applied to them. There are conditions in which inflammation is marked and is actually made worse by such drugs. This is demonstrated in ulcerative colitis, and for many years it has been a suspicion that psoriasis also can, on occasion, be exacerbated by indomethacin (90,95).

With the discovery by Samuelsson and co-workers (185) in 1980 of an alternative pathway of arachidonic acid metabolism by way of lipoxygenase to a series of highly active compounds, which they christened leukotrienes, came an important advance in understanding of the mechanisms of inflammation and a clue to why these exacerbations might occur. Among the leukotrienes, leukotriene B_4 has been found to be a potent chemotactic agent for leukocytes (164,183). Leukotriene C_4 and D_4 as a mixture represents the slow-reacting substance of guinea pig anaphylaxis (183). Leukotriene C_4 and D_4 are the mediators of allergic and asthmatic reactions (184). They are also thought to cause vasoconstriction (25), release thromboxanes from platelets (49) and increase vascular permeability (183). Blockage of the cyclooxygenase pathway may increase the formation of lipoxygenase products, and therefore, it is possible that a heightened production of leukotrienes is of significance in conditions exacerbated by nonsteroidal anti-inflammation drugs.

In a recent study, it was reported that although the topical administration of indomethacin in the bovine serum albumin uveitis model decreased the signs of inflammation, paradoxically it potentiated the migration of white cells into the aqueous humor. Higgs et al. (75) have also demonstrated in the rat that low doses of indomethacin potentiated the chemotactic response for white cells induced by intraperitoneal carageenin, whereas high doses inhibited this response. Since low doses of indomethacin inhibited cyclooxygenase but not lipoxygenase, Higgs et al. (75) suggested that the potentiation of chemotaxis by indomethacin was due to facilitation of chemotactic lipoxygenase product formation. To support this hypothesis further, these authors demonstrated that the chemotactic response was completely inhibited by BW755, an inhibitor of both cyclooxygenase and lipoxygenase enzymes (75). In the corneal epithelial denudation model, it was also shown that intraperitoneal administration of cyclooxygenase inhibitors (indomethacin, aspirin, and flurbiprofen) in high doses inhibited the release of polymorphonuclear (PMN) leukocytes into the tear fluids. In low doses, however, indomethacin and aspirin potentiated the release of PMNs into the tear fluid (200). Therefore, in this model it is possible that low doses of cyclooxygenase inhibitor would facilitate the formation of chemotactic lipoxygenase products, such as leukotriene B_4 from arachidonic acid by the lipoxygenase pathway, to potentiate the PMN response. Benoxaprofen, another nonsteroidal anti-inflammatory drug, inhibits the lipoxygenase-mediated conversion of arachidonic acid to HPETE (15-hydro-peroxy-arachidonic acid) (15-HPAA), an arachidonic acid analogue. Benoxaprofen differs significantly in its mode of action from other nonsteroidal anti-inflammatory drugs, showing relatively little ability to inhibit prostaglandin synthesis (28,57).

Benoxaprofen shows little ability to inhibit prostaglandin synthesis, according to Cashin et al. (28) but has a marked inhibitory effect on lipoxygenase activity (42). Benoxaprofen depresses the formation of leukotriene, particularly LTB_4, which is a potent stimulator of chemokinesis in leukocytes. Benoxaprofen also inhibits the accumulation of cells in inflammatory exudate. In view of these novel aspects of its pharmacology, it might have been predicted that clinical use would reveal differences between benoxaprofen and other nonsteroidal anti-inflammatory drugs (140).

There is some evidence that Behçet's syndrome might benefit from a drug such as benoxaprofen (1). If the effects seen in Behçet's syndrome are confirmed, it might suggest that the infiltrating PMN cells are actually participating in the pathologic physiology of that disorder, particularly if the inhibitory effect of benoxaprofen on the release of mediators such as SRS-A is verified as suggested by Boot et al. (21). Benoxaprofen has not had any significant trial in ophthalmology. It has been shown, however, to have some definite toxicity. It has great potential to produce increased sensitivity to sunlight. Sixty-five deaths have been linked to benoxaprofen. These were recorded subsequent to a paper recording five fatalities in elderly patients on the drug (203). Most of these patients had renal or hepatic impairment or both. Inevitably other drugs will be discovered that act in a similar way. The development will be hampered by not knowing the exact mode of action of benoxaprofen.

Tranylcypromine, an antidepressant drug, inhibits the conversion of cyclic endoperoxides PGI_2, and imidazole inhibits thromboxane synthesis. Most of these drugs inhibit early reactions in the synthetic pathways and therefore block the formation of more than one product. Imidazole and 15-HPA are exceptions to this rule and are not available for clinical use. No specific inhibitors of the conversion of HPETE to the leukotrienes or of the specific actions of the individual arachidonic acid metabolites have been identified. Lack of such antagonists is a barrier to elucidating the role of these metabolites in physiologic and pathophysiologic processes.

The fact that a drug inhibits the synthesis of a certain compound does not mean that a given drug effect is the direct result of a deficiency of that compound. For example, indomethacin not only inhibits the formation of cyclic endoperoxide by cyclooxygenase but also disrupts calcium flux across membranes, inhibits cyclic AMP-dependent protein kinase, phosphodiesterase, and inhibits one of the enzymes responsible for degradation of PGE_2.

Lipolysis

PGE_2 is synthesized by adipocytes and is a potent endogenous inhibitor of lipolysis. Since the formation of cyclic AMP is necessary in the action of hormones that stimulate lipolysis, the interactions between PGE and adenylate cyclase have been examined in considerable detail. PGE inhibits lipolysis by decreasing the formation of cyclic AMP in response to epinephrine, adreno-corticotropic hormone (ACTH), glucagon, and thyroid stimulating hormone (TSH). Consequently, PGE_2 may act as an endogenous antilipolytic substance interfering with the stimulation of cyclic AMP formation by hormones.

PENETRATION OF NONSTEROIDAL AGENTS

It is of interest to note that intraocular penetration of indomethacin is enhanced by the presence of an inflammatory state (71). Subconjunctival injection resulted in reduced penetration of indomethacin into ocular tissues and fluids compared to topical treatment. Topically applied indomethacin is known to enter the aqueous humor of phakic eyes as determined by gas chromatography (35), by using radioactive material (71), and by demonstration of the effectiveness of topical indomethacin in preventing the effects of prostaglandin precursor arachidonic acid (17,66,67,80,175). Studies by Green et al. (67) revealed the ocular penetration of topical indomethacin in both phakic and aphakic rabbit eyes after single- or multiple-dose drug applications.

Tissue and fluid concentrations were measured to determine any differences in the amount of drug penetration in the posterior pole between phakic and aphakic eyes, as might be anticipated from previous studies using labeled epinephrine hydrochloride (103,104). These studies also were done to see if the drug could be found in the posterior pole in therapeutically effective concentrations after topical application to the cornea. Green et al. (66,67) found that the amount of drug in the cornea of aphakic eyes was higher than that of phakic eyes at 2, 6, and 12 hr after administration. The aqueous humor concentrations were similar in both phakic and aphakic eyes, although the concentration in aphakic eyes at 2 hr was significantly greater than that of the phakic eyes.

The vitreous of the aphakic eye contained significantly greater drug concentrations than the phakic eye at 1, 6, and 12 hr after administration. The retinal and choroidal concentrations of indomethacin were not significantly different in either phakic or aphakic eyes, yet in both tissues the drug concentration was significantly greater than that in the vitreous.

The indomethacin concentrations in the retina and choroid were far less than those found to be therapeutic effectively in the anterior segment. Earlier data show that the dose of indomethacin that induced a 70% inhibitory effect on arachidonic acid metabolism was between 5 and 6 μg/ml (35). These concentrations were measured at 45 min after topical application of 0.5 ml indomethacin in 50 μl (1%) and correlate with data on microsomal fractions of ocular tissue where the concentration of indomethacin causing a 50% inhibition of prostaglandin formation from arachidonic acid was 18 μg/ml for the anterior uvea and 50 μg/ml for the retina (16).

Multiple-drop applications (every 12 hr for 3 days) did not result in tissue buildup of drug, which suggests that a regimen of a drop every 2 to 3 hr might be satisfactory to maintain an adequate anterior segment concentration of more than 4 μg/ml (66,67). This represents an increased frequency of drop administration compared with the currently recommended regimens that use the medication two to four times per day.

In the study of the ocular absorption elimination of a topically applied nonsteroidal anti-inflammatory drug, flurbiprofen, the compound was well absorbed in rabbit ocular tissues and was highly concentrated in the rabbit cornea (3). In aphakic eyes more drug penetrated to the vitreous and choroid retinal area than in the normal rabbit eyes, although corneal concentrations were still high. No ocular metabolism of flurbiprofen could be detected, and the ocular route of application did not lead to any changes in blood elimination rate or metabolism when compared with intravenously injected drugs.

The percentage of applied dose of flurbiprofen absorbed by ocular tissue is large when compared with the absorption of most commonly used ophthalmic drugs; for example, after application of 1% pilocarpine nitrate, about 1% of the dose was absorbed (114). After application of 0.5 or 2.5% cortisol, 1.6% of the dose was found in ocular tissue (86). After application of 0.05% epinephrine, 0.44% of the dose was found in the eye (217). The extent of ocular absorption of flurbiprofen is similar to that of dipivifrin, the lipophilic prodrug of epinephrine. After topical application of dipivifrin, 4% of the original dose was absorbed by ocular tissues.

Since no metabolism or degradation of flurbiprofen could be detected in ocular tissues, the amount of radioactive material in these tissues directly measures the amount of drug present. Prostaglandin synthetase in various human and animal sources is 50% inhibited in flurbiprofen concentrations ranging from 4 to 98 mg/ml (40). Drug concentrations in the ocular tissues treated by Anderson et al. (3) were sufficiently high to inhibit prostaglandin synthetase. Such inhibition has been demonstrated in the rabbit uvea and conjunctiva after topical flurbiprofen administration (108,200).

The high concentrations found in the cornea indicate that the drug should be especially efficacious in the treatment of corneal inflammations. The distribution in aphakic eyes is similar to the distribution seen in normal eyes, with the highest concentration of drug appearing in the cornea. However, the results indicate that more drug penetrates the posterior areas of the aphakic than the phakic eye, although the major portion of the absorbed drug still remains in the anterior segment of the eye even 3 hr after drug application. Anderson and co-workers (3) noted that there were larger variations in drug concentrations taken from aphakic eyes than those of control eyes, with the largest variations occurring in the iris tissues. This may be due to postsurgical inflammatory processes that varied in severity among the surgically treated animals, as it occurred less frequently in phakic animals.

PLATELET AGGREGATION

Although a physiologic role has not been established for PGE_2 and PGD_2 in platelet function, TXA_2 is a potent stimulator of platelet aggregation. In contrast, PGI_2 formed by the endothelial cells of blood vessel walls is a potent antagonist of platelet aggregation. Since decreases in cyclic AMP are associated with platelet aggregation, TXA_2 and PGI_2 may exert their opposing effects by influencing platelet generation of cyclic AMP (154).

Inhibitors of endogenous prostaglandin synthesis interfere with platelet aggregation. For example, a single dose of aspirin can suppress normal platelet aggregation for 48 hr. This effect is presumed to be the result of suppression of cyclooxygenase-mediated TXA_2 synthesis. Cyclooxygenase inhibition by a single dose of aspirin or indomethacin is of longer duration in platelets than in other tissues probably because the platelets, in contrast to nucleated cells that can synthesize new proteins, do not have the necessary machinery to form new enzymes. Consequently, the effect of the prostaglandin synthesis inhibitor persists until newly formed platelets have been released. Endothelial cells, on the other hand, rapidly recover cyclooxygenase activity following discontinuation of treatment with inhibitors of prostaglandin synthesis, and PGI_2 reduction is restored. This is one reason that patients taking these drugs are not predisposed to excessive formation of platelet thrombi. Another possible explanation is that the platelet is more sensitive than the endothelial cell to drugs that inhibit cyclooxygenase. Endothelial damage may lead to platelet aggregation along the blood vessel wall by causing a focal decrease in PGI_2 synthesis, thereby allowing unbridled platelet aggregation at the site of vessel wall damage.

VASCULAR EFFECTS

The vasoactive properties of the arachidonic acid metabolites are among their most important physiologic actions. Prostaglandins of the E and A series and PGI_2 are vasodilators, whereas $PGF_{2\alpha}$ and TXA_2 are vasoconstrictors. These effects appear to be the result of direct action on the smooth muscles of the vessel wall (105). If the systemic blood pressure is maintained, the vasodilatory arachidonic acid metabolites act to increase blood flow. If blood pressure falls, however, blood flow decreases even though the arterial bed is dilated, since the systemic-hypotension, catecholamine-induced vasoconstriction offsets the vasodilatory effect of the prostaglandin. For these reasons, significant alterations to systemic blood pressure must be excluded when evaluating the effect of arachidonic acid metabolites on organ blood flow.

NEUROTRANSMISSION

PGE inhibits egress of norepinephrine from sympathetic nerve terminals. The PGE effect on the norepinephrine secretion appears to be prejunctional—that is, at a site on the nerve terminal proximal to the synaptic cleft—and can be reversed by increases in calcium concentration in the perfusing medium. Therefore, PGE_2 may inhibit norepinephrine release by blocking calcium influx. Inhibitors of PGE_2 synthesis augment norepinephrine release in response to stimulation of adrenergic nerves.

In contrast, catecholamines can release PGE_2 from a variety of tissues, probably by an α-adrenergic-mediated mechanism. For example, in innervated tissue such as the eye, nerve stimulation or injection of norepinephrine causes release of PGE_2. This release is blocked after denervation or after administration of α-adrenergic blockers. A stimulus activates the nerve, causing release of norpinephrine, which in turn stimulates synthesis and release of PGE_2, which then feeds back at the prejunctional level of the nerve terminal to decrease the amount of norepinephrine released.

SUMMARY

Drugs such as aspirin have long been used as antipyretics and anti-inflammatory agents as well as analgesics. Several arguments have been marshaled to support a relation between inflammation and the arachidonic acid metabolites. Inflammatory stimuli release mediators such as histamine, bradykinin, and endogenous prostaglandins in apparent parallel.

Several arachidonic acid metabolites cause vasodilatation and hyperalgesia. Some arachidonic acid metabolites cause increased vascular permeability, a feature of the inflammatory response that gives rise to local edema.

Vasodilatation induced by PGE is not abolished by atropine, propranolol, methysergide, or antihistamines, known antagonists of the other possible mediators of the inflammatory response.

Prostaglandins are present in areas of inflammation, PMN cells release PGE during phagocytosis, and PGE is chemotactic for leukocytes. PGE can cause fever, usually after injection into the cerebral ventricles or into the hypothalamus of experimental animals. Pyrogens can cause increased concentration of prostaglandins in the cerebrospinal fluid, whereas prostaglandin synthesis inhibitors decrease fever and decrease release of prostaglandins into the cerebrospinal fluid.

Arachidonic acid metabolites have also been postulated to play a role in the immune response. Small amounts of PGE can suppress stimulation of the human lymphocytes by mitogens such as phytohemagglutinin. This observation and the fact that the inflammatory response is associated with a local release of arachidonic acid metabolites have led to the hypothesis that these substances act as negative modulators of lymphocyte function. The release of PGE by mitogen-stimulated lymphocytes may constitute a portion of the negative feedback mechanism by which lymphocyte activity is regulated. Sensitivity of lymphocytes to the inhibiting effect of PGE_2 increases with age, and indomethacin, flurbiprofen, and similar drugs augment lymphocyte responsiveness to mitogens to a degree in the elderly (169).

CORTICOSTEROIDS

Mechanisms of Anti-Inflammatory Action of Glucocorticoids

During the 30 years since cortisone was first reported to be effective for the treatment of rheumatoid arthritis (73), glucocorticoids have received wide clinical and experimental application as anti-inflammatory agents. Glucocorticoids are reported to be the only available chemotherapeutic agents that reverse all the clinical manifestations of inflammation, that is, pain, redness, heat, and swelling. Whether or not this is completely accurate, these hormones are useful clinically for treatment of a wide range of inflammatory processes that are associated with surgery. In spite of the years of extensive use, we still have considerable difficulty understanding the mechanisms by which these steroids act. Almost everyone has agreed that corticosteroids bind to intracellular receptors. This is followed by nuclear localization of the hormone-receptor complexes, then by successive steps requiring RNA and protein synthesis. There seems to be much evidence supporting a close relationship, at both the cellular and molecular level, between anti-inflammatory and physiologic effects and that the anti-inflammatory actions of glucocorticoids are many of the same cellular effects that give rise to immunosuppression (Table 2).

Recent advances in our understanding of the development of the immune responses by way of direct interaction between cells and through interactions mediated by soluble factors (factors ranging from established hormones through prostaglandins to the more recently recognized lymphokines and monokines) should lead to new insights concerning glucocorticoid mechanisms. For example, it now seems likely that an important component of the inhibition by glucocorticoids of the inductive phase of immune responses may be attributable to inhibition of production of certain of these soluble mediators (54,167).

The current view of the action of corticosteroids is that all physiologically significant effects of glucocorticoids are mediated by glucocorticoid receptors. The hormone is thought to pass freely through the membrane apparently by

TABLE 2. *Mechanism of action of steroid*

Receptor-mediated mechanism

Binding of glucocorticoid to intracellular receptors
Activation and translocation of the steroid-receptor complexes to the nucleus
RNA and protein synthesis

Effector protein formation → Glucocorticoid-induced proteins

Inhibition of production or effects of other vasoactive
    agents of immunologically active lymphokines
    and monokines that mediate immune response,
    e.g., phagocytosis → Inhibit biosynthesis and release
    Neutral protease secretion   inflammatory prostaglandins
    Antibody production
    Lymphokine-mediated movement of immune cells
    Lymphocyte proliferation
This could account for
    Intracellular liposomal stabilization
    Interference with degranulation of mast cells
    Interference with degranulation of granulocytes
    Interference with chemotaxis
    Inferference with maturation of lymphocytes
    Reduction in vascular permeability
    Suppression of fibroplasia

diffusion, then to bind noncovalently to soluble protein receptors to form the so-called cytoplasmic hormone receptor complex. These complexes are characterized by the fact that they are found in cytosol after cells are broken. Binding sites on the receptors have high stereochemical specificity and affinity for steroids with glucocorticoid activity, such as the naturally occurring glucocorticoids, corticosterone and cortisol, and the synthetic steroids, dexamethasone, prednisolone, and triamcinolone. Receptors also have a high affinity for certain closely related steroids such as progesterone, which have little glucocorticoid activity and can thus act as antiglucocorticods by competition with active steroids. These cytoplasmic and nuclear receptors for corticosteroids have been demonstrated in ocular tissues, e.g., trabecular meshwork outflow channels, Schlemm's canal outflow vessels, and scleral fibroblasts (181). These receptors have little or no affinity for androgens or estrogens or for cortisone and prednisone. These last two steroids were once thought to be glucocorticoids. They are now known to be inactive, but *in vivo* they become active through conversion to cortisol and prednisolone, respectively (53).

The steroid cytoplasmic complexes rapidly become activated or transformed, acquiring affinity for nuclear structures to which they become bound almost instantly. Activation involves a conformational rearrangement, perhaps irreversible, accompanied by redistribution of charges. At low temperatures activation is slow. Although the nature of the nuclear sites to which the complexes are bound is poorly understood, at least a substantial fraction of them are associated with chromatin. There is a definite time sequence to many of the events that happen after the arrival of the hormone-receptor complexes into the nucleus. The first general metabolic change that has been observed in thymus cells, for example, is inhibition of glucose uptake caused by a decreased rate of glucose transport. In thymus cells and other lymphocytes several inhibitory, metabolic effects start shortly thereafter (1 to 2 hr). These include a decrease in amino acid incorporation into proteins, probably a manifestation of general inhibition of protein synthesis, decreases in uridine incorporation into RNA, in adenosine triphosphate (ATP) levels, and in various transport processes, including transport of the amino acid analogue α-aminoisobutyric acid. About this time there is also an increase in so-called nuclear fragility measured by leakage of DNA from nuclei or by decreased recovery of nuclei after cells are broken by hypotonic shock. Thereafter, morphologic evidence of cell damage begins to appear, and measurable loss of viable cells can be detected in several hours. It seems that if one removes the cortisol from the receptor site some 5 min or longer after initial adherence, the effect of the cortisol carries on even though it has been removed.

There appears to be some evidence that corticosteroid increases RNA polymerase II activity and stimulates transcription of RNA. Several of the glucocorticoid effects that begin in the rat thymus cell by 1 hr, including the inhibition of uridine incorporation into RNA, the decrease in ATP levels, and the increase in nuclear fragility, are blocked by inhibitors of protein synthesis. The glucocorticoid inhibition of protein synthesis is blocked by actinomycin D; these latter effects are therefore also thought to be dependent on prior synthesis of messenger RNA effector proteins. How many such hormone-induced defective proteins there are in these experimental thymus cells and how many are related to each other are open questions. Similar questions remain for almost all the multitude of induced defector proteins that have been hypothesized to account for glucocorticoid effects in other systems (157).

There appear to be a number of factors that influence the glucocorticoid receptor levels. Low ATP levels have been correlated with a low receptor-site level in lymphocytes (156). Recent studies raised the possibility that dephosphorylation is associated with activation of the hormone-receptor complex (186). There is an increase in receptor levels that occurs in lymphocytes, for example, after antigen stimulation (197). Changes take place in glucocorticoid receptor levels in human peripheral lymphocytes after treatment with concanavalin A (Con A). How do these variations in receptor levels affect the sensitivity of cells to glucocorticoids? ATP-deprived thymus cells are insensitive to glucocorticoids, but it cannot be automatically concluded that the insensitivity is caused by absence of receptors, since other steps in the response to the hormones, such as the RNA or protein synthesis steps, are probably also blocked.

In regard to mitogen- and antigen-stimulated cells, the widely held view is that stimulated cells become insensitive to glucocorticoids. The evidence for this is not convincing. Glucocorticoid sensitivity and its relationship to receptors is a broad subject, being explored in many contexts. It is even being considered in glaucoma (181).

Cellular Mechanisms: Action of Glucocorticoid

As we have seen, inflammation results from a dynamic process involving several cell types, numerous mediators, and many physical and anatomical parameters. Changes in vascular caliber and blood flow, vascular permeability, and infiltration into the inflamed tissues by leukocytes result in the classic signs of acute inflammation, redness, swelling, heat, pain, and loss of function. Glucocorticoids appear to exert their anti-inflammatory action on the micro-circulation of inflamed tissues by inhibiting (a) the production and/or activity of vasoactive agents; (b) the movement of leukocytes to the inflamed area; and (c) the capability of immunocompetent cells to function once they enter the site of inflammation. During surgery, the vessels in the microcirculation near the injured tissue dilate, and the blood flow briefly increases before a relatively long period of retarded blood flow. Vascular permeability is enhanced, and fluid accumulates in the tissues. These initial vascular changes are largely caused by many vasoactive agents, among them prostaglandins, kinins, histamines, and slow-reacting substance of anaphylaxis (SRS-A).

Glucocorticoids reduce the production of prostaglandins (88). This glucocorticoid effect has been demonstrated convincingly within the past 5 years (153). The rate-limiting step in prostaglandin synthesis appears to be the phospholipase A_2 catalyzed release of arachidonic acid, the prostaglandin precursor for membrane phospholipids. Because the inhibitory effect of glucocorticoids on prostaglandin synthesis in whole cells could be prevented by addition of arachidonic acid, it was hypothesized that glucocorticoids reduced the availability of arachidonic acid (68,87). It is interesting also to note that inhibitors of protein and RNA synthesis interfere with the ability of glucocorticoids to inhibit prostaglandin biosynthesis. Cycloheximide and actinomycin D, inhibitors of protein and RNA synthesis, respectively, prevented or greatly reduced the ability of glucocorticoid to inhibit prostaglandin synthesis (20). These data imply that glucocorticoids induce the synthesis of a protein or a polypeptide that blocks prostaglandin production. Actually, Flower and Blackwell (56) demonstrate that infusion into guinea pig lungs of what appears to be a glucocorticoid-induced protein resulted in decreased prostaglandin synthesis. Recently, Blackwell and his colleagues characterized a specific glucocorticoid-induced protein with a molecular weight of 15,000, which they named macrocortin, that inhibits phospholipase A_2 activity and prostaglandin production (56).

Kinins—Glucocorticoid Effect

Bradykinin has the ability to affect smooth muscle in the vascular system and to attract leukocytes (89,101). Bradykinin is considered a potent inflammatory agent because of its effects on smooth muscle in the vascular system, its ability to attract leukocytes, and the interaction of the kinin system with other vascular regulatory processes, such as coagulation, fibrinolysin, and complement cascade. Recent research has implicated an essential role for prostaglandin metabolism in the mechanism of bradykinin action. Bradykinin induces the synthesis of prostaglandins in a variety of tissues and cultured cells. In addition, the bradykinin-induced increment in cyclic AMP of human synovial fibroblasts is inhibited by agents such as flurbiprofen, indomethacin, cyclooxygenase blockers, and by quinacrine, an inhibitor of phospholipase A_2 activity, as well as by cortisol. Since glucocorticoids decrease prostaglandin synthesis, it is not surprising that glucocorticoids inhibit bradykinin-induced inflammation that depends on arachidonic acid production and metabolism (159).

Histamine—Glucocorticoid Effect

Histamine released from mast cells and basophils in response to immune hypersensitivity reaction can cause vascular changes leading to inflammation. Cortisol has been shown to decrease histamine release in perfused lungs and mast cells of sensitized guinea pigs (69).

Glucocorticoids inhibit cyclic AMP phosphodiesterase, and this may cause an increase in cyclic AMP (129). An increase in mast cell cyclic AMP results in the decrease of histamine release. Since in human leukocytes glucocorticoids increase cyclic AMP and potentiate the increase in cyclic AMP induced by PGE_1, it has been suggested that glucocorticoid effects on cyclic AMP contribute to a reduction in histamine release (29).

Investigations have been carried out concerning the action in drugs affecting prostaglandin metabolism on histamine release following chemical immunological challenge. Most of these observations support the conclusion that nonsteroidal anti-inflammatory drugs augment histamine release (221).

Wojnar and co-workers (221) found this augmentation to take place with indomethacin, mefenamic acid, sodium salicylate, aspirin, sodium benzoate, and tartrazine. They believe that there is evidence that some of these agents might enhance histamine release in immediate-type hypersensitivity reactions. They might also be involved in the exacerbation of existing chronic urticaria (163). Okazaki and his co-workers (163) found that the addition of acetylsalicylic acid significantly enhanced histamine release and that this was simultaneously associated with an inhibition of prostaglandin E synthesis.

On the other hand, Thomas and Whittle (205) noted that certain nonsteroidal anti-inflammatory agents caused a 50% inhibition of submaximal histamine release. These were sodium meclofenamate, flufenamic acid, and indomethacin. These drugs also inhibited histamine liberation induced by antigen, either horse serum or egg albumin, from sensitized mast cells or that induced by ATP or crude phospholipase-A. Although these aspirin-like drugs had no consistent effect on nonspecific histamine liberation with surface active agents, such as Triton-X-100, the release of histamines following the incubation of mast cells with a calcium ionophore was markedly reduced. In contrast, the anti-inflammatory steroid betamethasone only slightly inhibited antigen or 48/80-induced histamine release. Polyphoretin phosphate also reduced histamine release. The authors note observations that nonsteroidal anti-inflammatory drugs inhibit histamine release support the finding that indomethacin reduces mast cell degranulation. The mechanism underlying this inhibitory activity is not known but may involve effects on cyclic AMP levels by way of phosphodiesterase inhibition, on membrane stability, or on calcium ion mobilization. Thus, the assessment of a role for endogenous prostaglandins in mast cells is made difficult by these possible actions of aspirin-like drugs, however, the ability of prostaglandins to produce mast cell histamine release could reflect a pathophysiologic modulator role during anaphylaxis. Further work must be done to clarify this problem (205).

SRS-A—Glucocorticoid Effect

SRS-A has recently been identified with arachidonic acid metabolites, especially leukotrienes C and D produced by mast cells and PMN leukocytes. Glucocorticoids may inhibit SRS-A through stimulation of a polypeptide macrocortin that blocks the phospholipid metabolism (122,166).

Cells—Glucocorticoid Effect

Glucocorticoids influence the movement of cells, inhibit leukocyte movement to the inflamed site, and may reduce the ability of leukocytes to remain in the inflamed area. There is a decrease in circulating lymphocytes following the use of corticosteroids brought about by the redistribution of circulating T-cells into extravascular compartments. Parillo and Faucia (167) have postulated that glucocorticoids cause alteration in the membranes of T-cells, thereby permitting them to leave the vasculature. Parrillo has shown that guinea pigs receiving cortisol have a reduced rate of bone marrow lymphocyte production (23,167). Glucocorticoids induce leukocytopenia, eosinophilia, basophilia, and monocytopenia. The mechanisms for this are not known, although alterations in traffic may also contribute to these effects. The increase in neutrophils after glucocorticoid therapy appears to be caused by enhanced release of neutrophils from bone marrow or by an increase of neutrophil circulating half-life and by reduced neutrophil movement out of the vasculature (167).

Although there is this alteration of traffic of cells, there is no definite evidence that redistribution of circulating cells contributes to anti-inflammatory effects. Macrophages and neutrophils are attracted by chemotactic factors produced at the site of inflammation. Chemotactic factor production by cultured guinea pig lymphocytes has been found to be inhibited by cortisol. Cortisol does not block the effect of exogenous chemotactic factor on macrophages (214). For example, plasminogen activator is an enzyme excreted by leukocytes that contributes to the migration of macrophages into inflammatory areas. Glucocorticoids inhibit the production of plasminogen activated by macrophages and human neutrophils (65,211).

The glucocorticoids may have an effect on the production of a migration inhibitory factor (MIF), but this is controversial. Almost everyone agrees, however, that the ability of MIF to reduce migration of macrophages is inhibited by glucocorticoids. The mechanism is unknown. MacGregor (127) has suggested that glucocorticoids induce a plasma protein in humans that decreases neutrophil adherence, and proteins of this nature could reduce the ability of neutrophils to remain at the site of inflammation.

Corticosteroids influence soluble mediators, such as lymphokines, and monokines, and have a direct effect on immune cells.

The mechanism for the death of lymphocytes induced by glucocorticoids has not been established. All effects appear to be initiated by receptor-mediated mechanisms. The morphologic changes are first seen to start in the nucleus. Similar morphologic changes have been found to accompany spontaneous death and death induced by other agents. Attempts to attribute this to inhibition of glucose uptake and alteration of protein synthesis have not been successful. These are cells that have developed a glucocorticoid resistance. This resistance can be accounted for by receptor defects, such as absence of receptor or drastically altered numbers of receptor sites, or the failure of the receptor to form nuclear complexes. It may be that glucocorticoids produce a number of defects, and it is this combination that leads to the death of the cell, for a definite obligatory pathway for cell death after exposure to glucocorticoids has not been identified. There are species differences among lymphocytes in that some are more susceptible to glucocorticoids than others. Man is a resistant species as far as his lymphocytes are concerned, but human lymphocytes are sensitive to glucocorticoids.

Effect of Glucocorticoids on T-Cell Mitogenesis

Glucocorticoids have been known for many years to inhibit induction by lectins, such as phytohemagglutinin (PHA) and Con-A of T-cell mitogenesis. This inhibition appears to be caused by inhibition of production of T-cell growth factor. T-cell growth factor is a lymphokine produced by T-cells, which in conjunction with antigen or lectin stimulates certain T-cells, such as murine T-cells, to proliferate. T-cell proliferation is T-cell growth factor dependent, and specific cytotoxic T-cells can be maintained in culture for long periods in the presence of T-cell growth factor (195). Glucocorticoids markedly suppress the production of T-cell growth factor, but exogenously supplied T-cell growth factor can overcome glucocorticoid-induced inhibition of mitogenesis. Inhibitory effects of glucocorticoids have long been known to be more pronounced on developing immune responses than on immunity previously established. The primary site for inhibition of T-cell growth factor production may not be the producer lymphocytes of T-cell growth factor themselves. To produce T-cell growth factor, these cells require not only lectins but also a signal in the form of a soluble factor or monokine derived from macrophages. Thus, it is possible that the primary action of glucocorticoids may be suppression of monokine production by macrophages (196).

The infiltration into the traumatized site of PMN cells and mononuclear phagocytes is an important aspect of inflammation that is impeded by glucocorticoid therapy. This action appears to be related to a decrease in the circulating pool of available cells, microvascular effects at the inflamed site, and perhaps direct effects on the phagocytes themselves (54). Although the direct effects of glucocorticoids on phagocyte function are potentially important, many—for example, decreased chemotaxis and bactericidal capacity and increased stability of lysosomal membranes—appear to be nonspecific effects caused by excessive steroid levels applied *in vitro*. However, physiologic levels of glucocorticoids have been shown to alter macrophage function. It has been shown that glucocorticoids decrease the *in vitro* tumoricidal activity of interferon on stimulated murine macrophages. This effect continues even after macrophages have reached full activation, and its magnitude correlates roughly with the relative anti-inflammatory potencies of the steroid tested (158). Nathan et al. (158) have reviewed the enormous variety of potential inflammatory substances produced by macrophages. These include neutral proteases, complement components, endogenous pyrogens, reactive oxygen metabolites, and bioactive lipids derived from arachidonic acid. In addition, macrophages and lymphocytes often collaborate to produce factors affecting the production of potentially harmful substances by other cells. One example is mononuclear cell factor, which is produced by macrophages and stimulates synovial cells to produce enzyme collagenase.

Studies in humans and animals suggesting that glucocorticoids influence Fc-receptor-dependent functions have been reviewed recently (167). A variety of *in vitro* immune responses are stimulated by Fc fragments of IGG. Fc fragments stimulate macrophages to produce both a stimulator of collagenase production and prostaglandins. Aberrant Fc receptor function seems to accompany chronic inflammatory disease such as seen in Sjögren's syndrome (70). Fahey and co-workers (53) have demonstrated that glucocorticoids influence macrophage Fc receptor levels by direct effect on the macrophage and by modulating production of the factor that greatly increases Fc receptor levels.

Acid hydrolases and neutral proteases are potentially destructive enzymes that are present in cells at inflammatory sites. These are released in response to a variety of inflammatory stimuli and may contribute to initiation and progression of inflammatory processes (41).

Glucocorticoids inhibit release of hydrolytic enzyme by acting on the cells directly or by acting on cells that aid in the release of these enzymes and indirectly by affecting other cells that produce stimulators of enzyme release. Glucocorticoids inhibit collagenase secretion, elastase and plasminogen activators but not lysozymes by macrophages (211). There is also evidence for inhibition of secretion of neutral proteases.

Effect of Corticoids in Antibody Production

Oral administration of glucocorticoids results in a decrease of total circulating immunoglobulin concentration in humans. Glucocorticoids may have an indirect effect on modulation of antibody production by altering production and activity of lymphokines and monokines. Glucocorticoids can inhibit T-cell growth factor production, which would tend to reduce specific helper-cell population, but also glucocorticoids could inhibit suppressor factors or suppressor cells, which could lead to enhanced antibody response.

Effect of Glucocorticoids on Lymphokines and Monokines

Cooperation between various lymphoid and accessory cells is now a major focus in cellular immunology. It is clear that in many cases communication between cells is achieved by soluble mediators (5). Recent advance in identification, separation, culture, and even cloning of functionally active lymphoid cells *in vitro* is allowing rapid elucidation of both the cellular origins and biological functions of many new factors (32,179).

It is possible that glucocorticoids can regulate lymphokine and monokine production, and this could explain many of their anti-inflammatory actions.

Corticosteroids may be used systemically in intraocular surgical management in the following: (a) intravenous corticosteroids just prior to surgery to the previously steroid treated patient to withstand the stress of surgery (to avoid adrenal insufficiency at the time of surgery); (b) sympathetic ophthalmia; (c) phacoanaphylactic uveitis; (d) lens-induced uveitis along with removal of lens or lens remnants; (e) nonspecific severe postoperative uveitis; (f) postoperative intraocular infection; (g) postoperative cystoid macular edema; and (h) graft rejection.

These ocular complications of topical and/or systemic steroid therapy may occur: (a) wound healing, particularly if steroids are used within the first few days of surgery; (b) opportunistic infections, herpes simplex, toxoplasmosis, fungi, bacteria, *Treponema;* (c) glaucoma; (d) cataract; (e) pseudopapilledema, pseudotumor cerebri; (f) exophthalmos; (g) ptosis; and (h) mydriasis.

Side effects of prolonged systemic corticosteroid administration include (a) Salt retention (less likely with prednisolone, prednisone, and methylprednisone);

(b) hypertension; (c) cardiovascular complications; (d) hyperglycemia; (e) gastric and duodenal ulceration; (f) re-exacerbation of tuberculosis; (g) psychoses; (h) muscle wasting; (i) osteoporosis; (j) pathologic fractures secondary to bone decalcification; (k) Cushing's syndrome; and (l) opportunistic infections.

The following are guidelines to minimize systemic side effects of corticosteroid therapy:

1. Appropriate dosage must be determined by trial and error for each patient.
2. Single dose of corticosteroid, even a large one, is virtually without harmful effects.
3. A few days of corticosteroid therapy, in the absence of specific contraindications, is unlikely to produce harmful side effects.
4. Prolonged therapy increases chances for harmful effects. Use the smallest dose to achieve the desired result.
5. Abrupt cessation of high-dose therapy should be avoided. The more prolonged the therapy the greater chance for adrenal insufficiency to occur.
6. Alternate-day therapy, i.e., a single dose every other day, will minimize the degree of suppression of the pituitary and adrenal cortex but may not be as effective.

CORNEAL INFLAMMATION

The suppression of corneal inflammation by anti-inflammatory corticosteroids, particularly on leukocyte accumulation in inflamed corneas, has been reported (94,109–111,116) (Table 3). Kenyon (94) has reviewed corneal inflammation, noting that it is characterized by infiltration of leukocytes, initially PMN leukocytes, into the tissue, together with edema and eventually neovascularization. All the therapeutic corticosteroid agents tried have shown effectiveness in the decrease in the number of PMN cells in the cornea. Some of these agents are more effective when the epithelium is removed than when the epithelium is intact. It is difficult to choose, on the basis of most of the

TABLE 3. *Ophthalmic topical corticosteroids*

Dexamethasone suspension (Maxidex®)
Dexamethasone sodium phosphate
   Ointment (Decadron®)
   Solution (Decadron®)
Fluorometholone suspension (FML Liquifilm®)
Hydrocortisone acetate
   Ointment (Cortamed® Hydrocortone)
   Suspension (Cortamed® Hydrocortone)
Medrysone suspension (HMS Liquifilm®)
Prednisolone acetate
   Suspension (Pred Forte®, Pred Mild®, Econopred®, Predulose®)
Presnisolone sodium phosphate (AK-pred®, Hydeltrasol®, Inflamase®, Metreton®)

experimentations and experiences, between prednisolone, prednisone, fluoro-metholone, and medrysone when the epithelium is gone, and in some experiments dexamethasone can be included with this group. Fluorometholone is an effective anti-inflammatory agent, and there is considerable clinical evidence that fluorometholone elevates intraocular pressure considerably less than the other anti-inflammatory corticosteroids (96,147).

There are many examples of the anti-inflammatory effects of corticosteroids. In experimental uveitis induced by bovine serum albumin, corticosteroids have alleviated the inflammatory signs of intraocular inflammation, such as the increase in protein in the aqueous, hyperemia of the anterior uvea, and leukocyte migration into the aqueous humor (106).

Similar experiments have shown that topical indomethacin and topical flurbiprofen can overcome increase of protein in the aqueous through the breakdown of the blood-aqueous barrier, increase in prostaglandin release into the aqueous humor, and dilatation of iris vessels in experimental uveitis models (108).

NEOVASCULARIZATION

Neovascularization after ocular surgery can occur in the cornea, iris, choroid, or retina. Nonsteroidal anti-inflammatory agents as well as the steroidal ones can play a role in eliminating the unwanted neovascularization. New corneal vessels arise from the activated limbal vascular plexuses and may invade the avascular cornea at all levels but show little tendency to breach limiting membranes and epithelial surfaces. Most corneal vessels, newly formed, display some degree of incompetence and leak dye during fluorescein angiography, particularly at their growing stage (132).

The precise factors promoting and governing vascular invasion are not known but probably include inflammatory cells, hypoxia, tissue compactness, loss of protease inhibitor activity, and prostaglandins (99). Experimental studies have shown that the new capillary sprouts are composed of proliferating endothelial cells and pericytes (139). Radioactive isotope studies confirm that the maximum mitotic activity occurs from three to four cells downstream from the growing frond (223).

Vascularization of the cornea usually occurs in pathologic states, perhaps initially as a defense mechanism against disease, and may be a beneficial process to resolve the inflammatory situation; however, vascularization also produces a loss of transparency and may, at times, cause an aggravation of symptoms and irritation. It of course can be disastrous in corneal grafts that are done for visual purposes. Once they are present, even though they may be subsequently cleared of blood in their lumen, the walls of the vessels may persist even though they have become obliterated almost to being invisible.

The cornea differs from other tissues of the eye in its compact nature. When the tissue compaction is reduced by edema secondary to surgical trauma, infections, toxins, or malnutrition pathways are opened up from the limbus and thus vascularization ingrowth can occur. Essentially there may be at least two factors in developing vascularization: (a) a release of normal tissue compaction and (b) an attractive factor or angiogenesis substance (30,31).

It is obvious that corneal edema is not the sole responsible factor. Vascular invasion may take place more markedly in areas that are not the most decompressed or swollen regions, and vascularization may be absent when gross swelling is present, both experimentally and in such clinical conditions as congenital endothelial dystrophy. There is also a possibility of there being a vasoinhibitory substance present in the cornea. Years ago, Meyer and Chaffee (144) suggested that the stromal-mucopolysaccharides might act in this way and that their depolymerization by hyaluronidase abolished their inhibitory influence. Michaelson was able to show that hyaluronidase had no effect on the growth of vessels in the cornea, nor is it necessary for corneal vascularization to be accompanied by a diminution of corneal mucoids (144,220).

There are many suggestions of a vasoformative factor being responsible for corneal vascularization (27,87,141,162). It was thought this was a product of an allergic reaction that stimulated vascularization; Bessey and Wolbach (14) suggested anoxia or hypoxia, as did Johnson and Eckardt (84) and later Ashton (7).

Iris neovascularization is unique in that it is typically the response of the normal tissue and vasculature to a remote disease process. The iris vessels are sensitive to a wide variety of stimuli, and neovascularization may be induced by inflammation (188). New iris vessels may also develop in ocular ischemia but are most common in retinal ischemia where there is a quantitative relationship between the extent of retinal ischemia and the presence of iris neovascularization (60,130). New iris vessels may ramify within the stroma for a time; however, they soon gain the anterior iris and freely proliferate on its surface. The mechanism of neovascular extension is not fully known. It has been suggested that progression is by a process of endothelial budding and migration in association with pericyte proliferation. The subsequent invasion of fibroblasts provides the new vessels with a supportive fibrous tissue mantle.

Vascularization can be an undesirable complication of ocular surgery. It becomes particularly annoying in corneal grafts and in the rubeosis iridis following vitrectomy. Rubeosis iridis occurs primarily in the diabetic eye, but some eyes with vascular occlusive diseases and other eyes with traumatic retinal detachment will also develop rubeosis. Eyes with minimal asymptomatic rubeosis preoperatively are likely to develop overt symptoms postoperatively, particularly if the intraocular pressure rises during the early postoperative period. Rubeosis after vitrectomy is most common in patients with diabetes mellitus. Such eyes are particularly resistant to therapy in which surgery has failed because of retinal detachment, recurrent hemorrhage, or residual inflammatory conditions.

Diabetic eyes are at risk for development of rubeosis after any type of surgery. Cataract surgery is followed by rubeosis iridis almost as frequently as is vitrectomy surgery in diabetic eyes. Aphakic diabetic eyes develop rubeosis much less frequently than those who undergo cataract extraction and vitrectomy at the same time. It has been suggested that if the diabetic eye has been able to withstand a cataract extraction without developing rubeosis, it also should be able to undergo a vitrectomy without developing rubeosis; however, if severe rubeosis develops following cataract extraction, the risk of rubeosis following vitrectomy is so great that it is usually not undertaken. For this reason, there are some surgeons who prefer to perform both procedures at the same time through a pars planum incision, particularly in the one-eyed patient. Statistics vary on the incidence of rubeosis iridis developing as a complication of vitrectomy, but this complication occurs in more than 20% of vitrectomized eyes (145,146,170).

There are many other causes or obvious associations with rubeosis iridis (2,188). There are those that fundamentally are primarily arterial insufficiencies, such as seen in aortic arch syndrome, carotid artery occlusion, giant cell artcritis, rctinal artery occlusion, sickle cell hemoglobinopathy, retrolental fibroplasia, and ciliary artery occlusion leading to anterior segment ischemia.

Rubeosis iridis may also follow evidence of arterial insufficiency with impaired venous drainage, such as carotid cavernous fistula, thrombotic retinal venous occlusion, Eale's disease, and diabetic microangiopathy. Proliferative vascular disease of the eye, such as hemangiomas, Coats' disease, persistent hyperplastic primary vitreous, could also lead to this complication. There are certain nonvascular diseases of the eye, such as tumor, choroidal melanoma, retinoblastomas, and some other conditions (uveitis, endophthalmitis, and retinal detachment) that can also produce this condition. Rubeosis iridis has been described after iris tumors, metastatic carcinoma, and radiation therapy.

As the nature of the disease is essentially an increase in vascularization, attention has to be directed to the causes of angiogenesis and particularly the causes of ocular neovascularization. Tissue hypoxia is essential, probably a triggering stimulus for neovascular response, but this may not be the only cause of vasculogenesis, for venous drainage seems to contribute to neovascularization; poor outflow of catabolites creates a sufficiently high concentration of vascogenic substances that cause endothelial cell proliferation and development of new vascular channels (8).

Choroid in Neovascularization

Choroidal neovascularization resembles a traditional type of vasoproliferation that is the hallmark of granulation tissue. The new vessels invade degenerating tissue. The stimulus for this vasoproliferation is not known. The presence of a low-grade inflammatory response, as indicated by the presence of macrophages, giant cells, lymphocytes, and activated retinal pigment epithelial cells, may be a key factor in inducement of new vessel infiltration (6,187).

Retinal Neovascularization

The normal retinal vasculature shows little tendency to proliferate, even in circumstances that are known to produce vasoproliferation elsewhere. Damage to the retina induced by chemical and surgical trauma, laser burns, hypoxia, and acute ischemia can stimulate some mitotic activity in endothelial cells of affected capillaries. A similar lack of response is noted in discrete inflammatory lesions. The normal retinal vasculature is also unresponsive to the chronic ischemia of the outer retina in widespread cellular degeneration and atrophy, as in glaucoma. Finkelstein and others believe that in some circumstances, normal retinal capillaries can respond if the angiogenic stimulus is sufficiently strong and close (55). It is often difficult to determine whether the angiogenic stimulus is ischemia or the effects of inflammatory products (74). Most conditions associated with retinal and papillary neovascularization are characterized by retinal vascular stasis. The exact circumstances that lead to vasoproliferation are not known.

Role of Components of the Inflammatory Response in Neovascularization

Corneal vascularization may be a manifestation of inflammatory response. Leukocytes may have an important pathogenetic role (98). Corneal vascularization induced by chemical injury may be severely suppressed under conditions that inhibit leukocytic infiltration into the cornea, such as corticosteroid therapy (59). The extent of vascularization in several models may be as much suppressed by anti-inflammatory agents, such as glucocorticoids, indomethacin, and flurbiprofen (37,43,59). Many experiments also have emphasized corneal vascularization associated with inflammatory responses and the intensity of new vessel formations directly related to the degree of leukocytic infiltration (13,51,52,59,194).

Available evidence implicates a variety of leukocytes, activated macrophages, and activated lymphocytes in neovascularization. These cells may be important in corneal surgery, which stimulates their invasion into the cornea. Although Fromer and Klintworth (59) suggest that leukocytes may be a prerequisite to corneal vascularization, others have shown that the cornea can be inundated by blood vessels in the absence of leukocytes (50,194).

Although corneal neovascularization can be initiated in the absence of leukocytes, the extent of vascular in-growth is decreased in experimental situations in which the number of leukocytes in the corneal stroma is diminished, that is, animals made leukopenic by whole body X-irradiation, antineutrophil serum, or ocular treatment with corticosteroids, and increased under conditions that provoke greater numbers of leukocytes to infiltrate the corneal tissue. Lutty et al. (125) have demonstrated that stimulated T-cells are a source of angiogenic material. There appears to be a potent lymphokine secreted by stimulated T-cells.

Prostaglandins appear to possess antigenic activity with prostaglandin E_1 being the most potent (12). That prostaglandins participate in the chain of events leading to corneal vascularization is supported by partial suppression of blood vessel proliferation by corticosteroids, inhibitors of phospholipase A_2, flurbiprofen, inhibitor of fatty acid cyclooxygenase, and indomethacin, a suppressor of prostaglandin synthetase (37).

Fibrin complement also may trigger neovascularization. There is evidence of apparent enhancement of corneal vascularization in the presence of antifibrinolysins, such as ϵ-amino-caproic acid (198). Increased permeability of the pericorneal blood vessels during the acute inflammatory episode allows the constituents of the plasma—insulin, epidermal growth factor, mesodermal growth factor, and fibroblast growth factor—to get into the cornea (12,64,100).

Therapy of Neovascularization

Vascularization of the cornea induced by a variety of stimuli can be inhibited by the use of corticosteroids. The more severe the stimulus, the larger the amount of steroid required for this inhibition. In other words, the activity of the steroid is graded and not absolute (9,36,78,85,124,138).

Systemic and topical corticosteroids may have a place in suppressing vasoproliferation that has an inflammatory or immunological basis (74). There is some laboratory evidence that vitamin E, a free radical scavenger, has an inhibitory effect on oxygen-induced retinopathy in kittens (174).

The antimitotic drugs perhaps could affect the dividing endothelial cells. Some recent experiments demonstrated that vasoproliferation following perforating injuries can be inhibited by combined topical and systemic administration of beta aminopropionitrile and penicillamine, which depressed the formation of vitreous scaffolding (155).

Corneal neovascularization is an important clinical function with a potential for good or harm. There is some suggestion that blood vessels growing into the cornea can act as a facilitator and accelerant of corneal wound healing. Experimentally produced thermal burns do not induce corneal ulceration as readily in corneas that are vascularized than in those that are not (34).

PUPILLARY CONSTRICTION

Most surgeons doing intraocular surgery, particularly intraocular lens surgery, desire to prevent the associated pupillary constriction. There is evidence that topical and systemic indomethacin can prevent pupillary constriction. At the present time a number of surgeons are using systemic indomethacin preoperatively in order to minimize the chances of pupillary constriction. Mishima and Masuda (134) were among the first to study this usage. They tried systemic aspirin or indomethacin, but large amounts were required and the effects were doubtful; however, they also pointed out that side effects cannot be disregarded in this mode of administration. They devoted most of their studies to the topical administration of indomethacin. They used indomethacin as 0.1% and

0.5% in an oil base. The oil base consisted of aluminum monostearate 10 g in purified sesame oil 490 g. It was prepared under sterile conditions. No pathologic changes were noted in rabbit eyes after an oil drop of 0.5% concentration instilled three times per day in rabbit eyes for 2 months. Similarly, in 3 human volunteers no deleterious side effects were found at the end of 2 months. In their studies they instilled indomethacin 3, 2, 1, and 0.5 hr before surgery. This provided them with a concentration that suppressed prostaglandin production after paracentesis (134).

In Mishima and Masuda's study (134) the pupils were routinely dilated by instillations of 1% atropine, 0.5% tropicamide and 10% phenylephrine hydrochloride. In spite of prior applications of these agents, pupillary constriction was found to occur during surgery to an extent that interfered with complete aspiration of cataractous material. The pupil diameter was measured with calipers before and after surgery, and those cases where the diameter at the end of surgery became half or less than the preoperative diameter were included in the miosis group. Cases with such extensive miosis were found in none of the indomethacin group but were seen in more than 50% of the nonindomethacin group. This was statistically significant. The degree of miosis was much less in the indomethacin group than in the nonindomethacin group.

In studies done on intracapsular cataract extractions, similar favorable effects on pupils were encountered following the use of topical 0.5% indomethacin. Some other interesting observations were made at the time. There was less flare, fewer floaters, and definitely less corneal edema in the first few days postsurgery than when eyes were treated with 0.5% indomethacin as compared to 0.1% dexamethasone. For these reasons it is suggested that the use of topical nonsteroidal anti-inflammatory agents can be helpful and have a beneficial effect in glaucoma surgery and penetrating keratoplasty as well as in retinal surgery.

It has been shown in rabbit eyes that laser irradiation of the iris initiates prostaglandin synthesis release, and that is likely to be the case in human eyes (207). The use of nonsteroidal anti-inflammatory agents preoperatively before retinal detachment surgery and photocoagulation or the use of the laser would seem advisable to help keep the pupil in a less miotic position, if desired.

CORNEAL AND CATARACT WOUND HEALING

Corneal wound healing is inhibited by a variety of factors, such as topical corticosteroids (9,62,120,123,131,202). There is evidence that antihistamines may delay wound healing (218), and nonsteroidal anti-inflammatory agents appear to inhibit corneal regeneration. There is some evidence that cyclic AMP may have an influence on wound healing. Epinephrine and prostaglandins appear to retard corneal epithelial cell regeneration and mitosis. It is postulated that they do so by increasing cyclic AMP.

There is no known drug therapy that can accelerate the healing of corneal stromal wounds. Perhaps work with growth factors might alter this concept. Soft contact lenses have been reported to increase the strength of limbal wounds.

For many years ascorbic acid has been thought to be important for the production of collagen in the healing of wounds. It functions as a co-factor in hydroxylation of proline. It may be required for the maturation of mononuclear cells into repair fibroblasts.

The cornea receives its ascorbic acid from the anterior chamber. The anterior chamber has a concentration of vitamin C, possibly 20 times the concentration of this substance in the plasma. This high level of ascorbic acid in the aqueous humor is maintained by transport occurring in and through the ciliary epithelium. Alkali burns damage this concentrating mechanism and thus produce a lower level of ascorbic acid in the aqueous humor as pointed out by Levinson et al. (121). Pfister and his co-workers have demonstrated that subconjunctival administration of ascorbic acid in rabbits with corneal lacerations significantly increased aqueous humor levels of ascorbic acid in control animals. However, such high levels did not increase the tensile strength in these otherwise normal animals; thus, the excess levels of ascorbic acid did not enhance wound healing. Many years ago, Boyd (22) reported that the healing of corneal wounds in aphakic animals' eyes, where corneal and aqueous humor levels in ascorbic acid are usually low, is generally slower than that in the contralateral phakic eye. The number of relapses during healing was greater in the aphakic eye than in the phakic eye. Pfister believes that the mechanism for this improvement in aphakic eyes and in alkali-burned eyes is the restoration toward the normal ascorbic acid concentration. Most likely this increase in ascorbate exerts its stable effect on the alkali burn and on the strength of corneal wounds in aphakic eyes by enhancing collagen production. Dietary dependence of humans on exogenous sources of ascorbic acid leads to specific clinical implications, especially in perforating ocular wounds. The ophthalmologist rarely has comprehensive knowledge of the nutritional status of his patient with perforating ocular trauma or in patients in whom surgery is planned. Pfister and his colleagues' observations suggest that an evaluation of the nutritional status of individuals after such trauma or before anticipated surgery, especially in the chronically ill, alcoholics, cancer victims, and even the elderly, might be rewarding if it permitted restoration of normal ascorbic acid levels in the aqueous humor (172,173).

Corticosteroids interfered somewhat with the proliferation of fibroblasts and new vessels in the corneas of rabbits with experimental wounds. The effect appeared to be less obvious with the topical application of the hormone than with subconjunctival injections (119). These studies suggested that various concentrations of cortisone may have a variable effect on the healing of wounds. Ashton and Cook (9) confirmed these applications and showed that the inhibition of fibroblastic activity in the cornea was marked but was related to the amount of cortisone given. This has been confirmed clinically, and it is now known that ocular surgery can be carried out while the patient is under treatment with an average dose of cortisone. There is some evidence that epithelial regeneration may be retarded by large doses of steroids and also that endothelial regeneration may be slowed by smaller doses. The dose for the slowing of regeneration of endothelium is in the range of that which would be employed therapeutically (9,119,160,165,199).

Corticosteroids have been known to be useful agents in the prevention of corneal neovascularization in a variety of surgical, clinical, and experimental circumstances (11,138,176,189). It was initially felt by Ashton and Cook (10) that these drugs worked by decreasing corneal edema as well as by promoting vasomotor tone and preventing an increase in capillary permeability. In contrast, prostaglandins, particularly of the E series, have been shown to produce and potentiate edema (209). Also, it was recently demonstrated by BenEzra (12) that many varieties of prostaglandins show a strong vasoformative tendency. It is now well established, as we have seen, that corticosteroids block prostaglandin formation by preventing the activation of phospholipase A_2, a key enzyme in the prostaglandin biosynthetic pathway. If these agents reduce neovascularization by inhibiting prostaglandin formation, other inhibitors of prostaglandin formation may have the same effect. One such inhibitor is flurbiprofen, a nonsteroidal anti-inflammatory agent that is thought to inhibit prostaglandin synthesis by inhibiting the fatty acid cyclooxygenase in a competitive time-dependent irreversible manner (180). Studies by Cooper et al. (37) demonstrate that flurbiprofen can block corneal neovascularization induced either by an alloxan injection or silver nitrate technique. Both prednisolone and 0.1% flurbiprofen were effective in inhibiting vessel growth when compared with controls in their experiments. Both were equally effective in the alloxan model. Flurbiprofen was more effective in the silver nitrate model. It may be that these agents are acting by inhibiting leukocyte migration, for Klintworth (99) has suggested that corneal vascularization is usually a manifestation of the inflammatory response mediated by leukocytes. It is possible that corticosteroids and flurbiprofen prevent leukocytic migration and subsequent release of prostaglandins from these cells into the cornea. This assumes, of course, that prostaglandins are manufactured by leukocytes in the cornea as in other tissues. Eliason's work (50) supports the view that leukocytes are not necessary for neovascularization. He suggests that an injured cornea is capable of producing an angiogenic factor from its native elements (50). Perhaps fatty acid substances are being released to be acted on by prostaglandin synthetic enzymes, which have been found in all tissues of the eye. Vascularization in this case is prevented not by leukocytic migration inhibition but by prevention of the substrate enzyme interaction (37).

UVEITIS

Iridocyclitis, which is usually minimal and self-limited, follows even the most uneventful cataract extractions. Clinically, aqueous cells and flares, engorgement of iris vessels, and miosis are best treated with topical cycloplegics.

The use of topical corticosteroids in uncomplicated cataract extractions does not usually decrease postoperative inflammation (24,135). However, topical corticosteroids administered more frequently, such as five times per day, do benefit some patients with significant postoperative inflammation (38).

Preoperative topical administration of indomethacin is reported to suppress postoperative inflammation. There is a suggestion that some of this inflammatory process may be prostaglandin mediated (152). Those postoperative inflammatory processes that are associated with vitreous loss and incarceration of vitreous or iris in the wound usually do not respond satisfactorily to either corticosteroids or nonsteroidal anti-inflammatory agents. Such chronic ocular inflammation may also be associated with epithelial or fibrous ingrowth, hyphema, and retinal detachment.

The chronic inflammatory state, such as uveitis, can eventually lead to pupillary membrane formation, secondary glaucoma due to peripheral anterior synechiae, and plugging the trabecular meshwork with inflammatory debris or adhesion of the iris to the vitreous face resulting in pupillary block or cystic macular degeneration, retinal detachment, and corneal endothelial decompensation. Such uveitis may be treated with topical, subtenons, or systemic corticosteroids to reduce the occurrence and severity of these complications.

POSTOPERATIVE INFECTIONS AND STEROID USAGE

The use of corticosteroids in the treatment of bacterial endophthalmitis has been controversial (120). Corticosteroid use is based on the assumption that damage from secondary reaction of inflammation can be reduced and thereby aid in reducing damage to vision. Most individuals use topical, subconjunctival and even systemic steroids in the management of suspected or proved intraocular postoperative infection. The use of steroids does reduce the inflammatory process and may interfere somewhat with the penetration of antibiotics that move from the blood stream into the eye. By returning the permeability of the aqueous blood vessel barrier toward normal, those antibiotics that have difficulty penetrating into the eye unless the permeability is increased would be reduced in quantity and thereby decrease their effect against the offending organism. Usually, the inflammatory process is sufficiently severe so that the corticosteroids do not seriously alter the penetrability of the antibiotic (118). To date nonsteroidal anti-inflammatory agents have not been used to any significant degree in the management of the inflammatory process associated with intraocular infection.

CORNEAL EDEMA

Corneal edema that results after intraocular surgery is usually iatrogenic, caused by mechanical or nonchemical injury to the endothelium of the cornea. The influence of nonsteroidal and steroidal anti-inflammatory agents on these changes is limited, as many factors appear to affect the corneal tissues during surgery.

Experimental studies on the corneal endothelium have shown that endothelial structure and function can be affected by the ionic composition of the perfusion media, ionic buffer capacity, substrate composition and pH. Studies have been done to determine the tolerance of the corneal endothelium for intraocular drugs, vehicles, and solutions that are used during intraocular surgery. Corneal edema has been reported following cataract extraction when a hypo-osmotic pilocarpine solution with a pH of 4.5 and an osmolality of 78 mOsm was used intracamerally (126).

Corneal edema has also been reported with acetylcholine and acetone used for miosis after delivery of the lens in cataract surgery (58). Vaughn and his co-workers (212) reported minimal corneal swelling following a 15-min endothelial perfusion of hyperosmotic acetylcholine in isolated perfused rabbit corneas. However, corneal swelling did result with isotonic carbachol.

Transient cataracts have been reported with the use of intraocular acetylcholine by Lazar and his co-workers (115,182). Cataracts have been attributed to the hyperosmolality of the acetylcholine, which has experimentally been shown to induce lens opacities in rabbits following intracameral injection (137,143).

Several criteria are usually used to evaluate the effects of these drugs, such as the degree of swelling of the cornea, the reversibility of the swelling, the degree of breakdown of endothelial cells (whether permanent or reparable), and the cell counts (whether or not any cells have been lost). The corneal endothelial cell viability is a crucial factor in the maintenance of corneal clarity. With the advent of biomicroscopic techniques of quantitative and qualitative evaluation of the endothelial monolayer, they become more critical of the manipulation of the cornea, more cognizant of the effect of this manipulation on the endothelial cells. Microsurgical techniques and attention to inflammation have reduced much of the trauma previously associated with surgical procedures in the anterior chamber. It is well known that living cells are particularly sensitive to narrow limits of pH, osmolality, and electrolyte composition in concentration. Much work has been done to determine the effects of these various factors on the corneal endothelium. Edelhauser et al. (47) described cytotoxic changes in the corneal endothelium due to phenylephrine used topically, changes that were greater after the epithelium was removed. This effect is reversible as the drug diffuses from the cornea. Jay and MacDonald (1978) demonstrated dose-related cytotoxic effect of pilocarpine and acetylcholine on cultured bovine endothelial cells and attributed them to extreme osmotic shock.

Leibowitz et al. (117) suggested that the replacement of aqueous by air produced morphologic endothelial changes compatible with local cell destruction, whereas Norn (161) has concluded from corneal pachymetry in human eyes after cataract extraction that air seems to protect the corneal endothelium. Harris and Hassard (72) reproduced Norn's findings of reduced corneal thickness in Leibowitz and colleagues' model.

In a recent study, Edelhauser and his co-workers (47) have demonstrated that changes in solution osmolality result in substantial alterations in corneal thickness without marked structural changes in the corneal endothelium. The alterations in the corneal thickness were reversible as shown by the effect of returning the perfusion media to isotonicity.

The degree to which the cornea swells or dehydrates will depend on the initial state of hydration before applying the solution. With the rabbit corneas, a normal state of hydration exists at the start of the experiment; therefore, the degree of thinning or swelling achieved with a change of 100 mOsm of hypo-osmotic or hyperosmotic solution is the same. By contrast, the human corneas, which have been stored under eye bank conditions, were started in the experiment in the hydrated state, and therefore a greater amount of dehydration occurred with the hyperosmotic solutions than with the hypo-osmotic solutions.

Sherrard (192) reported that 20% glycerin placed on the epithelial surface of an isolated perfused cornea will cause intracellular vacuoles in the endothelium that eventually rupture.

In the studies of Edelhauser (47) it is suggested that the osmotic stress on the corneal endothelium was minimized because the perfusion medium contained the necessary ions: sodium, potassium, calcium, magnesium, and chloride. If hypo-osmotic or hyperosmotic solutions were in contact with the endothelium without the necessary ions, the osmotic stress would be much greater, and endothelial cell destruction would occur as reported with intraocular miotics.

A solution that lacks calcium will cause endothelial cell junctional breakdown; therefore, a miotic or other intraocular drug or enzyme in a sodium chloride vehicle that is hypo-osmotic or hyperosmotic could be expected to cause greater endothelial damage due to the osmotic movement of water, since the endothelial junction would also be affected by the lack of calcium (92). In conclusion, Edelhauser's studies (47) indicated that the corneal endothelium could tolerate a wide range of solution osmolalities, 200 to 400 mOsm, without marked endothelial cell breakdown, provided the five essential ions are present in the perfusion medium or vehicle.

Recent studies by Lang and Hassard (112) have demonstrated that commonly used solutions introduced intraoperatively into the anterior chamber have predictable, and in some cases deleterious, effects on the corneal endothelium. In actual surgical procedures, they could find no demonstrable difference in endothelial cell loss in the late postoperative period when Miochol® as opposed to air was instilled to reconstitute the anterior chamber. Their observations would suggest that air may well have a deleterious, though short-lived effect on endothelial cells. Whether this is due to the mechanical effect of the bubble rubbing on the endothelium or the metabolic effect due to altered fluid content is difficult to determine. That it is short-lived is to be expected because of the movement of the bubble away from the endothelium when the patient is upright and walking the evening after the operation and because of the absorption of the air within 2 to 3 days.

Lang and Hassard's results with Miochol® (112) support those of Vaughn and colleagues (212) in indicating no demonstrable alteration in endothelial cell function with acetylcholine instillations. Nor were they able to demonstrate any of the cell events documented by Leibowitz and collaborators in their studies of eyes infused with air postmortem. When they placed phenylephrine into the anterior chamber during cataract extraction there was a striking difference in endothelial cell density, not only before and after the operation, but also compared with the density when phenylephrine is not used. Phenylephrine appeared to have an adverse effect regardless of what agent had been used to reconstitute the anterior chamber, but this effect appeared to be augmented when air was the reconstituent. The air/phenylephrine combination is the only one in which they saw a continuing cell loss in 20 days. They did see some loss of cells up to 6 days when air alone was used, and there may be some additive effect of the short-term effects of air and the more long-lasting effects of epinephrine when used together.

Effect of Reconstituents Instilled During Intracapsular Cataract Extraction on Corneal Endothelium

Corneal endothelial cell viability is a crucial factor in the maintenance of corneal clarity. With the advent of biomicroscopic techniques of quantitative and qualitative evaluation of the endothelial monolayer, we become more cognizant of the effects of manipulation on the endothelial cells. There are many factors that will affect the corneal endothelium, such as pH, osmolality, and electrolyte composition. With the infusion of replacement fluids into the anterior chamber during phacoemulsification procedures, intraocular lens insertion, and cataract extraction in general, a number of investigations have been done (48,137,177,212).

Rabbit eyes perfused with acetylcholine or carbachol produce endothelial swelling with carbachol but no permanent cell damage (212). Jay and Mac-Donald (83) demonstrated dose-related cytotoxic effects of pilocarpine and acetylcholine on cultured bovine endothelial cells and attributed them to extreme osmotic shock. Cohen et al. (33) and Edelhauser et al. (47) described cytotoxic changes in the corneal endothelium due to phenylephrine use topically.

Liebowitz and his associates (117) showed that the replacement of aqueous by air produced morphologic endothelial changes that they felt represented local cell destruction, whereas Norn (161) concluded that air seemed to protect the corneal endothelium. Norn's work has been confirmed by Harris and Hassard (72).

Recently, Lang and Hassard (112) evaluated the effects on corneal endothelium of commonly used intraocular reconstituents in the living human eye. They evaluated 77 patients in the hospital for cataract extraction. Their studies have demonstrated that commonly used solutions introduced intraocularly into the anterior chamber have demonstrated deleterious effects on the corneal endothelium in some cases. They could not demonstrate any endothelial cell loss when Miochol® was used to reconstitute the anterior chamber. Air, they found, had a deleterious but short-lived effect on endothelial cells. Their results were similar to those previously reported by Vaughn and his colleagues (212). They were not able to demonstrate any cell events documented by Leibowitz and collaborators, but they were able to demonstrate reduction in endothelial cell density after the use of phenylephrine. The combination of air plus phenylephrine had the most damaging effect. They did not consider the preservative in the phenylephrine in their studies, which may have been part of the adverse effect on the cells.

It is well known that endothelial cell counts decrease following uncomplicated cataract surgery. It could be related to corneal bending, surgical manipulation with endothelial contact, or the use of intraocular irrigating solutions. Fortunately, however, the cornea can remain clear in spite of significant reductions in endothelial cell count. The actual minimal number of central endothelial cells required to maintain corneal dehydration is not known. The drugs available for controlling resulting corneal edema when the endothelial function is inadequate are not very satisfactory. Drugs are used to lower intraocular pressure, to reduce inflammation, and to dehydrate the cornea, and soft contact lenses may also be helpful.

Tranexamic acid has been used in the treatment of hyphema, for certain types of corneal edema, and in patients with Fuchs endothelial dystrophy for long periods of time. Bramsen (23) feels that tranexamic acid can reduce corneal edema after surgery and have a favorable influence on traumatic hyphemas. Although this has not been confirmed by other investigators, it must still be considered a possibility. Tranexamic acid has been used systemically for hereditary angioneurotic edema (Quincke's edema), but when given to dogs in large doses, two investigations have demonstrated irreversible retinal atrophy, located both centrally and peripherally. In unpublished observations by Tonelli (206,207), however, 14 patients with hereditary angioneurotic edema treated for an average period of 6 years, ranging from 15 months to 8 years, with tranexamic acid were found by careful ophthalmologic study not to reveal any possible toxic damage caused by the treatment.

INTRAOCULAR PRESSURE AND NONSTEROIDAL DRUGS

Rich (178) reported that 25 ml indomethacin administered orally for six doses during 48 hr preceding cataract surgery significantly reduced the ocular pressure rise at 6 hr postoperatively as compared to the pressure rise of 20 patients in the control (no indomethacin) treated group. Although there are data showing that prostaglandins administered to the experimental animal eye can produce a rise in intraocular pressure associated with an alteration in the blood aqueous barrier, there is also evidence that in the eyes of monkeys, topical prostaglandins may lower intraocular pressure (19).

There are also studies that have demonstrated that the topical instillation of flurbiprofen four times a day for 30 days not only did not cause a rise in pressure but was followed by a few millimeters drop in intraocular pressure. This may or may not be a significant fall, however; most of the data that are available would suggest that topical indomethacin or topical flurbiprofen did not produce a rise in intraocular pressure in normal human eyes, nor has a rise in intraocular pressure been associated with the topical or systemic use of indomethacin in those cases that have been treated prophylactically or therapeutically for aphakic central macular edema (Leopold et al., *unpublished data*).

CYSTOID MACULAR EDEMA

It is well established that aphakic cystoid macular edema (ACME) (77) may occur in up to 60% or 70% of patients who have undergone intracapsular lens extraction (142,148). The evaluation of therapeutic intervention is difficult, since mild ACME may not affect vision, fluctuation in the severity of the ACME occurs, and the majority of patients with this entity show improvement or resolution of the edema without therapy (61,76,79). As pointed out by Jampol (82), carefully planned prospective randomized controlled clinical trials are necessary to determine the efficacy of agents like topical periocular, systemic corticosteroids, prostaglandin synthesis inhibitors, or others.

In evaluating previous and future studies it is also important to distinguish between prophylaxis of cystoid macular edema and the therapy of it once it is well established. It is unlikely that patients with advanced ACME and foveal damage will regain better visual acuity, even if a therapeutic agent reduces the amount of macular edema. Thus, if prophylaxis is not possible, early detection and treatment are desirable.

It has been suggested that inflammation could be responsible for ACME. The inflammation itself may be related to the release of several mediators— histamine, acetylcholine, small peptides such as substance P, bradykinin, and serotonin, as well as prostaglandins. Considerable attention has been directed to prostaglandins as possible mediators of the inflammation in the eye (190).

It has been well established that a wide variety of traumatic stimuli, such as anterior chamber paracentesis, laser irradiation of the iris, and mechanical stroking of the iris can produce prostaglandins in the anterior chamber (45). Prostaglandins have been shown to be increased in a number of other conditions, such as endotoxin-induced uveitis in the animal eye and in patients with uveitis, particularly Behçet's disease and glaucomatocyclitic crisis (45,46,133,207).

In 1974, Tennant proposed that prostaglandins produced by the iris during cataract surgery were causative in ACME. In 1981, following a review of the literature, Katz (91) concluded that sufficient controlled studies using consistent doses and modes of administration of indomethacin, with schedules that initiated therapy before surgery and maintained it for an adequate postoperative period, had not been conducted. He also concluded that without such studies it is difficult to determine if there was consistent benefit in the use of indomethacin to prevent ACME maintenance.

In 1982, Jampol (82) concluded that most prior studies suggest that topical prostaglandin synthesis inhibitors and perhaps systemic inhibitors are effective in the prophylaxis of ACME. In none of the studies to date, however, has a sustained significant effect of ACME or visual acuity been demonstrated.

Pecora (168) described one case of ACME that appeared to respond to oral ibuprofen 400 mg four times a day. Yannuzzi et al. (224) found that systemic indomethacin had no effect on patients with well-established ACME, that is, longer than 4 months duration.

Prophylactic studies by Klein, Katzin and Yannuzzi (97) found that systemic indomethacin 25 ml four times a day given to patients undergoing cataract extraction appeared to decrease the incidence of ACME 4 to 6 weeks after cataract extraction. However, the side effects of systemic indomethacin were significant and resulted in discontinuation of the medication in many patients. Sholiton et al. (193) were unable to demonstrate an effect of 25 ml indomethacin three times a day, beginning 1 day before surgery and continuing for 3 weeks after surgery, on the incidence of ACME in patients undergoing intracapsular cataract extraction. Shammas and Milkie (191) found no apparent effect of aspirin prophylaxis on the incidence of ACME in patients undergoing lens extraction and intraocular lens insertion.

Topical Prostaglandin Synthesis Inhibitors

Burnett et al. (26) have performed a small double-masked randomized trial of topical 1% fenoprofen for treatment of established ACME. No statistically significant effects of fenoprofen were demonstrable; however, several patients did show improvement while on fenoprofen therapy with recurrences following discontinuation of therapy.

Several investigators have used topical indomethacin for the prophylaxis of ACME. Miyake (148), for example, showed that 1% indomethacin given two to three times daily beginning the day before surgery and continuing to the 40th day after surgery resulted in a decrease in ACME in cases of intracapsular cataract surgery from 77% in control cases to 33% in the indomethacin-treated eye. More important, perhaps, is the fact that Miyake found that topical indomethacin given to one-eyed patients undergoing bilateral intracapsular cataract extraction could significantly decrease the occurrence of ACME in the treated eye (148,149).

Miyake demonstrated that analysis of aqueous humor in cataract patients during the postoperative period showed elevated levels of prostaglandin E_2 and $E_{2\alpha}$ and that these levels could be diminished by prior topical indomethacin therapy (151). In a randomized trial, Miyake determined the effects of 1%

indomethacin drops given from 1 day before surgery to 2 weeks post-cataract surgery on long-term incidence of ACME (150).

Miyake found a decreased incidence of edema 1 to 2 months after surgery in indomethacin-treated eyes and 4 to 7 months after surgery, but not 1 to 1.5 years after surgery. Only during the early 1 to 2 months postoperative periods was a difference in visual acuity noted between the control and indomethacin-treated eyes. Yannuzzi (225) also reported a series of studies in the role of topical indomethacin in the prophylaxis of ACME.

A 1% aqueous suspension of indomethacin was administered to patients undergoing intracapsular lens extraction, and the incidence of ACME in the indomethacin-treated group was significantly less than in the control group 5 weeks after cataract surgery, 19% versus 36%; however, only a small number of patients were followed beyond 5 weeks. There was no significant difference between the groups 10 weeks after surgery. No adverse effects from the drug were reported. It is apparent that although topical indomethacin was effective in the immediate postoperative period, decreasing angiographically proved ACME, no sustained effect on ACME or its visual acuity was confirmed.

In a group of patients undergoing extracapsular lens extraction with posterior lens insertion, Kraff et al. (102) reported the effect of topical indomethacin 1% on incidence of ACME. In this randomized trial, indomethacin reduced the angiographic incidence of ACME from 18.5% to 9.6%. No effect on vision was apparent (102).

Value of Prophylaxis in CME

The data available suggest that prophylactic therapy with either topical indomethacin 1% or systemic indomethacin may reduce the angiographic incidence of ACME by as much as 50%. This prophylactic treatment does not appear to have any eventual influence on visual acuity, but it does reduce the incidence and severity of edema during the period of therapy. Side effects of systemic medication can be significant and may require cessation of medication in many patients. It would appear, therefore, that the greatest promise may reside in the topical form of therapy.

Further therapeutic trials are clearly necessary in the attempt to determine the real advantages or justification for the use of indomethacin or other cyclooxygenase inhibitors in ACME. Therapy should be started at least 24 hr prior to surgery and continued for some time after the surgery has been completed. The optimum duration of postoperative treatment has not been determined. Many other possibilities for therapy exist. Only a few of the other cyclooxygenase inhibitors have been tried, such as fenoprofen and ibuprofen, and studies are currently underway with flurbiprofen. It may be that one of these will produce more significant and favorable results than have been seen with indomethacin. Certainly further investigations of the use of topical corticosteroids, as well as other anti-inflammatory agents (such as H_1 and H_2 blockers) and antineuropeptides (such as anti-substance P) can also be studied.

Most of the data available would suggest that there is little effect on preexisting ACME with the use of systemic or topical indomethacin; however, since it has been recognized that most, if not all, patients with ACME have signs of ocular inflammation and that aphakic patients with inflamed eyes (that is, after surgical complications such as iris prolapse or vitreous loss) have a higher incidence of ACME than those who have eyes without inflammation, efforts to treat ACME using anti-inflammatory agents, including corticosteroids, prostaglandin synthetase, or cyclooxygenase inhibitors, can be tried. Usually the response to anti-inflammatory therapy is reasonably prompt, within a few days or a week. Prolonged therapy for 3 or 4 weeks or longer usually does not bring about improvement where it did not occur in an earlier interval.

Almost all of the nonsteroidal anti-inflammatory drugs can be made into a form for periocular injection, but there are no data concerning their value in this condition. There are very few penetration data following subconjunctival administration of any of these agents. Almost all of these drugs have been designed for oral use, but one can make up solutions of drugs, such as flurbiprofen, that theoretically could be given subconjunctivally. There has been no reported experience with this approach, and it cannot be recommended except for investigation.

Shammas and Milkie (191) found no apparent effect of aspirin prophylaxis on the incidence of ACME in patients undergoing lens extraction and intraocular lens insertion. It may be that other agents would succeed where aspirin has failed. Aspirin in sufficiently large doses can block experimentally induced breakdown of the blood-aqueous barrier in the anterior segment and might possibly do so in the posterior segment with large enough doses. At the present time there are insufficient data in the literature to suggest that aspirin would not do as well as other agents. Indomethacin has been used in more trials. Other agents might be more useful than indomethacin; however, all of this will depend on future well-controlled studies.

Attempts to halt an established ACME process have not been very successful. It is quite possible, however, that treatment would prevent fresh formation of prostaglandins, while metabolic breakdown and the active transfer out of the eye of prostaglandins that already exist would take place. In time, the amount of prostaglandins in the eye might be reduced considerably, but of course other mediators or agents present would not be affected. Perhaps one would be justified in trying these agents for a few weeks before assuming that they would be of no value.

In 1967 and 1968 a series of studies with topically administered indomethacin in a variety of external ocular inflammatory disorders were tried (for review see refs. 91 and 120). Aqueous suspensions of 0.25%, 0.5%, and 1% indomethacin were administered into the conjunctival sac of 107 patients in five studies in which indomethacin was compared with a placebo. Each strength was given four times daily for up to 76 days. In the variety of conditions treated, no significant suppression of established inflammatory disorders occurred. Repeated measurements of intraocular pressure in 11 patients did not demonstrate significant changes in intraocular pressure. Topical flurbiprofen 0.03% did not alter intraocular pressure in known high corticosteroid responders, nor did it block corticosteroid-induced ocular hypertension (63).

There is some evidence in ophthalmology, based solely on clinical criteria, that the anti-inflammatory effect of indomethacin is significant enough to permit a reduction of the amount of steroids required (18).

Although the classical aspirin-like drugs, salicylates, indomethacin, etc., block prostaglandin biosynthesis, they do not inhibit the formation of the major chemotactic metabolite of arachidonic acid, namely, HETE. They may even increase concentration of this compound in tissues. It is not clear whether treatment with these drugs enhances the migration of leukocytes in clinical situations. Clearly, a drug that blocks the formation of HETE by the lipoxygenases, in addition to prostaglandin formation by the cyclooxygenases may have advantages. Leukocytic infiltration, a consequence of the lipoxygenase metabolite LTB_4, is perhaps responsible for much of the damage done in many ocular inflammations.

Ingestion of aspirin by normal individuals causes a definite prolongation of bleeding time. It can occur with a dose as small as 0.3 g. A dose of 0.65 g aspirin approximately doubles the mean bleeding time of normal persons for a period of 4 to 7 days. This effect is probably due to acetylation of platelet cyclooxygenase. Aspirin therapy should be stopped for at least 1 week prior to surgery and certainly should be avoided in patients with severe hepatic damage, hypoprothrombinemia, macroglobulinemia, and vitamin K deficiency in disorders of connective tissue (e.g., amyloidosis, scurvy), disorders of platelet adhesion (e.g., uremia, Von Willebrandt's disease), and disorders of platelet interaction and platelet release. In such patients, inhibition of platelet hemostasis can result in hemorrhage.

There is no carefully controlled study that would give the specifics concerning vitreous hemorrhage and aspirin, but certainly the general considerations would favor avoidance of aspirin intake for a reasonable period prior to any planned or elective surgery. It has been suggested that aspirin should not be used as an analgesic in patients who have hyphemas, because of the danger of rebleeding (39). This would suggest that where there may be a threat of hemorrhage or rebleeding, one probably should use agents such as Tylenol®, Demerol®, or codeine, which may be more suitable analgesics, in order to reduce the possibilities of rebleeding.

Studies that have been done with topical indomethacin have employed 1% indomethacin given two or three times daily beginning the day before surgery and continuing for 6 or more weeks after surgery. Other studies have used 1% indomethacin given from 1 day before surgery to 2 weeks after cataract surgery. Penetration studies of topical indomethacin in phakic and aphakic rabbit eyes by Green, Bowman, Luxenberg and Friberg (67) suggest that the indomethacin concentrations in the retina and choroid are far less than those found to be therapeutically effective in the anterior segment.

They actually found that the highest retina and choroidal concentrations of indomethacin were about 100 times less than those required to induce a 50% inhibition of prostaglandin formation. These data support the notion that topically applied indomethacin affects anterior segment inflammation and indicates that the drug may influence cystoid macular edema by actions at the blood-aqueous barrier rather than at the posterior pole. This is especially true of the retina, where concentrations of indomethacin needed to inhibit biotransformation of arachidonic acid are at least three times greater than that needed in the anterior uvea (16).

Multiple-drop application every 12 hr for 3 days does not result in tissue buildup of drug. This indicates that each topical drug application might be considered separately at the frequency used and suggests that a regimen of 1 drop every 2 or 3 hr might be satisfactory to maintain an adequate anterior segment concentration of more than 4 μg/ml. Based on the pharmacokinetic data found in the studies of Green et al. (67) this represents an increased frequency of drop administration compared with currently recommended regimens of medication two to four times per day.

The regimen for flurbiprofen 0.03% based on the penetration studies of Anderson et al. (3) would also show that flurbiprofen penetrates well, but it should be applied also at least every 2 to 3 hr, as it is metabolized rapidly.

REFERENCES

1. Allen, B. R. (1983): Benoxaprofen and the skin. *Br. J. Dermatol.,* 109:361–364.
2. Anderson, D. M., Morin, J. D., and Hunter, W. S. (1971): Rubeosis iridis. *Can. J. Ophthalmol.,* 6:183.
3. Anderson, J., Chen, C. C., Brasil-Vita, J., and Shackelton, M. (1982): Disposition of topical flurbiprofen in normal and aphakic rabbit eyes. *Arch. Ophthalmol.,* 100:642–645.
4. Anggard, E., and Samuelsson, B. (1964): Smooth muscle stimulating lipids in sheep iris. *Biochem. Pharmacol.,* 13:281.
5. Apestin, R. J., and Hughes, W. F. (1981): Lymphocyte-induced corneal neovascularization: A morphologic assessment. *Invest. Ophthalmol. Vis. Sci.,* 21:87.
6. Archer, D. B., and Gardiner, T. A. (1981): Electron microscopic features of experimental choroidal neovascularization. *Am. J. Ophthalmol.,* 91:433–457.
7. Ashton, N. (1957): Retinal vascularization in health and disease. *Am. J. Ophthalmol.,* 44:7.
8. Ashton, N. (1961): Neovascularization in ocular disease. *Trans. Ophthalmol. Soc. U. K.,* 81:145.
9. Ashton, N., and Cook, C. (1951): Effect of cortisone healing of corneal wounds. *Br. J. Ophthalmol.,* 35:708.
10. Ashton, N., and Cook, C. (1953): Mechanisms of corneal neovascularization. *Br. J. Ophthalmol.,* 37:193–209.
11. Ashton, N., Cook, C., and Langham, M. (1951): Effect of cortisone on vascularization and opacification of the cornea induced by Alloxan. *Br. J. Ophthalmol.,* 35:718.
12. BenEzra, D. (1978): Neovasculogenic ability of prostaglandins growth factors and synthetic chemoattractants. *Am. J. Ophthalmol.,* 86:455–462.
13. Berman, W., Ausprunk, D., Rose, J., Langer, R., et al. (1981): Plasminogen activator causes neovascularization of the cornea. *Proc. Int. Soc. Eye Res.,* 1:75.

14. Bessey, O. A., and Wolbach, S. B. (1939): Vascularization of cornea of rat in riboflavin deficiency, with note on corneal vascularization in vitamin A deficiency. *J. Exp. Med.,* 69:1–12.
15. Deleted in proof.
16. Bhattacherjee, T., and Eakins, K. (1974): Inhibition of the prostaglandin synthetase systems in ocular tissue by indomethacin. *Br. J. Pharmacol.,* 50:227–230.
17. Bhattacherjee, P., Eakins, K. E., and Hammond, B. (1981): Chemotactic activity of arachidonic acid lipoxygenase products in the rabbit eye. *Br. J. Pharmacol.,* 73:254P–255P.
18. Bikoff, G., Cherbonnel, B., and Kremer, M. (1981): Prostaglandin assay in human aqueous humor after intraocular implantation: Effects of indomethacin. *J. Fr. Ophtalmol.,* 4:593–595.
19. Bito, L. Z., Danga, A., Blanco, J., and Camras, C. B. (1983): Long-term maintenance of reduced intraocular pressure by daily and twice daily topical application of prostaglandins to cat or rhesus monkey eyes. *Invest. Ophthalmol. Vis. Sci.,* 24:312.
20. Blackwell, G. J., Carnuccio, R., DiRosa, M., Flower, R. J., Parente, L., and Bersico, P. (1980): Macrocortin, a polypeptide causing the anti-phospholipase activity of glucocorticoids. *Nature,* 287:147–149.
21. Boot, J. R., Sweatman, J. F., Cox, B. A., Stone, K., and Dolfin, W. (1982): The anti-allergic effect of benoxaprofen, a lipooxygenase inhibitor. *National Archives of Allergy and Applied Immunology,* 67:340.
22. Boyd, T. A. S., and Campbell, F. W. (1955): Influence of ascorbic acid and healing of corneal ulcers in man. *Br. Med. J.,* 2:1145.
23. Bramsen, S. (1978): Marrow lymphocyte production during chronic hydrocortisone administration. *J. Reticuloendothel. Soc.,* 23:111–118.
24. Burde, R. M., and Waltman, S. R. (1972): Topical corticosteroids after cataract surgery. *Ann. Ophthalmol.,* 4:290.
25. Burke, J. A., Levi, R., Guo, Z. G., and Corey, E. (1980): Leukotriene C-4, D-4, and E-4: Effect on human and guinea pig cardiac preparations in vitro. *J. Pharmacol. Exp. Ther.,* 22:230.
26. Burnett, J., Tessler, H., Isenberg, S., and Tso, M. O. M. (1983): Double-masked trial of fenoprofen sodium: Treatment of chronic aphakic cystoid macular edema. *Ophthalmic Surg.,* 14:150–152.
27. Campbell, D. G., and Michaelson, I. C. (1949): Blood vessel formation in the cornea. *Br. J. Ophthalmol.,* 33:248–255.
28. Cashin, C. H., Dawson, W., and Kitchen, E. A. (1977): The pharmacology of benoxaprofen. *J. Pharm. Pharmacol.,* 29:330.
29. Claman, H. N. (1975): How corticosteroids work. *J. Allergy Clin. Immunol.,* 55:145–151.
30. Cogan, D. G. (1948): Vascularization of the cornea, its experimental induction by small lesions and new theory of its pathogenesis. *Trans. Am. Ophthalmol. Soc.,* 46:457.
31. Cogan, D. G. (1949): Vascularization of cornea: Its experimental induction by small lesions and new theory of its pathogenesis. *Arch. Ophthalmol.,* 41:406–416.
32. Cohen, S., Pick, E., Oppenheim, J. J. (eds.). (1979): *Biology of the Lymphokines,* Academic Press, New York.
33. Cohen, K. L., Van Horn, D. L., Edelhauser, H. F., and Schultz, R. O. (1979): The effect of phenylephrine on normal and regenerated endothelial cells in cat cornea. *Invest. Ophthalmol. Vis. Sci.,* 18:242.
34. Conn, H., Berman, M., Kenyon, K., Langer, R., and Gage, J. (1980): Stromal vascularization prevents corneal ulceration. *Invest. Ophthalmol. Vis. Sci.,* 19:362.
35. Conquet, G., Plazonnet, B., and Le Douarec, J. C. (1975): Arachidonic acid induced elevation of intraocular pressure and anti-inflammatory agents. *Invest. Ophthalmol. Vis. Sci.,* 14:772–775.
36. Cook, C., and McDonald, R. K. (1951): Effect of cortisone on the permeability of the blood-aqueous barrier to fluorescein. *Br. J. Ophthalmol.,* 35:730.
37. Cooper, C. A., Bergamini, M. V. W., and Leopold, I. H. (1980): Use of flurbiprofen to inhibit corneal neovascularization. *Arch. Ophthalmol.,* 98:1102.
38. Corboy, J. M. (1976): Corticosteroid therapy for the reduction of postoperative inflammation after cataract extraction. *Am. J. Ophthalmol.,* 82:923.
39. Crawford, J. S. (1977): The effect of aspirin on rebleeding of traumatic hyphema. *Trans. Am. Ophthalmol. Soc.,* 74:357–362.

40. Crook, D., Collins, A. J., and Rose, A. J. (1976): A comparison of the effects of flurbiprofen on prostaglandin synthetase from human rheumatoid synovium and enzymatically active animal tissues. *J. Pharm. Pharmacol.,* 28:535.

41. Davies, P., and Allison, A. C. (1970): The release of hydrolytic enzyme from phagocytic and other cells participating in acute and chronic inflammation. In: *Inflammation,* 267–294. Springer-Verlag, Berlin.

42. Dawson, W., Boot, J. R., Harvey, Y., and Walker, J. R. (1982): The pharmacology of benoxaprofen with particular reference to effects on lipooxygenase products formation. *Eur. J. Rheumatol. Inflamm.,* 5:61.

43. Deutsch, D. A., and Hughes, W. F. (1979): Suppressive effects of indomethacin on thermally induced neovascularization of rabbit corneas. *Am. J. Ophthalmol.,* 87:536.

44. Douglas, W. W. (1980): Autacoids. In: *The Pharmacological Basis of Therapeutics,* edited by L. S. Goodman and A. G. Gilman, pp. 608–609. Macmillan, New York.

45. Eakins, K. E. (1977): Prostaglandin and non-prostaglandin mediated breakdown of the blood-aqueous barrier. *Exp. Eye Res.,* 25(Suppl):483–498.

46. Eakins, K. E., Whitelocke, R. A. F., Bennett, A., and Martenet, A. C. (1972): Prostaglandin-like activity in ocular inflammation. *Br. Med. J.,* 3:452–453.

47. Edelhauser, H. F., Hine, J. E., Pederson, H., Van Horn, D. S., and Schultz, R. O. (1979): Effect of phenylephrine on the cornea. *Arch. Ophthalmol.,* 97:937.

48. Edelhauser, H. F., Van Horn, D. L., Schultz, R. O., and Hyndiuk, R. A. (1976): Comparative toxicity of intraocular irrigating solutions on the corneal endothelium. *Am. J. Ophthalmol.,* 81:473.

49. Ehinger, D. A., Morris, A. R., Piper, P. J., and Sirois, P. (1978): The release of prostaglandins and thromboxanes from guinea pig lung by slow reacting substance of anaphylaxis inhibition. *Br. J. Pharmacol.,* 64:211.

50. Eliason, J. A. (1978): Leukocytes in experimental corneal vascularization. *Invest. Ophthalmol. Vis. Sci.,* 17:1087–1095.

51. Eliason, J. A. (1979): Stimulation of vascular endothelium by an epithelial homogenate. *Invest. Ophthalmol. Vis. Sci.,* 18(Suppl):75.

52. Epstein, R. J., and Hughes, W. F. (1981): Lymphocyte-induced corneal neovascularization. A morphologic assessment. *Invest. Ophthalmol. Vis. Sci.,* 21:87.

53. Fahey, J. E., Guyre, P. M., and Munck, A. (1981): Mechanisms of anti-inflammatory actions of corticosteroids. In: *Advances in Inflammation Research,* vol. 2, edited by G. Weissman, p. 21. Raven Press, New York.

54. Faucia, A. F. (1979): Mechanisms of the immunosuppressive and anti-inflammatory effects of glucocorticoids. *J. Immunopharmacol.,* 1:25.

55. Finkelstein, D., Clarkson, J., Dibbie, K., Hillis, A., Kimball, A., Orth, D., and Tremp, C. (1982): A branched vein occlusion study group—retinal neovascularization outside with involved segment. *Ophthalmology,* 89:1357–1361.

56. Flower, R. J., and Blackwell, G. J. (1979): An anti-inflammatory steroid-induced biosynthesis of a phospholipase A_2 inhibitor which prevents prostaglandin generation. *Nature,* 278:456–459.

57. Ford-Hutchinson, A. W., Walker, J. R., Connor, N. S., Oliver, A. M., and Smith, M. J. N. (1977): Separate anti-inflammatory effects of indomethacin, flurbiprofen and benoxaprofen. *J. Pharm. Pharmacol.,* 29:372.

58. Fraunfelder, F. T., editor (1976): *Drug-Induced Ocular Side Effects and Drug Interactions.* Lea and Febiger, Philadelphia.

59. Fromer, C. H., and Klintworth, G. K. (1975): Evaluation of the role of leukocytes in the pathogenesis of experimentally-induced corneal vascularization. Studies on the effect of leukocyte elimination on corneal vascularization. *Am. J. Pathol.,* 81:531.

60. Gartner, S., and Henkind, P. (1978): Neovascularization of the iris. *Surv. Ophthalmol.,* 22:291–312.

61. Gass, J. B. M., and Northon, E. W. D. (1969): A follow-up study of cystoid macular edema following cataract extractions. *Trans. Am. Acad. Ophthalmol. Otolaryngol.,* 73:665–682.

62. Gasset, A. R., and Katzen, B. (1975): Antiviral drugs in wound healing. *Invest. Ophthalmol. Vis. Sci.,* 14:628.

63. Gieser, D. K., Hodapp, E., Goldbery, I., Kass, M., and Becker, B. (1981): Flurbiprofen and intraocular pressure. *Ann. Ophthalmol.,* 13:831–833.

64. Gospodarowicz, B., Brown, K. D., Birdwell, D. R., and Zetter, B. R. (1978): Control of proliferation of human vascular endothelial cells: Characterization of the response of human umbilical vein endothelial cells to fibroblast growth factor, epidermal growth factor. *J. Cell. Biol.,* 77:774.

65. Granelli-Piperno, A., Vassalli, J. D., and Reich, E. (1977): Secretion of plasminogen activator by human polymorphonuclear leukocytes modulation by glucocorticoids and other effectors. *J. Exp. Med.,* 146:1693–1706.

66. Green, K., Bowman, K., Luxenberg, M. N., and Friberg, T. R. (1983): Penetration of topical indomethacin into phakic and aphakic eyes. *Arch. Ophthalmol.,* 2:284–288.

67. Green, K., Bowman, K., Luxenberg, M. N., and Friberg, T. R. Penetration of topical indomethacin into phakic and aphakic rabbit eyes. *Arch. Ophthalmol.,* 101:384–388.

68. Gryglewski, R. J. (1976): Steroid hormones, anti-inflammatory steroids and prostaglandins. *Pharmacol. Res. Commun.,* 8:337–349.

68a. Gryglewski, R. J., Panzuenko, B., Korbut, R., Grodyinsk, A. L., and Ocetkiewicz, A. (1975): Corticosteroids inhibit prostaglandin release from perfused mesenteric blood vessels of rabbits and perfused lungs of sensitized guinea pigs. *Prostaglandins,* 10:343–355.

69. Hamberg, M. (1976): On the formation of thromboxane B and 12-L-hydroxy-5,8,10,14-eicosatetraneoic acid in tissues from the guinea pig. *Biochim. Biophys. Acta,* 431:651.

70. Hamburger, G. H., Harlamps, M. M., Hawley, T. J., and Faulk, M. M. (1979): Sjögren's syndrome; A defect in the reticuloendothelial system Fc receptor specific clearance. *Ann. Intern. Med.,* 91:534–538.

71. Hanna, C., and Sharp, J. D. (1972): Ocular absorption of indomethacin by the rabbit. *Arch. Ophthalmol.,* 88:196–198.

72. Harris, R. A., and Hassard, D. T. R. (1978): Corneal effects of intraocular air. *Can. J. Ophthalmol.,* 13:262.

73. Hench, P. S., Kendall, E. C., Slocumb, C. H., and Polley, H. S. (1949): Effect of hormone of adrenal cortex 17-hydroxy-11-d-hydro corticosterone, compound E, and of pituitary adrenocorticotropic hormone on rheumatoid arthritis. Preliminary Report. *Mayo Clin. Proc.,* 24:181–197.

74. Henkind, P. (1978): Ocular neovascularization. *Am. J. Ophthalmol.,* 85:287–301.

75. Higgs, G. A., Flower, R. J., and Vane, J. R. (1979): A new approach to anti-inflammatory drugs. *Biochem. Pharmacol.,* 28:1959.

76. Hitchings, R. A. (1977): Aphakic macular edema: A two-year follow-up study. *Br. J. Ophthalmol.,* 61:628–630.

77. Irvine, A. R. (1976): Cystoid maculopathy. *Surv. Ophthalmol.,* 21:1–17.

78. Irvine, S. R., and Irvine, M. D. (1951): The effect of cortisone on the primary and secondary aqueous and on corneal vascularization in rabbits. *Bulletin of Johns Hopkins Hospital,* 89:288.

79. Jacobson, D. R., and Dellaport, A. (1974): A natural history of cystoid macular edema after cataract extraction. *Am. J. Ophthalmol.,* 77:445–447.

80. Jaffe, D., Podos, S. M., and Becker, B. (1973): Indomethacin blocks arachidonic acid associated elevations of aqueous humor prostaglandins E$_1$. *Invest. Ophthalmol. Vis. Sci.,* 12:621–622.

81. Jaffe, N. S. (1981): *Cataract Surgery and Its Complications,* 3rd ed., pp. 357–373. C. V. Mosby, St. Louis.

82. Jampol, L. M. (1982): Pharmacologic therapy in aphakic cystoid macular edema: A review. *Ophthalmology,* 89:891–897.

83. Jay, J. L., and Macdonald, M. (1978): Effects of intraocular miotics on cultured bovine corneal endothelium. *Br. J. Ophthalmol.,* 62:815.

84. Johnson, L. V., and Eckardt, R. E. (1940): Rosacea keratitis and conditions with vascularization of cornea treated with riboflavin. *Arch. Ophthalmol.,* 23:899–907.

85. Jones, I. S., and Meyer, K. (1950): Inhibition of vascularization of the rabbit cornea by local application of cortisone. *Proc. Soc. Exp. Biol. Med.,* 74:102.

86. Jones, R. G., and Stiles, J. S. (1963): The penetration of cortisol into normal and pathologic rabbit eyes. *Am. J. Ophthalmol.,* 56:84–90.

87. Julianelle, L. A., Morris, M. L., and Harrison, R. W. (1963): Experimental study of corneal vascularization. *Am. J. Ophthalmol.,* 16:962.

88. Kantrowitz, S., Robinson, D. R., McGuire, M. D., and Levine, L. (1975): Cortisone inhibits prostaglandin production by rheumatoid synovia. *Nature,* 258:738–739.

89. Kaplan, A. P., Kaye, A. B., and Austen, K. S. (1972): A pre-albumin activator of pre-kallikerin appearance of chemotactic activity for human neutrophiles by the conversion of human pre-kallikerin to kallikerin. *J. Exp. Med.,* 135:81–97.

90. Katamoya, H., and Kawada, A. (1981): Exacerbation of psoriasis induced by indomethacin. *J. Dermatol.,* 8:323.

91. Katz, I. M. (1981): Indomethacin. *Ophthalmology,* 88:455–458.

92. Kaye, G. E., Mishima, S., Cole, J. D. et al. (1968): Studies in the cornea VII: Effects of perfusion with a calcium-free medium on the corneal endothelium. *Invest. Ophthalmol. Vis. Sci.,* 7:53.

93. Keller, H. U., and Sorkin, E. (1957): On the chemotactic effect of bacteria. *Int. Arch. Allergy Appl. Immunol.,* 31:505–517.

94. Kenyon, K. R. (1983): Morphology and pathologic responses of cornea to disease. In: *The Cornea, Scientific Foundations in Clinical Practice,* edited by G. Smolin and R. Thoft, pp. 43–75. Little Brown & Company, Boston, Toronto.

95. Kern, A. B. (1966): Indomethacin for psoriasis. *Arch. Dermatol.,* 96:239.

96. Kitazawa, Y. (1976): Increased intraocular pressure induced by corticosteroids. *Am. J. Ophthalmol.,* 82:492–495.

97. Klein, R. M., Katzin, H. M., and Yannuzzi, L. A. (1979): The effect of indomethacin pretreatment on aphakic cystoid macular edema. *Am. J. Ophthalmol.,* 84:487–489.

98. Klintworth, G. K. (1973): The hamster cheek pouch: An experimental model of corneal vascularization. *Am. J. Pathol.,* 73:691.

99. Klintworth, G. K. (1977): The contribution of morphology to our understanding of the pathogenesis of experimentally produced corneal vascularization. *Invest. Ophthalmol. Vis. Sci.,* 16:281–285.

100. Klintworth, G. K., and Berger, P. C. (1981): Neovascularization of the cornea. Current concepts of its pathogenesis. In: *Int. Ophthalmol. Clin.,*

101. Konzet, T. H., and Sturmer, E. (1960): Biological activity of synthetic polypeptides with bradykinin-like properties. *Br. J. Clin. Pharmacol.,* 15:544–551.

102. Kraff, M. C., Sanders, D. R., Jampol, L. M. et al. (1982): Prophylaxis of pseudophakic cystoid macular edema with topical indomethacin. *Ophthalmology,* 89:885–890.

103. Kramer, S. G. (1976): Retinal uptake of topical epinephrine in aphakia. In: *Symposium on Ocular Therapy,* vol. 9, edited by I. H. Leopold and R. P. Burns, chap. 7. John Wiley, New York.

104. Kramer, S. G. (1980): Epinephrine distribution after topical administration in phakic and aphakic eyes. *Trans. Am. Ophthalmol. Soc.,* 78:947–982.

105. Kuehl, F. A., and Egan, R. W. (1980): Prostaglandins, arachidonic acid and inflammation. *Science,* 210:978–984.

106. Kulkarni, P. S., Bhattacherjee, P., Eakins, K. E., and Srinivasan, B. B. (1981): Anti-inflammatory effects of betamethazone phosphate, dexamethasone phosphate and indomethacin on rabbit ocular inflammation induced by bovine serum albumin. *Curr. Eye Res.,* 1:43.

107. Kulkarni, P. S., and Srinivasan, B. D. (1980): Effects of topical and interperitoneal indomethacin and flurbiprofen on prostaglandin biosynthesis of rabbit anterior uvea. *Invest. Ophthalmol. Vis. Sci.,* 19(Arvo Suppl):17.

108. Kulkarni, P. S., and Srinivasan, B. B. (1983): Steroidal and non-steroidal anti-inflammatory drugs in ocular inflammation. *Ocular Inflam. Ther.,* 1:11–18.

109. Kupferman, A., and Leibowitz, H. M. (1974): Pharmacology of topically applied dexamethasone. *Trans. Am. Acad. Ophthalmol. Otolaryngol.,* 78:856.

110. Kupferman, A., and Leibowitz, H. M. (1975): Anti-inflammatory effectiveness of topically administered corticosteroids in the cornea without epithelium. *Invest. Ophthalmol. Vis. Sci.,* 14:252–255.

111. Kupferman, A., and Leibowitz, H. M. (1975): Therapeutic effectiveness of fluorometholone in inflammatory keratitis. *Arch. Ophthalmol.,* 93:1011–1014.

112. Lang, R. M., and Hassard, D. P. R. (1981): Effects on the corneal endothelium of anterior chamber reconstituents instilled during intracapsular cataract extraction. *Can. J. Ophthalmol.,* 16:70.

113. Larsen, G. L., and Henson, P. M. (1983): Mediators of inflammation. *Annu. Rev. Immunol.,* 1:335–359.

114. Lazar, E. R., and Horlington, M. (1975): Pilocarpine that was in the eyes of rabbits following topical application. *Exp. Eye Res.,* 21:281–287.
115. Lazar, M., Rosen, N., and Nemet, P. (1977): Miochol-induced transient cataract. *Ann. Ophthalmol.,* 9:1142.
116. Leibowitz, H. M., and Kupferman, A. (1974): Anti-inflammatory effectiveness in the cornea of topically administered prednisolone. *Invest. Ophthalmol. Vis. Sci.,* 13:757–763.
117. Leibowitz, H. M., Lang, R. A., and Sandstrom, M. (1974): Corneal endothelium; the effect of air in the anterior chamber. *Arch. Ophthalmol.,* 92:227.
118. Deleted in proof.
119. Leopold, I. H., Purnell, J. E., Cannon, E. J., Steinmetz, C. G., and McDonald, P. R. (1951): Local and systemic cortisone in ocular disease. *Am. J. Ophthalmol.,* 34:361–371.
120. Leopold, I. H., and Sacks, E. B. (1977): The medical approach to complications of intraocular surgery and trauma. In: *Eye Surgery,* edited by R. N. Fasanella, Charles C Thomas, Springfield, IL.
121. Levinson, R. A., Patterson, C. A., and Pfister, R. R. (1976): Ascorbic acid prevents corneal ulceration and perforation following experimental alkali burns. *Invest. Ophthalmol. Vis. Sci.,* 15:986.
122. Lewis, R. A., Austen, K. F., Drazen, J. M., Clark, D. A., Morfat, A., and Corey, E. J. (1980): Slow reacting substances of anaphylaxis: Identification of leukotrienes C-1 and D from human and rat sources. *Proc. Natl. Acad. Sci. U.S.A.,* 77:3710–3714.
123. Liebowitz, M., and Elliott, J. H. (1966): Chemotherapeutic immunosuppression of the corneal graft reaction. *Arch. Ophthalmol.,* 76:338.
124. Lister, A., and Greaves, D. P. (1951): Effect of cortisone upon the vascularization which follows corneal burns. *Br. J. Ophthalmol.,* 35:725.
125. Lutty, G. A., Liu, S. H., and Pendergast, R. H. (1984): Angiogenic lymphokines of activated T-cell origin. *Invest. Ophthalmol. Vis. Sci.,* 24:1595–1601.
126. MacDonald, M. (1978): Effects of intraocular miotics on cultured bovine corneal endothelium. *Br. J. Ophthalmol.,* 62:815.
127. MacGregor, R. R. (1977): Granulocyte adherence changes induced by hemodialysis, endotoxin, epinephrine and glucocorticoids. *Ann. Intern. Med.,* 86:35–39.
128. Malmon, K. L., Roklin, R. E., and Rosenkranz, R. P. (1981): Autocoids as modulators of the inflammatory and immune response. *Am. J. Med.,* 71:100–106.
129. Manganiello, V., and Vaughan, M. (1972): An effect of dexamethasone on adenosine 3′,5′-monophosphate content and adenosine 3′,5′-monophosphodiesterase activity of cultured hepatoma cells. *J. Clin. Invest.,* 51:2763–2767.
130. Margargall, E., Brown, G. C., Augsberger, J. J., and Donoso, L. A. (1982): Efficacy of panretinal photocoagulation in preventing neovascular glaucoma following ischemic central retinal vein obstruction. *Ophthalmology,* 89:780–784.
131. Marsen, D. R., Kanai, A., and Gasset, A. R. Beta irradiation inhibition of corneal healing, tensile strength and ultrastructural change. *Invest. Ophthalmol. Vis. Sci.,* 10:826.
132. Marsh, R. J., and Ford, S. M. (1980): Blood flow in the anterior segment of the eye. *Trans. Ophthalmol. Soc. U.K.,* 100:388–397.
133. Masuda, K., Izawa, Y., and Mishima, S. (1973): Prostaglandins in uveitis: A preliminary report. *Jpn. J. Ophthalmol.,* 17:166–170.
134. Masuda, K., Izawa, Y., and Mishima, S. (1976): Breakdown of the blood aqueous barrier and prostaglandin. Presented at the IX World Congress of the European Microcirculation Society.
135. Maustakallio, A., Kaufman, H., Johnston, G. et al. (1973): Corticosteroid efficacy in postoperative uveitis. *Ann. Ophthalmol.,* 5:519.
136. McCarey, B. E., Edelhauser, H. F., and Van Horn, D. L. (1973): Functional and structural changes in the corneal endothelium during in vitro perfusion. *Invest. Ophthalmol. Vis. Sci.,* 12:410.
137. McCarey, B. M., Polack, F. M., and Marshall, W. (1976): The phacoemulsification procedure. The effect of irrigating solutions on the corneal endothelium. *Invest. Ophthalmol. Vis. Sci.,* 15:449.
138. McCoy, C. A., and Leopold, I. H. (1960): Steroid treatment of Alloxan-induced corneal opacification and vascularization. *Am. J. Ophthalmol.,* 49:906–908.
139. McCracken, J. S., Berger, P. C., and Klintworth, G. K. (1979): Morphologic observations on experimental corneal vascularization in the rat. *Lab. Invest.,* 45:519–530.

140. Meacock, S. C. R., and Kitchen, E. A. Effects of the nonsteroidal anti-inflammatory drug, benoxaprofen, on leukocyte migration. *J. Pharm. Pharmacol.*, 31:366.
141. Menkin, V. (1941): Cellular injury in relation to proliferative and neoplastic response. *Cancer Res.*, 1:548–556.
142. Meredith, T. A., Kenyon, K. R., Singerman, L. J., and Fine, S. L. (1976): Perifovial vascular leakage in macular edema after intracapsular cataract extraction. *Br. J. Ophthalmol.*, 60:765–769.
143. Mester, V., Stein, H. J., and Koch, H. R. (1977): Experimental lens opacities in rabbits induced by intraocular application of acetylcholine. *Ophthalmic. Res.*, 9:99.
144. Meyer, K., and Chaffee, E. (1940): Mucopolysaccharide acid of cornea and its enzymatic hydrolysis. *Am. J. Ophthalmol.*, 23:1320.
145. Michel, R. G. (1976): Vitreal/retinal and anterior segment surgery through the pars planum, Part II. *Ann. Ophthalmol.*, 8:1497.
146. Michel, R. G., and Ryan, S. J., Jr. (1975): Results and complications of 100 consecutive cases of pars planum vitrectomy. *Am. J. Ophthalmol.*, 80:24.
147. Mindel, J. S., Tavitian, H. O., Smith, H., and Walker, E. C. (1980): Comparative ocular pressure elevation by medrysone, fluorometholone and dexamethasone phosphate. *Arch. Ophthalmol.*, 98:1577–1578.
148. Miyake, K. (1977): Prevention of cystoid macular edema after lens extraction by topical indomethacin: A preliminary report. *Albrecht von Graefes Arch. Klin. Exp. Ophthalmol.*, 203:81–88.
149. Miyake, K. (1978): Prevention of cystoid macular edema after lens extraction by topical indomethacin. II. A control study in bilateral extractions. *Jpn. J. Ophthalmol.*, 22:80–94.
150. Miyake, K., Sakamura, S., and Miura, H. (1980): Long-term follow-up study on prevention of aphakic cystoid macular edema by topical indomethacin. *Br. J. Ophthalmol.*, 64:324–328.
151. Miyake, K., Sugiyama, S., Norimatsu, I., and Ozawa, T. (1978): Prevention of cystoid macular edema after lens extraction by topical indomethacin: III. Radioimmunoassay measurement of prostaglandins in the aqueous during and after lens extraction procedures. *Albrecht von Graefes Arch. Klin. Exp. Ophthalmol.*, 209:83–88.
152. Mochizuki, M., Sawa, M., and Masuda, K. (1977): Topical indomethacin in intracapsular extraction of senile cataract. *J. Ophthalmol. (Tokyo)*, 21:215.
153. Moncada, S., Needleman, P., Bunting, S., and Vane, J. R. (1976): Prostaglandins endoperoxide and thromboxane generating system and their selective inhibition. *Prostaglandins*, 12:323.
154. Moncada, S., and Vane, J. R. (1978): Unstable metabolites of arachidonic acid and their role in hemostasis and thrombosis. *Br. Med. Bull.*, 34:129.
155. Moorehead, L. C. (1983): Effects of beta aminopropionitrile after posterior penetrating injury in the rabbit. *Am. J. Ophthalmol.*, 93:97–109.
156. Munck, A., and Brinck-Johnsen, R. (1968): Specific and non-specific physiochemical inter-actions of glucocorticoids and related steroids with rat thymus cells *in vitro. J. Biol. Chem.*, 243:5556–5565.
157. Munck, A., and Leung, K. (1977): Glucocorticoid receptors in the mechanisms of actions. In: *Receptors and Mechanisms of Actions of Steroid Hormones*, Part 2, edited by J. R. Pasqualini, pp. 311–397. Marcel Decker, New York.
158. Nathan, C. F., Murray, H. W., and Cohn, Z. A. (1980): The macrophage as an effector cell. *N. Engl. J. Med.*, 303:622–626.
159. Newcombe, D. S., Fahuy, J. D., and Ishikawa, Y. (1977): Hydrocortisone inhibition of bradykinin activation of human synovial fibreblasts. *Prostaglandins*, 13:235–244.
160. Newell, F. W., and Dixon, J. M. (1951): The effect of subconjunctival cortisone upon the immediate union of experimental corneal graft. *Am. J. Ophthalmol.*, 34:977.
161. Norn, M. S. (1975): Corneal thickness after cataract extraction with air in the anterior chamber. *Acta Ophthalmol. (Copenh.)*, 53:747.
162. Offret, G., and Chauvet, P. (1950): Contribution a l'étude du traitement de la vascularization de la cornée. *Arch. Ophthalmol.* (Paris) 10:344–366, 480–494, 593–612.
163. Okazaki, T., Ilea, V. S., Rosario, N. A., Reisman, R. E., Arbesman, C. E., Lee, J. L., and Middleton, E. Jr. (1977): Regulatory role of prostaglandin E in the allergic histamine release with observations on the responsiveness of basophil leukocytes and the effect of acetylsalicylic acid. *J. Allergy Clin. Immunol.*, 60:360–366.
164. Palmer, R. M. T., Stepney, R., Higgs, T. A., and Eakins, K. E. (1980): Chemotactic activity of arachidonic acid lipooxygenase products on leukocytes from different species. *Prostaglandins*, 20:411.

165. Palmerton, E. S. (1955): The effect of local cortisone on wound healing in rabbit corneas. *Am. J. Ophthalmol.,* 40:344.
166. Parker, C. W., Jachik, B. A., Huber, M. G., and Falkenhein, S. F. (1979): Characterization of the slow reacting substance as a family of thiolipids derived from arachidonic acid. *Biochem. Biophys. Res. Commun.,* 89:1186–1192.
167. Parrillo, J. E., and Faucia, A. S. (1979): Mechanisms of glucocorticoid action on human processes. *Annu. Rev. Pharmacol. Toxicol.,* 19:179–201.
168. Pecora, J. L. (1978): Ibuprofen in the treatment of central serous chorioretinopathy. *Ann. Ophthalmol.,* 10:1481–1483.
169. Pelus, L. M., and Strausser, H. R. (1977): Prostaglandins and the immune response. *Life Sci.,* 20:903.
170. Peyman, G. A., Huamonte, S. U., and Goldberg, M. F. (1976): 100 consecutive pars planum vitrectomies using the vitrophage. *Am. J. Ophthalmol.,* 81:263.
171. Pfister, R. R. et al. (1980): The efficacy of ascorbate after severe experimental alkali burns—depends upon the route of administration. *Invest. Ophthalmol. Vis. Sci.,* 19:1526.
172. Pfister, R. R., Nocolaro, M. L., and Patterson, C. A. (1981): Sodium citrate reduces the incidence of corneal ulceration and perforation in extreme alkal-burned eyes. Acetyl, ceptaine and ascorbate have no favorable effect. *Invest. Ophthalmol. Vis. Sci.,* 21:786.
173. Pfister, R. R., Patterson, C. A., and Hayso, S. A. (1978): Topical ascorbic decreases in the incidence of corneal ulceration after experimental alkali burns. *Invest. Ophthalmol. Vis. Sci.,* 17:1019.
174. Phelps, D. L., and Rosenbaum, A. L. (1979): Vitamin E in kitten oxygen induced retinopathy: Blockage of vitreal neovascularization. *Arch. Ophthalmol.,* 97:1522–1526.
175. Podos, S. M., Becker, B., and Kass, M. (1973): Prostaglandin inhibition and intraocular pressure. *Invest. Ophthalmol. Vis. Sci.,* 12:426–433.
176. Polack, F. M. (1965): The effect of ocular inflammation on corneal graft. *Am. J. Ophthalmol.,* 62:59.
177. Polack, F. M., and Sugar, A. (1976): The phacoemulsification procedure: Corneal endothelial changes. *Invest. Ophthalmol. Vis. Sci.,* 15:458.
178. Rich, W. J. (1977): Prevention of post-operative ocular hypertension by prostaglandin inhibitors. *Trans. Ophthalmol. Soc. U.K.,* 97:168–171.
179. Rocklan, R. E., Bentzen, K., and Greinder, D. (1980): Mediators of immunity, lymphokines and monokines. *Adv. Immunol.,* 29:55–136.
180. Rome, L. H., and Lands, W. E. M. (1975): Structural requirements for the time dependent inhibition of prostaglandin biosynthesis by anti-inflammatory drugs. *Proc. Natl. Acad. Sci. U.S.A.,* 72:4863–4865.
181. Rosario Hernandez, M., Wenk, E. J., Weinstein, B. I., Abumabar, P. et al. (1984): Glucocorticoid target cells in human outflow pathway: Autopsy and surgical specimens. *Invest. Ophthalmol. Vis. Sci.,* 24:1612–1616.
182. Rosen, N., and Lazar, M. (1978): The mechanism of the michol lens opacity. *Am. J. Ophthalmol.,* 86:57.
183. Samuelsson, B. (1980): Leukotrienes, a new group of biologically active compounds including SRS-A. *Trends Pharmacol.,* 5:227.
184. Samuelsson, B. (1981): Leukotrienes: Mediators of allergic reactions and inflammation. *Int. Arch. Allergy Appl. Immunol.,* 56(Suppl. 1):98.
185. Samuelsson, B., Borgeat, P., Hammarstom, S., and Murphy, R. C. (1980): Leukotrienes, a new group of biologically active compounds. In: *Advances in Prostaglandin and Thromboxane Research,* vol. 6, Raven Press, New York.
186. Sardo, J. J., Hammond, M. D., Stratford, C. A., and Pratt, W. B. (1979): Activation of thymocyte glucocorticoid receptors the steroid binding form; the roles of reducing agents ATP and stable factors. *J. Biol. Chem.,* 254:4779–4789.
187. Sarks, F., Van Driel, D., Maxwell, S., and Killingsworth, M. (1980): Softening of drusen and subretinal neovascularization. *Trans. Ophthalmol. Soc. U.K.,* 100:414–422.
188. Schulze, R. R. (1967): Rubeosis iridis. *Am. J. Ophthalmol.,* 63:487–495.
189. Schwartz, D. (ed.). (1966): Corticosteroids in the eye. *Int. Ophthalmol. Clin.,* 6:753–797.
190. Sears, M. L., Neufeld, A. H., and Jampol, L. M. (1973): Prostaglandins. *Invest. Ophthalmol. Vis. Sci.,* 12:161–164.
191. Shammas, H. J. F., and Milkie, C. F. (1979): Does aspirin prevent postoperative cystoid macular edema? *Am. Intraocul. Implant Soc. J.,* 5:337.

192. Sherrard, E. S. (1978): Characterization of changes observed in the corneal endothelium with a specular microscope. *Invest. Ophthalmol. Vis. Sci.,* 17:322.
193. Sholiton, D. B., Reinhart, W. J., and Frank, K. E. (1979): Indomethacin as a means of preventing cystoid macular edema following intracapsular cataract extraction. *Am. Intraocul. Implant Soc. J.,* 5:137–140.
194. Sholley, M. M., Gimbrone, M. A., Jr., and Cotran, R. S. (1978): The effects of leukocyte depletion on corneal neovascularization. *Lab. Invest.,* 38:32.
195. Smith, K. A. (1980): T-cell growth factor. *Immunol. Rev.,* 51:337–357.
196. Smith, K. A., Crabtree, G. R., Gillis, F., and Munck, A. (1980): Glucocorticoid control of T-cell proliferation. *Prog. Cancer Res. Ther.,* 14:125–134.
197. Smith, K. A., Crabtree, G. R., Kennedy, S. J., and Munck, A. (1977): Glucocorticoid receptors and glucocorticoid sensitivity of mitogen stimulated and unstimulated human lymphocytes. *Nature,* 267:523–526.
198. Smith, R. S., and Smith, L. A. (1980): Effects of BP961 on corneal wound healing. *Invest. Ophthalmol. Vis. Sci.,* 19(Suppl.):254.
199. Spink, A. I., and Baras, I. (1956): Effect of steroids on tensile strength of corneal wounds. *Am. J. Ophthalmol.,* 42:759.
200. Srinivasan, B. D., and Kulkarni, B. S. (1980): The effect of indomethacin, flurbiprofen and prednisolone acetate on conjunctival prostaglandin biosynthesis and polymorphonuclear leukocyte release following corneal injury. *Invest. Ophthalmol. Vis. Sci.,* 19(Arvo suppl.):228.
201. Srinivasan, B. D., Kulkarni, P. S. (1980): The role of arachidonic acid metabolites in the mediation of polymorphonuclear leukocyte response following corneal injury. *Invest. Ophthalmol. Vis. Sci.,* 19:1087.
202. Sugar, J., and Chandler, J. W. (1974): Experimental wound strength. *Arch. Ophthalmol.,* 92:270.
203. Taggart, H. M., and Alderdice, J. M. (1982): Fatal cholestatic jaundice in patients taking benoxaprofen. *Br. Med. J.,* 284:1372.
204. Tennant, J. L. (1978): Prostaglandins in ophthalmology. In: *Current Concepts in Cataract Surgery. Selected Proceedings of the Fifth Biennial Cataract Congress,* edited by J. M. Emery, St. Louis. C. V. Mosby, 360:2.
205. Thomas, R. V., and Whittle, B. J. R. (1976): Prostaglandins and the release of histamine from rat peritoneal mast cells. *Br. J. Pharmacol.,* 57:474–475.
206. Tonelli, G. (1972): *Lederle Laboratories Confidential Report,* 11:210–222.
206a.Tonelli, G. (1972): Tranexamic acid one year oral study in dogs. *Lederle Laboratories Confidential Report,* 9:137–209.
207. Unger, W. G., Perkins, E. S., and Bass, M. S. (1974): Response of the rabbit eye to laser irradiation of the iris. *Exp. Eye Res.,* 19:367.
208. Deleted in proof.
209. Vane, J. R. (1976): Prostaglandins as mediators of inflammation. *Adv. Prostaglandin Thromboxane Res.,* 2:791–801.
210. Vane, J. R. (1983): Prostacyclin. (Editorial). *Royal Soc. Med.,* 76:245–249.
211. Vassali, J. D., Hamilton, J., and Reich, E. (1976): Macrophage plasminogen activator modulation of enzyme production by anti-inflammatory steroids, mitotic inhibitors and cyclic nucleotides. *Cell,* 8:271–281.
212. Vaughn, E. D., Hull, D. S., and Green, K. (1978): Effective intraocular miotics on the corneal endothelium. *Arch. Ophthalmol.,* 96:1897.
213. Von Euler, U. S. (1935): A depressor substance in the vesicular gland. *J. Physiol. (Lond.),* 84:21.
214. Wahl, S. M., Altman, L. C., and Rosenstreich, D. L. (1975): Inhibition of in vitro lymphokine synthesis by glucocorticoids. *J. Immunol.,* 115:476–481.
215. Waitzman, M. D. (1970): Possible new concepts relating prostaglandins to various ocular functions. *Surv. Ophthalmol.,* 14:301.
216. Ward, P. A., Leopold, I. H., and Newman, L. J. (1968): Bacterial factors chemotactic for polymorphonuclear leukocytes. *Am. J. Pathol.,* 52:725–736.
217. Wei, C. P., Anderson, J. A., and Leopold, I. H. (1978): Ocular absorption and metabolism of topically applied epinephrine and a dipivalyl ester of epinephrine. *Invest. Ophthalmol. Vis. Sci.,* 17:315–321.

218. Weil, V. J., Elisoph, I., and Laval, J. (1958): Cataract wound healing in the rabbit eye. *Arch. Ophthalmol.,* 59:551.
219. Deleted in proof.
220. Wise, G. (1943): Ocular rosacea. *Am. J. Ophthalmol.,* 26:591.
221. Wojnar, R. J., Herarn, T., and Starkweather, S. (1980): Augmentation of allergic histamine release from human leukocytes by nonsteroidal anti-inflammatory analgesic agents. *J. Allergy Clin. Immunol.,* 66:37–45.
222. Worst, J. G. F. (1975): Biotoxizitat des Kammerwassers. Eine vereinheitlichende pathologische Theorie, begrundet auf hypothetische biotoxische kammerwasserfaktoren. *Klin. Monatsbl. Augenheilk.,* 167:376–384.
223. Yamagami, I. (1970): Electron microscopic study of the cornea. The mechanism of experimental new vessel formation. *Jpn. J. Ophthalmol.,* 14:41–58.
224. Yanuzzi, L. A., Klein, R. M., Wallyn, R. H. et al. (1977): Ineffectiveness of Indomethacin in the treatment of chronic cystoid macular edema. *Am. J. Ophthalmol.,* 84:527–529.
225. Yanuzzi, L. A., Landau, A. N., and Turtz, A. L. (1981): Incidence of aphakic cystoid macular edema with the use of topical indomethacin. *Ophthalmology,* 88:947–954.

Commentary

Immunosuppressants in Corneal Transplantation

Cyclosporin A (CS-A) is an exciting discovery. It is a very powerful immunosuppressant that could provide an adjunct or alternative to the customary paths to immunosuppression. CS-A is a cyclic undecapeptide product of the fungi cylindrocarpon lucidium and trichoderma polysporum. The compound has a selective effect on lymphocytes, mainly T cells. It seems that there may be considerable nephrotoxicity, less hepatotoxicity, and perhaps gingival hyperplasia, hirsutism or tremor. The issue of increased incidence of lymphoma requires continued study. After topical application of CS-A, as after corneal graft, remarkable suppression of the immune tissue can occur, but, can be monitored. Hoffmann and his associates have made an important contribution that will doubtless be put to clinical trial in several institutions.

The Editors

Surgical Pharmacology of the Eye,
edited by M. Sears and A. Tarkkanen.
Raven Press, New York © 1985.

Immunosuppressants in Corneal Transplantation

*F. Hoffmann and **M. Wiederholt

*Department of Ophthalmology and **Department of Clinical Physiology, Klinikum
Steglitz, Free University of Berlin, 1000 Berlin 45, Federal Republic of Germany

SUMMARY: The endothelial immunoreaction represents the main cause for
failure of a corneal transplant. The following groups of drugs can be used to
prevent an immune reaction: steroids, cytostatics, antilymphocyte sera and
cyclosporin A. Cytostatics and antilymphocyte sera are limited to use in a
small number of difficult cases with unfavorable prognosis because of their
serious side effects. After experience with 22 transplants with a follow-up
period of from 3 weeks to 15 months we think that the combination of
topically applied steroids and topically applied cyclosporin A may be the best
treatment available today. The side effects of the steroids can be reduced with
a lower dosage, and, the sutures can be removed after 5 months if necessary.
The side effect of the combined treatment of steroids and cyclosporin A can
be an intensive epithelial alteration in the first weeks after surgery, when both
drugs are applied as frequently as 5 times per day.

Immunoreaction currently represents the main cause for failure of a corneal transplant. Since improvement of the microsurgical operation techniques as well as of the preparation and conservation of donor corneas in the past two decades has brought the rate of surgical success of a clear transplant up to approximately 100% 1 to 2 weeks after the operation, prevention of an immunoreaction is becoming more and more important. Though it is possible to prevent immunoreactions in animal experiments by systemic administration of prednisolone 0.75 mg/kg body weight (50), the known side effects would render it unjustifiable to apply such a high steroid dose in humans for the long postoperative healing phase. Instead, most ophthalmologists apply water-soluble 0.1% dexamethasone drops for immunoprophylaxis. With this therapy, however, 15% to 30% (1,15,17,24) of the patients still develop immunoreactions, and this rate is even markedly higher (40% to 65%) in patients with an unfavorable prognosis (32,42,51), e.g., in those with inflamed eyes or strongly vascularized corneas. The concept of immunoprophylaxis through steroids therefore requires improvement. The discussion concerning the application of new forms of therapy will be preceded by a description of immunoreactions to transplanted corneas.

The immunoreaction can be roughly divided into four steps (13):

1. Recognition of the exogenous histocompatibility antigens. Certain constituents of the cell surface function as antigens. These are the gene products of the so-called serologically defined major histocompatibility complex (MHC) and the so-called leukocyte-defined weaker histocompatibility antigens. The incidence of immunoreaction after keratoplasty is reduced when three or four HLA antigens are compatible, particularly in cases where the initial situation is unfavorable (53,54).

The immune system recognizes transplanted cells that are not completely compatible genetically as antigenic foreign substances, much like pathogenic organisms or malignant body cells. While the HLA A- and B-antigens of the MHC are evident in endothelial cells, stroma cells, and epithelial cells (37), the D- and DR-antigens of the weaker histocompatibility complex appear to be present only in the Langerhans cells of the epithelial cell layer. In the avascular human cornea, these Langerhans cells are found only in the region near the limbus (23). According to other investigations (20), Langerhans cells are definitely present, though in small numbers, in the midperiphery of the cornea.

2. B- and T-lymphocytes activated by antigen contact. Immunoglobulin-producing plasma cells develop from the stimulated B-lymphocytes (humoral immunity) and immunocytes from the T-lymphocytes (cellular immunity). At this stage of the immunoreaction, the recipient is sensitized to the histocompatibility antigens of the donor, but no sign of an immunoreaction is recognizable.

3. Localization of the donor cells by immunocompetent cells. It is not known how the immunocompetent cells of the host reach the donor cells, probably by chance. However, once the immunoreaction has begun, it is intensified by manifold mechanisms and becomes clinically recognizable.

4. Destruction of the transplant by the immunoreaction. At least two different mechanisms can lead to destruction of the transplant. In vascularized transplants, antibodies against the main histocompatibility complex can reach the donor cells and induce a hyperacute immunoreaction by means of a complement activation and an antibody-dependent, cell-mediated cytotoxicity (ADCC). Whereas the hyperacute defense reaction is mainly of importance in vascularized transplants, e.g., heart and kidney, the primary mechanism for the immunoreaction in corneal transplants appears to be the T-cell-mediated immunoreaction to histocompatibility antigens on the cell surface.

STEROIDS

Steroids do not appear to influence any of the specific steps of the immunoreaction. There is no definite evidence that steroids exert a significant influence on the concentrations of circulating antibodies such as IgG and IgE nor that they have an influence on the normal course of development of a cell-mediated immunity (22). Of decisive significance is the antiphlogistic effect of steroids in corneal transplantation. In this way, they reduce the chance of information concerning the implantation of foreign tissue and its sensitization. During an immunoreaction, they suppress the inflammation that accompanies and intensifies it. Steroids destroy the T-lymphocytes at the site of the immunoreaction. They prevent the accumulation of macrophages at the site of the immunoreaction by blocking the macrophage-motility-inhibiting factor (MIF) of the lymphokines that is released by the lymphocytes (2).

In the direct postoperative phase, the antiphlogistic effect of steroids is of importance inasmuch as edema formation and fibrinogenesis are reduced, capillary dilatation is restricted, migration of leukocytes into the transplant is prevented, and capillary proliferation is inhibited (22). During a mean follow-up period of 20 months (10 to 42 months) after keratoplasty, we found (24) an immunoreaction in 19 of 86 transplants. In the first postoperative days, 17 patients had blood or fibrin in the anterior chamber; 11 of these 17 patients (65%), as opposed to only 8 of the other 69 patients (12%), later had an immunoreaction.

The antiphlogistic effect of steroids is of decisive significance for transplantation surgery. As a rule, steroids are applied as eye drops (dexamethasone 0.1%) five times daily in the first 1 to 3 weeks, then reduced to 2 drops after 1 to 3 months, and discontinued altogether 4 to 8 weeks after removal of the suture (46,51). Frequently 4 mg dexamethasone is injected subconjunctivally during the operation. A systemic steroid application directly following the operation or after an immunoreaction has occurred is not necessary, since local steroids also eliminate lymphocyte accumulation in the endothelium (51). Nevertheless, steroids cannot prevent immunoreactions and do, on the other hand, lead to side effects that make a reduction of the steroid dose seem desirable. The following side effects are of importance:

1. The hypertensive effect of steroids has been known for about 20 years (3) and frequently occurs in the postoperative phase after keratoplasty. Intraocular pressure can be considerably increased by steroids, particularly in patients with a concomitant history of glaucoma. In numerous studies (33,38,43,45), equal importance is attached to glaucoma and the immunoreaction as the main problems in the postoperative treatment of keratoplasty.

2. The cataractogenic effect of steroids has also been known for some time (6) but is frequently underestimated due to the fact that it cannot be measured very easily. Donshik et al. (16) found a dose-dependent cataract formation in about 30% of their keratoconus patients at a mean total dose of less than 40 mg dexamethasone locally applied. This dose is attained in the postoperative treatment of many keratoplasties and even exceeded when immunoreactions occur.

3. Steroids delay epithelial wound healing (39). The keratitis filiformis (46)

and keratitis punctata (24) observed in 27% to 40% of patients following keratoplasty can probably at least partially be interpreted as a side effect of steroids.

4. Steroids inhibit resistance to infection (29) and facilitate infection by bacteria or fungi (44). Infections occur particularly after epithelial lesions (29) and are more frequently observed on corneal transplants with a keratopathia punctata (24).

5. Steroids inhibit fibroblast proliferations (22) and thus delay wound healing of the transplant. The result is that the suture material must remain in the transplant for 6 to 12 months, producing a foreign-body stimulus that again requires steroid application.

CYTOSTATICS

Some cytostatics, systemically applied, have been successfully used for the prophylaxis or treatment of immunoreactions. Their effect lies in a reduction of cell proliferation. These drugs can lead to serious side effects, such as bone marrow depression, hepatic and renal dysfunctions, lowered resistance to infection, and increased tumor formation (18). These side effects restrict the application of cytostatics in cases of keratoplasty to a small number of particularly difficult situations. The drugs used to combat the immunoreaction are subdivided into alkylating substances such as chlorambucil, procarbazine, and cyclophosphamide and the antimetabolites azathioprine, mercaptopurine, and methotrexate (52).

The cytostatics produce leukopenia with a reduction of the T- and B-cells, resulting in a marked decrease of the inflammations that accompany the immunoreaction. However, there does not appear to be any specific influence on the immunoreaction (52). Azathioprine is the antimetabolite most frequently used for keratoplasty. It is used alone or in combination with steroids (19,25,41,53). In some patients, chlorambucil or mercaptopurine (34) is combined with steroids, or cyclophosphamide and procarbazine are combined with local steroid therapy (21) either concomitantly (35) or alternating weekly.

Cytostatics have been used in only a few cases and only when the prognosis was unfavorable; thus, there is hardly any statistical information to be reported. Cytostatics are not suitable for treatment of an immunoreaction that has already begun. Local or subconjunctival therapy with antimetabolites is not successful (18,40).

ANTILYMPHOCYTE SERA

Whereas antimetabolites inhibit the proliferation of lymphocytes, antilymphocyte sera (ALS) or antilymphocyte globulin (ALG) deplete the circulating lymphocytes (52). Favorable results have been obtained by the application of ALS, particularly in the area of kidney transplantation (36). In animal experiments, the immunoreaction after keratoplasty could be delayed or suppressed (49,55), but the concomitant suppression of the resistance to infections restricts the clinical application of ALS for keratoplasty. In cases of keratoplasty with a particularly unfavorable prognosis, it was not possible to achieve a favorable result by the application of ALS in 5 patients receiving concomitant doses of steroids and azathioprine. In animal experiments, it was possible to achieve a delay in the immunoreaction by preoperative treatment of the donor cornea with heterologous (5) or homologous (12) blocking antibodies.

CYCLOSPORIN A

Cyclosporin A (CS-A) is a new immunosuppressive drug that has excited some interest in recent years. In a screening program of fungal products in a cell-mediated cytolysis assay, it was discovered in 1976 that CS-A has a powerful immunosuppressive activity (7). The fungal extract is a neutral cyclic polypeptide of 11 amino acids (consisting of a characteristic unsaturated C-9 amino acid) and is highly soluble in alcohol and fat solvents but totally insoluble in aqueous solutions. Further studies showed an immunosuppressive effect of CS-A following either parenteral or oral administration in rats, mice, and guinea pigs (8). There was very little toxicity to the hematopoietic system, which was an important difference from the other immunosuppressive drugs. Obviously it was suggested that this drug might be worthy of investigation in organ allograft models.

In animal studies, it was observed that CS-A prolonged survival of kidney grafts in dogs (10) and orthotopic heart grafts in pigs (11). In the following years, extensive animal studies performed in the common laboratory species with various organ grafts demonstrated the powerful and relatively nontoxic immunosuppressive activity of CS-A. Especially in animals treated with azathioprine and/or methylprednisolone, survival time of transplanted organs was considerably shorter than in CS-A-treated animals (for review, see ref. 56). These results were sufficiently encouraging to perform clinical trials. CS-A has been under investigation in organ transplant centers all over the world, and its general introduction, especially in kidney, liver, pancreas, and bone marrow transplantation, is now imminent (56). Calne et al. (9) first treated patients who received kidneys from cadaver donors with CS-A, given initially as the sole immunosuppressant. Several side effects not seen in animal models considerably complicated the clinical management of the allograft recipients. Nephrotoxicity, hepatotoxicity, hirsutism, tremor, hyperesthesia, gum hyperplasia, nausea, and diarrhea were recorded. By monitoring CS-A blood levels and manipulating the oral dose within the limits of toxicity, the side effects of CS-A can be prevented to some extent (56). Thus, CS-A is effective in preventing acute allograft rejection in man, and in most studies, the patients given CS-A did better than the control group treated with other immunosuppressive drugs. However, the precise dose and length of treatment will need to be established to avoid some toxic side effects and to obtain optimal therapeutic response.

The attainment of optimal results in corneal transplantation depends on skillful surgical procedure and a consistently effective and safe immunosuppression. It is, therefore, self-evident that CS-A has been tried for transplantation of corneal allografts. In the animal model, penetrating or interlamellar keratoplasties were performed in rabbits (Table 1). To ensure rejection of the corneal allograft, it is necessary to perform additional skin grafts (4,14,30,31,48) or to vascularize the cornea (26,27,28,47). Systemic (intramuscular) administration of CS-A in high doses of 25 mg/kg/day for 14 to 28 days has been shown to considerably delay the onset of immunogenic rejection of corneal grafts (4,14,27,48). However, due to the possible side effects with long-term CS-A administration, a systemic immunosuppression by CS-A is not justified in clinical corneal transplantation. Thus, the effects of topical administration of CS-A on corneal allografts were investigated. Although the subconjunctival injection of CS-A was shown to prolong corneal graft survival (30,31), severe local irritations like lid edema, chemosis, hemorrhages, and drug residues limited the practicability of this route of administration. Interestingly, a single retrobulbar injection of 5 to 20 mg CS-A was sufficient to produce a dose-dependent tolerance of vascularized corneal grafts (47). However, a retrobulbar injection of CS-A is not preferable in clinical keratoplasty.

In a first report on topically applied 1% CS-A oil solution, no significant effect of CS-A on corneal graft survival was reported (48). It was suggested that the highly hydrophobic, lipid-soluble compound does not easily penetrate corneal tissue. However, in a rabbit model without skin sensitization, topical 1% CS-A oil solution effectively prevented corneal graft rejection (26,27,28). These data seem to contradict each other, but the difference in the experimental models used may explain the discrepancy. In corneal allografts without additional sensitization by skin grafts, corneal graft antigens alone induce an immune response, and suppression of such a mild antigen induction could be presumed to be due to local action of CS-A. Since the routes of reabsorption and the metabolism of topically applied CS-A are not known at present, the access of CS-A to the various tissues of the eye and to the draining lymph nodes is unpredictable. In our studies (30,31), topical instillation of a 5% water-soluble preparation of CS-A delayed corneal graft rejection in a model with large antigen load, sensitizing the rabbit with additional skin grafts. Local or systemic side effects of CS-A could not be observed. Since skin allograft survival was not prolonged by CS-A eye drops, a direct local effect of topical CS-A on the immunologic reactivity of the eye is very likely. Thus, systemically and—what is more important for the clinical situation in man—topically administered CS-A was effective in preventing and supressing corneal allograft reactions in rabbits.

TABLE 1. *Treatment of corneal allograft (penetrating keratoplasty) with cyclosporin A (CS-A)*

Species	Model	Application of CS-A	Results	References
Rabbit	Additional skin graft	25 mg/kg/dy, i.m., for 28 dy	Prolonged graft survival; 50% clear 20 wk after surgery	14
Rabbit	Additional skin graft	25 mg/kg/dy, i.m., for 14 or 28 dy	Prolonged graft survival	48
		1% in arachis oil eye drops 5 times/dy for 28 dy	No effect on graft survival	
Rabbit	Allografts with vascularization	1% in arachis oil eye drops 5 times/dy for 4 wk	Prolonged graft survival	26,28
		1% in arachis oil eye drops 5 times/dy for 1 mo, then 1–2 times/dy for 2 mo	Further increase of graft survival	
Rabbit	Nonvascularized recipient	Single retrobulbar injection, 5 mg in 0.25 ml olive oil	Prolonged graft survival	47
	Vascularized recipient	Single retrobulbar injection, 5, 10, or 20 mg in olive oil	Prolonged graft survival, dose dependent, 5 mg less effective than in nonvascularized recipient	
Rabbit	Additional skin graft	3 mg/kg/dy in oil subconjunctivally for 28 dy	Prolonged graft survival	30,31
		5% water-soluble preparation eye drops 5 times/dy for 28 dy	Prolonged graft survival	
Rabbit	Allografts with vascularization	15–25 mg/kg/dy, i.m., for 14 dy	Prolonged graft survival	27
		1% in arachis oil eye drops 5 times/dy for 28 dy		
		1% in arachis oil eye drops 5 times/dy for 4 wk, twice/dy for 5 wk, once/dy for 4 wk		
Rabbit	Interlamellar corneal grafting, additional skin graft	25 mg/kg/dy, i.m., for 14 dy	Prolonged graft survival	4
Man	High-risk patients with glaucoma	2% in miglyol 812 oil eye drops every 2 hr for 3 wk, then 5 times/dy for 4 wk, 3 times/dy for 4 wk, twice dy for 6 mo	No signs of graft rejection in 3 out of 4 patients	*Klin. Monatsbl. Augenheilk. (in press)*
Man	Regular keratoplasties	2% in castor oil eye drops 5 times/dy for 3 mo, 3 times/dy for 3 mo, 2 times/dy for 1 mo, 1 times/dy for 1 mo	No signs of graft rejection in 15 of 18 patients	*Klin. Monatsbl. Augenheilk. (in press)*
		0.1% dexamethasone eye drops 5 times/dy for 10 dy, 3 times/dy for 10 dy, 2 times/dy for 10 dy, 1 times/dy for 5 mo		

The precise mode of action of CS-A has not yet been determined, but it appears to be most effective when given at the time of immunization. This indicates that CS-A interferes at an early stage of antigenic triggering of lymphocytes and production of antibody by lymphocytes (56,57). There is general agreement that CS-A inhibits predominantly T-lymphocyte-dependent immune responses and does not interfere with macrophages, granulocytes, and hematopoietic tissue. CS-A inhibits the capacity of T-lymphocytes to synthesize and release lymphokines. There is disagreement about the differential effect of CS-A among T-lymphocyte subpopulations. In addition, recent studies indicate that this agent may be affecting B-cell function in a manner similar to the mode of action on T-cells (56,57). CS-A supresses both humoral and cellular immunity. Although the remarkable immunosuppressive properties of CS-A *in vivo* are well described, its mechanism of action in preventing allograft rejection is not clear. This is partly due to the fact that the events leading to graft rejection are much debated. CS-A probably inhibits T-cell activation and thus prevents the activation of the allograft-specific T-cell response. Besides this major inhibitory effect of CS-A on the T-lymphocytes, additional specific and/or nonspecific effects of CS-A cannot be excluded, especially in long-term tolerance of allografts. In corneal allograft experiments in rabbits, systemic or locally applied CS-A was effective in delaying allograft rejection in spite of strong antigenic sensitization by vascularization or additional skin grafting (4,14,26,27,28,30,31,47,48). The effect of systemic CS-A therapy is probably based primarily on the inhibition of the antigen induction of T-lymphocytes. Whether such a mechanism—suppression of antigen induction of lymphocytes *in situ*—applies to local drug therapy needs to be investigated.

The significance of the above-mentioned studies lies in the observation that CS-A, especially as eye drops, can be used effectively in corneal transplants. Up to now, topically applied corticosteroids have been the most effective drugs to prevent corneal graft reaction. However, immune corneal graft rejections are frequently observed, and corticosteroid therapy is associated with serious complications, such as delayed wound healing and development of glaucoma and cataract. Thus, in a first clinical trial, we applied CS-A locally in 4 glaucoma patients undergoing penetrating keratoplasty (*unpublished observations*). CS-A 2% (in miglyol 812 oil) eye drops were applied every 2 hr for 3 weeks, then five times daily for 4 weeks and three times daily for 4 weeks. After removal of the first running suture of the cross-stitch suture, CS-A was administered once or twice daily for 6 months. The second running suture was removed 6 months after the operation. During the 24-month follow-up period after the penetrating keratoplasty, no signs of graft rejection could be observed in 3 patients. In particular, one corneal transplant with severe epithelial and stromal vascularization showed no indications of corneal rejection. The only graft that failed to clear occurred in a young illiterate patient with questionable drug compliance. A significant plasma level of CS-A (by radioimmunoassay method) could not be detected in the 4 patients. Due to the adverse reactions to the miglyol oil (discomfort, redness of the eye, and keratitis punctata), which have not been reported in rabbit eyes, a new formula of CS-A eye drops in oil is under investigation. In 18 patients cyclosporin eye drops (2% in castor oil) were given in combination with low dose dexamethasone eye drops (0.1%). During the follow-up period of 3 to 8 months after keratoplasty 15 transplanted corneas are still clear, three corneas have become opacified and exhibited signs of an immunoreaction. Intraocular pressure was normal in all patients. Side effects probably ascribed to cyclosporin were punctate keratitis and red eye syndrome. In summary, topically applied CS-A has been shown to produce ocular immunosuppression and thus inhibit corneal graft rejection in man. Clearly the effects of CS-A on corneal grafts need to be investigated further.

REFERENCES

1. Abbot, R. L., and Forster, R. K. (1979): Determinants of graft clarity in penetrating keratoplasty. *Arch. Ophthalmol.,* 97:1071–1075.
2. Balow, J., and Rosenthal, A. S. (1973): Glucocorticoid suppression of macrophage migration inhibiting factor. *J. Exp. Med.,* 137:1031–1039.
3. Becker, B., and Mills, D. W. (1963): Elevated intraocular pressure following corticosteroid eye drops. *J.A.M.A.,* 185:884–886.
4. Bell, T. A. G., Easty, D. L., and McCullagh, K. G. (1982): A placebo-controlled blind trial of cyclosporin-A in prevention of corneal graft rejection in rabbits. *Br. J. Ophthalmol.,* 66:303–308.
5. Binder, P. S., Gebhardt, B. M., Chandler, J. W., and Kaufman, H. E. (1975): Immunologic protection of rabbit corneal allografts with heterologous blocking antibody. *Am. J. Ophthalmol.,* 79:949–954.
6. Black, R. L., Oglesby, R. B., von Sallmann, L., and Bunim, J. (1960): Posterior subcapsular cataracts induced by corticosteroids in patients with rheumatoid arthritis. *J.A.M.A.,* 174:166–172.
7. Borel, J. F. (1976): Comparative study of in vitro and in vivo drug effects on cell-mediated cytotoxicity. *Immunology,* 31:631–641.
8. Borel, J. F., Feurer, C., Magnee, C., and Stahelin, H. (1977): Effects of the new antilymphocytic peptide cyclosporin A in animals. *Immunology,* 32:1017–1025.
9. Calne, R. Y., Thiru, S., McMaster, P., Craddock, G. N., White, D. J. G., Evans, D. B., Dunn, D. C., Pentlow, B. D., and Rolles, K. (1978): Cyclosporin A in patients receiving renal allograft from cadaver donors. *Lancet,* 2:1323–1327.
10. Calne, R. Y., and White, D. J. G. (1977): Cyclosporin A. A powerful immunosuppressant in dogs with renal allografts. *IRCS Med. Sci.,* 5:595.
11. Calne, R. Y., White, D. J. G., Rolles, K., Smith, D. P., and Herbertson, B. M. (1978): Prolonged survival of pig orthotopic heart grafts treated with cyclosporin A. *Lancet,* 1:1183–1185.
12. Chandler, J. W. (1976): Immunologic protection of rabbit corneal allografts: prolonged survival of allografts pretreated with homologous antibody against transplantation antigens. *Invest. Ophthalmol. Vis. Sci.,* 15:213–216.
13. Chandler, J. W. (1982): Symposium: Pathophysiology of graft failure. Immunology—new approaches. *Cornea,* 1:281–286.
14. Coster, D. J., Shephard, W. F. I., Chin Fook, T., Rice, N. S. C., and Jones, B. R. (1979): Prolonged survival of corneal allografts in rabbits treated with cyclosporin A. *Lancet,* 2:688–689.
15. Donshik, P. C., Cavanagh, H. D., Boruchoff, S. A., and Dohlman, C. H. (1979): Effect of bilateral and unilateral grafts on the incidence of rejections in keratoconus. *Am. J. Ophthalmol.,* 87:823–826.
16. Donshik, P. C., Cavanagh, H. D., Boruchoff, S. A., and Dohlman, C. H. (1981): Posterior

subcapsular cataracts induced by topical corticosteroids following keratoplasty for keratoconus. *Ann. Ophthalmol.,* 13:29–32.

17. Ehlers, N., and Bramsen, Th. (1978): Management of late corneal graft problems. *Acta Ophthalmol. (Copenh),* 56:984–997.

18. Elliot, J. E., and Leibowitz, H. M. (1966): Chemotherapeutic immunosuppression of the corneal graft reaction. *Arch. Ophthalmol.,* 76:709–711.

19. Elliot, J. H., Leibowitz, H. M., Boruchoff, S. A., and Bounds, G. W. (1970): Penetrating keratoplasty with adjunctive azathioprine therapy—a preliminary report. In: *Ocular Anti-Inflammatory Therapy,* edited by H. E. Kaufman, pp. 169–191. Charles C Thomas, Springfield, IL.

20. Gillette, Th. E., Chandler, J. W., and v. Greiner, J. (1982): Langerhans cells of the ocular surface. *Ophthalmology,* 89:700–711.

21. Gnad, H. D. (1980): Immunosuppressive Therapie nach perforierender Keratoplastik. *Ophthalmologica,* 180:9–14.

22. Goodman, L. S., and Gilman, A. (1980): *The Pharmacological Basis of Therapeutics,* pp. 1479–1480. Macmillan, New York.

23. Gronemeyer, U., Stein, H., and Gerdes, J. (1983): Vorkommen von HLA-DR Antigenen in der Hornhaut. *Fortschr. Ophthalmol.,* 80:345–347.

24. Hoffmann, F. (1981): Keratoplasty with cross-stitch suture. In: *Proceedings of the VIth Congress, European Society of Ophthalmologists,* pp. 567–571. Grune and Stratton, New York.

25. Hughes, W. F., and Kallmeyer, J. (1967): Aetiology and treatment of the corneal homograft reaction including azathioprine. *S. Afr. Med. J.,* 41:548–551.

26. Hunter, P. A. (1981): Potential role of cyclosporin A in corneal grafting. *J. R. Soc. Med.,* 74:810–813.

27. Hunter, P. A., Garner, A., Wilhelmus, K. R., Rice, N. S. C., and Jones, B. R. (1982): Corneal graft rejection: A new rabbit model on cyclosporin A. *Br. J. Ophthalmol.,* 66:292–302.

28. Hunter, P. A., Wilhelmus, K. R., Rice, N. S. C., and Jones, B. R. (1981): Cyclosporin A applied topically to the recipient eye inhibts corneal graft rejection. *Clin. Exp. Immunol.,* 45:173–177.

29. Jones, B. R. (1975): Principles in the management of oculomycosis. *Am. J. Ophthalmol.,* 79:719–751.

30. Kana, J. S., Hoffmann, F., Buchen, R., Krolik, A., and Wiederholt, M. (1982): Rabbit corneal allograft survival following topical administration of cyclosporin A. *Invest. Ophthalmol. Vis. Sci.,* 22:686–690.

31. Kana, J. S., Hoffmann, F., Buchen, R., Krolik, A., and Wiederholt, M. (1982): Der Effekt der lokalen Gabe von Cyclosporin A auf die Überlebenszeit von Hornhauttransplantaten beim Kaninchen. *Fortschr. Ophthalmol.,* 79:132–134.

32. Khodadoust, A. A. (1973): The allograft reaction: The leading cause of late failure of clinical corneal grafts. In: *Corneal Graft Failure, Ciba Foundation Symposium,* edited by B. R. Jones, pp. 151–163. Elsevier, Amsterdam.

33. Kok-Van Alphen, C. C., and Völker-Dieben, H. J. M. (1979): Diagnosis and treatment of complications in the follow-up period after corneal transplantation. *Doc. Ophthalmol.,* 46:227–235.

34. Kok-Van Alphen, C. C., Völker-Dieben, H. J. M., v. d. Heuvel, J. E. A., Otto, A. J., and Dake, C. L. (1981): Die Abstossung des Hornhauttransplantates: Eine immunologische Krankheit. *Ber. Zusammenkunft Dtsch. Ophthalmol. Ges.,* 78:443–446.

35. Martenet, A. C. (1980): Echecs des cytostatiques en ophthalmologie. *Klin. Monatsbl. Augenheilkd.,* 176:648–651.

36. Monaco, A. F., and Codish, S. D. (1976): Survey of the current status of the clinical use of antilymphocyte serum. *Surg. Gynecol. Obstet.,* 142:417–428.

37. Newsome, D. A., Takasugi, M., Kenyon, K. R., Stark, W. J., and Opelz, G. (1974): Human corneal cells in vitro: Morphology and histocompatibility (HLA) antigen of pure cell populations. *Invest. Ophthalmol. Vis. Sci.,* 13:23–32.

38. Olson, R. J., and Kaufman, H. E. (1977): A mathematical description of causative factors and prevention of elevated intraocular pressure after keratoplasty. *Invest. Ophthalmol. Vis. Sci.,* 16:1085–1092.

39. Petroutsos, G., Guimaraes, R., Giraud, J. P., and Pouliquen, Y. (1982): Corticosteroids and corneal epithelial wound healing. *Br. J. Ophthalmol.,* 66:705–708.

40. Polack, F. M. (1965): Inhibition of immune corneal graft rejection by azathioprine. *Arch. Ophthalmol.,* 74:683–689.
41. Polack, F. M. (1967): Effect of azathioprine on corneal graft reaction. *Am. J. Ophthalmol.,* 64:233–244.
42. Polack, F. M. (1973): Clinical and pathological aspects of the corneal graft reaction. *Trans. Am. Acad. Ophthalmol.,* 77:418–432.
43. Polack, F. M. (1977): *Corneal Transplantation.* Grune and Stratton, New York.
44. Rao, G. H., and Aquavella, J. V. (1979): Cephalosporium endophthalmitis following penetrating keratoplasty. *Ophthalmic Surg.,* 10:34–37.
45. Robinson, C. H. (1979): Indications, complications and prognosis for repeat penetrating keratoplasty. *Ophthalmic Surg.,* 10:27–34.
46. Rotkis, W. M., Chandler, J. W., and Forstot, S. L. (1982): Filamentary keratitis following penetrating keratoplasty. *Ophthalmology,* 89:946–949.
47. Salisbury, J. D., and Gebhardt, B. M. (1981): Suppression of corneal allograft rejection by cyclosporin A. *Arch. Ophthalmol.,* 99:1640–1643.
48. Shephard, W. F. I., Coster, D. J., Chin Fook, T., Rice, N. S. C., and Jones, B. R. (1980): Effect of cyclosporin on the survival of corneal grafts in rabbits. *Br. J. Ophthalmol.,* 148–153.
49. Smolin, G. (1969): Suppression of the corneal homograft reaction by antilymphocytic serum. *Arch. Ophthalmol.,* 81:571–576.
50. Sugar, A., Benson, W., Burde, R. M., and Waltman, S. R. (1973): Alternate day versus daily systemic corticosteroids in corneal homograft rejection. *Am. J. Ophthalmol.,* 75:486–489.
51. Sundmacher, R. (1977): Immunreaktionen nach Keratoplastik. *Klin. Monatsbl. Augenheilkd.,* 171:705–722.
52. Vane. J. R., and Ferreira, S. H. (1979): Anti-inflammatory Drugs. In: *Handbook of Experimental Pharmacology,* Vol. 50, pp. 531–547. Springer Verlag, Berlin.
53. Vannas, S., Karjalainen, K., Ruusuvaara, P., and Tiilikainen, A. (1976): HLA-compatible donor cornea for prevention of allograft reaction. *Albrecht v. Graefes Arch. Ophthalmol.,* 198:217–222.
54. Völker-Dieben, H. J. M., Kok-Van Alphen, C. C., and Kruit, P. J. (1979): Advances and disappointments, indications and restrictions regarding HLA-matched corneal grafts in high-risk cases. *Doc. Ophthalmol.,* 46:219–226.
55. Waltman, S., Faulkner, H. W., and Burde, R. M. (1969): Modification of the ocular immune response. I. Use of antilymphocytic serum to prevent immune rejection of penetrating homografts. *Invest. Ophthalmol. Vis. Sci.,* 8:196–200.
56. White, D. J. G., editor (1982): *Cyclosporin A.* Elsevier Biomedical Press, Amsterdam, New York, Oxford.
57. Wiesinger, D., and Borel, J. F. (1979): Studies on the mechanism of action of cyclosporin A. *Immunobiology,* 156:454–463.

Commentary

Toxicology of Intraoperative Pharmacologic Agents

With characteristic thoroughness Woog and Albert have given us a complete description of the toxicology of drugs used by the ophthalmic surgeon. This chapter is replete with valuable cautionary information for the surgeon who wants to use drugs in a manner that will reduce adverse effects.

Information about the cellular and subcellular sites of action of drugs gives clues about the mechanism of their toxic action. Compared to what is known in other tissues, knowledge of drug metabolism in the eye is very limited. After systemic administration of drugs, the role of drug metabolizing and detoxifying systems in protecting the eye is important. The uveal tract is the obvious point of defense for the eye. Failure of a uveal system results in damage to the internal avascular tissues of the eye. More work on ocular drug metabolizing systems is required. Such studies might well be valuable in drug design and in the development of animal models of human disease. After ocular administration, the demonstrations of selective toxicities on a cellular level, as in the case of ornithine (2), or, on a subcellular level (lysosomes), as in the case of the aminoglycosides, like gentamicin (1), have important clinical impact.

As certain categories of drugs are considered for the protection of surgically traumatized ocular tissue, we must know more about their toxicology. For example, increased agreement has developed about the value of preoperative use of steroidal and/or nonsteroidal prophylaxis in the surgical patient. Toxicology of ocular perfusates that include these agents in appropriate concentrations might provide information useful for modifications of current perfusion fluids for vitrectomy and/or anterior segment surgery.

The Editors

REFERENCES

1. D'Amico, D. J., Libert, J., Kenyon, K. R., Hanninen, L. A., and Caspers-Velu, L. (1984): Retinal toxicity of intravitreal gentamicin. *Invest. Ophthalmol. Vis. Sci.,* 25:564–572.
2. Kuwabara, T., Ishikawa, Y., Kaiser-Kupfer, M. I. (1981): Experimental models of gyrate atrophy on pyridoxine and low-protein, low arginine diets. *Ophthalmology,* 88:311–315, 1981.

Surgical Pharmacology of the Eye,
edited by M. Sears and A. Tarkkanen.
Raven Press, New York © 1985.

Toxicology of Intraoperative Pharmacologic Agents

John J. Woog and Daniel M. Albert

*Department of Ophthalmology, Harvard Medical School, Massachusetts Eye
and Ear Infirmary, Boston, Massachusetts 02114*

SUMMARY: The horizons of intraocular surgery have been broadened by the use of certain pharmacological agents but adverse reactions and toxicity still occur. Adverse effects from usual doses of retrobulbar anesthetics, particularly lidocaine or bupivacaine, are extremely uncommon. Balanced salt solution to which glutathione, bicarbonate, or glucose has been added or Ringer's solution with glutathione or bicarbonate added, are probably the most suitable irrigating solutions. From a review of the literature and personal experience, a satisfactory replacement for vitreous remains to be developed, and, where possible, intraocular injection of air or gas is still advised. The uniformly grim prognosis with systemically treated endophthalmitis justifies the use of intravitreal antibiotics—particularly in association with vitrectomy—despite retinal toxicity. Choice of drug depends on the causative organism. The greatest experience has been with gentamycin. Miconazole appears to be a less toxic agent than amphotericin B. The well described toxicity of periocularly administered corticosteroids inadvertently injected into the vitreous is probably from the accompanying vehicle. Injection of dexamethasone and triamcinolone is well tolerated. The use of intraocular injections of 5-fluorouracil to inhibit proliferative vitreoretinopathy or maintain patent filtering blebs is feasible only if low doses are used and administration can be discontinued before toxic changes to retina and corneal endothelium become irreversible. It is not clear if the processes of scarring of filtration blebs or continual proliferative vitreoretinopathy will remain significantly inhibited once therapy with 5-fluorouracil has been discontinued.

Recent years have witnessed a tremendous broadening of therapeutic horizons in ophthalmic surgery, achieved largely through numerous advances in surgical instrumentation and technique. These advances have been facilitated in many instances by the incorporation into surgical procedure of various pharmacologic agents, inert substances, and mechanical devices. It is important to note, however, that each addition to the surgical armamentarium is associated with the potential for unfavorable and occasionally vision- or life-threatening reactions to intervention. In this chapter, we focus on adverse reactions resulting from the application of pharmacologic agents in or around the eye during selected surgical procedures.

151

PERIOCULAR AGENTS
Local Anesthetics
Topical Agents

Topical anesthetics are often used intraoperatively in preparation for the administration of local anesthetics by injection into the periorbital and retrobulbar tissues. Adverse reactions to the small dosages of topical anesthetics applied preoperatively are uncommon and are generally self-limited. Instillation of proparacaine 0.5%, for example, is associated with only mild conjunctival injection, pain, and tearing in most cases, although superficial punctate keratitis, punctal occlusion, and allergic reactions with pronounced chemosis and conjunctival injection have been reported (1). A similarly low incidence of significant toxicity has been noted following administration of benoxinate, another popular topical anesthetic, in one large series (2). Cocaine, on the other hand, is considerably more toxic to the corneal epithelium (1) and is used, in fact, to remove the epithelium in a variety of surgical procedures (1). As an indirect sympathomimetic agent, cocaine may also precipitate angle-closure glaucoma in susceptible individuals through pupillary dilatation (1).

Long-term administration of topical anesthetics may result in delayed healing of corneal epithelial defects through (a) inhibition of epithelial mitosis and migration (3), and (b) interference with epithelial oxidative metabolism mediated by the accumulation of highly toxic lactic acid (4). The persistent epithelial defects, stromal infiltration and ulceration, and complete corneal anesthesia associated with chronic self-administration of topical anesthetics (5,6) are unlikely sequellae of one-time use in the operating room.

Intravenous injection of anesthetic agents intended for topical use may result in serious systemic reactions. Intravenous administration of tetracaine, for example, may precipitate total cardiorespiratory collapse, typically without antecedent convulsive activity; a systemic dose of 100 mg tetracaine (5 ml of a 2% solution) is potentially fatal (1). Parenteral injection of cocaine may result in the development of a "cocaine reaction" characterized by anxiety, agitation, convulsions, and ultimately, cardiorespiratory arrest. Dosages of cocaine as small as 20 mg (1 ml of 2% solution) have been associated with the appearance of this constellation of findings, and a total dose exceeding one g may be fatal (1). Other local anesthetics (including procaine, lidocaine, prilocaine, mepivacaine, and bupivacaine) possess a significantly higher therapeutic index and are the preferred agents for periocular administration; adverse reactions noted with the use of these injectable agents are discussed briefly below.

Injectable Agents

General comments

Numerous visual complications ranging from transient visual impairment to permanent loss of light perception have been documented following local injection of anesthetics or other agents during various ophthalmic procedures (7–21). Retrobulbar injection, for example, is one well-utilized method of drug delivery that has been associated with visual loss in a number of cases through a variety of mechanisms. Optic atrophy has been documented following retrobulbar injection (11) and has been attributed to direct nerve injury from the needle and/or to hemorrhage within the nerve sheath. Perforation of the globe may occur (13). Retrobulbar hemorrhage is noted in approximately 1% to 2% of retrobulbar injections and is probably the most common complication of this technique (14); although increased intraorbital pressure with proptosis, elevated intraocular pressure, optic nerve compression, and vascular occlusion may develop secondarily, the visual prognosis in retrobulbar hermorrhage is usually good (9,12). Central retinal artery occlusion is probably the most feared complication of retrobulbar injection, and may occur in association with retrobulbar hemorrhage (12) or in its absence (14); in the latter circumstance, visual loss may be transient and may be related to direct arterial injury during injection, to arterial compression by the injected material, or to pharmacologic effect of the injected compounds (14). Central retinal artery occlusion may also presumably occur on an embolic basis, as in one reported case following retrobulbar corticosteroid injection in which steroid particles were visualized in the retinal vascular system (15). Combined central retinal artery and vein occlusion has also developed in several patients as a result of postinjection optic nerve sheath hematoma, as documented by computed tomographic and ultrasonographic studies (10,12). The onset of visual loss may be delayed in such patients (10).

Visual complications have also occurred following injection into the anterior orbit or into the lids (7–9), generally as a result of intraorbital hemorrhage, elevated intraorbital pressure, and vascular occlusion, as described above. In summary, it is important to note that visual loss following periocular injection generally occurs as a consequence of trauma to the globe or orbital soft tissues, including the optic nerve and opthalmic artery, and with the possible exception of the group of patients with transient central retinal artery occlusion described above, not on the basis of adverse pharmacologically mediated reactions to the injected agents per se. Important pharmacologically mediated systemic complications of local anesthetic administration may indeed occur, however, as discussed below.

Systemic complications of local anesthetic administration

Several factors influence the toxicity of local anesthetic injections: (a) the quantity and concentration of anesthetic solution; (b) the presence or absence of epinephrine in the anesthetic mixture; (c) vascularity of the injection site; (d) rate of drug metabolism; (e) anesthetic allergy; and (f) miscellaneous patient factors, including age and body weight. Adverse effects are often dose- or blood-level-dependent; blood-level-dependent adverse reactions may occur, in turn, as a result of simple overdosage or inadvertent intravascular injection or as a result of patient hypersensitivity to normal anesthetic dosage (16). In the special case of retrobulbar anesthesia, direct injection into the ophthalmic artery or into the optic nerve sheaths with retrograde passage of the anesthetic agent to the central nervous system may constitute yet another mechanism through which apparent anesthetic overdosage or hypersensitivity may occur (17,18). Similar mechanisms have been postulated in instances of adverse systemic reactions to local injection of lidocaine (and mepivacaine) in dental anesthesia (19,20).

Untoward anesthetic reactions are conveniently classified according to the predominant manifestation of toxicity, as noted below:

Central nervous system. Central nervous system toxicity of local anesthetics is characterized by central stimulation with anxiety, apprehension, delirium, ataxia, vertigo, nausea and vomiting, tremors, fasciculations, and seizures, followed by central depression with drowsiness, coma, and ultimately respiratory failure (1,16,19,22).

Cardiovascular system. Adverse cardiovascular reactions resulting from local anesthetic injection include pallor, diaphoresis, bradycardia, and postural hypotension. Rapid intravenous injection of even moderate dosages of local anesthetic agents may precipitate total cardiovascular collapse in the absence of premonitory central nervous system signs (16).

Respiratory system. Apnea may occur following anesthetic administration on the basis of direct medullary depression, respiratory muscle paralysis during convulsive activity, or primary cardiac arrest (16).

Allergic reactions. Allergic reactions to local anesthetic agents are said to be uncommon, although attempts to define the true incidence of anesthetic allergy are confounded by the inclusion in various series of cases of drug overdosage, patient hypersensitivity to normal dosage, occult intravascular injection, reactions to vasoconstrictors present in the injection mixture, and vasovagal reactions following anesthetic administration. At any rate, signs of anesthetic allergy range from urticaria and angioneurotic edema to laryngeal edema, bronchospasm, and systemic vasodilatation with hypotension (23). Most instances of apparent allergy are associated with the use of ester-linked agents (including cocaine, procaine, chloroprocaine, and amethacaine); allergic reactions to amide-linked compounds have been documented but are extremely rare (24).

The use of multidose vials of anesthetic containing methylparaben as a preservative may result in patient sensitization to this compound, and an allergic reaction to this preservative may develop on subsequent challenge with a methylparaben-containing anesthetic agent (25).

Miscellaneous. The addition of epinephrine to local anesthetic mixtures will decrease the rate of anesthetic absorption and may thus prolong the duration of anesthesia and minimize apparent drug toxicity. Adverse reactions to the vasoconstrictor component of the anesthetic mixture may occur, however, and include pallor, diaphoresis, agitation, hypertension, tachypnea, tachycardia, and increased myocardial irritability (1,16,26). There is evidence to suggest that the incorporation of epinephrine in local anesthetic mixtures should be limited in patients receiving general anesthetic agents that increase cardiac sensitivity to circulating catecholamines (including cyclopropane and halothane) (1) in patients receiving tricyclic antidepressants (1) and in patients with hypertension, thyrotoxicosis (16,27), or coronary artery disease (16,28). Epinephrine may be contraindicated in patients with glaucoma as well, as its presence in the retrobulbar mixture may be associated with a decrease in ophthalmic artery pulse pressure (26).

Hyaluronidase is another agent commonly added to ophthalmic injections of local anesthetics. Hyaluronidase is relatively nontoxic (1), although mild orbital edema was associated with the periocular injection of early preparations of this enzyme (30). The use of hyaluronidase may result in a shortening of duration of anesthetic action (30).

Toxicity of specific local anesthetic agents

Specific anesthetic agents are considered briefly:

Procaine. Procaine, the para-aminobenzoic acid ester of diethylaminoethanol, is the drug of preference for discussion of potency and toxicity of injectable local agents (25). Procaine has one-fourth the toxicity of cocaine as assessed by the effects of standard drug dosage on survival of white mice following subcutaneous or intraperitoneal injection (25). Five hundred milligrams (50 ml of 1% solution) is considered a safe injectable dosage, and a higher dosage might be administered safely following addition of epinephrine to the anesthetic mixture (1). Manifestations of procaine toxicity include agitation, delirium, seizures, allergic phenomena, and cardiorespiratory arrest, as described above.

Lidocaine. Lidocaine (diethylamino 2,6 acetoxylidide) is a common ingredient of injectable mixtures used for lid block and retrobulbar anesthesia. Lidocaine is nonirritating to tissues in concentrations up to 88%; concentrations recommended for clinical use, however, are significantly lower, ranging from 1% to 2% (31). The toxicity of this agent is one-fifth that of cocaine and 50% greater than that of procaine (1,25). The maximal safe dosage of lidocaine without epinephrine is 500 mg (50 ml of 1% solution) (1). Proper technique for injection of lidocaine and other local agents calls for aspiration and examination of the syringe for reflux of blood prior to injection and movement of the needle during injection, if possible, to avoid inadvertent intravascular administration of anesthetic with the systemic complications thereof outlined above. Blood was noted in the syringe following anesthetic injection in a patient who subsequently developed grand mal seizures following the administration of 60 mg lidocaine with 0.0005% epinephrine; intra-arterial injection was similarly postulated as the etiologic factor in a second patient who developed convulsions following the injection of 7.5 mg bupivacaine and 72.5 mg lidocaine with

0.0005% epinephrine. Both patients did well with administration of oxygen and intravenous diazepam (17). Interestingly, lidocaine is given in dosages approaching 100 mg (the equivalent of 10 ml of 1% solution) by rapid intravenous infusion in the standard treatment of ventricular tachyarrhythmias without untoward consequences (32).

Mepivacaine. Studies of the toxicity of mepivacaine (D-1-N-methyl pipecolic acid 2,6 dimethylanide hydrochloride) have yielded conflicting results. Local tissue irritation (cytotoxicity) following injection of mepivacaine has been said to be intermediate between that of lidocaine and procaine (21), or significantly less than that of both of the latter agents (25). Inflammation, neovascularization, fibroblastic proliferation, and necrosis of cutaneous muscle have been noted following intracutaneous injection (25). Estimates of the systemic toxicity of this compound are similarly variable. In one study, mepivacaine induced less drowsiness, ataxia, and vomiting in dogs than equivalent dosages of lidocaine and procaine. Measurement of the actual mean lethal intravenous dosages of these agents, however, revealed that mepivacaine was 50% more toxic than procaine (21). Yet another study demonstrated that procaine, lidocaine, and mepivacaine were of equal systemic toxicity (1).

Recommended maximal dosages of mepivacaine range from 625 to 725 mg. Serious systemic reactions are uncommon with this agent, although drowsiness, ataxia, tachycardia, facial twitching, and mild hypertension or hypotension may be seen (1,33). Mepivacaine induces less vasodilatation than procaine (33) and may be used for most purposes without added epinephrine (25). Mepivacaine may thus be particularly suitable for use in those patient groups described above for whom vasoconstrictor injection is contraindicated.

Bupivacaine. Bupivacaine (1-N-butyl-D,L-piperidine-2-carboxylic acid 2,6 dimethylanilide) is an amide-linked anesthetic that has found considerable popular use at present due to the profound and prolonged sensory anesthesia obtained following retrobulbar injection (25,34). Bupivacaine is customarily used in concentrations varying from 0.25% to 0.75% with a maximum safe dosage for systemic administration of 200 mg; the addition of a vasoconstrictor increases the duration of drug activity only slightly but decreases bleeding somewhat and significantly reduces peak blood levels (25), enhancing drug safety. In general, anesthesiologic usage adverse reactions including hypotension, bradycardia, and convulsions following accidental intravascular injection are no more frequent with bupivacaine than with equipotent dosages of lidocaine or mepivacaine. Recently, however, a series of reports in the ophthalmic literature has raised concern over the safety of this drug as utilized for retrobulbar anesthesia (18,35,36). In one report, four patients experienced confusion followed by sudden respiratory arrest after retrobulbar injection of 6 ml of 0.75% bupivacaine without epinephrine (18,36). Intubation and mechanical ventilation were required, although uneventful recovery ensued within 20 min of injection in each case. No reflux of blood was noted on attempted aspiration prior to injection in these cases; inadvertent intravascular injection was thus considered unlikely. In addition, the authors noted that the dosage of bupivacaine administered was far less than had been given intravenously in other cases without untoward consequences (36). The authors postulated instead that the apneic episodes may have resulted from injection of bupivacaine into the optic nerve sheath with retrograde passage of the agent in high concentration through the cerebrospinal fluid to the brain. In a second report, unconsciousness, respiratory arrest, and, ultimately, total cardiopulmonary arrest developed in a patient with arteriosclerotic cardiovascular disease, congestive heart failure, hypertension, chronic renal failure, and anemia following the retrobulbar injection of 2 ml of a mixture of 0.5% bupivacaine and 2% mepivacaine. The pathophysiologic mechanism underlying the development of cardiac arrest in this case was not clear, but the numerous medical problems listed above may have been contributory. The patient did well with supportive therapy (35).

These reports have led one author to contend that the risk of cardiac or of respiratory arrest may be disproportionately high with bupivacaine and to suggest that usage of this agent be discontinued (36). This recommendation has been disputed by other investigators who note that bupivacaine and the other local agents are of equal toxicity when given in equipotent doses (18); in a recent study, these investigators encountered no anesthetic-related complications in a series of 96 procedures utilizing retrobulbar injection of bupivacaine (34).

Prilocaine. Prilocaine (alpha-N-propylamine-2-methyl-proprioanilide) is an amide-linked agent with approximately 60% of the toxicity of lidocaine (25). This relative lack of toxicity has been attributed to drug-related inhibition of vasodilatation and decreased drug absorption (37) and to a rapid rate of drug metabolism (25). Prilocaine is used in a concentration of 0.5% to 5.0% with a maximal safe systemic dosage of 800 mg. Adverse systemic reactions are extremely uncommon with this agent and are qualitatively similar to those noted with other local anesthetics (25). Prilocaine is unique in that administration of dosages exceeding 600 mg may result in the development of methemoglobinemia (25). This complication is thought to be clinically insignificant except for those patients with preexistent methemoglobinemia, severe anemia, or cardiac failure who may develop cyanosis (37); treatment with intravenous methylene blue 1 mg/kg is effective when indicated (25).

Summary. The precise incidence of serious systemic reactions to ophthalmic injections of local anesthetics is difficult to determine. In one series of 1,000 patients receiving retrobulbar anesthesia for retinal detachment repair one patient developed convulsions and respiratory muscle spasm responding to intravenous barbiturate therapy (38). In a recent study of 128 retrobulbar anesthetic procedures utilizing either 2% lidocaine or 0.75% bupivacaine with and without epinephrine no drug-related complications were noted (34).

Little information is available concerning the effects on ocular structure and function of inadvertent intraocular injection of local anesthetics. In one study intravitreal injection in rabbits of 10 mg lidocaine resulted in suppression of the B-wave of the electroretinogram, with partial recovery noted within 5 to 8 hr of injection. Histopathologically, lesions were observed in the outer plexiform layer (including disruption of synapses between photoreceptors, bipolar cells, and horizontal cells) (39).

Periocular Antibiotics and Steroids

Periocular injections of antimicrobial agents and anti-inflammatory agents are widely employed in the treatment of active ocular disease and in the prophylaxis of postoperative infection and inflammation. Although periocular injections are generally well tolerated, adverse reactions of varying severity and clinical significance have been reported in association with this mode of drug delivery. Several clinical and experimental reports describing various complications of periocular injections of antimicrobial agents are summarized in Table 1.

Numerous real and theoretical complications of periocular corticosteroid injection have been described, including: (a) transient pain and chemosis following injection; (b) orbital infection; (c) orbital scarring with secondary strabismus; (d) ptosis; (e) acceleration of cataract formation; (f) elevation of intraocular pressure (40); (g) inhibition of corneal wound healing (41); (h) local immunosuppression with exacerbation or reactivation of intraocular infection (e.g., toxoplasmic retinochoroiditis) (42); (i) corneal perforation in patients with peripheral ulcerative keratitis; (j) central retinal artery occlusion (15); and (k) induction of an iatrogenic Cushing's syndrome with adrenal suppression (43,44). Perforation of the globe and inadvertent intraocular injection are additional risks of subconjunctival or retrobulbar corticosteroid injection. Signs and symptoms of intraocular injection may include sudden onset of eye pain and visual loss, hypotony or immediate elevation of intraocular pressure, vitreous hemorrhage, retinal breaks, retinal detachment, retinal degeneration, appearance of steroid deposits in the subretinal space or in the vitreous cavity, and a pseudohypopyon composed of steroid particles in aphakic patients (44–47). The onset of ocular pain and visual dysfunction may on occasion be delayed for several days following inadvertent intraocular administration of steroids (45). Glaucoma, glaucomatous and nonglaucomatous optic atrophy, and proliferative vitreoretinopathy are well-recognized sequellae of inadvertent intraocular steroid injection; the latter complication may be a manifestation of toxicity of the injection vehicle and not of corticosteroid toxicity per se (45). Patients suffering the complications of bulbar perforation and intraocular steroid injection may do well with conservative therapy, including careful monitoring of the intraocular pressure and closure of retinal breaks (47,48), although heroic surgical efforts including pars plana vitrectomy, endophotocoagulation, air-fluid exchange, and scleral buckling may be necessary to achieve a satisfactory visual result (46).

TABLE 1. *Toxicity associated with subconjunctival administration of antimicrobial agents*

Agent	Species studied	Observations
Amphotericin B (49)	Human	125 μg injection well-tolerated
Amphotericin B (50)	Human	Yellow pigmentation of conjunctiva, and subconjunctival nodules composed of histiocontaining eosinophilic PAS-positive material following subconjunctival injection of 5.5 mg
Carbenicillin (51)	Monkey	Transient hyperemia and chemosis following injection
		Focal lymphocytic and polymorphonuclear leucocytic infiltrates in conjunctiva; cornea, sclera, uveal tract, and retina normal
Carbenicillin (52)	Human	Pain lasting for several minutes following injection; conjunctival hyperemia and chemosis lasting up to 11 days post-injection
Cephalothin (53)	Human	Pain, chemosis, and hyperemia lasting 35 min, 2.5 hr, and 4 dy following injection, respectively
Cephalothin (54)	Human	50-mg dose well-tolerated; potential allergic cross-reactivity in penicillin-allergic patients (55)
Clindamycin (42)	Human	Total dose of 550 mg over 3 wk by subconjunctival injection well tolerated
Clindamycin (56)	Human	150 mg by subtenon's injection well tolerated
		450 mg by subtenon's injection followed by transient diplopia
		450 mg by retrobulbar injection followed by papillitis with optic atrophy
Gentamicin (57)	Rabbit Rat Human	Membrane-bound lamellar osmiophilic inclusions in conjunctival fibroblasts following subconjunctival injection; abnormalities similar to those in proximal renal tubular epithelial cells following systemic aminoglycoside therapy
Penicillin (58)	Human	50 mg subconjunctival injection irritating but well tolerated; potentially hazardous in penicillin-allergic patients
Tobramycin (59)	Rabbit	Transient conjunctival hyperemia and chemosis following injection

INTRAOCULAR AGENTS

Irrigating Solutions

Irrigating solutions are required for the performance of numerous intraocular surgical procedures, including intracapsular and extracapsular cataract extraction, intraocular lens implantation, phacoemulsification, filtration surgery, penetrating keratoplasty, anterior segment reconstruction, and pars plana vitrectomy. Most of the studies exploring the ocular toxicity of these irrigants have focused on the effects of these solutions on the corneal endothelium as assessed in various *in vitro* perfusion (61–69) systems, although retinal function following intravitreal irrigation with various solutions has also been the subject of investigation (70). A brief review of the corneal and retinal toxicities of several available irrigating solutions will perhaps be of value to the pharmacologist in the formulation of the ideal irrigant and to the ophthalmic surgeon in the modification of surgical technique.

Normal Saline Solution

Normal saline solution (NSS) (0.9%) contains the two principal ionic constituents of aqueous humor (71) (Table 2). Persistent corneal clouding has been observed following *in vivo* perfusion of rabbits with NSS (72), and this irrigant is associated with the highest rate of endothelial swelling (98 μm/hr) of several solutions studied by *in vitro* perfusion of human and rabbit corneal buttons (62–64) (Fig. 1). Ultrastructural studies of specimen perfused with NSS have revealed loss of endothelial cell plasma membranes (63). Cytologic correlates of endothelial toxicity noted in tissue culture studies include rounding of individual endothelial cells with retraction of cytoplasmic processes and inhibition of endothelial cell movement (72).

Intravitreal irrigation with NSS in rabbits is associated with a decrement in electroretinographic B-wave amplitude (70) and with the development of a progressive posterior subcapsular cataract (73).

Plasmalyte 148

Plasmalyte (a solution containing sodium, potassium, chloride, magnesium, acetate, and gluconate, as shown in Table 2) was the standard solution used during phacoemulsification between 1971 and 1976. Initial studies of the effect of Plasmalyte on the endothelium utilized approximately 300 ml of this

TABLE 2. *Composition of selected intraocular irrigating solutions (mEq/l)*

Solution	Na	K	Ca	Mg	Cl	HCO_3	HPO_4	Ascorbate	Lactate	Other
Extracellular fluid	142	4	5	3	103	27	3			
Aqueous humor (rabbit) (105)	146.5	4.7			105.1	27.7	0.89	0.96	12.1	
Normal saline solution	154				154					
Ringer's lactate	130	4	2.7		109				28	
Plasmalyte 148	140	5		3	98					Acetate 27 Gluconate 23
BSS + T (84)	122	5	1	1	122	25	3			GSH 0.3 Dextrose 5

Modified after Schwartz.

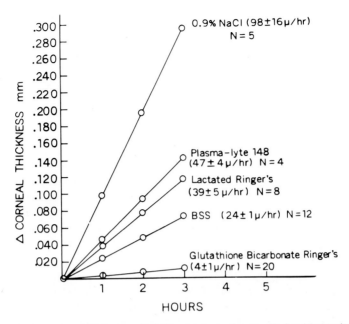

FIG. 1. Changes in corneal thickness of rabbit corneas perfused with five intraocular irrigating solutions. (From ref. 75 with permission © The Ophthalmic Publishing Company.)

solution in a 10-min irrigation-aspiration procedure in the cat anterior chamber. Scanning electron microscopy of specimens thus perfused revealed no evidence of endothelial injury (74). Similarly, in a second study a 10-min irrigation-aspiration with Plasmalyte in rabbit and cat anterior chambers produced no endothelial damage as assessed by scanning electron microscopy and nitroblue tetrazolium staining (75). *In vitro* perfusion studies were confirmatory, with no corneal swelling evident following a 20-min perfusion period (76). Subsequent studies, however, suggested that Plasmalyte was not the ideal irrigating solution for anterior segment surgery. A 15-min irrigation-aspiration procedure with Plasmalyte in the *in vivo* feline model resulted in corneal edema and endothelial disruption in five of 10 eyes examined (88). In a study by Edelhauser and associates (64) a human corneal button perfused *in vitro* for 30 minutes with Plasmalyte demonstrated numerous ultrastructural abnormalities including irregularities of the endothelial surface with loss of tight junctions, vacuolation of cytoplasm, and swelling of endothelial cell nuclei and cytoplasmic organelles. In a second experiment, a 4-hr perfusion of human corneal button with Plasmalyte resulted in complete disruption of the endothelium with destruction of the cell plasma membrane, dilation of the endoplasmic reticulum, cytoplasmic vacuolation, and mitochondrial swelling evident on transmission electron microscopy (64).

As is evident from Fig. 1, the corneal swelling rate of 47 μm/hr associated with *in vitro* perfusion with Plasmalyte is significantly better than that found with NSS perfusion but is worse than that seen with perfusion with Ringer's lactate, balanced salt solution, or enriched balanced salt solution. The apparent superiority of the latter solutions in the maintenance of corneal thickness and the observation that corneal swelling rates exceeding 33 μm/hr are correlated with endothelial degeneration (78) suggest that irrigation with Plasmalyte should probably be avoided when possible.

Ringer's Lactate Solution

Ringer's lactate (RL) contains sodium, potassium, chloride, lactate (a bicarbonate precursor), and calcium (Table 2) (79). The latter ion has been implicated in the maintenance of endothelial tight junctions and thus plays an important role in the preservation of stromal deturgescence. Ringer's lactate lacks a satisfactory substrate for the glucose-bicarbonate dependent endothelial pump (65–67), however, and is somewhat acidic and hypotonic relative to aqueous humor. As seen in Fig. 1, *in vitro* perfusion with RL is associated with rapid corneal swelling (albeit less rapid than that observed with NSS or Plasmalyte) and with several alterations in the ultrastructural appearance of the endothelium, including dilatation of the rough endoplasmic reticulum, cytoplasmic vacuolation, and nuclear pyknosis (63).

Balanced Salt Solutions

Several products containing many of the ions and buffer systems essential for normal cellular metabolism are available; the ingredients of one such product are listed in Table 2. Ionic magnesium enhances the efficiency of the magnesium-dependent ATPase of the endothelial pump and is thus an important component of physiologic balanced salt solutions (64). Short-term application of balanced salt solution to tissue culture preparations of rabbit endothelium results in no morphologic evidence of cellular injury (72). *In vivo* perfusion of rabbit corneal buttons with balanced salt solution produces transient corneal edema (72), however, and perfusion chamber experiments confirm the development of progressive corneal swelling following perfusion with balanced salt solution. Dilation of the rough endoplasmic reticulum and rupture of endothelial cell plasma membranes have been noted on electron microscopic study of perfused corneas (64).

Other studies have demonstrated that lens clarity is maintained in rabbits during model vitrectomy procedures and during *in vitro* lens perfusion utilizing balanced salt solution as the intraocular irrigant and perfusate, respectively (73).

Enriched Balanced Salt Solutions

The addition of glutathione, bicarbonate, and glucose to balanced salt solution permits *in vitro* perfusion of rabbit (63,64,68,69) and human (62,64) corneas with a minimal increase in corneal thickness (Fig. 1) and with essentially no disruption of the ultrastructural integrity of the endothelium. *In vivo* rabbit studies similarly demonstrate relative preservation of the electro-retinographic B-wave following irrigation with balanced salt solution containing glutathione, bicarbonate, and glucose during vitrectomy (70). Glucose (or other high-energy compounds such as adenosine) is required for aerobic metabolism of the endothelium (60) and for maintenance of the endothelial (65–67) pump. Bicarbonate ion is also important in the maintenance of endothelial pump function (65,66) and constitutes in addition a component of the normal buffer system of the aqueous humor (69), whereas glutathione plays a major role in the preservation of endothelial cell membrane integrity via its antioxidative (60,63,64,68,69) effects. Clinical studies evaluating the incidence of corneal edema following vitrectomy in normal (81) and diabetic (82) patients confirm the superiority of balanced salt solutions containing glutathione, bicarbonate, and glucose in the maintenance of corneal endothelial function.

Balanced salt solutions with glutathione, bicarbonate, and glucose are effective in preserving lenticular clarity during *in vitro* perfusion of normal rabbit (73) and monkey (83) lenses and during *in vivo* vitrectomy procedures in rabbits (73). Lenses from diabetic rabbits demonstrate opacification when perfused with these solutions, but cataract formation can be inhibited by the addition of more glucose to the irrigant (73).

Preservatives in Intraocular Irrigating Solutions

One of the drawbacks associated with the use of currently available enriched balanced salt solutions is the need to reconstitute the irrigant immediately prior to surgery and to discard unused material 6 hr after preparation (84). The addition of a nontoxic preservative would allow manufacturer packaging of a complete solution and reuse of a bottle of solution during several procedures. Several studies evaluating the toxicity of preservatives in intraocular solutions, however, have failed to identify the ideal nontoxic preservative. Intraocular benzalkonium chloride, for example, is associated with conjunctival erythema, exudate, chemosis, corneal epithelial defects, corneal edema, and iritis when instilled in concentrations exceeding 0.01% in rabbits (85). Benzalkonium chloride in a concentration of 0.01% was well tolerated on one rabbit study (85), but its use in another study resulted in profound corneal edema (86). Scanning and transmission electron microscopy in the latter group of animals revealed endothelial swelling, cytoplasmic vacuolation, and disruption of organelles with concentrations of benzalkonium chloride as low as 6.5×10^{-4} T. Endothelial ultrastructural integrity was maintained during perfusion with benzalkonium chloride in a concentration of $6.5 \times 10^{-6}\%$, but the preservative efficacy of this dilute solution is questionable (85).

Other preservatives including thimerosal (87) and chlorhexidine (88) have also been associated with pronounced endothelial toxicity. The observation that instillation during phacoemulsification procedures of two drops of undiluted 0.1% epinephrine containing 0.1% sodium bisulfite caused endothelial toxicity prompted investigation of the toxicologic effects of this widely used agent (74). Morphologic evidence of endothelial injury including cytoplasmic vacuolation and loss of organelles was documented by electron microscopy following a 5-min perfusion of isolated rabbit corneas with 0.1% epinephrine containing 0.1% sodium bisulfite. Perfusion studies with unpreserved epinephrine and with 0.1% sodium bisulfite alone implicated sodium bisulfite as the toxic agent in this combination (89). Perfusion with 0.05% sodium bisulfite or with 0.02% epinephrine containing 0.02% sodium bisulfite was associated with preservation of corneal thickness and normal endothelial cytoarchitecture (89,90). Specular microscopic studies of feline corneas following *in vivo* perfusion with 0.02% epinephrine, 0.1% sodium bisulfite, and chlorobutanol 0.1% to 0.5% were nontoxic as well (91). Nonetheless, unpreserved epinephrine is preferred by many surgeons for use in irrigating solutions for extracapsular cataract extraction and phacoemulsification (92). The pH and osmolality of the epinephrine-containing irrigant are also of importance in the preservation of corneal clarity. Use of the appropriate diluent and a weak buffer system (as in balanced salt solution) will facilitate maintenance of an acceptable pH and osmolality (200 to 450 mOsm/liter) (93,94). Commercially available epinephrine products formulated at a low pH (4.0) with an antioxidant (sodium bisulfite) and a strong buffer system may be associated with endothelial disruption and corneal edema following intracameral administration (95).

Pupilloactive Agents in Intraocular Surgery

Mydriatics

As mentioned above, epinephrine 0.02% was well tolerated when administered intracamerally in clinical and experimental studies (89,91). Experimentally, topical application of phenylephrine 2.5% in rabbits results in vacuolation of the corneal epithelium and in endothelial disruption with corneal edema when applied following epithelial denudation (96). These findings are consistent with the clinical observation that phenylephrine applied intracamerally for mydriasis during vitreous surgery results in stromal edema and opacification (97). Topical cyclopentolate hydrochloride has also been implicated in the development of corneal edema when administered topically in eyes in which the epithelium has been removed (98).

Miotics

In vitro perfusion of rabbit corneas with pilocarpine in concentrations of 0.25% or greater was associated with progressive corneal swelling in one study. Ultrastructural abnormalities in perfused specimens included endothelial shrinkage with disruption of tight junctions and intracellular vacuolation with margination of nuclear chromatin and fragmentation of nucleoli (99). Intraocular administration of carbachol 0.01%, a direct and indirect parasympathomimetic agonist (1), produced no specular microscopic (100) or scanning electron microscopic (89) evidence of endothelial injury in cats. Perfusion of isolated rabbit corneas, on the other hand, with carbachol 0.01% was associated with progressive corneal swelling at a rate of 53 μm/hr for the first 2 hr following perfusion with a decrease in the swelling rate thereafter. The perfused specimens were ultrastructurally normal, however, and the endothelial dysfunction noted following carbachol perfusion was attributed to the low pH of the perfusate (100).

Acetylcholine 1% solution was well tolerated intracamerally in perfusion studies in rabbits (100) and cats (91), although a tendency for lens opacification (presumed secondary to the hyperosmolality of the acetylcholine solution) has been noted in the former species. This compound is frequently used clinically during intraocular lens implantation following cataract extraction (102). There have been two reports of adverse systemic reactions following intracameral administration of acetylcholine. In one case, hypotension, bradycardia, facial flushing, dyspnea, and diaphoresis were noted following instillation of an undisclosed amount of acetylcholine into the anterior chamber. The episode was terminated by the intravenous administration of atropine and ephedrine (103). A second patient developed similar manifestations of cholinergic hyperactivity including hypotension, bradycardia, and transient ventricular dysrhythmias upon intracameral administration of 20 mg acetylcholine; the patient in this case as well responded favorably to intravenous atropine (104). The paucity of reports in the literature describing adverse systemic reactions to intraocular acetylcholine despite the widespread use of this agent may reflect a truly low incidence of systemic side effects (related, perhaps, to the extremely rapid metabolism of acetylcholine by acetylcholinesterase) or may be related to the limited monitoring of vital signs during procedures performed without anesthesiologic supervision.

As noted above, benzalkonium chloride appears to be extremely toxic to the endothelium when applied intracamerally (85,86), and topical medications (including pupilloactive agents) containing this preservative should probably be avoided during intraocular procedures.

Vitreous Substitutes

Numerous substances have been introduced into the eye in an attempt to preserve anterior or posterior segment volume during various intraocular and extraocular surgical procedures. These substances have facilitated the performance of relatively common ophthalmic procedures such as intraocular lens implantation and have even served as a basis for successful intervention in a smaller group of patients with previously inoperable ocular disease such as proliferative vitreoretinopathy. Several problems may be encountered in the clinical usage of the agents, however, as discussed in the section that follows.

Intraocular Gases

Air

Intraocular injection of air is used (a) during intraocular lens implantation to maintain anterior chamber depth and prevent contact of the pseudophakos with the corneal endothelium and (b) during retinal reattachment surgery as a mechanical tamponade to promote closure of retinal breaks and subsequent chorioretinal scar formation. Several experimental studies have been performed to clarify the effects of air on various ocular structures, as noted below.

Corneal endothelium. Injection of 0.15 ml of air into the anterior chambers of rabbits was associated with the development of corneal edema in one study (106); in another study, injection of air into the cat anterior chamber resulted in a 7% decrease in endothelial cell density compared to control animals, as assessed by specular microscopy two months following injection. This effect was noted despite a mean persistence of intracameral air of only 4 days, prompting the author to recommend removal of intracameral air immediately after use, when possible (107). Other investigators have described the presence of endothelial cell membrane lesions of varying severity following *in vivo* exposure of rabbit corneal endothelium to air (108). Rabbit endothelium is said to assume a "peau d'orange" appearance by slit-lamp biomicroscopy following air exposure, and transmission electron microscopy of specimens thus treated reveals evidence of corneal endothelial degeneration (109).

Uveal tract. In early studies air was noted to be extremely "irritating" when placed in the anterior chamber of rabbit eyes (110), leading to the development of a chronic fibrinous iritis with iris atrophy and formation of peripheral anterior and posterior synechiae (106,111). More recent studies in monkeys have confirmed an increase in ocular vascular permeability following air injection as measured by the passage of (119) I-labelled protein into the vitreous and aqueous humor. This disruption of the blood-ocular barrier was found to be transient and was correlated temporally with the persistence of the air bubble; in most animals ocular vascular permeability had returned to normal within one month of injection (112).

Lens. Opacification of the anterior lens capsule was noted in 20% of rabbit eyes receiving 0.15 ml of air by intracameral injection (106). Posterior subcapsular cataract development has been described in owl monkeys within 12 to 14 hr after air injection if the air bubble was allowed to impinge on the posterior lens capsule. These lens changes were to some extent reversible following the removal of air. Lens clarity was maintained in 11 of 12 animals in which air-lens tough was absent; one animal in this study demonstrated minor and completely reversible lens opacification (113). The presence of air-lens contact thus appears to be the critical factor in cataractogenesis following intraocular air injection. Further observations concerning cataract formation during the use of air-gas mixtures will be outlined in the discussion of intraocular gases below.

Glaucoma. Experimental glaucoma has been induced in normal rabbits by the posterior segment injection of air with resultant forward displacement of the lens-iris diaphragm, pupillary block, and angle closure (111). In a series of rabbits undergoing removal of 40% of the vitreous body; however, posterior segment injection of equal volumes of air was not associated with elevation of intraocular pressure or further loss of vitreous (114).

Posterior segment. Studies with owl monkeys reveal no clinical or histopathologic abnormalities following intravitreal injection of air (115).

The risks and complications of intraocular air injection in humans have been summarized by several investigators (116–122) and include the following:

Ocular injuries resulting from traumatic injection. Lens injury, retinal tears, and injection site bleeding may occur as a result of traumatic injection technique (116).

Ocular injuries resulting from misplaced air injection. Subretinal air injection may result in retinal tear formation with development of exacerbation of retinal detachment (116). Air injection into the potential space between the pigmented and nonpigmented layers of the ciliary pigment epithelium has also been documented, with subsequent loss of the nonpigmented layer, avulsion of the vitreous base (116), and retinal dialysis (118). This complication may be prevented by the use of indirect ophthalmoscopic control during air injection (121).

Intraocular infection. Endophthalmitis may follow the intravitreal injection of contaminated materials, including air. Millipore filters are effective in reducing the incidence of this complication of air injection (111). Sterile vitriitis has also been noted following air injection (120).

Cataract. Lens opacification may occur as a result of lens trauma during injection as noted above, or as a result of air bubble contact with the lens epithelium. Opacities following intravitreal injection of air are characteristically posterior subcapsular in location and are often at least partially reversible upon removal of air (124).

Glaucoma. The use of air in phakic (116,122) and aphakic (116,117) patients has been associated with the development of pupillary and angle block glaucoma, respectively. Traditional signs and symptoms of elevated intraocular pressure such as eye pain, nausea and vomiting, decrease in visual acuity, and ocular injection may be present but may be misinterpreted in these postoperative patients. This group of patients may thus be at a higher risk for development of complications of sustained elevation of intraocular pressure such as vascular occlusion, wound rupture, or rupture of the globe (90,119,123). These considerations have led several clinicians to recommend careful and regular monitoring of intraocular pressure following air injection with release of air by paracentesis for intraocular pressures exceeding 40 mm Hg (119). Prone positioning of the patient may also be of value in the prevention of air block glaucoma and its sequellae (119).

Other intraocular gases

The use of air in retinal reattachment surgery is limited by its relatively rapid absorption in the posterior segment. The use of other intraocular gases has been advocated when a tamponade effect of greater than 2 days' duration is required (123). Complications associated with the use of these agents have been defined in several laboratory and clinical studies and are reviewed briefly below.

Sulfur hexafluoride. Numerous investigators have assessed experimentally the effects of sulfur hexafluoride (SF_6) on ocular structure and function (112,114,125–129).

1. Corneal endothelium: Instillation of a sulfur hexafluoride-air mixture into the anterior chamber of rabbits resulted in endothelial abnormalities including a "peau d'orange" appearance on slit-lamp biomicroscopy, with endothelial cell degeneration noted on ultrastructural examination. These changes were transient, however, and no permanent endothelial lesions were noted (126). The ability of rabbit corneal endothelium to undergo mitosis following injury might limit the applicability of this study in terms of the clinical usage of SF_6.

2. Uveal tract: A transient uveitis with cell and tension elevation was found to occur, and was maximal within 24 hr of injection. These observations led the authors of this study to recommend careful monitoring of intraocular pressure beginning six hours after surgery (114).

3. Cataract: Lens opacities developing in owl monkeys following injection of SF_6 were related to gas bubble-lens contact, as in the case of intraocular air-induced cataract (113). Typically, posterior subcapsular changes evolved and progressed following a 12-hr period of gas-lens contact; partial clearing of the opacities was noted upon absorption or removal of the gas bubble (121).

4. Retinal function: No differences in electroretinographic B-wave amplitude or threshold responses were noted in owl monkeys undergoing intraocular injection of SF_6 as compared with control animals (113).

5. Ocular histopathology: Histopathologic examination of monkey eyes enucleated following injection of air or SF_6 was remarkable only for mild retinal edema (113). No histopathologic lesions were noted in rabbit eyes examined after intravitreal injection of 0.1 ml of SF_6 (128).

The current clinical experience with SF_6 is limited and the adverse effects encountered during the use of this agent are listed below:

1. Glaucoma: In one series intraocular pressures exceeding 30 mm Hg were noted in 45 of 101 patients receiving intravitreal SF_6 (129). Intraocular pressure elevations were more pronounced in patients receiving 100% SF_6. This observation confirmed the findings of previous investigators (114). Eleven of the 101 patients in this series developed central retinal artery occlusion with loss of light perception; the fact that 10 of these 11 patients had postoperative elevations of intraocular pressure underscores the potential gravity of glaucoma following gas injection. Use of a mixture containing 40% SF_6 and 60% air has been recommended to minimize bubble expansion and forestall the development of elevations of intraocular pressure (125).

2. Cataract: Between 27% (120) and 60% (119) of patients undergoing intraocular SF_6 injection in reported series developed significant lens opacities within 6 months of surgery. Interpreting these statistics is difficult, however, as cataract formation in this patient population may also reflect trauma at the time of surgery or underlying ocular disease such as persistent retinal detachment.

3. Iritis: Twenty-six of 101 patients in the study cited above developed a transient fibrinous iritis, attributed to iris-gas bubble contact. Iritis was more severe in diabetic patients. Fibrinous exudation into the anterior chamber was associated with a higher incidence of elevated intraocular pressure in this study (129).

4. Miscellaneous: Intravitreal injection of the SF_6 in pseudophakic patients may result in forward displacement of the implant with endothelial touch and corneal decompensation (131). This complication may be prevented by simultaneous intracameral injection of SF_6 (131) or by placement of a transcorneal suture to limit forward movement of the implant (132). Iatrogenic retinal breaks, inadvertent subretinal injection of gas, and injection site hemorrhage are also documented complications of SF_6 injection (129).

Perfluorocarbon gases. Animal studies have defined the ocular toxicity associated with anterior segment and posterior segment injection of these highly insoluble and long-lasting gases.

1. Anterior segment injection: Rabbits receiving 0.15 ml of a mixture of SF_6 and C_4F_8 by intracameral injection developed marked conjunctival hyperemia, corneal opacification with edema, exudative iritis, iris atrophy, cataract, and profound glaucoma with optic disc cupping. These changes were less severe when bubble volume was reduced to 0.1 ml or when a mixture of 40% SF_6-C_4F_8 and 60% air was used; anterior lens capsule opacification and iritis with peripheral anterior synechia formation were noted even in these animals, however (125). In a study utilizing owl monkeys intracameral injection of either pure C_4F_8 or a mixture of 40% C_4F_8 and 60% air was associated with the development of mature cataract (115).

The anterior segment toxicity of another perfluorocarbon, perfluoropentane, has also been investigated. Injection of 2 μl of this agent into the anterior chamber of rabbit eyes was followed by the rapid development of glaucoma with chamber deepening (secondary to bubble expansion), iritis with posterior synechiae formation, corneal edema, and cataract. Injection instead of 0.5 μl of perfluoropentane resulted in no immediate reaction, with the exception of a mild transient iritis; 1 week following injection, however, there were noted areas of localized corneal haze and localized opacification of the anterior lens capsule in 60% and 20% of treated animals, respectively, corresponding to areas of gas bubble contact. These changes regressed with bubble resorption (133).

2. Posterior segment injection: Cataract formation similar to that encountered with SF_6 has been described with the experimental use of various perfluorocarbon gases, including perfluoroethane, perfluoropentane, and octafluorocyclobutane. Early changes included a fine posterior subcapsular granularity; later typical posterior subcapsular cataracts developed (104,134). Lens opacification following gas injection has been attributed to mechanical interference by the gas bubble with nutrient and waste product transport across the posterior capsule (133). In support of this hypothesis is the observation that cataract incidence increases in direct relation to the volume of the gas bubble and the area of the bubble-lens interface (115). Lens opacities may clear with bubble (113,134) resorption, as in the case of SF_6- and air-associated lens changes.

Intravitreal injection of 1 to 2 μl of perfluoropentane in rabbits resulted in cataract formation along with forward movement of the lens-iris diaphragm, shallowing of the anterior chamber, glaucoma, and corneal edema. No significant anterior segment complications were observed following intravitreal injection of 0.5 μl of this agent (133).

Intraocular pressure elevation following perfluorocarbon injection during vitrectomy is related to the percentage of vitreous volume replaced with gas and the concentration of gas injected, as noted in the discussion of intraocular pressure elevation associated with SF_6.

Intravitreal injection of C_4F_8 in monkeys is associated with temporary disruption of the blood-ocular barrier. Vascular permeability normalizes with gas absorption (112).

Numerous histopathologic studies have failed to reveal significant lesions in animal eyes following injection of perfluorocarbon gases, with the possible exception of posterior cortical vacuolation of the lens (112,115,128,132).

The manifestations of perfluorocarbon toxicity noted in the limited clinical usage of these agents are qualitatively similar to the adverse effects noted in the animal studies described above. In one report, injection of a mixture of 40% C_4F_8 and 60% air resulted in mild iritis with a transient elevation of intraocular pressure (135).

Other considerations

Intraocular gas injection and general anesthesia. As noted above, intraocular injection of insoluble gases will be associated with a postoperative increase in bubble volume. The expansion in bubble volume is mediated by the diffusion of soluble blood-borne gases (particularly nitrogen) into the newly created ocular cavity until the partial pressures in the eye and in the bloodstream are equal for each gas; diffusion of the injected gas out of the eye is limited by low gas solubility. It follows that injection of room air should not be associated with bubble expansion, as the components of the injected gas in this case (i.e., air) are already in toric equilibrium with blood-borne gases. This prediction has been borne out experimentally (114). It also follows that alterations in the gaseous composition of the bloodstream will result in a disequilibrium with an intraocular air bubble and a secondary change in bubble volume. These theoretical considerations achieve clinical relevance in the case of nitrous oxide inhalation anesthesia. Administration of nitrous oxide during or after the injection of intraocular gas will allow anesthetic diffusion into the intraocular gas bubble with a rapid increase in bubble volume and elevation of the intraocular pressure. It has been calculated in an elegant computer simulation of the interaction between intraocular gases and anesthetic agents that continuation of 70% nitrous oxide inhalation anesthesia after gas injection would result in a rapid threefold increase in bubble volume (136). Cessation of nitrous oxide anesthesia at the time of injection and 15 min prior to injection would be associated with a 35% or 15% increase in bubble volume, respectively. The resultant changes in intraocular pressure depend on other factors (including scleral rigidity, anterior chamber depth, and preoperative outflow facility) in addition to changes in bubble volume, and are less easily calculated. At any rate, experimental studies in monkeys have confirmed the results of this computer simulation; intraocular administration of 0.5 ml of air in an animal receiving 75% nitrous oxide inhalation anesthesia is associated with a 16 mm Hg increment in intraocular pressure returned to a normal level within 27 min of cessation of anesthesia, presumably with a rapid (and undesirable) decrease in bubble volume (137). These considerations have led several authors to suggest that nitrous oxide be withheld during procedures calling for intraocular gas injection (138), or that nitrous oxide administration be discontinued at or prior to the time of injection (136).

Atmospheric pressure. Several investigators have pointed out that a drop in environmental atmospheric pressure may result in the expansion of an intraocular gas bubble with the development of acute glaucoma (119,138). Air travel in nonpressurized aircraft should thus perhaps be avoided in the immediate postoperative period.

Silicone Oils

Silicone oils constitute another large group of materials employed in vitreoretinal surgery. Although these compounds have been investigated experimentally and clinically for over 20 years (139,140), their use has remained controversial due to concerns about the long-term toxicity of these agents. In this section, we will summarize the results of clinical and experimental studies addressing the question of silicone oil toxicity.

Experimental studies

In one study, intravitreal injection of silicone oil in rabbits was well tolerated over an unspecified follow-up period, with no evidence of retinal injury, cataract formation, glaucoma, or intraocular inflammation (141). Similarly, no complications of oil injection were observed in a second rabbit study after a 2-year postinjection follow-up period (139). These results were confirmed in a third series of experiments using rabbits, cats, and monkeys; no anterior or posterior segment lesions were noted at the time the experiment concluded 15 months following injection (142). One author, however, reported the development of keratopathy in rabbits following migration of the oil bubble into the anterior chamber after intravitreal injection (143). This finding contrasts with the observation in another study that intracameral injection of silicone oil was well tolerated in 35 of 36 rabbit eyes. One eye in this series developed pupillary block glaucoma due, presumably, to occlusion of the pupil by the oil bubble; no changes in tonographic facility of outflow or aqueous humor biochemistry were evident (141).

Mild-to-moderate anterior uveitis and cataract formation have been described in animal eyes following intravitreal oil injection (144). Retinal toxicity has been of perhaps special concern, as these agents are used in patients with severe preexistent retinal disease, in whom further retinal injury should be avoided. In one study only transient inner nuclear layer edema was present in rabbit eyes following the injection of silicone oil during a 6-month follow-up period. The same finding was noted in saline-injected control eyes. "Bubbles" noted in the retina and sclera upon histopathologic examination of these eyes were thought to represent artifacts of tissue processing (145). One author, however, has described retinal ganglion cell degeneration following oil injection (144). A second investigator has demonstrated migration of silicone oil droplets into the retina through openings in the inner limiting membrane; histochemical techniques revealed aggregates of retinal phospholipids around silicone oil globules within minutes of injection (146).

Clinical studies

Reports of adverse reactions to silicone oil injection abound in the literature, and are summarized in Table 3. Specific lesions attributed to silicone oil toxicity are discussed briefly below.

Operative complications of silicone oil injection. Operative complications of oil injection include iatrogenic retinal tears, inadvertent subretinal injection of silicone, injection site hemorrhage, and development of pupillary block glaucoma. The latter may be associated with herniation of vitreous or retinal tissue through the injection site or surgical wound, migration of silicone into the anterior chamber, or vascular occlusion (147).

Late complications of silicone oil injection. Intraocular silicone oil is generally

TABLE 3. *Complications of silicone oil injection*

Author	Complications
Cibis (140)	Massive periretinal proliferation, endophthalmitis, retinal detachment, keratopathy, fibrous ingrowth at injection site
Okun (147)	Keratopathy, cataract, glaucoma, retinal detachment
Grey and Leaver (148)	Keratopathy, cataract
Scott (149)	Keratopathy
Leaver et al. (150)	Keratopathy, cataract, glaucoma
Watzke (151)	Cataract, glaucoma, macular pucker
Scott (152)	Glaucoma
Watzke (153)	Massive periretinal proliferation
Sugar and Okamura (154)	Anterior segment necrosis
Everett (155)	Panophthalmitis

well tolerated for up to 5 years postinjection (140), but numerous late complications of oil injection have been reported, including the following:

1. Keratopathy: Corneal changes following silicone oil injection range from mild haze (145) to progressive stromal opacification with vascularization and the development of bullous (140,147–149) keratopathy. A brownish discoloration of Bowman's membrane may also be noted (140), and frank band keratopathy may occur (150). The severity of corneal damage correlates directly with the extent of contact of silicone with the posterior corneal surface; keratopathy is said to be most pronounced in aphakic patients with large oil droplets resting against the endothelium (148). Trauma may also result in anterior migration of intravitreal silicone and subsequent corneal decompensation (140).

2. Cataract: The incidence of cataract following silicone injection varies from 49% to 57% (147,148,150) after 1 year to 74% to 85% (148,150) after 2 years. The lens opacities are initially posterior subcapsular in location and later progress to involve the entire lens (148). It has been stated that lens opacification will occur in every patient undergoing silicone oil injection given an adequate period of follow-up (151). Other investigators have noted, however, that the underlying vitreoretinal disease necessitating silicone oil injection in this patient population is associated with a high incidence of cataract development even in the absence of surgical intervention (152).

3. Glaucoma: Glaucoma has been reported in 2% to 15% (146,148,150) of oil recipients and is associated with the presence of silicone oil droplets in the superior angle in 63% to 100% (148,150) of cases. The observations of oil droplets in the superior angle is not, however, predictive of a subsequent elevation of intraocular pressure. This finding was present in 25% to 40% (148,150) of patients following silicone oil injection, but only 25% to 42% (148,150) of patients with oil droplets in the superior angle develop glaucoma.

4. Retinal dysfunction: Inferior retinal detachment may follow silicone oil injection as a result of inferior subretinal injection or localization of oil and

subsequent superior migration of this buoyant material (147). Recurrent detachment and macular pucker may occur on the basis of continued vitreoretinal proliferation, as well (140,143). The effect of silicone on retinal function is difficult to ascertain, as intraocular silicone acts as an insulating substance and interferes with the performance of conventional electrophysiological studies (150). The existence of a functional "silicone retinopathy" (154) per se is thus still open to question (150).

5. Miscellaneous: Anterior segment necrosis occurred in one eye 4 months following injection of silicone oil during repair of a giant retinal tear (154). In two cases violent intraocular inflammation simulating endophthalmitis was noted shortly after oil injection (140,155). Fibrous ingrowth at the site of oil injection has also been documented (140).

Pathologic correlates. Histopathologic findings have been reported in several instances where enucleation followed silicone injection, and these observations are summarized in Table 4. Of special interest is the description by several authors (147,150) of silicone-globule laden macrophages in the anterior chamber and trabecular meshwork. This finding suggests that the glaucoma associated with silicone oil injection may be due in part to a cellular reaction to this foreign material and not to specific toxic properties of silicone itself. In addition, numerous silicone bubbles were observed in the glaucomatous optic nerve of an eye studied in our laboratory twelve years following injection of silicone oil. Intraneural migration of silicone may thus constitute yet another

TABLE 4. *Histopathologic findings following silicone oil injection*

Report	Site of silicone deposition	Comments
Okun (147)	Retina, anterior chamber	Macrophagic response in anterior chamber; minimal intraretinal inflammation
Leaver (150)	Corneal endothelium, anterior and posterior lens cortex, trabecular endothelium, retina (Müller cells and extracellular space)	Enucleation 2 yr postinjection; globule-laden macrophages in trabecular meshwork; neurosensory retina largely spared
Sugar & Okamura (154)	Vitreous, retina	Enucleation 4 mo postinjection; minimal intraretinal inflammation
Blodi (156)	Iris, retina, corneal scar	Enucleation 7 yr postinjection
Watzke (157)	Preretinal membrane, retina, subretinal space, trabeculum, iris root	Enucleation 2 yr postinjection
Ni (157a)	Corneal scar, iris stroma trabeculum, ciliary body, retina, preretinal and subretinal membranes	Enucleation 12 yr postinjection

mechanism through which silicone oil-related optic nerve damage may develop (157).

The presence of intraretinal silicone in all enucleated human eyes studied confirms (147,149,154,156,157) the results of the animal experiments cited above (146). There was surprisingly little inflammation or tissue disruption associated with intraretinal silicone in the human specimens examined, however. The precise significance of intraretinal migration of silicone thus remains uncertain.

Recently routine removal of silicone oil 8 weeks following injection has been advocated as a means of avoiding the sequellae associated with the long-term presence of intraocular oil (158). Complications associated with the temporary use of intraocular silicone await further definition.

Miscellaneous Vitreous Substitutes

Several other substances have been introduced into the anterior chamber or vitreous cavity as volume supplements, with occasional adverse reactions, as noted below.

Hyaluronic acid

Hyaluronic acid has been used in the replacement of vitreous since 1960 and has been generally well tolerated (159). In early studies intravitreal injection of hyaluronic acid resulted in transient vitreous haze (159) and mild iritis and vitritis, possibly related to the pH of the preparation used (160). As currently formulated sodium hyaluronate is iso-osmotic and has a physiologic pH.

Recently sodium hyaluronate 1% has achieved widespread use as an adjunct in intraocular lens implantation. As an aqueous substitute this viscoelastic substance provides endothelial protection from mechanical trauma during lens implantation (161–164). Several studies utilizing specular microscopy (162), pachometry (162–164), light microscopy with trypan blue staining (164), and scanning and transmission electron microscopy of corneal specimens following *in vivo* instillation of sodium hyaluronate into the rabbit anterior chamber (162,163) and *in vitro* perfusion of isolated rabbit corneal buttons with hyaluronate (164) have demonstrated that this agent is nontoxic to the corneal endothelium.

Several reports have indicated that the use of sodium hyaluronate in the anterior chamber during surgery may be associated with a postoperative elevation of intraocular pressure (165,166). In one experimental study, maximal intraocular pressures of 48 and 67 mm Hg were noted in rabbit and monkey eyes at periods of 3 hr and 90 min, respectively, following hyaluronate injection. Intraocular pressure elevation was of lesser magnitude and of shorter duration in eyes undergoing balanced salt solution irrigation at the conclusion of the surgical procedure (164). In a second study, instillation of sodium hyaluronate into the anterior chambers of enucleated human eyes caused a 65% decrease in outflow facility in unoperated eyes and a 76% decrease in facility in eyes in which corneal or limbal sutures were placed prior to a hyaluronate perfusion. Obstruction to aqueous outflow was not relieved in either group of eyes by irrigation with BSS; irrigation with hyaluronidase, however, was successful in restoring outflow facility to baseline values (167). Clinically, the tendency for pressure elevation is especially pronounced in eyes containing a mixture of hyaluronate, lens material, and blood (166).

Despite initial concerns to the contrary (168), there is no apparent inhibition by sodium hyaluronate of corneoscleral wound healing in experimental studies (169).

In marked contrast to hyaluronic acid is hyaluronic acid sulfate, which is highly toxic to ocular tissues. Intravitreal administration of this agent is followed by rapid corneal opacification, elevation of intraocular pressure, cataract formation, zonulolysis with subluxation of the lens, rubeosis iridis with hyphema, vitreous liquefaction, vitreous membrane formation, and retinal detachment (170,171).

Chondroitin sulfate

This mucopolysaccharide has also been employed in the protection of the endothelium during intraocular lens surgery (172). In one study, 20% chondroitin sulfate provided excellent endothelial protection during intraocular lens implantation in rabbits, as assessed with trypan blue staining and light microscopy. *In vitro* corneal perfusion studies, however, revealed marked, albeit reversible, decreases in corneal thickness following perfusion with 20% chondroitin sulfate alone or dissolved in balanced salt solution; these changes were attributed to the hyperosmolality of these solutions (656 and 1,052 mOsm, respectively). Scanning electron microscopy of corneas perfused with 20% chondroitin sulfate with balanced salt solution revealed loss of endothelial cell microvilli and mild loosening of endothelial cell junctions. Transmission electron microscopy of corneas perfused with 20% chondroitin sulfate alone demonstrated mild endothelial edema (164).

Clearance of this agent from the anterior chamber occurs in 24 to 30 hr following surgery, as compared with the 1- to 2-week period occasionally needed for clearance of sodium hyaluronate (165). One group of investigators found no significant elevations in intraocular pressure in animals 24 hr following intracameral injection of chondroitin sulfate (173). In a second study, however, anterior chamber administration of 20% chondroitin sulfate resulted in intraocular pressure peaks of 50 and 55 mm Hg 2 hr and 90 min after injection in rabbits and monkeys, respectively; intracameral irrigation of monkey eyes with BSS following chondroitin sulfate administration resulted in a less marked elevation of intraocular pressure at 90 min (30 mm Hg). An intraocular pressure peak of 37 mm Hg was noted 90 min following the instillation of 10% chondroitin sulfate in rabbit eyes (164).

Mild anterior subcapsular lens vacuolation was noted three months after instillation of 20% chondroitin sulfate in three of four monkey eyes studied (164).

Methylcellulose

This highly viscous compound has also been proposed for use in the protection of the endothelium during lens implantation. In one study an elevation in intraocular pressure of 45 mm Hg was noted 1 day following use of methylcellulose during intraocular lens implantation in patients (174). In a second study, a maximal intraocular pressure of 36 mm Hg was observed 2 hr following intracameral injection. Methylcellulose provided only moderate protection of the endothelium from mechanical trauma, although perfusion studies revealed no ultrastructural evidence of endothelial toxicity. No tendency for late lens opacification was noted (164).

Whole vitreous implants

Implantation of centrifuged whole vitreous into cat eyes resulted in a high incidence of vitreous opacification and retinal detachment (175). Several complications were noted in a series of vitreous implants in 72 human eyes, including cataract (2 patients), glaucoma (3 patients), rubeosis iridis, and vitreous hemorrhage (1 patient each). Vitreous haze was commonly present following implantation but generally cleared within 10 days of surgery (176). Endophthalmitis is another acknowledged risk of whole vitreous implantation (177,178).

Polygeline

This colloidal plasma volume expander has been instilled in rabbit eyes in concentrations up to 3.5% without incident. Higher concentrations were associated with iritis, vitritis, and mild elevation of intraocular pressure (179). In limited clinical studies, intravitreal polygeline was similarly well tolerated, with one of 13 patients in the treatment group developing an elevation of intraocular pressure of uncertain etiology (180).

Glyceryl methacrylate hydrogel

Transient vitreous opacification was observed following experimental implantation of glyceryl methacrylate hydrogel in the vitreous cavity. No evidence of uveitis or intraretinal inflammation was noted (193).

Polyethylene sulfonic acid

Intravitreal administration of this highly toxic substance in rabbits resulted in severe disorganization of the globe, with band keratopathy, cataract, lens dislocation, vitreous liquefaction and membrane formation, and retinal detachment (182).

Dextran and dextran sulfate

Dextran 500 and dextran sulfate 500 were well tolerated in the vitreous cavities of cats. Instillation of progressively higher molecular weight dextrans, however, was associated with progressive vitreous opacification and ocular inflammation. Instillation of a 0.08% solution of dextran sulfate 2000 resulted in phthisis bulbi. Vitreous liquefaction occurred in all treated animals, including those receiving low molecular weight dextrans (175).

Acrylamide

In one experimental study, intravitreal implantation of acrylamide was associated with anterior uveitis of 10 days' duration, vitritis of 6 weeks' duration, and a significant incidence of cataract, retinal break formation, and retinal detachment. In limited clinical studies with six patients, one patient developed severe vitritis following acrylamide implantation while vitreoretinal proliferation occurred in a second patient (183). In a second experimental study, intracameral injection of poly(2-hydroxy ethyl acrylate) (PHEA) resulted in fibrinous iritis with membrane formation, increased intraocular pressure, corneal edema, and lens opacification. Findings after posterior segment injection of PHEA included vitreous haze, vitreous membrane formation, localized chorioretinal atrophy, and development of posterior subcapsular cataracts. Chronic nongranulomatous anterior vitritis and retinal disorganization with gliosis and chorioretinal scarring were observed histopathologically (183).

Collagen gel

Anterior uveitis was noted in approximately one-third of patients in a clinical study of 16 human eyes; this reaction was severe and was associated with the development of a hypopyon in two of the 16 eyes treated. Biomicroscopic observation revealed rapid fragmentation and degradation of the collagen gel even in cases in which gel implantation was apparently well tolerated (184).

Intravitreal Antimicrobial Agents

Bacterial and fungal endophthalmitis have long represented a major source of visual morbidity in postoperative patients and in debilitated or immunocompromised patients predisposed to disseminated systemic infection. In the past successful management of this difficult problem has been limited by several factors including delay in specific bacteriologic diagnosis and inability to achieve adequate intraocular antimicrobial levels through periocular or systemic administration. The uniformly grim prognosis associated with end-ophthalmitis has in recent times been modified somewhat by the introduction of new therapeutic modalities including pars plana vitrectomy and instillation of intravitreal antibiotics (185). Numerous experimental and clinical studies, however, have demonstrated that this mode of drug delivery may itself be associated with the potential for significant ocular injury. Several reports outlining the toxicity of individual intravitreal antimicrobial agents are reviewed below.

Gentamicin

In one study intravitreal administration of 500 μg of this aminoglycoside antibiotic in noninfected albino rabbits resulted in no evidence of toxicity by histopathologic or electroretinographic criteria. Instillation of 1,000 μg of gentamicin resulted in electrophysiologic abnormalities with focal retinal destruction noted on histopathologic examination. Cataract formation and development of band keratopathy were noted at dosages exceeding 2,000 and 8,000 μg, respectively. Intracameral administration of a dosage of 8,000 μg was well tolerated, with only a transient postoperative iritis (186). In a second report, clinical and pathologic abnormalities following intravitreal administration of gentamicin in dosages up to 500 μg were limited to fine posterior subcapsular lens vacuolation which regressed within 5 weeks of injection (187). These findings contrast markedly, however, with those of other studies. In one report, intravitreal administration of 500 μg of gentamicin was associated with posterior subcapsular lens vacuolation in 10 of 10 eyes, choroiditis in 6 of 10 eyes, and vitritis, severe chorioretinitis, and retinal degeneration and scarring in 1 of 10 eyes treated (188). In another study intravitreal injection of 400 μg was followed by extinction of the electroretinogram; retinal edema, disorganization of the nuclear layers, disruption of the photoreceptor outer segments, and degeneration of the retinal pigment epithelium were noted histopathologically. Several animals demonstrated electroretinographic abnormalities and focal retinal lesions on light microscopy following administration of 100 μg of gentamicin. A further reduction of dosage to 50 μg was associated with no evidence of drug toxicity (189).

The apparent discrepancies between the results of these studies may be due in part to differences in location and technique of intravitreal injection (189,190). In a study designed to test this hypothesis injection into the posterior part of the rabbit vitreous cavity with the needle bevel facing the retina was associated with histopathologic evidence of toxicity at dosages as low as 30 μg. On the other hand, dosages up to 200 μg were well tolerated when administered into the anterior vitreous with the needle bevel facing the anterior chamber. The latter finding prompted the authors of this study to recommend this technique of intravitreal antibiotic administration in the treatment of patients with endophthalmitis. A dosage of gentamicin of 400 μg was recommended on the basis of this study, in view of the fact that the volume of the vitreous cavity in the human eye is more than twice that of the rabbit eye (190). Other authors, however, have suggested a gentamicin dosage of 100 μg for clinical use (191).

Incorporation of gentamicin in irrigation solutions used during vitrectomy procedures in rabbits resulted in retinal damage when drug concentration equalled or exceeded 25 μg/ml of irrigant (190).

Tobramycin

In one report, intravitreal administration of 500 μg of tobramycin was well tolerated in nine of 10 eyes, with chorioretinal scarring noted in 1 eye (188). In another study retinal structure and function were preserved following intravitreal injection of tobramycin in dosages up to 750 μg. Focal retinal disorganization was observed with dosages equalling or exceeding 1,000 μg. Transient posterior subcapsular vacuolation was noted at the 1,000 μg dosage level as well, and progression of these opacities to mature cataracts occurred with dosages of 4,000 to 8,000 μg. In addition, administration of 4,000 μg of tobramycin was associated with the development of uveitis and extinction of the electroretinogram.

Irrigating solutions containing 10 μg/ml tobramycin resulted in no evidence of toxicity when instilled during vitrectomy procedures in rabbit eyes. Focal retinal lesions could be demonstrated histopathologically in animals receiving irrigants containing 20 μg/ml, although the electroretinogram remained normal in this group. Extinction of the electroretinogram and profound disruption of the retinal architecture were noted following intravitreal irrigation with solutions containing 50 μg/ml of tobramycin (192).

Amikacin

Studies investigating the potential use of this new aminoglycoside antibiotic in vitrectomy irrigating solutions have revealed a pattern of toxicity similar to that of tobramycin. Incorporation of amikacin in the irrigant in concentrations up to 10 μg/ml resulted in no evident retinal toxicity. Infusate concentrations of 20 and 50 μg/ml were associated with focal retinal disorganization and with extensive retinal destruction and compromise of retinal function, respectively (192).

The precise mechanism through which aminoglycoside antibiotics exert their toxic effects on the retina and retinal pigment epithelium remains to be defined. In one rabbit study, however, numerous abnormal intracytoplasmic inclusions were noted in the retinal pigment epithelium and in the inner plexiform layer following intravitreal administration of gentamicin. Disruption of photoreceptor outer segments with relative sparing of the inner segments was also observed, and subsequent ophthalmoscopic examination revealed a pigmentary retinopathy with areas of retinal pigment epithelial disorganization and retinal atrophy. These observations have led the authors of this study to postulate an alteration of retinal pigment epithelial lysosomal metabolism as a possible pathogenetic mechanism of aminoglycoside retinal toxicity (193).

Cephaloridine

No histopathologic or electrophysiologic manifestations of toxicity were noted following intravitreal administration of 250 µg of cephaloridine in rabbit eyes. Disruption of photoreceptor outer segments, RPE degeneration, and retinal hemorrhage were observed with increasing frequency as drug dosage was advanced from 500 to 5,000 µg. Intravitreal administration of 10,000 µg of cephaloridine resulted in marked anterior and posterior segment inflammation with extinction of the electroretinogram within 24 hours of injection (188,196).

Penicillin

Incorporation of penicillin in vitrectomy irrigating solutions in a concentration of 80 µg/ml was compatible with the preservation of normal retinal architecture and function. Electroretinographic findings remained normal when the drug concentration was raised to 100 µg/ml, although histopathologic abnormalities including cytoplasmic vacuolation and ganglion cell nuclear pyknosis were evident (195).

Carbenicillin

Cataract formation was evident in rabbits receiving intravitreal injections of this semisynthetic penicillin in dosages exceeding ten milligrams. Retinal attenuation, disorganization of nuclear layers, and retinal destruction were noted in animals receiving dosages of 15 to 20 mg; dosages of 8 to 10 mg were associated with relatively circumscribed areas of retinal thinning and less profound disruption of the retinal architecture. A dosage of 7 mg was thus considered to be the maximal nontoxic dosage of carbenicillin for intravitreal administration in this study (196).

Oxacillin

Infusion of irrigating solutions containing oxacillin in a concentration of 10 µg/ml was associated with no anatomic or electrophysiologic evidence of retinal toxicity (195).

Methicillin

No morphologic or electrophysiologic abnormalities were noted in rabbit eyes receiving up to 10 mg of methicillin by intravitreal injection (197). The infusion of irrigating fluid containing 25 μg/ml of methicillin was also well tolerated during vitrectomy procedures in rabbits. Histopathologic evidence of retinal injury was apparent following infusion of a solution containing 50 μg/ml of methicillin in combination with gentamicin 8 μg/ml (195).

Vancomycin

Intravitreal administration of 1 mg of vancomycin produced no appreciable evidence of ocular toxicity. Dosages of 2 to 5 mg of vancomycin were associated with the development of focal retinal lesions, and a profound vitritis was noted with dosages exceeding 5 mg. Intravitreal injection of vancomycin in dosages exceeding 10 mg was followed by total retinal destruction and disorganization (198).

Lincomycin

No histopathologic or electroretinographic abnormalities were observed following intravitreal injection of lincomycin in dosages up to 1500 μg. Neuroretinal lesions ranging from focal disruption to panretinal necrosis were noted with dosages of 5,000 to 10,000 μg. The outer retinal layers including the photoreceptors were thought to be more susceptible to the toxic effects of this agent. Lens opacification was noted at higher lincomycin dosages as well (199).

Clindamycin

Infusion of a clindamycin-containing solution into rabbit eyes was well tolerated at a drug concentration of 10 μg/ml alone or in combination with gentamicin 8 μg/ml. Higher concentrations of clindamycin were associated with progressive ocular injury as assessed by electroretinography and histo-pathologic examination of treated eyes (192).

Chloramphenicol

No lesions were noted ophthalmoscopically in rabbits receiving intravitreal injections of chloramphenicol in dosages up to 5 mg. Dosages exceeding 2 mg, however, were associated with electrophysiologic abnormalities, with extinction of the electroretinogram noted at a dosage of 5 mg. Focal retinal destruction was evident histopathologically at this dosage as well (200). Chloramphenicol was nontoxic when used in vitrectomy irrigating solutions in concentrations up to 20 μg/ml (192).

Moxalactam

The toxicity of this third-generation cephalosporin was investigated in a study assessing the efficacy of this agent in the treatment of experimental staphylococcal endophthalmitis in rabbits. Electroretinographic and histopathologic findings suggested that 2 mg was the maximal nontoxic intravitreal dosage of moxalactam. Focal retinal abnormalities were noted in two eyes receiving lower dosages (250 to 500 μg) of moxalactam, but these lesions were ascribed to mechanical trauma at the time of injection. Instillation of higher dosages of this antibiotic resulted in progressive retinal destruction. All eyes demonstrated transient conjunctival hyperemia and chemosis following injection (201).

Amphotericin B

Adverse effects associated with the intravitreal administration of this antifungal agent vary somewhat from report to report. In one study intravitreal injection of amphotericin B in dosages as low as 1 to 10 μg resulted in pronounced vitreal inflammation. Injection of dosages of 75 to 100 μg was followed by severe vitritis, retinal detachment, and lens opacification. Dosages exceeding 1,000 μg resulted in the rapid development of mature cataracts. Histopathologic studies in this series of animals revealed retinal necrosis and retinal breaks at the 1 μg dosage level and confirmed the presence of cataract, choroiditis, and chorioretinal scarring at higher dosage levels (202). In a second set of experiments, however, no ophthalmoscopic, histopathologic, or electroretinographic manifestations of toxicity were noted in animals treated with 5 to 10 μg of intravitreal amphotericin B. Vitritis, retinal necrosis, and retinal detachment were observed in this study at dosage levels exceeding 25 μg (203).

Intracameral application of amphotericin B was performed in a third set of rabbit experiments designed to evaluate the toxicity of this modality in the adjunctive therapy of fungal corneal ulcers. Instillation of 25 μg amphotericin B resulted in conjunctival injection, dilation of iris blood vessels, and lens opacities. These changes resolved within 36 hr of injection. Injection of 50 μg resulted in conjunctival injection, iris hyperemia, cataract, and corneal edema, all resolving within 96 hr of injection. Administration of 125 μg amphotericin B, however, was associated with a severe and persistent uveitis, cataract formation, and irreversible corneal opacification (204).

Experience with intraocular administration of amphotericin B in the therapy of fungal ocular infections in humans is limited. In one report, a patient receiving a total dosage of 77.5 μg amphotericin B by intracameral administration developed a corneal pannus, vitreous membrane formation, total retinal detachment, and loss of light perception (204). Bare light perception only was preserved in a second patient with postoperative *Cephalosporium* sp. endophthalmitis treated with a total of 40 μg amphotericin B by anterior chamber injection in addition to topical, subconjunctival, and intravenous antifungal therapy (205). It must be noted that the relatively poor visual outcome in these cases may have reflected the extent and virulence of the underlying infection rather than the toxicity of amphotericin B itself.

Miconazole

In one study miconazole nitrate and its vehicle chremophor-EL were associated with significant ocular toxicity including lens opacification, vitritis, and retinal edema, necrosis, and detachment when injected intravitreally in rabbit eyes in dosages exceeding 100 μg. Mild to moderate retinal changes were noted following administration of dosages ranging from 10 to 80 μg. No ophthalmoscopic, electrophysiologic, or histopathologic abnormalities were evident in owl monkeys receiving up to 80 μg of miconazole. On the basis of these findings a maximal dosage of 40 micrograms was recommended for clinical use (206). In one report intravitreal injection of 10 μg of miconazole nitrate was apparently well tolerated in the treatment of endophthalmitis caused by amphotericin B and flucytosine-resistant *Paecilomyces lilacinus.*

Enzymes of Use in Ophthalmic Surgery

Alpha-Chymotrypsin (ACT)

Alpha-chymotrypsin is an endopeptidase of molecular weight 2,500 derived from pancreatic exocrine tissue and capable of hydrolyzing specific peptide bonds involving the amino acids L-tyrosine, L-phenylalanine, L-tryptophan, L-methionine, and L-leucine as well as ester, amide, hydroxyamide, hydrazide, and carbon-carbon bonds (208). In the monkey eye ACT acts at a poorly defined site on the zonule to produce zonular fragmentation at 1000-A intervals, and clinically this enzyme is widely employed in intracapsular cataract extraction to enhance zonulolysis and facilitate lens removal (210,211). Numerous clinical and experimental studies have been performed in an attempt to further define the adverse effects associated with the use of this agent, and these studies are summarized below.

Cornea

Alpha-chymotrypsin is minimally toxic to the corneal endothelium. In one monkey study, for example, intracameral injection of ACT was well tolerated, with no evidence of corneal endothelial injury on histopathologic examination (212). Corneal edema, opacification, and even perforation have been observed following enzyme administration in other animal studies, but these changes have always been associated with extreme elevations in intraocular pressure (212–214). In other studies, 3-min *in vivo* perfusion of rabbit corneas with ACT resulted in varying degrees of endothelial disruption and corneal opacification; similar changes were noted, however, in controls following perfusion in NSS (215). Intracorneal injection of ACT may result in true corneal swelling and opacification (214).

In early reports administration of ACT was associated with inhibition of corneoscleral wound healing, with an attendant increased incidence of complications including wound leaks, flat chamber, striate keratopathy, and uveal prolapse (216). One experimental study indicated that administration of ACT in the clinically employed dilutions of 1:5000 or 1:10,000 resulted in derangement of corneal stromal metabolism in organ cultures of calf corneas, as reflected by decreased ^{35}S incorporation in ground substance mucopolysaccharide synthesis (217). Later studies, however, revealed that the tensile strength of healing corneoscleral wounds was equal in control rabbits and in animals receiving intracameral enzyme injection (214,218,219). The apparent inhibition of wound healing mentioned above may in fact have been related to the effects of unrecognized and untreated elevations of intraocular pressure in many eyes receiving ACT.

Glaucoma

The occurrence of "enzyme-glaucoma" was first recognized in 1964 in a study describing elevations in intraocular pressure above 24.4 mm Hg in 72.5% and 23.6% of 343 eyes undergoing intracapsular cataract extraction with and without ACT, respectively (220). Typical signs and symptoms include headache, eye pain, and corneal edema in an eye with an elevated tension, deep anterior chamber, minimal anterior chamber inflammation, patent iridectomy, and gonioscopically open angle (220). The intraocular pressure elevation in these patients has been correlated in several studies with a decrease in aqueous outflow facility (221,222). The onset of intraocular pressure elevation occurs within two days of enzyme administration, and the intraocular pressure is maximal within two to five days following surgery. Without treatment, the tension generally normalizes between 7 and 19 days postoperatively; in one study of 210 eyes with ACT glaucoma only 1 eye had a persistent elevation of intraocular pressure (221). Long-term follow-up studies of treated patients reveal no evidence of permanent trabecular meshwork injury on gonioscopic or tonographic examination (221,222).

As mentioned above, intraocular pressures exceeding 24.4 mm Hg may occur in over 70% of eyes undergoing cataract extraction with ACT. Other studies, however, suggest that an elevation of intraocular pressure of 6 mm Hg or more above baseline occurs in only 17% of eyes receiving enzyme, as compared with 8% of non-enzyme-treated controls (223). Attempts to define patient groups at special risk for the development of enzyme-glaucoma through analysis of host factors including steroid-responsiveness of aqueous outflow facility and aqueous humor levels of anti-ACT have been generally unsuccessful (223). It has been demonstrated, however, that both the incidence and severity of enzyme-glaucoma are related to the total dosage of ACT injected. In one study, for example, only 55% of patients receiving 0.25 ml of ACT developed intraocular pressures exceeding 24.4 mm Hg, as compared with 70% of patients receiving 1.5 ml of enzyme (213). This observation supports the common clinical practice of using a small volume of a 1:5000 or 1:10,000 dilution of alpha-chymotrypsin.

Aqueous suppressants including carbonic anhydrase inhibitors and timolol and hyperosmotic agents constitute the mainstays of treatment of ACT glaucoma. Prophylactic efforts including preoperative acetazolamide and mannitol (224) and intraoperative administration of miotics and subconjunctival corticosteroids (221) have been largely unsuccessful.

Enzyme-glaucoma has been studied extensively in a number of animal species and has even been proposed as an experimental model for glaucoma by several authors (209,213,225,226). Several animal studies have served to elucidate the probable pathogenesis of ACT glaucoma. First, it was noted in one series of owl monkey experiments that posterior chamber injection of ACT was a prerequisite for the subsequent occurrence of enzyme-glaucoma; this observation implicated the posterior chamber structures (zonules, ciliary body, or lens itself) in the development of ACT glaucoma. As mentioned in the clinical discussion above, the rate of onset, severity, and duration of intraocular pressure elevation were all directly related in animal studies to the dosage of enzyme employed (212). In early studies no histopathologic abnormalities were noted in the outflow structures in various species in which ACT glaucoma had been induced (219,225). In one experiment utilizing owl monkeys, however, scanning electron microscopy disclosed the presence of zonular fragments apparently blocking the outflow channels in animals with elevated intraocular pressure following ACT administration (209). The relationship of enzyme-glaucoma to trabecular obstruction by zonular fragments was substantiated in a second study in which glaucoma was produced in owl monkeys by the intracameral injection of unfiltered aqueous humor from other animals previously treated with ACT (228).

Investigators have also proposed other mechanisms for the development of enzyme glaucoma, including enzyme-induced necrosis and atrophy of the ciliary muscle with resultant collapse of the trabecular meshwork and obstruction to outflow, or inhibition of "unconventional" aqueous outflow across the ciliary body (213). The prolonged elevation of intraocular pressure occurring in rabbits following enzyme administration is reduced by indomethacin, leading several authors to postulate a prostaglandin-mediated disruption of the blood-ocular barrier by ACT as another mechanism underlying the development of enzyme-glaucoma (229).

Lens

Lens subluxation presumably secondary to complete zonulolysis has been described following posterior chamber (212,213,225) or intravitreal injection of ACT in experimental models. The incidence of lens dislocation correlated directly with the extent of intraocular pressure elevation in one study (212).

Uveal tract

Transient iridocyclitis has been noted in dogs following posterior chamber administration of enzyme in dosages as low as 100 U (225,226). No morphologic evidence of ciliary body injury was apparent in 18 canine eyes undergoing intravitreal injection of 0.4 ml of 1:5000 solution of ACT. As mentioned above, however, ciliary muscle atrophy was a prominent and potentially important histopathologic finding in a series of owl monkeys undergoing posterior chamber injection of enzyme (213).

Retina and vitreous

In canine studies posterior chamber or intravitreal injection of ACT has been associated with various posterior segment abnormalities, including vitriitis, vitreous liquefaction, vitreous hemorrhage, vitreous band formation, retinal hemorrhages, intraretinal edema, and retinal detachment (212,213,225–227). Corresponding histopathologic changes include degeneration of the photoreceptor outer segments and of the retinal pigment epithelium, intraretinal fibrosis, chorioretinal scarring, retinal thinning, and loss of the ganglion cell, nerve fiber, and outer nuclear layers (212,213,230–234). The severity of the vitreous reaction to ACT injection may reflect similarities in biochemical composition of the zonules and of the vitreous gel (222). Chorioretinal lesions associated with ACT may similarly be more pronounced at the ora serrata near the zonular insertion (232). At any rate, the potential retinal complications of enzyme administration have led several authors to recommend caution in using ACT in patients with vitreous liquefaction, a ruptured anterior hyaloid, or disinsertion of the vitreous base, in whom substances injected into the posterior chamber would have direct access to the retina (232). Clinically, however, ACT has been employed in patients with ruptured anterior hyaloid membranes without complication (235).

Several studies have demonstrated that enzyme has no effect on the anterior hyaloid membrane or lenticulo-vitreous adhesions (the so-called "hyaloideo-capsular ligament") (236,237). Alpha-chymotrypsin will not, therefore, prevent vitreous loss in young patients with lenticulo-vitreous adhesions undergoing intracapsular cataract extraction, and its use for this purpose should probably be avoided (237–239).

Optic nerve

Optic atrophy, glaucomatous cupping, and gliosis of the optic nerve head have been induced in experimental animals following administration of ACT (212,213,225,230). The histopathologic changes associated with these clinical findings have been well described in an elegant study by Zimmerman and co-workers using owl monkeys and posterior chamber injection of ACT (225). During days 1 to 4 postinjection there was noted progressive hydropic degeneration of the optic nerve head at the lamina cribrosa with demyelination, axonal swelling, and papilledema. Beginning on day 4, cavernous changes were seen in the optic nerve posterior to the lamina cribrosa, and on day 7 optic atrophy and early cupping were evident. By 2 to 4 weeks, glaucomatous cupping was pronounced and microglial proliferation was noted in the optic nerve head.

The optic nerve lesions described above following enzyme administration have been attributed to the effects of elevated intraocular pressure and not to specific optic neurotoxicity associated with ACT per se. Similar alterations in optic nerve morphology have been reported, for example, following the induction of experimental glaucoma by intracameral injection of talc or dental cement (226).

Fibrinolytic Agents

Plasmin (fibrinolysin) is an enzyme which catalyzes the degradation of fibrin to fibrin degradation products. The generation of plasmin is in turn mediated by several substances including the enzymes streptokinase (SK) and urokinase (UK) and various tissue factors which accelerate the conversion of the circulating plasmin precursor plasmin to the active fibrinolytic enzyme (Fig. 2). Plasmin and various plasminogen activators have been found by several investigators to enhance the clearance of anterior chamber blood and fibrin and to decrease the incidence of secondary glaucoma, and have thus been considered useful in the management of traumatic hyphema (240–242). Significant ocular toxicity may be associated with the use of these agents, however, as discussed below.

Experimental studies

In one rabbit study, anterior chamber irrigation with solutions containing 15,000 to 30,000 units of SK was associated with a 70% incidence of transient corneal clouding and a 23% incidence of permanent corneal opacification (243). In other studies, intracameral instillation of 50,000 units of SK resulted in a severe anterior chamber reaction with profound corneal edema (244,245). Corneal opacification and swelling and anterior uveitis were similarly observed following intracameral (246) or intravitreal (247) administration of UK in concentrations from 2,500 to 5,000 U/ml in the management of experimental hyphema or vitreous hemorrhage, respectively. It is important to note, however, that in other studies *in vitro* perfusion of rabbit corneal buttons with solutions containing 1,000 to 5,000 U/ml UK resulted in no evidence of corneal endothelial injury as assessed by specular microscopy and scanning electron microscopy. This observation has led one author to suggest that the corneal

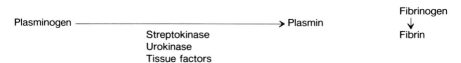

FIG. 2. Method of action of fibrinolytic agents.

changes associated with the use of plasminogen activators may reflect intense intraocular inflammation following the initiation of fibrinolysis and not inherent toxicity of the plasminogen activating substances themselves (243).

Several studies have been performed to evaluate the safety and efficacy of plasmin in the management of experimental hyphema. In one rabbit study, intracameral injection of 750 U plasmin was apparently well tolerated (248), while in another study corneal opacification and elevation of intraocular pressure were noted following plasmin administration (249). In a third study mild striate keratopathy occurred in 50% of rabbit eyes following a 30-min incubation of a blood-enzyme mixture in the anterior chamber. Histopathologic examination of treated eyes confirmed the presence of endothelial disruption and stromal edema. These corneal changes resolved within 5 days of administration of fibrinolysin in a concentration of 1,250 U/ml but persisted indefinitely following administration of enzyme in a concentration exceeding 5,000 U/ml (250).

Clinical Studies

Clinical experience with plasmin and plasminogen activators is limited. In one report, the treatment of hyphema with intracameral injections of 5,000 U SK and 200 U streptodornase was followed by severe secondary glaucoma and corneal edema in all eyes treated (n = 5) (251). In another small series, intracameral injection of SK in dosages between 25,000 and 35,000 U was associated with the development of phthisis bulbi in two patients and with the onset of pain and loss of light perception necessitating enucleation in a third eye (252). Chemosis, corneal opacification, and anterior uveitis varying in severity from mild aqueous flare to hypopyon formation have been described following intraocular administration of plasmin itself (249,253). Subconjunctival injection of plasmin has also been performed in the treatment of fibrinous iritis and has been associated with profound lid edema and chemosis (254).

Antimetabolites

Intraocular or periocular administration of antimetabolites and cytotoxic agents has been proposed as an adjunct to surgical management of various ophthalmic disorders including proliferative vitreoretinopathy, subconjunctival fibrosis following filtration surgery, and proliferation of the lens epithelium following extracapsular cataract extraction. Adverse ocular side effects associated with the systemic use of antineoplastic agents have been well-summarized in several recent reports (255,256). The more limited data available concerning the ocular toxicity of these agents following local application is reviewed below.

Intravitreal Steroid Injections

Intravitreal injection of 400 μg of dexamethasone resulted in no clinical, histopathologic, or electroretinographic evidence of toxicity in one rabbit (257) study. Intravitreal administration of 1 mg triamcinolone acetonide without a vehicle was similarly well tolerated (258).

5-Fluorouracil

This synthetic pyrimidine analogue was nontoxic when administered intravitreally in dosages up to one milligram in several studies using a rabbit model of proliferative vitreoretinopathy (259–261). In another study, however, administration of multiple 1.25-mg doses of 5-fluorouracil intravitreally resulted in corneal opacification and extinction of the electroretinogram, with photoreceptor disruption and loss of ribosomes in retinal cells noted on histopathologic and ultrastructural examination of treated eyes. Corneal changes and electrophysiologic abnormalities were reversible when the frequency of 5-fluorouracil administration was diminished, and no evidence of corneal endothelial or retinal toxicity was noted when daily 5-fluorouracil dosage was decreased to 0.5 mg (261,262).

In yet another study intravitreal 5-fluorouracil in concentrations of 10^{-5} g/ml had no effect on the electroretinographic B-wave amplitude. Diminution of the B-wave was noted at concentrations of 10^{-3}–10^{-4} g/ml, and B-wave extinction was noted at concentrations exceeding 5×10^{-3} g/ml but was reversible following replacement of the test solution with a 5-fluorouracil free medium (264).

Early clinical studies utilizing subconjunctival injections of 5-fluorouracil after trabeculectomy to minimize postoperative scarring of the filtration bleb have demonstrated an increased incidence of wound leaks, delayed wound healing, and persistent corneal epithelial defects in patients treated with this modality. These complications were reversible and resolved with discontinuation of 5-fluorouracil therapy (265). Injection of 5-fluorouracil into skin tumors involving the eyelids may be associated with subsequent scar formation and cicatricial ectropion requiring surgical correction (255).

Vinca Alkaloids

Fusiform degeneration of ganglion cell dendrites and agglutination of neurofibrils with vacuolation of perikaryon cytoplasm were noted following intravitreal injection of vincristine. The photoreceptors were reportedly unaffected, as were amacrine and bipolar cells (266). Vinblastine administration was also associated with blockage of orthograde and retrograde axonal transport in retinal ganglion cells (267). This blockage of axoplasmic flow is thought to be mediated by the binding of the vinca alkaloids to tubulin, the protein

TABLE 5. *Adverse ocular effects associated with local administration of antimetabolites and cytotoxic agents*

Agent	Observation
Thiotepa (269)	Intravitreal injection of 6 mg associated with transient lens opacification and vitreous clouding
Nitrogen mustard (269)	Intravitreal injection of dosages as low as 9 μg resulted in aqueous flare, vitreous membrane formation, and retinal hemorrhages
Cyclophosphamide (269)	Intravitreal injection of 3 mg well tolerated; injection of 6 mg followed by vitreous membrane formation
Daunorubicin (271, 272)	No electroretinographic evidence of toxicity at a vitreous concentration of 10 nmol/eye in a rabbit model of proliferative vitreoretinopathy; retinal detachment in all eyes following injection of 85 nmol/eye
Chlorambucil (273)	Extensive disruption of the neuroretina following transplacental exposure of the human fetus
Actinomycin D (274)	Marked decrease in protein synthesis in embryonic chick neuroretina exposed to actinomycin D in tissue culture

subunit of cytoplasmic microtubules, with subsequent depolymerization of formed microtubules. Disruption of rapid axonal transport may occur with intravitreal dosages of vinblastine as low as 10 μg; administration of vinblastine in dosages exceeding 500 μg may also be associated with direct suppression of ganglion cell protein synthesis (268).

Methotrexate

Intravitreal injection of 3 mg methotrexate resulted in vitreous membrane formation but not electroretinographic evidence of toxicity in a study performed to evaluate the potential toxicity of this agent in the chemotherapy of retinoblastoma (266). In another study, exposure of explants of chick embryonic neuroretina to methotrexate was followed by a decline in the regenerative capacity of proliferating cohorts of cells (259). The relevance of this observation to the possible use of this agent in the adult human is unclear.

Reports of adverse ocular effects associated with local administration of other antimetabolites and cytotoxic agents are summarized in Table 5.

REFERENCES

1. Havener, W. H. (1978): *Ocular Pharmacology,* 4th ed., C. V. Mosby, St. Louis.
2. Schlege, H. E., and Swan, K. C. (1954): Benoxinate (dorsacaine) for rapid corneal anesthesia. *Arch. Ophthalmol.,* 51:663–670.
3. Gundersen, T., and Liebman, S. D. (1944): Effect of local anesthetics on regeneration of corneal epithelium. *Arch. Ophthalmol.,* 31:29–33.
4. Kinoshita, J. H. (1962): Some aspects of carbohydrate metabolism of the cornea. *Invest. Ophthalmol. Vis. Sci.,* 1:178–186.
5. Behrendt, T. (1956): Experimental study of corneal lesions produced by topical lesions. *Am. J. Ophthalmol.,* 41:99–105.
6. Behrendt, T. (1957): Experimental secondary effects of topical anesthesia of the cornea. *Am. J. Ophthalmol.,* 44:74–77.

7. Goldsmith, M. O. (1967): Occlusion of the central retinal artery following retrobulbar hemorrhage. *Ophthalmologica,* 153:191–196.
8. Waller, R. R. (1978): Is blindness a realistic complication in blepharoplasty procedures? *Ophthalmology,* 85:730–735.
9. Carroll, R. P. (1982): Blindness following lacrimal nerve block. *Ophthalmic Surg.,* 13:812–814.
10. Sullivan, K. L., Brown, G. C., Forman, A. R., Sergott, R. C., and Flanagan, J. C. (1983): Retrobulbar anesthesia and retinal vascular obstruction. *Ophthalmology,* 90:373–377.
11. Ellis, P. P. (1974): Retrobulbar injections. *Surv. Ophthalmol.,* 18:425–430.
12. Kraushar, M. F., Seelenfreund, M. H., and Freilich, D. B. (1974): Central retinal artery closure during orbital hemorrhage from retrobulbar injection. *Trans. Am. Acad. Ophthalmol. Otolaryngol.,* 78:65–70.
13. Schlaegel, T. F., and Wilson, T. M. (1974): Accidental intraocular injection of depot corticosteroids. *Trans. Am. Acad. Ophthalmol. Otolaryngol.,* 78:847–855.
14. Klein, M. L., Jampol, L. M., Condon, P. I., Rice T. A., and Serjeant, G. R. (1982): Central retinal artery occlusion without retrobulbar hemorrhage after retrobulbar anesthesia. *Am. J. Ophthalmol.,* 93:573–577.
15. Ellis, P. P. (1978): Occlusion of the central retinal artery after retrobulbar corticosteroid injection. *Am. J. Ophthalmol.,* 85:352–356.
16. Atkinson, R. S., Rushman, G. B., and Lee, J. A. (1982): *Synopsis of Anesthesia,* pp. 656–657. John Wright & Sons, Bristol, England.
17. Meyers, E. F., Ramirez, R. C., and Boniuk, I. (1978): Grand mal seizures after retrobulbar block. *Arch. Ophthalmol.,* 96:847.
18. Beltranena, H. P., Vega, M. J., Kirk, N., and Blankenship, G. (1981): Inadvertent intravascular bupivacaine injection following retrobulbar block: Report of three cases. *Regional Anesthesia,* 6:149–151.
19. Aldrete, J. A., Roma-Salas, F., Arora, S., Wilson, R., and Rutherford, R. (1978): Reverse arterial blood flow as a pathway for central nervous system toxic responses following injection of local anesthetics. *Anesth. Analg.,* 57:428–433.
20. Aldrete, J. A., Narang, R., Sada, T., Tan Liem, S., and Miller, G. P. (1977): Reverse carotid blood flow—a possible explanation for some reactions to local anesthetics. *J. Am. Dent. Assoc.,* 94:1142–1145.
21. Vey, E. K., Finlay, J., and Everett, W. G. (1962): A clinical evaluation of mepivacaine for retrobulbar anesthesia. *Am. J. Ophthalmol.,* 53:827–832.
22. El-Shewy, T. M., Amin, E., and El-Khateaeb, M. S. (1969): Evaluation of mepivacaine (Carbocaine) as a local anesthetic in ophthalmic surgery. *Bull. Ophthal. Soc. Egypt,* 62:253–260.
23. Noble, D. S., and Pierce, G. F. M. (1961): Allergy to lignocaine. *Lancet,* 2:1436.
24. Brown, D. T., Beamish, D., Wildsmith, J. A. W. (1981): Allergic reaction to an amide local anaesthetic. *Br. J. Anesth.,* 53:435–437.
25. Collins, V. J. (1976): *Principles of Anesthesiology.* Lea & Febiger, Philadelphia.
26. Svedmyr, N. (1968): The influence of a tricyclic anti-depressive agent (protriptyline) on some of the circulatory effects of noradrenaline and adrenaline in man. *Life Sci.,* 7:77–84.
27. Svedmyr, N. (1966): Studies on the relationships between some metabolic effects of thyroid hormones and catecholamines in animals and man. *Acta Physiol. Scand.,* 68(Suppl. 274):1–46.
28. Laaka, V., Nikki, P., and Tarkkanen, A. (1972): Comparison of bupivacaine with and without adrenalin and mepivacaine with adrenalin in intraocular surgery. *Acta Ophthalmol. (Copenh.),* 50:229–239.
29. Horven, I. (1978): Ophthalmic artery pressure in retrobulbar anesthesia. *Acta Ophthalmol. (Copenh.),* 56:574–586.
30. Russell, D. A., and Guyton, J. S. (1954): Retrobulbar injection of lidocaine for anesthesia and akinesis. *Am. J. Ophthalmol.,* 38:78–84.
31. King, J. H., and Wadsworth, J. A. C. (1981): *An Atlas of Ophthalmic Surgery,* 3rd ed. J. B. Lippincott, Philadelphia.
32. Freitag, J. J., and Miller, L. W., eds. (1980): *Manual of Medical Therapeutics.* Little Brown & Co., Boston.
33. Young, I. (1960): Upper arm block with carbocaine (mepivacaine). *Anesth. Analg.,* 39:451–455.

34. Chin, G. N., and Almquist, H. T. (1983): Bupivacaine and lidocaine retrobulbar anesthesia. *Ophthalmology,* 90:369–372.
35. Rosenblatt, R. M., May, D. R., and Barsoumian, K. (1980): Cardiopulmonary arrest after retrobulbar block. *Am. J. Ophthalmol.,* 90:425–427.
36. Smith, J. L. (1982): Retrobulbar bupivacaine can cause respiratory arrest. *Ann. Ophthalmol.,* 14:1005–1006.
37. Moorman, L. T., and Kenny, G. S. (1971): Prilocaine as a local anesthetic useful in ophthalmic surgery. *Am. J. Ophthalmol.,* 72:468–471.
38. Cibis, P. A. (1965): In: *Controversial Aspects of the Management of Retinal Detachment,* vol. 3, edited by C. L. Schepens and C. D. J. Regan pp. 222–223. Little Brown & Co., Boston.
39. Stangos, N., Rey, P., Leuenberger, P., and Korel, S. (1971): The effect of xylocaine injections on the rabbits' retina: Averaged ERG and electron microscopy. *Vision Res.,* 11:1208–1209.
40. Kalina, R. E. (1969): Increased intraocular pressure following subconjunctival corticosteroid administration. *Arch. Ophthalmol.,* 81:788–790.
41. Aquavella, J. V., Gasset, A. R., and Dohlman, C. H. (1964): Corticosteroids in corneal wound healing. *Am. J. Ophthalmol.,* 58:621–626.
42. Tabban, K. F. (1980): Treatment of ocular toxoplasmosis with clindamycin and sulfadiazine. *Ophthalmology,* 87:129–134.
43. Nozik, R. A. (1972): Periocular injection of steroids. *Trans. Am. Acad. Ophthalmol. Otolaryngol.,* 76:695–705.
44. O'Connor, G. R. (1976): Periocular corticosteroid injections: Uses and abuses. *Eye Ear Nose Throat Monthly,* 55:83–88.
45. Schlaegel, T. F., Jr., and Wilson, F. M. (1974): Accidental intraocular injection of depot corticosteroids. *Trans. Am. Acad. Ophthalmol. Otolaryngol.,* 78:847–855.
46. Zinn, K. M. (1981): Iatrogenic intraocular injection of depot corticosteroid and its surgical removal using the pars plana approach. *Ophthalmology,* 88:13–17.
47. Giles, C. L. (1974): Bulbar perforation during periocular injection of corticosteroids. *Am. J. Ophthalmol.,* 77:438–441.
48. McLean, E. B. (1975): Inadvertent injection of corticosteroid into the choroidal vasculature. *Am. J. Ophthalmol.,* 80:835–837.
49. Theodore, F. H., Littman, M. L., and Almedi, E. (1961): The diagnosis and management of fungal endophthalmitis following cataract extraction. *Arch. Ophthalmol.,* 66:163–175.
50. Bell, R. W., and Ritchey, J. P. (1971): Subconjunctival nodules after amphotericin B injection. Medical therapy for aspergillas corneal ulcer. *Arch. Ophthalmol.,* 90:402–404.
51. Rich, A. M., Dunlap, W. A., and Patridge, J. R. (1973): The effectiveness, safety, and use of carbenicillin in ophthalmology. *Am. J. Ophthalmol.,* 75:490–495.
52. Boyle, G. L., Gwon, A. E., Zinn, K. M., and Leopold, I. H. (1972): Intraocular penetration of carbenicillin after subconjunctival injection in man. *Am. J. Ophthalmol.,* 73:754–759.
53. Boyle, G. L., Abel, R., Jr., Lazachek, G. W., and Leopold, I. H. (1972): Intraocular penetration of sodium cephalothin in man after subconjunctival injection. *Am. J. Ophthalmol.,* 74:868–874.
54. Records, R. E. (1969): The cephalosporins in ophthalmology. *Surv. Ophthalmol.,* 13:207–214, 345–354.
55. Batchelor, F. R., Dewdney, J. M., Weston, R. D., and Wheeler, A. C. (1966): The immunogenicity of cephalosporin derivatives and their cross-reaction with penicillin. *Immunology,* 10:21–33.
56. Tate, G. W., and Martin, R. G. (1977): Clindamycin in the treatment of human ocular toxoplasmosis. *Can. J. Ophthalmol.,* 12:188–195.
57. Libert, J., Ketelbant-Balasse, P. E., Van Hoof, F., Aubert-Tulkens, G., and Tulkens, P. (1979): Cellular toxicity of gentamicin. *Am. J. Ophthalmol.,* 87:405–411.
58. Records, R. E. (1969): The penicillins in ophthalmology. *Surv. Ophthalmol.,* 13:207–214.
59. Purnell, W. D., and McPherson, S. D. (1974): The effect of tobramycin on rabbit eyes. *Am. J. Ophthalmol.,* 77:578–582.
60. Burke, M. J., Parks, M. M., Calhoun, J. H., Diamond, J. G., and deFaller, J. M. (1981): Safety evaluation of BSS Plus in pediatric intraocular surgery. *J. Pediatr. Ophthalmol. Strabismus,* 18:45–49.
61. Harper, J. Y., and Pomerat, C. M. (1958): In vitro observations on the behavior of conjunctival and corneal cells in relation to electrolytes. *Am. J. Ophthalmol.,* 46(5, Part II):269–275.

62. Edelhauser, H. F., Gonnering, R., and Van Horn, D. L. (1978): Intraocular irrigation solutions. *Arch. Ophthalmol.,* 96:516–520.
63. Edelhauser, H. F., Van Horn, D. L., Hyndiuk, R. A., and Schultz, R. O. (1975): Intraocular irrigating solutions: Their effect on the corneal endothelium. *Arch. Ophthalmol.,* 93:648–657.
64. Edelhauser, H. F., Van Horn, D. L., Schultz, R. O., and Hyndiuk, R. A. (1976): Comparative toxicity of intraocular irrigating solutions on the corneal endothelium. *Am. J. Ophthalmol.,* 81:473–481.
65. Hodson, S. (1971): Evidence of a bicarbonate-dependent sodium pump in corneal endothelium. *Exp. Eye Res.,* 11:20–29.
66. Hodson, S., Miller, F., and Riley, M. F. (1971): The electrogenic pump of rabbit corneal endothelium. *Exp. Eye Res.,* 24:245–253.
67. Riley, M. V., Miller, F., Hodson, S., and Linz, D. (1977): Elimination of anions derived from glucose metabolism or substrates for the fluid pump of rabbit corneal endothelium. *Exp. Eye Res.,* 24:255–261.
68. Dikstein, S., and Maurice, D. M. (1972): The metabolic basis for the fluid pump in the cornea. *J. Physiol.,* 221:29–41.
69. McCarey, B. E., Edelhauser, H. F., and Van Horn, D. L. (1973): Functional and structural changes in the corneal endothelium during in vitro perfusion. *Invest. Ophthalmol. Vis. Sci.,* 12:410–417.
70. Moorhead, L. C., Redburn, D. A., Merritt, J., and Garcia, C. A. (1979): The effects of intravitreal irrigation during vitrectomy on the electroretinogram. *Am. J. Ophthalmol.,* 88: 239–245.
71. Kinsey, V. E., and Reddy, D. V. N. (1966): Chemistry and dynamics of aqueous humor. In: *The Rabbit in Eye Research,* edited by J. H. Prince. Charles C Thomas, Springfield, IL.
72. Merrill, D. L., Fleming, T. C., and Girard, L. J. (1960): The effects of physiologic balanced salt solutions and normal saline on intraocular and extraocular tissues. *Am. J. Ophthalmol.,* 49:895–898.
73. Haimann, M. H., Abrams, G. W., Edelhauser, H. F., and Hatchell, D. L. (1982): The effect of intraocular irrigating solutions on lens clarity in normal and diabetic rabbits. *Am. J. Ophthalmol.,* 94:594–605.
74. Emery, J. M., Landes, D. J., and Bendken, R. M. (1974): The phacoemulsifier: An evaluation of performance safety margins. In: *Current Concepts in Cataract Surgery. Selected Proceedings of the Third Biennial Cataract Surgical Congress,* edited by J. M. Emery and D. Paton, pp. 208–222. C. V. Mosby, St. Louis.
75. Polack, F. M., and Sugar, A. (1976): The phacoemulsification procedure. II. Corneal endothelial changes. *Invest. Ophthalmol. Vis. Sci.,* 15:458–469.
76. McCarey, B. D., Polack, F. M., and Marshall, W. (1976): The phacoemulsification procedure. I. The effect of intraocular irrigating solutions on the corneal endothelium. *Invest. Ophthalmol. Vis. Sci.,* 15:449–457.
77. Binder, P. S., Sternberg, H., Wickham, M. A., and Worthen, D. M. (1976): Corneal endothelial damage associated with phacoemulsification. *Am. J. Ophthalmol.,* 82:48–54.
78. McCarey, B. E., Edelhauser, H. F., and Van Horn, D. L. (1973): Functional and structural changes in the corneal endothelium during in vitro perfusion. *Invest. Ophthalmol. Vis. Sci.,* 12:410–417.
79. Schwartz, S. I., Shires, G. I., Spencer, F. C., and Storer, E. H. (1983): *Principles of Surgery,* 4th ed. McGraw-Hill, New York.
80. Kaye, G. I., Mishima, S., Cole, J. D., and Kaye, N. W. (1968): Effects of perfusion with a calcium-free medium on the corneal endothelium. *Invest. Ophthalmol.,* 7:53–66.
81. Waltman, S. R., Carrol, D., Schommelpfenning, W., and Okun, E. (1975): Intraocular irrigating solution for vitrectomy. *Ophthalmol. Surg.,* 6:90–94.
82. Benson, W. E., Diamond, J. G., and Tasman, W. (1981): Intraocular irrigating solutions for pars plana vitrectomy. *Arch. Ophthalmol.,* 99:1013–1015.
83. Christiansen, J. M., Kollaritz, C. R., Fukui, H., Fishman, M. L., Michels, R. G., and Mikuni, L. (1976): Intraocular irrigating solutions and lens clarity. *Am. J. Ophthalmol.,* 82:594–597.
84. Alcon Laboratories, Surgical Products Division, Fort Worth, TX. July 1982.
85. Britton, B., Hervey, R., Kasten, K., Gregg, S., and McDonald, T. (1976): Intraocular irritation evaluation of benzalkonium chloride in rabbits. *Ophthalmic Surg.,* 7(3):46–55.
86. Green, K., Hull, D. S., Vaugh, E. D., Malizia, A. A., and Bowman, K. (1977): Response to ophthalmic preservatives. *Arch. Ophthalmol.,* 95:2218–2221.

87. Van Horn, D. L., Edelhauser, A. F., Prodanovich, G., Eiferman, R., and Pederson, H. J. (1977): Effect of the ophthalmic preservative thimerosal on rabbit and human corneal endothelium. *Invest. Ophthalmol. Vis. Sci.,* 16:273–280.

88. Green, K., Livingston, V., Bowman, K., and Hull, D. S. (1980): Chlorhexidine effects on the corneal epithelium and endothelium. *Arch. Ophthalmol.,* 98:1273–1278.

89. Hull, D. S., Chemotti, M. T., Edelhauser, H. F., Van Horn, D. L., and Hyndiuk, R. A. (1975): Effect of epinephrine on the corneal endothelium. *Am. J. Ophthalmol.,* 79:245–250.

90. Hull, D. S. (1979): Effects of epinephrine, benzalkonium chloride, and intraocular miotics on corneal endothelium. *South. Med. J.,* 72:1380–1381.

91. Olson, R. J., Kolodner, H., Riddle, P., and Escapini, H., Jr. (1980): Commonly used intraocular medications and the corneal endothelium. *Arch. Ophthalmol.,* 98:2224–2226.

92. Jaffe, N. S. (1981): *Cataract Surgery and Its Complications,* 3rd ed. C. V. Mosby, St. Louis.

93. Gonnering, R., Edelhauser, H. F., Van Horn, D. L., and Durant, W. (1979): The pH tolerance of rabbit and human corneal endothelium. *Invest. Ophthalmol. Vis. Sci.,* 18:373–390.

94. Edelhauser, H. F., Hanneken, A. M., Pederson, H. J., and Van Horn, D. L. (1981): Osmotic tolerance of the rabbit and human corneal endothelium. *Arch. Ophthalmol.,* 99:1281–1287.

95. Edelhauser, H. F., Hyndiuk, R. A., Zeeb, A., and Schultz, R. O. (1982): Corneal edema and the intraocular use of epinephrine. *Am. J. Ophthalmol.,* 93:327–333.

96. Edelhauser, H. F., Hine, J. E., Pederson, H., Van Horn, D. L., and Schultz, R. O. (1979): The effect of phenylephrine on the cornea. *Arch. Ophthalmol.,* 97:937–947.

97. Machemer, R. (1975): *Vitrectomy: A Pars Plana Approach.* Grune & Stratton, New York.

98. MacRae, S. M., and Edelhauser, H. F. (1983): Post-operative corneal edema. *Am. J. Ophthalmol.,* 95:552–554.

99. Coles, W. H. (1975): Pilocarpine toxicity effects on the rabbit corneal endothelium. *Arch. Ophthalmol.,* 93:36–41.

100. Vaughn, E., Hall, D. S., and Green, K. (1978): Effect of intraocular miotics on the corneal endothelium. *Arch. Ophthalmol.,* 96:1897–1900.

101. Rosen, N., and Lazar, M. (1978): The mechanism of the Miochol lens opacity. *Am. J. Ophthalmol.,* 86:570–571.

102. Emery, J. M., and Little, J. A. (1979): *Phacoemulsification and Aspiration of Cataracts.* C. V. Mosby, St. Louis.

103. Gombos, G. M. (1982): Systemic reactions following intraocular acetylcholine instillation. *Ann. Ophthalmol.,* 14:529–530.

104. Babinski, M., Smith, B., and Wickerham, E. P. (1976): Hypotension and bradycardia following intraocular acetylcholine injection. Report of a case. *Arch. Ophthalmol.,* 94:675–676.

105. Sears, M. L. (1981): The aqueous. In: *Adler's Physiology of the Eye,* edited by R. Moses, p. 218. Mosby, St. Louis.

106. Brubaker, S., Peyman, G. A., and Vygantas, C. (1974): Toxicity of octafluorocyclobutane after intracameral injection. *Arch. Ophthalmol.,* 92:324–328.

107. Olson, R. J. (1980): Air and the corneal endothelium: An in vivo specular microscopy study in cats. *Arch. Ophthalmol.,* 98:1283–1284.

108. Leibowitz, H. M., Laing, R. N., and Sandstrom, M. (1974): Corneal endothelium: The effect of air in the anterior chamber. *Arch. Ophthalmol.,* 92:227–230.

109. Van Horn, D. L., Edelhauser, H. F., Aaberg, T. M., and Pederson, H. J. (1972): In vivo effects of air and sulfur hexafluoride gas on rabbit corneal endothelium. *Invest. Ophthalmol. Vis. Sci.,* 11:1028–1036.

110. Von Sallmann, L. (1946): Discussion: Technical uses of air in ophthalmology. *Trans. Am. Ophthalmol. Soc.,* 35:525–536.

111. Stallard, H. B. (1955): The use of air in eye surgery. *Trans. Ophthalmol. Soc. U.K.,* 75:33–41.

112. Constable, I. J., and Swan, D. A. (1975): Vitreous substitution with gases. *Arch. Ophthalmol.,* 93:416–419.

113. Fineberg, E., Machemer, R., Sullivan, P., Norton, E. W. D., Hamasaki, D., and Anderson, D. (1975): Sulfur hexafluoride in owl monkey vitreous cavity. *Am. J. Ophthalmol.,* 79:67–76.

114. Killey, F. P., Edelhauser, H. F., and Aaberg, T. M. (1978): Intraocular sulfur hexafluoride

and octafluorocyclobutane—effects on intraocular pressure and vitreous volume. *Arch. Ophthalmol.,* 96:511–515.

115. Peyman, G. A., Vygantas, C. M., Bennett, T. O., Vygantas, A. M., and Brubaker, S. (1975): Octafluorocyclobutane in vitreous and aqueous humor replacement. *Arch. Ophthalmol.,* 93: 514–517.

116. Chawla, H., and Birchall, C. H. (1973): Intravitreal air in retinal detachment surgery. *Br. J. Ophthalmol.,* 57:60–70.

117. Chawla, H. (1973): Intravitreal air in aphakic retinal detachment. *Br. J. Ophthalmol.,* 57:58–59.

118. Norton, E. W., Aaberg, T., Fung, W., and Curtin, V. T. (1969): Giant retinal tears. I. Clinical management with intravitreal air. *Am. J. Ophthalmol.,* 68:1011–1021.

119. Machemer, R., and Allen, A. W. (1976): Retinal tears 180 degrees and greater: Management with vitrectomy and intravitreal gas. *Arch. Ophthalmol.,* 94:1340–1346.

120. O'Connor, P. R. (1976): Intravitreous air injection and the Custodis procedure. *Ophthalmic Surg.,* 7(2):86–89.

121. Brubaker, S. J., Peyman, G. A., and Vygantas, C. M. (1974): Toxicity of octafluorocyclobutane after intracameral injection. *Arch. Ophthalmol.,* 92:324–328.

122. Scheie, H. G., and Frayer, W. (1950): Ocular hypertension induced by air in the anterior chamber. *Trans. Am. Ophthalmol. Soc.,* 48:88–95.

123. Spaeth, G. L., ed. (1982): *Ophthalmic Surgery,* W. B. Saunders, Philadelphia.

124. Rosengem, B. (1938): Results of treatment of detachment of the retina with diathermy and injection of air into the vitreous. *Acta Ophthalmol. (Copenh.),* 16:573–579.

125. Schepens, C. L., Freeman, H. M., and Thompson, R. F. (1965): A power driven multipositional operating table. *Arch. Ophthalmol.,* 73:671–673.

126. Van Horn, D. L., Edelhauser, H. F., Aaberg, T. M., and Pederson, H. J. (1972): In vivo effects of air and sulfur hexafluoride gas on rabbit corneal endothelium. *Invest. Ophthalmol. Vis. Sci.,* 11:1028–1036.

127. Vygantas, C. M., Peyman, G. A., Daily, M. J., and Ericson, E. S. (1973): Octafluorocyclobutane and other gases for vitreous replacement. *Arch. Ophthalmol.,* 90:235–236.

128. Norton, E. W. D. (1973): Intraocular gas in the management of selected retinal detachments. *Trans. Am. Acad. Ophthalmol. Otolaryngol.,* 77:85–97.

129. Abrams, G. W., Swanson, D. E., Sabates, W. I., and Goldman, A. I. (1982): The results of sulfur hexafluoride gas in vitreous surgery. *Am. J. Ophthalmol.,* 94:165–171.

130. Sabates, W. I., Abrams, G. W., Swanson, D. E., and Norton, E. W. D. (1981): The use of intraocular gases. The results of sulfur hexafluoride gas in retinal detachment surgery. *Ophthalmology,* 88:447–454.

131. Diddie, K. R., and Smith, R. E. (1980): Intraocular gas injection in the pseudophakic patient. *Am. J. Ophthalmol.,* 89:659–661.

132. Fuller, D. G., and Hutton, W. L. (1980): Anterior chamber suture in pseudophakic retinal detachments requiring intraocular gas. *Arch. Ophthalmol.,* 98:1101.

133. Constable, I. J. (1974): Perfluoropentane in experimental ocular surgery. *Invest. Ophthalmol. Vis. Sci.,* 13:627–629.

134. Lincoff, H., Madirossian, J., Lincoff, A., Liggett, P., Iwamoto, T., and Jakobiec, F. (1980): Intravitreal longevity of three perfluorocarbon gases. *Arch. Ophthalmol.,* 98:1610.

135. Peyman, G. A., Namperumalsamy, P., and Vygantas, C. (1975): Clinical trial of intravitreal C_4F_8 in retinal detachment surgery. *Can. J. Ophthalmol.,* 10:218–221.

136. Stinson, T. W., 3rd, and Donlon, J. V., Jr. (1982): Interaction of intraocular air and sulfur hexafluoride with nitrous oxide: A computer simulation. *Anesthesiology,* 56:385–388.

137. Smith, R. B., Carl, B., Linn, J. G., Jr., and Nemoto, E. (1974): Effect of nitrous oxide on air in vitreous. *Am. J. Ophthalmol.,* 78:314–317.

138. Aronowitz, J. D., and Brubaker, R. F. (1976): Effect of intraocular gases on intraocular pressure. *Arch. Ophthalmol.,* 94:1191–1196.

139. Stone, W., Jr. (1956): Alloplasty in surgery of the eye. *N. Engl. J. Med.,* 258:486–490.

140. Cibis, P. A. (1965): *Vitreoretinal Pathology and Surgery in Retinal Detachment.* C. V. Mosby, St. Louis.

141. Cibis, P. A., Becker, B., Okun, E., and Canaan, S. (1962): The use of liquid silicone in retinal detachment surgery. *Arch. Ophthalmol.,* 68:590–599.

142. Armaly, M. F. (1962): Ocular tolerance to silicones I—replacement of aqueous and vitreous by silicone fluids. *Arch. Ophthalmol.,* 68:390–395.

143. McPherson, A. R., cited by C. L. Schepens and C. D. J. Regan. (1960): *Controversial Aspects of the Management of Retinal Detachment.* Little Brown & Company, Boston.
144. Lee, P. F., Donovan, R. H., Mukai, N., Schepens, C. L., and Freeman, H. F. (1969): Intravitreous injection of silcone: An experimental study. *Ann. Ophthalmol.,* 1(2):15–25.
145. Labelle, P., and Okun, E. (1972): Ocular tolerance to liquid silicone: An experimental study. *Can. J. Ophthalmol.,* 7:199–204.
146. Mukai, N., Lee, P. F., and Schepens, C. L. (1972): Intravitreous injection of silicone: An experimental study II. *Ann. Ophthalmol.,* 4:273–277.
147. Okun, E. (1968): Intravitreal surgery utilizing liquid silicone—a long-term follow-up. *Trans. Pacif. Coast Oto. Ophthalmol. Soc.,* 49:141–159.
148. Grey, R. H. B., and Leaver, P. K. (1977): Results of silicone oil injection in massive preretinal retraction. *Trans. Ophthalmol. Soc. U.K.,* 97:238–241.
149. Scott, J. D. (1977): A rationale for the use of liquid silicone. *Trans. Ophthalmol. Soc. U.K.,* 97:235–237.
150. Leaver, P. K., Grey, R. H. B., and Garner, A. (1979): Silicone oil injection in the treatment of massive preretinal retraction. II. Late complications in 93 eyes. *Br. J. Ophthalmol.,* 63:361–367.
151. Watzke, R. C. (1967): Silicone retinopoiesis for retinal detachment. A long-term clinical evaluation. *Arch. Ophthalmol.,* 77:185–196.
152. Scott, J. D. (1974): The treatment of massive vitreous retraction by the separation of preretinal membranes using liquid silicone. *Mod. Probl. Ophthalmol.,* 15:285–290.
153. Watzke, R. C. (1982): Use of silicone oil. *Arch. Ophthalmol.,* 100:1354–1355.
154. Sugar, H. S., and Okamura, I. D. (1976): Ocular findings six years after intravitreal silicone injection. *Arch. Ophthalmol.,* 94:612–615.
155. Everett, W. G., cited by C. L. Schepens and C. D. J. Regan (1960): *Controversial Aspects of the Management of Retinal Detachment.* Little Brown and Company, Boston.
156. Blodi, F. C. (1971): Injection and impregnation of liquid silicone into ocular tissues. *Am. J. Ophthalmol.,* 71:1044–1051.
157. Watzke, R. C. (1967): Silicone retinopoiesis for retinal detachment. *Surv. Ophthalmol.,* 12:333–337.
157a.Ni, C., Wang, W. J., Albert, D. M., and Schepens, C. L. (1983): Intravitreous silicone injection: Histopathological findings in a human eye after 12 years. *Arch Ophthalmol.,* 101:1399–1401.
158. Gonuers, M. (1982): Temporary use of intraocular silicone oil in the treatment of detachment with massive periretinal proliferation. Preliminary report. *Ophthalmologics,* 184:210–218.
159. Balazs, E. A. (1960): Discussion. In: *Importance of the Vitreous Body in Retina Surgery with Special Emphasis on Reoperations,* edited by C. L. Schepens, pp. 114–146. C. V. Mosby, St. Louis.
160. Castren, J. A. (1964): Intrabulbar vitreous and hyaluronic acid injections. *Acta Ophthalmol. (Copenh.),* 42:427–434.
161. Miller, D., O'Connor, P., and Williams, T. (1977): Use of sodium hyalurinate during intraocular lens implantation in rabbits. *Ophthalmic Surg.,* 8:58–61.
162. Grave, E. L., Polcak, F. M., and Balazs, E. A. (1980): The protective effect of sodium hyalurenate to corneal endothelium. *Exp. Eye Res.,* 31:119–127.
163. Stauncter, R., and Kretzcr, F. (1982): Protective effect of hyaluronic acid in anterior segment surgery in the rabbit model. In: *Cataract Surgery. Selected Proceedings of the Seventh Biennial Cataract Surgery Congress,* edited by J. M. Emery and A. C. Jacobson, pp. 65–68. Appleton-Century-Croft, New York.
164. MacRae, S. M., Edelhauser, H. F., Hyndiuk, R. A., Burd, E. M., and Schultz, R. O. (1983): The effects of sodium hyaluronate chondroitin sulfate, and methylcellulose on the corneal endothelium and intraocular pressure. *Am. J. Ophthalmol.,* 95:332–341.
165. Miller, D., and Stegmann, R. (1981): Use of sodium hyaluronate in human intraocular lens implantation. *Ann. Ophthalmol.,* 13:811–815.
166. Rashid, E. R., and Waring, G. O. (1982): Use of Healon in anterior segment trauma. *Ophthalmic Surg.,* 13:201–203.
167. Berson, F. G., Patterson, M. M., and Epstein, D. L. (1983): Obstruction of aqueous outflow by sodium hyaluronate in enucleated human eyes. *Am. J. Ophthalmol.,* 95:668–672.
168. Pinkus, H., and Perry, E. T. (1953): The influence of hyaluronic acid and other substances on tensile strength of healing wounds. *J. Invest. Dermatol.,* 21:365–369.

169. Arzeno, G., and Miller, D. (1982): Effect of sodium hyaluronate on corneal wound healing. *Arch. Ophthalmol.,* 100:152.
170. Landholm, W. M., and Watzke, R. C. (1965): Experimental retinal detachment with a sulfated polysaccharide. *Invest. Ophthalmol. Vis. Sci.,* 4:42–50.
171. Talman, E. L., and Harris, J. E. (1959): Ocular changes induced by polysaccharides. II. Detection of hyaluronic acid sulfite after injection into ocular tissues. *Am. J. Ophthalmol.,* 47:428–437.
172. Soll, D., Harrison, S., Artuos, F., and Clinch, T. (1980): Evaluation and protection of corneal endothelium. *Am. Intraoc. Implant Soc. J.,* 6:239–242.
173. Soll, D., and Harrison, S. (1981): The use of chondroitin sulfite in protection of the corneal endothelium. *Ophthalmology,* 88(Suppl):51.
174. Fechner, P. U. (1977): Methylcellulose in lens implantation. *Am. Intraocular Implant Soc. J.,* 3:180–181.
175. Gombos, G. M., and Berman, E. R. (1967): Chemical and clinical observations on the fate of various vitreous substitutes. *Acta Ophthalmol.,* (Copenh.), 45:794–806.
176. Shafer, D. M. (1957): The treatment of retinal detachment by vitreous implant. *Trans. Am. Acad. Ophthalmol. Otolaryngol.,* 81:194–200.
177. Hudson, J. R. (1968): Internal tamponage with donor vitreous. In: *New and Controversial Aspects of Retinal Detachment,* edited by A. McPherson, pp. 365–370. Harper and Row, New York.
178. Hruby, K. (1961): Hyaluronic acid as vitreous body substitute in retinal detachment, *Klin Monatsbl. Augenheilk.,* 138:484–496.
179. Oosterhuis, J. A., van Haeringen, N. J., Jeltes, I. G., and Glasius, E. (1966): Polygeline as a vitreous substitute. I. Observations in rabbits. *Arch. Ophthalmol.,* 76:258–265.
180. Oosterhuis, J. A. (1966): Polygeline as a vitreous substitute. II. Clinical results. *Arch. Ophthalmol.,* 76:374–377.
181. Daniele, S., Refojo, M. F., Schepens, C. L., and Freeman, H. M. (1968): Glyceryl methacrylate hydrogel as a vitreous implant—an experimental study. *Arch. Ophthalmol.,* 80:120–127.
182. Doughman, D. J., Watzke, R. C., and Burian, H. M. (1969): The ocular effects of intravitreal injection of polyethylene sulfonic acid. *Am. J. Ophthalmol.,* 67:571–580.
183. Muller-Jensen, K. (1974): Alloplastic vitreous replacement with acrylamide—a preliminary report. *Med. Probl. Ophthalmol.,* 12:385–389.
184. Pruett, R. C. (1974): Collagen vitreous substitute. II. Preliminary clinical trials. *Arch. Ophthalmol.,* 91:29–32.
185. Baum, J., Peyman, G. A., and Barza, M. (1982): Intravitreal administration of antibiotics in the treatment of bacterial endophthalmitis. III. Consensus. *Surv. Ophthalmol.,* 26:204–206.
186. Peyman, G. A., May, D. R., Ericson, E. S., and Apple, D. J. (1974): Intraocular injection of gentamicin: Toxic effects and clearance. *Arch. Ophthalmol.,* 92:42–47.
187. May, D. R., Ericson, E. S., Peyman, G. A., and Axelrod, A. J. (1974): Intraocular injection of gentamicin—single injection therapy of experimental bacterial endophthalmitis. *Arch. Ophthalmol.,* 91:487–489.
188. Atkins, W. S., and McPherson, S. D., Jr. (1975): Intravitreal injection of ampicillin, cephaloridine, gentamicin, and tobramycin. *Surg. Forum,* 26:542–544.
189. Zachary, I. G., and Forster, R. K. (1976): Experimental intravitreal gentamicin. *Am. J. Ophthalmol.,* 82:604–611.
190. Peyman, G. A., Paque, J. T., Meisels, H. I., and Bennet, T. O. (1975): Post-operative endophthalmitis: A comparison of methods for treatment and prophylaxis with gentamicin. *Ophthalmic Surg.,* 6(2):45–55.
191. Forster, R. K., Cachary, I. G., Cottingham, A. J., and Norton, E. W. D. (1976): Further observations on the diagnosis, cause, and treatment of endophthalmitis. *Am. J. Ophthalmol.,* 81:52–56.
192. Stainer, G. A., Peyman, G. A., Meisels, H., and Fishman, G. (1977): Toxicity of selected antibiotics in vitreous replacement fluid. *Ann. Ophthalmol.,* 9:615–618.
193. D'Amico, D. J., Kenyon, K. R., and Hanninen, L. A. (1983): Retinal toxicity of gentamicin after intravitreal injection: Evidence of lysosomal involvement in RPE and retina. *Invest. Ophthalmol. Vis. Sci.,* 24(Suppl.):292.
194. Graham, R. O., Peyman, G. A., and Fishman, G. (1975): Intravitreal injection of cephaloridine in the treatment of endophthalmitis. *Arch. Ophthalmol.,* 93:56–61.
195. Morgan, B. S., Larson, B., Peyman, G. A., and West, C. S. (1979): Toxicity of antibiotic combinations for vitrectomy infusion fluid. *Ophthalmic Surg.,* 10(10):74–77.

196. Schenk, A. G., Peyman, G. A., and Paque, J. T. (1974): The intravitreal use of carbenicillin (Geopen) for treatment of Pseudomonas endophthalmitis. *Acta Ophthalmol. (Copenh.)*, 52:707–717.
197. Daily, M. J., Peyman, G. A., and Fishman, G. (1973): Intravitreal injection of methicillin for treatment of endophthalmitis. *Am. J. Ophthalmol.*, 76:343–350.
198. Homer, P., Peyman, G. A., Koziol, J., and Sanders, D. (1975): Intravitreal injection of vancomycin in experimental staphylococcal endophthalmitis. *Acta Ophthalmol. (Copenh.)*, 53:311–320.
199. Schenk, A. G., and Peyman, G. A. (1974): Lincomycin by direct intravitreal injection in the treatment of experimental bacterial endophthalmitis. *Albrecht von Graefes. Arch. Klin. Ophthalmol.*, 190:281–291.
200. Koziol, J., and Peyman, G. (1974): Intraocular chloramphenicol and bacterial endophthalmitis. *Can. J. Ophthalmol.*, 9:316–321.
201. Leeds, N. H., Peyman, G. A., and House, B. (1982): Moxolactam (Moxam) in the treatment of experimental staphylococcal endophthalmitis. *Ophthalmic Surg.*, 13:653–656.
202. Souri, E. N., and Green, W. R. (1974): Intravitreal amphotericin B toxicity. *Am. J. Ophthalmol.*, 78:77–81.
203. Axelrod, A. J., Peyman, G. A., and Apple, D. J. (1974): Intravitreal amphotericin B toxicity. *Am. J. Ophthalmol.*, 78:875–876.
204. Foster, J. B., Almeda, E., Littman, M. L., and Wilson, M. E. (1958): Some intraocular and conjunctival effects of amphotericin B in man and in the rabbit. *Arch. Ophthalmol.*, 60:555–564.
205. Green, W. R., Bennet, J. E., and Goos, R. D. (1965): Ocular penetration of amphotericin B. *Arch. Ophthalmol.*, 73:769–775.
206. Tolentino, F. I., Foster, C. S., Lahav, M., Liu, L. H. S., and Rabin, A. R. (1982): Toxicity of intravitreous miconazole. *Arch. Ophthalmol.*, 100:1504–1509.
207. Miller, G. R., Rebell, G., and Magoon, R. C. (1978): Intravitreal antimycotic therapy and care of mycotic endophthalmitis caused by a *Paecilomyces lilacanus* contaminated pseudephakos. *Ophthalmic Surg.*, 9:54–63.
208. Schwartz, B., and Schwartz, J. B. (1960): A review of the biochemistry and pharmacology of alpha-chymotrypsin. *Trans. Am. Acad. Ophthalmol. Otolaryngol.*, 64:17–24.
209. Anderson, D. R. (1971): Experimental alpha chymotrypsin glaucoma studied by scanning electron microscopy. *Am. J. Ophthalmol.*, 71:470–476.
210. Barraquer, J. (1958): Totale Linsenextraktion nach Aufloesung der Zonula durch alpha Chymotrypsin/enzymatische Zonulyse. *Klin. Mbl. Augenh.*, 133:609–615.
211. Schwartz, B., Corwin, M., and Israel R. (1968): A double-blind therapeutic trial of the effect of alpha-chymotrypsin on the facility of cataract extraction. *Trans. Am. Acad. Ophthalmol. Otolaryngol.*, 64:46–57.
212. Kalvin, N. H., Hamasaki, D. I., and Gass, J. D. M. (1966): Experimental glaucoma in monkeys. I. Relationship between intraocular pressure and cupping of the optic disc and cavernous atrophy of the optic nerve. *Arch. Ophthalmol.*, 76:82–93.
213. Lessell, S., and Kuwabara, T. (1969): Experimental alpha-chymotrypsin glaucoma. *Arch. Ophthalmol.*, 81:853–864.
214. Bedrossian, R. H., and Calli, R. A. (1962): Clinical application of new laboratory data on alpha chymotrypsin. *Arch. Ophthalmol.*, 67:616–621.
215. von Sallman, L. (1960): Experimental studies of some ocular effects of alpha chymotrypsin. *Trans. Am. Acad. Ophthalmol. Otolaryngol.*, 64:25–32.
216. Townes, C. D. (1960): Unfavorable effects of alpha chymotrypsin in cataract surgery. *Arch. Ophthalmol.*, 64:108–113.
217. Munich, W. (1961): Studies on the influence of alpha chymotrypsin on the uptake of radioactive sulphur in the tissues of the cornea. *Graefe Arch. Ophthalmol.*, 104:145–150.
218. Fink, A., Bernstein, H. N., and Binkhorst, D. (1962): Effect of alpha chymotrypsin on corneal wound healing. *Arch. Ophthalmol.*, 67:616–621.
219. Wind, C. A., and Gasset, A. R. (1972): The effect of alpha chymotrypsin on intraocular pressure and corneal wound healing. *Am. Ophthalmol.*, 4:32–39.
220. Kirsch, R. E. (1964): Use of alpha chymotrypsin in cataract extraction followed by transient glaucoma. *Arch. Ophthalmol.*, 72:612–660.
221. Galin, M. A., Barasch, K. R., and Harris, L. S. (1966): Enzymatic zonulolysis and intraocular pressure. *Am. J. Ophthalmol.*, 61:690–696.
222. Kirsch, R. E. (1965): Further studies on glaucoma following cataract extraction associated

with the use of alpha chymotrypsin. *Trans. Am. Acad. Ophthalmol. Otolaryngol.,* 69:1011–1023.

223. Kirsch, R. E. (1966): Dose relationship of alpha chymotrypsin in production of glaucoma after cataract extraction. *Arch. Ophthalmol.,* 75:774–775.

224. Lantz, J. M., and Quigley, J. H. (1973): Intraocular pressure after cataract extraction: Effects of alpha chymotrypsin. *Can. J. Ophthalmol.,* 8:339–343.

225. Zimmerman, L. E., DeVenecia, G., and Hamasaki, D. I. (1967): Pathology of the optic nerve in experimental acute glaucoma. *Invest. Ophthalmol.,* 6:109–125.

226. Kalvin, N. H., Hamasaki, D. I., and Gass, J. D. M. (1966): Experimental glaucoma in monkeys. II. Studies of intraocular vascularity during glaucoma. *Arch. Ophthalmol.,* 76:94–103.

227. Leydhecker, W., and Dardenne, U. (1963): Histologische Untersuchangen am Trabekel System Nach Kurzfristiger Einwirkuna von Alpha-Chymotrypsin. *Klin Monatsbl Augenheilk,* 142:554–559.

228. Chee, P., and Hamasaki, T. (1971): The basis of chymotrypsin-induced glaucoma. *Arch. Ophthalmol.,* 85:103–106.

229. Sears, D., and Sears, M. (1974): Blood aqueous barrier and alpha chymotrypsin glaucoma in rabbits. *Am. J. Ophthalmol.,* 77:378–383.

230. Bawie, K. P., Gelalt, K. N., Gumm, G. G., and Samuelson, D. A. (1982): Effects of alpha-chymotrypsin on the canine eye. *Am. J. Vet. Res.,* 43:207–216.

231. Papadopoulies, P., and Formstron, C. (1966): Observations of the reclinatum of the crystalline lens in the dog by means of the intravitreal injection of alpha-chymotrypsin and on the effect of that agent on the ocular tissues, with special reference to the retina. In: *Aspects of Comparative Ophthalmology,* edited by G. Jones. p. 329. Pergamon Press, New York.

232. O'Malley, C., Moskovitz, M., and Stratsma, B. R. (1961): Experimentally induced adverse effects of alpha-chymotrypsin. *Arch. Ophthalmol.,* 66:539–544.

233. Maumenee, A. E. (1960): Effect of alpha-chymotrypsin on the retina. *Trans. Am. Acad. Ophthalmol. Otolaryngol.,* 64:33–36.

234. Raduct, M., and Pajor, R. (1960): Histological investigations on the effect exerted by alpha-chymotrypsin on the retina. *Acta Ophthalmol. (Copenh.),* 38:583–586.

235. Flom, L. (1960): Alpha-chymotrypsin and ruptured hyaloid. *Am. J. Ophthalmol.,* 49:357–358.

236. Geeraetz, W. J., Ghan, G., and Guerny, D. III. (1960): The effect of alpha-chymotrypsin on zonular fibres and anterior hyaloid membrane: Experiments on eyes in the human, rabbit, and dog. *South. Med. J.,* 53:82–85.

237. Troutman, R. C. (1966): Effects of alpha-chymotrypsin. *Arch. Ophthalmol.,* 76:764.

238. Girard, L. J., Neely, W., and Sampson, W. G. (1962): The use of alpha-chymotrypsin in infants and children. *Am. J. Ophthalmol.,* 54:95–101.

239. Cogan, J. E., Symans, H. M., and Gibbs, D. C. (1959): Intracapsular cataract extraction using alpha-chymotrypsin. *Br. J. Ophthalmol.,* 43:193–199.

240. Scheie, H. G., Ashley, B. J., Jr., and Weiner, A. (1961): The treatment of total hyphema with fibrinolysin (plasma). *Arch. Ophthalmol.,* 66:226–231.

241. Rakusen, W. (1972): Traumatic hyphema. *Am. J. Ophthalmol.,* 74:284–292.

242. Leet, D. M. (1977): Treatment of total hyphemas with urokinase. *Am. J. Ophthalmol.,* 84:79–84.

243. Smillie, J. W. (1954): The effect of streptokinase on simulated hyphema. *Am. J. Ophthalmol.,* 37:911–917.

244. Jukotsky, S. L. (1951): A new technique in the treatment of hyphema. *Am. J. Ophthalmol.,* 34:1692–1696.

245. O'Rourke, J. F. (1955): An evaluation of intraocular streptokinase. *Am. J. Ophthalmol.,* 39:119–136.

246. Horven, I., and Opsahl, R. (1964): Fibrinolysis and Hyphema. *Acta Ophthalmol. (Copenh.),* 42:957–961.

247. Bramsen, T. (1978): Effect of urokinase on central corneal thickness and vitreous hemorrhage. *Acta Ophthalmol. (Copenh.),* 56:1006–1012.

248. Drance, S. M. (1961): An ophthalmologist's approach to fibrinolysis. *Angiology,* 12:149–151.

249. Horven, I. (1961): The effect of fibrinolysis on blood injected into the anterior chamber of the eye in rabbits. *Acta Ophthalmol (Copenh.),* 39:44–49.

250. Morton, W. R., and Turnbull, W. (1964): Effect of intracameral fibrinolysis on rabbit cornea. *Am. J. Ophthalmol.,* 57:280–287.
251. Braley, A. E. (1955): Discussion: An evaluation of intraocular streptokinase. *Am. J. Ophthalmol.,* 39:119–136.
252. Friedman, M. W. (1952): Streptokinase in ophthalmology. *Am. J. Ophthalmol.,* 35:1184– 1187.
253. Scheie, H. G., Ashley, B. J., and Weiner, A. (1961): The treatment of total hyphema in fibrinolysis (Plasmin). A preliminary report. *Arch. Ophthalmol.,* 66:226–231.
254. Binder, R. F., Binder, H. F., and Skelly, J. R. (1961): Fibrinolysis in the human eye. *Arch. Ophthalmol.,* 65:648–651.
255. Fraunfelder, F. T., and Meyer, S. M. (1983): Ocular toxicity of anti-neoplastic agents. *Ophthalmology,* 90:1–3.
256. Shingleton, B. J., Breifang, D. C., Albert, D. M., Ensmonger, W. D., Chandler, W. F., and Greenberg, H. S. (1982): Ocular toxicity associated with high-dose carmustine. *Arch. Ophthalmol.,* 100:1766–1772.
257. Graham, R. O., and Peyman, G. A. (1974): Intravitreal injection of dexamethasone treatment of experimentally induced endophthalmitis. *Arch. Ophthalmol.,* 92:149–154.
258. McCuen, B. W., 2nd, Bessler, M., Tano, Y., Chandler, D., and Machemer, R. (1981): The lack of toxicity of intravitreally administered triamcinolone acetonide. *Am. J. Ophthalmol.,* 91:785–788.
259. Blumenkranz, M. S., Ophir, A., Claflin, A. J., and Hajed, A. (1982): Fluorouracil for the treatment of massive periretinal proliferation. *Am. J. Ophthalmol.,* 94:458–467.
260. Belkin, M., Avni, I., and Naveh-Floman, N. (1983): Prevention of post-traumatic vitreous proliferation. *Invest. Ophthalmol. Vis. Sci.,* 24(Suppl.):241.
261. Opher, A. (1983): Prevention of experimental massive peri-retinal proliferation by 5-fluorouracil. *Metab. Pediatr. Syst. Ophthalmol.,* 7:109–113.
262. Lewis, G. P., Guerin, C. J., Erickson, P. A., and Stern, W. H. (1983): Reversible toxicity of 5-FU treatment for proliferative vitreoretinopathy. *Invest. Ophthalmol. Vis. Sci.,* 24(Suppl.):241.
263. Stern, W. H., Guer, C. J., Erickson, P. A., Lewis, G. A., Anderson, D. H., and Fisher, S. K. (1983): *Ocular toxicity of fluorouracil after vitrectomy. Am. J. Ophthalmol.,* 96:43–51.
264. Nao, I., and Honda, Y. (1983): Toxic effect of fluorouracil on the rabbit retina. *Am. J. Ophthalmol.,* 96:641–643.
265. Parrish, R. K., Heuer, D., Gressel, M., Anderson, D. R., Paulmberg, P. F., and Hodapp, E. (1983): 5-Fluorouracil and glaucoma filtration surgery—a clinical study. *Invest. Ophthalmol. Vis. Sci.* 24(Suppl.):2.
266. Vrabec, F., Obenberger, J., and Bolkova, A. (1968): Effect of intravitreous vincristine sulfate on the rabbit retina. *Am. J. Ophthalmol.,* 66:199–204.
267. Bunt, A. H., and Lund, R. D. (1974): Vinblastine-induced blockage of orthograde and retrograde axonal transport of protein in retinal ganglion cells. *Exp. Neurol.,* 45:288–297.
268. Bunt, A. H. (1973): Protein synthesis in ganglion cells of rabbit retina after intravitreous injection of vinblastine. *Invest. Ophthalmol.,* 12:467–469.
269. Ericson, L., Karlberg, B., and Rosengren, B. H. O. (1964): Trials of intravitreal injections of chemotherapeutic agents in rabbits. *Acta Ophthalmol. (Copenh.),* 42:721–726.
270. Daniels, E., and Moore, K. L. (1976): Early chick neuroretinal responses following direct exposure to methotrexate. *J. Morphol.,* 150:307–319.
271. Kirmani, M., Santana, M., Sorjente, N., Wiedemann, P., and Ryan, S. J. (1983): Drug treatment of MPP. *Invest. Ophthalmol. Vis. Sci.,* 24(Suppl.):241.
272. Santana, M., Kiömani, M., Sorgent, N., Wiedemann, P., and Ryan, S. J. (1983): Ocular toxicity of intravitreal daunorubicin. *Invest. Ophthalmol. Vis. Sci.,* 24(Suppl.):291.
273. Rugh, R. (1965): Radiation and radiomionetic chlorambucil and the fetal retina. *Arch. Ophthalmol.,* 74:382–393.
274. Schwartz, R. J. (1973): Control of glutamine synthetase synthesis in the embryonic chick neural retina. *J. Biol. Chem.,* 248:6426–6435.

Commentary

Retinal Phototoxicity in Ocular Surgery

Initial observations of environmental light damage to the retina were made in 1966 by Werner Noell. Documented reports of retinal light damage in subhuman primates and patients after exposure to the illumination of ordinary surgical microscopes during intraocular surgery have awakened the ophthalmologist to the toxicity of light for the human retina. Tso and other workers in the field have shown that even very short exposures to the coaxial beam of the surgical microscope may induce foveal damage, particularly in senescent patients. Additional factors that predispose to damage or worsen injury from light are: dark adaptation before light exposure, elevated body temperature, pigmented retinas as compared with albinos, the shorter wavelengths of light of the visible spectrum, and continuous exposure as compared with short intermittent exposures.

A few minutes of exposure to visible light can damage the human retina. Interestingly, the retina is the only tissue in the body where light is highly focused on oxygenated cells. Possible mechanisms for photochemical toxicity of the retina must therefore include not only the formation of free radicals from sensitized endogenous molecules but also the possibility that by a photodynamic reaction the molecules sensitized by light react with oxygen to provide a superoxide radical which then attacks other molecules within the cell. These photochemical mechanisms do depend on wavelength, intensity, and duration of exposure, but are different from thermal or mechanical lesions induced by light, and, importantly, are different from the lesion of cystoid macula edema. The photochemical damage created by short wavelengths is seen in stages in the retinal pigment epithelium and the photoreceptor layers. (The lesion of solar retinopathy may also be caused by the short wavelengths of the solar spectrum.)

Recent excellent articles dealing with protective mechanisms in the retina as well as the specificity and cause of the photochemical lesions have been published by Irvine et al. (1) and Parver et al. (2). Certainly the cell biology of photic injury to the retina requires further work. The retina has its own defense mechanisms, but pretreatment with steroids may decrease susceptibility to light injury. Protective antioxidants include ascorbic acid (Tso is particularly interested in its action), glutathione, vitamin E (alpha tocopherol), and especially beta carotenes. Standards of illumination intensity and spectral standards for our surgical microscopes are necessary. Filters may turn out to be useful. For the moment, however, the surgeon can easily cover the cornea conveniently during anterior segment surgery done under coaxial illumination to protect the patient during otherwise perfect surgery.

The Editors

REFERENCES

1. Irvine, A. R., et al. (1984): *Arch. Ophthalmol.,* 102:1358.
2. Parver, L., et al. (1984): *Arch. Ophthalmol.,* 102:772.

Surgical Pharmacology of the Eye,
edited by M. Sears and A. Tarkkanen.
Raven Press, New York © 1985.

Retinal Phototoxicity in Ocular Surgery

Mark O. M. Tso

*Georgiana Theobald Ophthalmic Pathology Laboratory, University of Illinois
Eye and Ear Infirmary, Chicago, Illinois 60612*

SUMMARY: Light toxicity is definitely a serious complication in intraocular surgery. From the physical parameters of the ophthalmic instruments measured by Calkins et al. (13), photic maculopathy may be relatively common, even though the retinal damage may be subtle. Because of the ability of the photoreceptor cells to regenerate, impaired visual acuity may partially recover. The alarming aspect of this iatrogenic disease is that the remarkable susceptibility of the retina to the light of the operating microscope may be as short as 1 min. Mechanisms of damage must be investigated in order to assist the redesign of illuminating systems. Meanwhile, the most important step ophthalmologists may take to protect their patients is to cover the cornea with a sponge or similar material to shield the retina from the operating microscope light. In the aging macula, exposure to the operating light, ophthalmic instruments, or excessively ambient illumination may accelerate the degenerative process. Certain pharmacologic agents may ameliorate or exaggerate this disease process.

With the advent of microsurgery in ophthalmology in the last two decades, illumination engineers have installed various innovative light sources in ophthalmic instruments and operating microscopes. They have acted on the precept that the brighter the illuminating system (1), the more precise and the more pleased the ophthalmic surgeons will be in their clinical and surgical procedures.

In 1966, Noell (2) observed that apparently harmless environmental lighting such as that of a fluorescent lamp may cause permanent damage to the photoreceptors of rodents. Following this lead, many visual scientists have examined photic injury to the retina, defining (a) the physical characteristics of the light that causes retinal damage, (b) the physiological parameters of the animals, which will influence light toxicity in the retina, and (c) the possible pathogenetic mechanisms of retinal light toxicity. However, because of marked differences in species susceptibility and the paucity of human reports of retinal light toxicity, the findings in the animal experiments have not influenced the illumination engineers in their design of the ophthalmic instruments. However, the recently well-documented reports of retinal light damage (3–5) in patients during routine intraocular surgery have awakened ophthalmic surgeons to the importance of light toxicity for the human retina.

CLINICAL STUDIES

McDonald and Irvine (3) first reported light-induced maculopathy in 6 patients after extracapsular cataract extraction with implantation of posterior chamber lens. The patients were operated on with a ceiling-mount Zeiss operating microscope with a 30-W bulb. The surgical procedure consisted of anterior capsulotomy, expression of the lens nucleus, removal of cortical material, and polish of the posterior lens capsule. Under an air bubble, the posterior chamber lens was inserted and the wound was closed with interrupted sutures.

The surgical operating time varied from 1 hr 15 min to 1½ hr. Postoperatively, the best corrected visual acuity of the patients ranged from 20/30 to 20/100. In the three cases, a subtle pale retinal area with fine granularity was noted around the macula 1 week, 2 weeks, and 11 days after surgery, respectively. Three other cases were not noted ophthalmoscopically until fluorescein angiography was performed in an attempt to explain the poor vision. Fluorescein angiograms showed a discrete chorioretinal lesion with mottling in the center and irregular marginal staining. One of the 6 patients developed, in addition, cystoid macular edema; others had no clinical evidence of cystoid macular edema. Visual field done by computer directed "octopus" examination documented dense paracentral scotoma in 3 of 6 patients.

To confirm that these retinal lesions were indeed induced by the operating microscope, McDonald and Irvine did the same surgical procedure of lens extraction and implantation of intraocular lens on an adult rhesus monkey under the operating microscope and obtained similar retinal lesions noted by ophthalmoscopy and fluorescein angiography. This lesion also appeared "identical" to the lesions reported by Hochheimer and co-workers in phakic monkeys after exposure to the light of the operating microscope for 60 min. These well-documented cases raised the warning of the phototoxic potential of light from the operating microscopes and ophthalmic instruments.

A second report (4) of light-induced maculopathy from the operating microscope in patients after implanting intraocular lens was presented at the poster session of the 1983 American Academy of Ophthalmology meeting by Ho et al., who were able to document the absence of macula diseases in patients 1 to 2 years prior to surgery by fundus photographs, and the subsequent appearance of discrete macular lesions after cataract extraction, comparable to those described by McDonald and Irvine.

Recently Berler and Peyser (5) studied 310 cataract operations performed under two operating microscopes with different light intensities. The two operating microscopes, Zeiss OM-6 and OM-7 models with incandescent coaxial illumination, emitted light intensity at the visible spectrum (450 to 950 nm) of 0.046 W/cm^2 and 0.016 W/cm^2 at the corneal surface and ultraviolet output of 110 $\mu W/cm^2$ and 2 $\mu W/cm^2$, respectively. The study included only relatively healthy patients with uncomplicated cataract operations and no known retinopathy or diseases in the ocular media. Patients with surgical complications, corneal opacities, glaucoma, diabetes mellitus, uveitis, and retinopathy were excluded. Seventy-one eyes were operated on under the high-intensity microscope, and 62 were operated on under the low-intensity microscope. Patients were followed for 1 to 6 months. Only visual acuity was evaluated, and ophthalmoscopic and fluorescein angiographic findings were not included in the study. Reduced visual acuity of 20/40 or worse was considerably more prevalent in patients operated on with the high-intensity microscope. It is interesting to note that 6 months after operation, visual acuity of 20/40 or worse was observed in 19% of the patients operated on with the high-intensity microscope but in only 5% of those operated on with the low intensity light. It is difficult to draw a conclusion from this study because of the absence of detailed ophthalmoscopic findings. The possibility that some of these patients may suffer from photic injury to the macula under the high-intensity operating microscope was considered.

The above three studies of possible light toxicity in the retina after routine cataract extraction serve as an important bridge between the large volume of experimental work in light damage in animal models and lighting toxicity in surgical procedures on human patients.

EXPERIMENTAL STUDIES IN NONHUMAN PRIMATES

In the last two decades, experimental work on light injury to the retina has been performed on rats, rabbits, hamsters, frogs, pigeons, cats, dogs, monkeys, and baboons. Species differences make it difficult to compare the human cases of light toxicity after intraocular surgery with the photic injury of the lower animals, particularly rodents. Furthermore, the human cases of retinal light toxicity have well-documented clinical features, but histopathologic, electrophysiologic, and biochemical studies have not yet been reported. On the other hand, most of the animal studies presented well-documented histopathologic, electrophysiologic, and biochemical observations, but few have carefully described the clinical features of the retina after light injury, especially in the lower animals. The experimental studies discussed in this report are confined to nonhuman primates.

Hochheimer, D'Anna, and Calkins (6) demonstrated that the exposure of the retina of phakic rhesus monkeys to an operating microscope with an estimated retinal irradiance of 750 μW/cm^2 for 1 hr produced a whitening lesion of the retina that persisted for more than 1 year. McDonald and Irvine (3) produced a similar retinal lesion in a rhesus monkey that underwent extracapsular lens extraction and implantation of a posterior chamber lens. In both reports, no histopathologic study was described. Parver, Auker, and Fine (7) exposed the retina of cynomolgus monkeys to the light of an operating microscope with or without filter, with calculated retinal irradiance of 1.06 W/cm^2 and 0.89 W/cm^2, respectively, for 1 hr. They noted slight clouding of the retina after exposure to the unfiltered light ophthalmoscopically, but no fluorescein angiography was done. Histologically, they noted vacuolation and liquefaction necrosis of retinal pigment epithelium. Photoreceptor outer segments showed tubular vesicular degeneration and necrosis. Swollen axons contained microtubules in disarray and densification of Mueller cell cytoplasm. In none of the above reports was sequential study of the pathologic process of retinal light toxicity done.

Clinical features of the human patients with photic injury after cataract extraction are remarkably similar to that of the photic maculopathy in the rhesus monkeys (8,9) produced by the light of an indirect ophthalmoscope, which helped to illustrate the sequential pathologic process of this iatrogenic disease.

The manifestations of the photic maculopathy in rhesus monkey after exposure to the indirect ophthalmoscope were divided into three phases: (a) the initial response in the first week, (b) the subsequent and pigmentary changes associated with macrophagic response in the first month, and (c) the reparative phase extending from the first month to 5 years after injury. In phase 1, immediately after exposure to the light of an indirect ophthalmoscope for 1 to 2 hr, the maculas showed no abnormality by ophthalmoscopy. In the second to the seventh days after exposure, the animals developed whitening of the outer layers of the retina, which was initially subtle and difficult to detect by ophthalmoscopy. By fluorescein angiography, diffuse leakage from the retinal pigment epithelium was evident (Fig. 1A). Similarly, the fundus changes in the human patients developing retinal light toxicity after lens extraction were too subtle to detect by ophthalmoscopy but could be easily seen by fluorescein angiography.

In the histopathologic study of the animal model, the retinal pigment epithelium showed mild derangement of the pigment granules. The photoreceptor outer segments were disoriented. Focal pyknosis of the nuclei of the photoreceptor cells was seen, and edema of the inner plexiform layers was noted (Fig. 2).

In phase 2, the retinal edema gradually subsided and the macula became irregularly pigmented, ophthalmoscopically. The retina was initially flat. In some eyes, however, the center of the lesion became mildly elevated and appeared yellowish. Fluorescein angiography showed staining of the damaged pigment epithelium with focal area of hypofluorescence (Fig. 1B). The irregular mottling of macula in the monkeys closely mimicked that described in the human patients. In the human cases, the irregular pigmentation was easily missed as an aging change.

Histopathologic study of the monkey in phase 2 showed infiltration of macrophages into subretinal space, clustering around the damaged outer segment of photoreceptor cells and the retinal pigment epithelium (Fig. 3). In the more severe areas, focal loss of photoreceptor cells was observed, and the

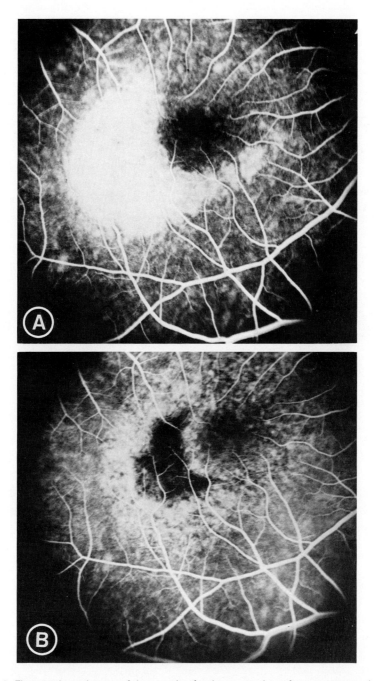

FIG. 1. A: Fluorescein angiogram of the macula of a rhesus monkey after exposure to the light of an indirect ophthalmoscope 3 days earlier, showing extensive leakage in the macula area. **B:** Fluorescein angiogram of the same monkey 4 weeks after exposure to the light of an indirect ophthalmoscope, showing an irregular pigmented area in the macula and an area of mottled hypofluorescence, very much similar to the lesion shown in light-induced maculopathy in human patients.

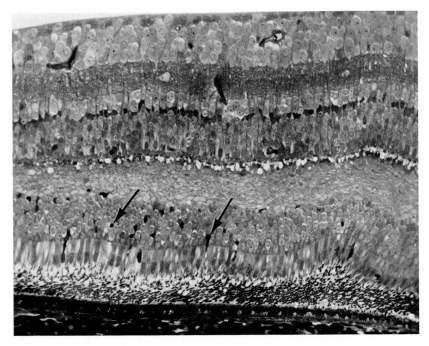

FIG. 2. In the acute stage after photic injury, focal pyknosis of photoreceptor cells (*arrows*), derangement of photoreceptor elements, and edema of the retina are seen. Methylene blue, × 145.

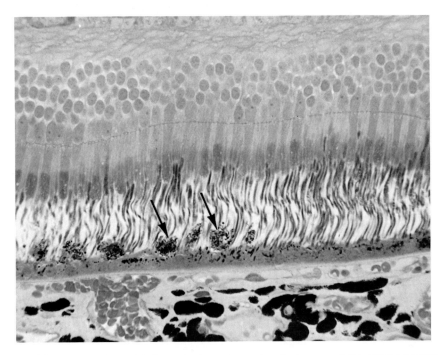

FIG. 3. Macrophages (*arrows*) laden with pigment granules cluster around the damaged outer segments. The retinal pigment epithelium is extensively depigmented. Methylene blue, × 440.

outer nuclear layer became 1 to 2 nuclei thick. A placoid proliferation of retinal pigment epithelium was noted in the center of the lesions (Fig. 4A).

In phase 3, a reparative process developed. The irregular macular pigmentation persisted clinically. A placoid proliferation of retinal pigment epithelium resulted in an elevated depigmented yellowish lesion, ophthalmoscopically, and showed persistent staining in fluorescein angiograms even 5 years after initial light exposure. Pathologically, the retinal pigment epithelium resumed its cuboidal shape but remained irregularly depigmented. The photoreceptor elements overlying the pigment epithelium were partially regenerated. In some cases, the outer segments remained abnormally short. The inner segments of the photoreceptor cells showed hypertrophy (Fig. 4B). The number of photoreceptor cell nuclei in the outer nuclear layer remained diminished. Neovascularization was seen extending from the choroid into the proliferated retinal pigment epithelium plaque. Patients described by McDonald and Irvine did not have a long follow-up, and the yellowish raised plaque of the monkeys was not noted.

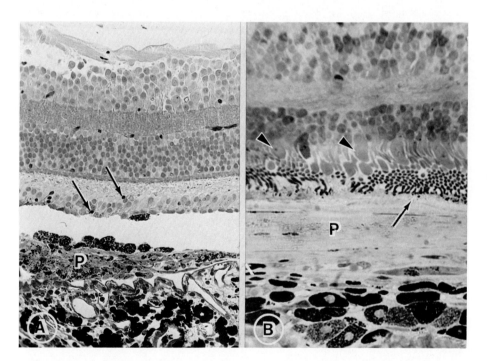

FIG. 4. A: In the more severe lesions, marked loss of photoreceptor cells (*single arrow*) is seen with placoid proliferation of retinal pigment epithelium (P). Methylene blue, × 150. **B:** In the chronic phase, shortening of outer segments and hypertrophy of inner segments of photoreceptor cells (*arrowheads*) are noted. Retinal pigment epithelium (*single arrow*) is extensively depigmented, and a proliferative plaque of spindly cells (P) is present anterior to the choroid. Methylene blue, × 300.

The visual acuity of the rhesus monkeys with placoid proliferation and photic maculopathy has been tested by psychophysical studies (10). Two animals with characteristic photic maculopathy showed visual acuity of 20/40 and 20/30 in the injured eyes, compared with 20/15 and 20/18 in the control opposite eyes, respectively. Histologic study of these maculas showed regeneration of the photoreceptor elements over the macula with considerable loss of photoreceptor cell nuclei. We concluded that the photoreceptor cells in photic maculopathy in the rhesus monkey were capable of partial regeneration with some recovery of visual function. However, the recovery was incomplete because of mild loss of photoreceptor cells, which in some focal retinal areas showed as much as 50% to 70% reduction in cells. This experiment provided further explanation for the observations of McDonald and Irvine in human patients with light-induced maculopathy. Due to the regenerative ability of the photoreceptor elements, the maculopathy induced by the operating microscope might have been missed clinically because of the gradual recovery of visual function.

Fuller, Machemer, and Knighton (11) examined the effect of intraocular fiberoptic light used for pars plana vitrectomy on the macula of adult owl monkeys. The eyes were exposed to the intraocular light for 5, 10, 15, 20, and 30 min. The animals were examined 1 hr, 24 hr, 1 week, and 4 weeks after exposure. In the initial phase, such as 24 hr after light exposure of 15 to 20 min, whitening of the outer retina and retinal pigment epithelium was noted ophthalmoscopically, with leakage of fluorescein. One month after exposure, irregular hypopigmentation and hyperpigmentation were observed ophthalmoscopically. Histologically, damage to outer layers of the retina with focal loss of photoreceptor cells was noted. The retinal irradiance was calculated to be 0.22 W/cm^2. They believed that the threshold of an ophthalmoscopically visible lesion was 15 min of intraocular light exposure and that microscopic changes could be seen in the macula as little as 10 min after light exposure.

Friedman and Kuwabara (12) exposed the retina of rhesus monkeys to the light of a direct ophthalmoscope for 15 min and observed whitening of the retinal pigment epithelium 24 hr later, which faded and became irregularly pigmented. They noted that the initial changes consisted of dilatation of the villi of the pigment epithelial cells and disruption of photoreceptor outer segments, and they believed that this photic injury might be potentiated by the increase of body temperature.

In summary, ophthalmic instruments, including the direct and indirect ophthalmoscopes, operating microscopes, intraocular fiberoptic light and slit lamps, could damage the retina. Damage was not seen immediately after exposure but could be observed a few hours to a few days after exposure, as edema of the outer layer of the retina developed, and could be easily demonstrated by fluorescein angiography as leakage from retinal pigment epithelium. Subsequently, the retina became depigmented, and in severe cases a raised retinal pigment epithelial scar could be seen. In the chronic phase, there was regeneration of the photoreceptor elements resulting in partial recovery of vision.

The ophthalmoscopic appearance, fluorescein angiographic findings, histopathologic features, and clinical course of the photic maculopathy are totally different from those of aphakic cystoid macular edema or Irvine-Gass syndrome. In the photic maculopathy, the retinal edema was diffused, and the macula did not appear cystic. The fluorescein leakage appeared in the first week after exposure and was diffuse, without a petaloid staining pattern. Histologically, photic maculopathy showed damage of retinal pigment epithelium and photoreceptor cells, whereas cystoid macular edema exhibited cysts in the outer plexiform layer and inner nuclear layer of the retina. It is doubtful that these two entities are causally related.

PHYSICAL PARAMETERS OF THE LIGHT FROM SOME OPHTHALMIC INSTRUMENTS

The retinal irradiances of various ophthalmic instruments were correlated by Calkins, Hochheimer, and D'Anna (13) with recommended maximal permissible exposures from the American National Standards Institute laser safety guidelines. They calculated the retinal irradiance that patients might receive from direct or indirect ophthalmoscopes, slit lamps, surgical microscopes, and overhead surgical lamps. The average retinal irradiance from an American Optical (AO) or a Frigi Xonix indirect ophthalmoscope was 69 μW/cm^2 when the transformer was at 6.5 V and 125 μW/cm^2 when the transformer was at maximum setting. Direct ophthalmoscopes tested included the AO giantscope and Welch Allyn ophthalmoscope with a standard bulb, and they gave a retinal irradiance of 29 μW/cm^2, approximately half that of the indirect ophthalmoscope. A slit lamp with a plano contact lens using medium-intensity settings produced a retinal irradiance of 217 μW/cm^2, approximately three times that produced by the indirect ophthalmoscope. Overhead surgical lamps yielded a retinal irradiance of 25 μW/cm^2 at a level comparable to that from a direct ophthalmoscope. The Zeiss OpMi I operating microscope with various external fiberoptic sources produced in phakic patients with various refractive errors a retinal irradiance of 100 μW/cm^2 to 970 μW/cm^2. For aphakic patients, the irradiance ranged from 85 μW/cm^2 to 590 μW/cm^2. The operating microscope produced a retinal irradiance of two to ten times more than that of an indirect ophthalmoscope. Using the laser safety standards, Calkins believed that the operating microscope light would be unsafe after 1 min!

In consideration of the physical parameters resulting in damage to the retina, we must evaluate spectrum of wavelengths, intensity, duration, intermittent or continuous exposure, and focused or nonfocused light, as well as the visual angle of light directed at the retina. Many of these variables were altered from time to time during the use of various clinical instruments for examination of patients, so many of the measured and calculated retinal irradiances varied considerably in the clinical setting.

PHYSIOLOGIC FACTORS AFFECTING LIGHT TOXICITY TO THE RETINA

The physiologic factors affecting light toxicity to the retina were derived from animal experiments, mostly done in rodents. Many of the physiologic factors may be species dependent but may apply to human light-toxicity reactions in some degree. The factors that influence the light-toxicity reactions include the following:

1. *Location in the retina.* Different regions of the retina exhibited various susceptibility to photic injury. Howell, Rapp, and Williams (14) noted that the central superior region of the hooded rat retina was more susceptible, whereas Noell (15) observed that the retina in the peripapillary region and near the ora serrata appeared to be more resistant. Carter-Dawson and co-workers (16) described the inferonasal region of the normal and vitamin-A-deficient rat retina as more susceptible to light injury.

2. *Dark adaptation.* Rats that were adapted to the dark for 2 weeks before light exposure appeared to be more severely injured when exposed to light (17).

3. *Body temperature.* In both rodents and monkeys, the photic injury of the retina may be exaggerated when the body temperature is raised during exposure (2,12).

4. *Pigmentation.* Although it was generally suspected that albino rat is more susceptible to photic injury, Rapp and Williams (18) exposed albino and pigmented rats with dilated pupils to light that was controlled to produce equal steady-state bleaching and compared retinal damage in both species. They suspected that pigmented rats appeared to be less susceptible because the iris pigmentation lowered the retinal irradiance. However, the albino and pigmented rats were of different strains. The possibility of different strains' susceptibilities to photic injury must be considered.

5. *Age.* Lai et al. (19) reported that light damage appeared to increase with advancing age in rats. More severe photic injury was observed in retinas of 7-week-old rats when compared to those of 3- to 4-week-olds. The retina of newborn rhesus monkey was examined by Messner and was believed to be very susceptible to light damage.

6. *Species difference.* Rats, rabbits, frogs, pigeons, dogs, monkeys, and humans show marked differences in susceptibility. Lawwill et al. (20) found that hamsters were more prone to light damage when compared to rabbits and cats, and threshold injuries of monkeys, rabbits, and humans were considerably higher than that of rats.

7. *Nutritional state.* Vitamin A deficiency ameliorated light damage in rats

(21). The possibility that ascorbate, vitamin E, and selenium may effect photic injury in retina will be considered in the following sections.

8. *Different wavelengths.* Exposure to short wavelengths of the visible spectrum appears to result in more severe retinal injury. In general, the action spectrum of the inflicting light was a decreasing function of wavelengths (22,23).

9. *Dose rate.* Higher intensity of the inflicting light will result in more severe retinal lesions.

10. *Continuous or intermittent exposure.* Sperling and co-workers (23,24) noted that intermittent blue or green light produced damage to the cone cells of monkeys. Continuous exposure under similar conditions inflicted more severe damage to retinal pigment epithelium. In humans, cataractous lens or an implanted intraocular lens will filter light of different wavelengths into the retina. Since injury varies with wavelengths, the changes in the ocular media will alter the light injury.

Thus, the physiologic state of the patients will definitively affect the photic injury. Since patients who undergo intraocular lens implantation with operating microscope frequently have different physiologic states, so the photic maculopathy in these patients would be expected to vary.

POSSIBLE MECHANISMS OF LIGHT TOXICITY

Whereas radiant energy damage to retina is frequently grouped by three basic mechanisms, namely, mechanical (for example, YAG laser injury), photocoagulative (for example, Ruby laser injury), and photic injuries, the light toxic reaction in patients after intraocular surgery is most likely an example of photic injury, since the retinal irradiance is too low to cause a significant temperature rise. A number of theories have been proposed to explain photic injury on the retina by light of low intensity.

1. In some animal experiments, the light-toxicity response is related to rhodopsin absorption, which has been studied by Noell in rodents (15,21). In these lesions there was loss of retinal pigment epithelium, disruption of outer segments of photoreceptor cells, pyknosis of the photoreceptor nuclei, and eventual atrophy of the entire retina. Deficiency of vitamin A appeared to protect the animals. This type of injury has the action spectrum of rhodopsin absorption. It is not certain whether this mechanism of light damage can be demonstrated in the primate models.

2. The most probable mechanism in the light toxicity reaction of the primates is that described by Ham (25,26) and Lawwill (27). The toxic effects seemed to be most severe when the retina was exposed to short wavelengths in the visual spectrum (400 to 550 nm). The power density was too low to produce significant temperature rise and was therefore not a thermal injury. In this type of light damage, the most prominent pathologic feature was

necrosis and subsequent reactive proliferation of the retinal pigment epithelium. Although some of the outer segment photoreceptor cells were grossly disrupted, some of the photoreceptor cells survived. Ham suspected that this may be a photo-oxidative reaction, and Lawwill showed that the phototoxic effect was oxygen dependent. Ham further postulated that chronic exposure to the short wavelengths might be a contributing factor to senile macular degeneration.

3. The third mechanism is color-blinding light toxicity, described by Sperling and co-workers (23). They demonstrated that the posterior pole and macula of nonhuman primates showed selective loss of blue-sensitive cones to blue light and green-sensitive cones to green after intermittent exposure. He further compared the color-blinding retinal lesion with that of continuous exposure to blue light for 120 continuous min. In the latter lesion, distinct disruption of retinal pigment epithelial and mild photoreceptor cell degeneration were observed.

PHARMACOLOGIC AGENTS AFFECTING RETINAL LIGHT TOXICITY

Since the exact mechanisms of light toxicity to the retina have not been definitively determined, only a few pharmacologic agents have been found or suspected to affect light toxicity reaction in the retina. The agents that will be discussed include ascorbate, selenium and vitamin E, corticosteroids, photosensitizing drugs such as psoralen, chlorpromazine, thioridazine, tetracycline, and hematoporphyria.

Vitamin C

One of the possible mechanisms of photic injury to the retina is the production of superoxide radicals induced by light (28,29). These radicals may damage cell membranes of the retinal cells causing lipid peroxidation and disruption of plasmalemma. Ascorbate is known to be present in the retina in large quantity, but its function has not been determined. Recently it has been postulated that ascorbate may be an important antioxidant in the eye, providing protective function to the retina against superoxide radicals produced by light. In our recent studies of normal guinea pig and baboon retinas, we noted that ascorbate was largely present in the reduced form in the neural retina but in the oxidized form in the pigment epithelium. When guinea pigs, which, like humans and monkeys, depend on exogenous vitamin C, were exposed to fluorescent light, more severe damage was observed in scorbutic animals when compared with the normals (30). When one eye of 6 normal baboons was exposed to the light of an indirect ophthalmoscope for 30 min with the opposite eye covered, mild photic injury was noted in the pigment epithelium and photoreceptor elements (29). After light exposure, the reduced ascorbate decreased in neural retina of the posterior pole, whereas the level of ascorbate in the peripheral retina remained unchanged. Although the changes in the retina and the mechanisms of phototoxic injury are very complex, the possibility that ascorbate may indeed play an important part in amelioration of photic injury to retina should be entertained.

The study by Organisciak, Wang, and Kou (31) on the effect of ascorbate in the normal rat retina after light exposure further confirms this direction of research. Even though the rat produces endogenous ascorbate and does not require exogenous ascorbate, Organisciak and co-workers observed that ascorbate decreased in normal rat after exposure to intense light for 24 hr in an age- and light-dependent fashion. When ascorbate was given to the rats before exposure, the rhodopsin in the retina after light exposure was consistently higher than in rats that had no supplement of ascorbate in their diet. This experiment suggested that ascorbate supplement may ameliorate light exposure in the rat. In contrast, glutathione in the rat retina was unaffected after intense light exposure.

Vitamin E and Selenium

Vitamin E and selenium, which are important components of glutathione peroxidase, are important antioxidants in the retina. Kagan et al. (32) noted a significant accumulation of lipid hydroperoxide in rod outer segments after exposure to light of wavelengths that bleach rhodopsin. Vitamin E was found to inhibit this accumulation of lipid hydroperoxide. However, the exact role of vitamin E glutathione peroxidase in protective function of light-induced retinopathy is uncertain. Stone and co-workers (33) found that rats deficient in vitamin E and selenium did not show exaggerated photic injury. No experiments on primates have yet been reported.

Corticosteroids

The effect of corticosteroids on photic injury has recently been investigated by Ham and co-workers (34). They exposed the retina of 2 anesthetized monkeys to light of wavelengths peaked at 440 nm. Using minimal ophthalmoscopic retinal changes at 24 hr after exposure as the biological end point, they observed that 125 mg methylprednisolone given intravenously 1 hr before exposure raised the threshold by a factor of 2. They also injected methylprednisolone 1 hr after exposure and produced marginal elevation of the blue-light threshold. These investigators did not provide explanations for their observation, but the possibility that the corticosteroid simply delayed the edema of the retina after photic injury and was not actually elevating the threshold of photic injury must be considered.

Photosensitizing drugs such as the phenothiazine derivatives chlorpromazine and thioridazine have been known to produce retinopathy after prolonged usage (35,36). However, whether the disease so produced is related to light-induced toxicity is not known. Whether drugs such as 8-methoxypsoralen and others used for treatment of vitiligo would exaggerate light toxicity in the retina has not been determined and should be investigated.

ACKNOWLEDGMENTS

This work is supported in part by Public Health Service grant EY1903 and Core grant IP30 EY01792.

REFERENCES

1. Cogan, D. C. (1968): Lighting and health hazards. *Arch. Ophthalmol.,* 79:2.
2. Noell, W. K., Walker, V. S., Kang, B. S., Berman, S. (1966): Retinal damage by light in rats. *Invest. Ophthalmol.,* 5:450–473.
3. McDonald, H. R., and Irvine, A. R. (1983): Light-induced maculopathy from the operating microscope in extracapsular cataract extraction and intraocular lens implantation. *Ophthalmology,* 90:945.
4. Ho, B. (1983): Poster session, American Academy of Ophthalmology Annual Meeting, Chicago.
5. Berler, D. K., and Peyser R. (1983): Light intensity and visual acuity following cataract surgery. *Ophthalmology,* 80:933.
6. Hochheimer, B. F., D'Anna, S. A., and Calkins, J. L. (1979): Retinal damage from light. *Am. J. Ophthalmol.,* 88:1039.
7. Parver, L. M., Auker, C. R., and Fine, B. S. (1983): Observations on monkey eyes exposed to light from an operating microscope. *Ophthalmology,* 80:964.
8. Tso, M. O. M. (1973): Photic maculopathy in rhesus monkey: A light and electron microscopic study. *Invest. Ophthalmol. Vis. Sci.,* 12:17.
9. Tso, M. O. M., Fine, B. S., and Zimmerman, L. E. (1972): Photic maculopathy produced by the indirect ophthalmoscope. I. Clinical and histopathologic study. *Am. J. Ophthalmol.,* 73:686.
10. Tso, M. O. M., Robbins, D. O., and Zimmerman, L. E. (1974): Photic maculopathy: A study of functional and pathologic correlation. *Mod. Probl. Ophthalmol.,* 12:220.
11. Fuller, D., Machemer, R., and Knighton, R. W. (1978): Retinal damage produced by intraocular fiberoptic light. *Am. J. Ophthalmol.,* 85:519.
12. Friedman, E., and Kuwabara, T. (1968): The retinal pigment epithelium. IV. The damaging effects of radiant energy. *Arch. Ophthalmol.,* 80:265.
13. Calkins, J. L., Hochheimer, B. F., and D'Anna, S. A. (1980): Potential hazards from specific ophthalmic devices. *Vision Res.,* 20:1039.
14. Howell, W. L., Rapp, L. M., and Williams, T. P. (1982): Distribution of melanosomes across the retinal pigment epithelium of a hooded rat: Implications for light damage. *Invest. Ophthalmol. Vis. Sci.,* 22:139.
15. Noell, W. K. (1980): Possible mechanisms of photoreceptor damage by light in mammalian eyes. *Vision Res.,* 20:1163.
16. Carter-Dawson, L., Kuwabara, T., and Bieri, J. G. (1982): Intrinsic, light-independent, regional differences in photoreceptor cell degeneration in vitamin A deficient rat retinas. *Invest. Ophthalmol. Vis. Sci.,* 22:249.
17. Noell, W. K. (1979): Effects of environmental lighting and dietary vitamin A on the vulnerability of the retina to light damage. *Photochem. Photobiol.,* 29:717.
18. Rapp, L. M., and Williams, T. P. (1980): The role of ocular pigmentation in protecting against retinal light damage. *Vision Res.,* 20:1127.
19. Lai, Y. L., Jacoby, R. O., and Jonas, A. M. (1978): Age-related and light-associated retinal changes in Fischer rats. *Invest. Ophthalmol. Vis. Sci.,* 17:634.
20. Lawwill, T., Crockett, S., and Currier, G. (1977): Retinal damage secondary to chronic light exposure, thresholds and mechanisms. *Doc. Ophthalmol.,* 44:379.
21. Noell, W. K., and Albrecht, R. (1971): Irreversible effects of visible light on the retina: Role of vitamin A. *Science,* 172:76.

22. Ham, W. T., Jr., Mueller, H. A., Ruffolo, J. J., Jr., and Clark, A. M. (1979): Sensitivity of the retina to radiation damage as a function of wavelength. *Photochem. Photobiol.,* 29:735.
23. Sperling, H. G., Johnson, C., and Harwerth, R. S. (1980): Differential spectral photic damage to primate cones. *Vision Res.,* 20:1117.
24. Harwerth, R. S., and Sperling, H. G. (1975): Effects of intense visible radiation on the increment-threshold spectral sensitivity of the rhesus monkey eye. *Vision Res.,* 15:1193.
25. Ham, W. T., Jr., Mueller, H. A., and Sliney, D. H. (1976): Retinal sensitivity to damage from short wavelength light. *Nature,* 260:153.
26. Ham, W. T., Jr., Mueller, H. A., Ruffolo, J. J., Jr., and Clarke, A. M. (1979): Sensitivity of the retina to radiation damage as a function of wavelength. *Photochem. Photobiol.,* 29:735.
27. Lawwill, T., Crockett, R. S., and Currier, G. (1977): Retinal damage secondary to chronic light exposure, thresholds and mechanisms. *Doc. Ophthalmol.,* 44:379.
28. Woodford, B. J., Tso, M. O. M., and Lam, K. W. (1983): Reduced and oxidized ascorbates in guinea pig retinas under normal and light-exposed conditions. *Invest. Ophthalmol. Vis. Sci.,* 24:862.
29. Tso, M. O. M., Woodford, B. J., and Lam, K. W. (1984): Distribution of ascorbate in normal primate retina and after photic injury: a biochemical, morphological correlated study. *Curr. Eye Res.,* 3:181.
30. Woodford, B. J., and Tso, M. O. M. (1984): Exaggeration of photic injury in scorbutic guinea pig retinas. *Invest. Ophthalmol. Vis. Sci.,* 25(Suppl.):90.
31. Organisciak, D. T., Wang, H. M., and Kou, A. L. (1984): Ascorbate and glutathione levels in the developing normal and dystrophysical rat retina: Effect of intense light exposure. *Curr. Eye Res.,* 3:257.
32. Kagan, V. E., Shvedova, A. A., Norikou, K. N., and Kozlor, Y. P. (1973): Light-induced free radical oxidation of membrane lipids in photoreceptors of frog retina. *Biochim. Biophys. Acta,* 330:76.
33. Stone, W. L., Katz, M. L., Lurie, M., Marmor, M. F., and Dratz, E. A. (1979): Effects of dietary Vit E and selenium on light damage to the rat retina. *Photochem. Photobiol.,* 29:725.
34. Ham, W. T., Jr., Mueller, H. A., Ruffolo, J. J., et al (1984): Basic mechanisms underlying the production of photochemical lesions in the mammalian retina. *Curr. Eye Res.,* 3:165.
35. Meredith, T. A., Aaberg, T. M., and Willerson, W. D. (1978): Progressive chorioretinopathy after receiving thioridazine. *Arch. Ophthalmol.,* 96:1172.
36. Siddal, J. R. (1966): Ocular toxic changes associated with chlorpromazine and thioridazine. *Can. J. Ophthalmol.,* 1:190.

Commentary

Tissue Adhesives in Ophthalmology

Progress in the application of tissue glues to the solution of clinical problems such as wound approximation and leaks has been accomplished, albeit slowly. Dr. Khodadoust spells out the needs and requirements. The glues are easy to apply, requiring a dry field to produce a strong swift bond and tissue adherence. They can be used to seal corneal or even orbital perforations (CSF leaks) and to produce tarsorrhaphies. Usually these glues are cyanoacrylates that polymerize in the presence of hydroxyl ions creating a bond after contact with tissue water. The longer complex alkyl side chain, the less biodegradable, but, the less tissue toxic is the compound. A neat fibroplastic layer is produced under the bond to cover the defect. Closer collaboration with the polymer chemist and encouragement from industry and the FDA for these "orphan" compounds might prove useful.

Recently Dr. Buschmann from Würzburg (1) has reported the successful application of a fibrinogen tissue adhesive to promote sealing of perforations in the capsule of the crystalline lens after injury.

The Editors

REFERENCE

1. Buschmann, W. (1983): *Klin. Monatsbl. Augenheilkd.,* 183:241–245.

Surgical Pharmacology of the Eye,
edited by M. Sears and A. Tarkkanen.
Raven Press, New York © 1985.

Tissue Adhesives in Ophthalmology

Ali A. Khodadoust

Yale University School of Medicine, New Haven, Connecticut 06510

SUMMARY: The potential of sutureless surgery provided by surgical glue is an attractive concept because it can be used for repair of certain wounds that are difficult to repair by conventional suturing techniques. These include perforated corneal ulcers, fistula of filtering blebs, leaking surgical wounds or scleromalacia, as well as for ordinary surgery. An ideal tissue adhesive should rapidly bind two wound surfaces with an adequate tensile strength and be nontoxic. Various monomers of cyanoacrylates have been tried. They rapidly bind wound edges with an adequate strength, are noncarcinogenic, but still are too toxic and are nonbiodegradable. Despite these limitations, the medical grade of cyanoacrylates (*n*-butyl alpha cyanoacrylate or histacryl glue) has been shown to be effective in emergency management of perforated or impending perforation of corneal ulcers, temporary tarsorrhaphy, various leaking filtering blebs and wounds as well as reinforcement of the sclera in patients with thin sclera or staphyloma. Although none of the existing monomers of cyanoacrylates have fulfilled the criteria for an ideal glue, they have provided a step toward sutureless surgery.

Surgical glue is attractive because it can potentially be used for sutureless surgery, to stop bleeding or seal off leaking wounds, and, above all, to glue tissue that would otherwise be difficult to repair by conventional suturing techniques (such as liver, spleen, kidney, and small vessels or nerves). An ideal tissue adhesive should rapidly bind two wound surfaces with an adequate tensile strength and be nontoxic, noncarcinogenic, and, above all, biodegradable. Such a surgical glue could have a wide clinical application in ophthalmology as an alternative to the suturing technique for repair of wounds that are difficult to manage, such as perforated corneal ulcers, fistulae of filtering blebs, scleromalacia, or leaking surgical wounds.

In the past, several attempts have been made to use blood-clotting factors such as fibrin and thrombin as biological glue for repair of conjunctival wounds, corneoscleral incisions, plastic surgery, and keratoplasty (41–55). None of the agents provided adequate tensile strength and the idea was abandoned. In early 1960, the cyanoacrylate adhesives became available, and the concept of surgical glue gained new momentum. The initial compound (methyl-cyanoacrylate or Krazy Glue®), although it provided a rapid adhesion of two surfaces with adequate tensile strength, was too toxic for clinical application. Other monomers were synthesized, and numerous reports have appeared in literature comparing the toxicity, biodegradability, and hemostatic properties of these agents. Most of the reports in literature dealing with surgical glues have been on experimental animals, and their clinical usage remains controversial. Despite marked reduction of toxicity in newer compounds, none are biodegradable, and they cannot replace the suturing technique. Eventual necrosis of tissue at the interface interrupts the natural process of wound healing. These agents, however, have been used for selected clinical conditions such as perforated corneal ulcers and leaking wounds. In these problems, the glue temporarily maintains the integrity of the globe while the natural process of healing takes place beneath the adhesion. In this chapter, our present knowledge of surgical glues will be reviewed briefly, and the potential clinical applications will be discussed.

HISTORY

The adhesive action of cyanoacrylate polymers was reported by Coover and his co-workers in 1959 (11). Methyl-2-cyanoacrylates (Eastman 910 adhesive) became commercially available and were known as Krazy Glue®. This agent was used as tissue adhesive in experimental vascular surgery in dogs in 1960 (10). Soon thereafter, it was used for bronchial closure and applied in a wide variety of general surgical procedures involving the intestine, liver, spleen, kidney, and genitourinary tract (22).

In 1963, Krazy Glue® was experimentally used as a tissue adhesive in ophthalmology. It was tested on rabbit eyes as an alternative method for lid suture, conjunctival flaps, limbal closure, muscle surgery, and other conditions (5,6,17,53,57). The glue was found to be too toxic—leading to irritation, edema, and necrosis of the tissue—thus limiting its clinical use. Other monomers were synthesized and tested. Alkyl derivatives of cyanoacrylates, developed by Leonard and his co-workers (33), were found to be less toxic and were better tolerated by living tissue [Refojo et al. (45)]. Numerous reports of its use for many surgical procedures on experimental animals and for selected cases in humans have appeared in the literature. Although none of the existing monomers of the cyanoacrylates have fulfilled the criteria of the ideal glue, they have been a step toward the concept of sutureless surgery (20,34).

CHEMISTRY

The cyanoacrylate monomers are transparent, colorless liquids with low molecular weight. The monomer of alkyl-2-cyanoacrylates are derivatives of ethylene combined with nitride (CN) and an alkyloxycarbonyl group (COOR) (Fig. 1). R can be either methyl, ethyl, butyl, pentyl, n-heptyl, hexyl, octyl, decyl, trifluoroisopropyl (C3H4F3), or isobutyl. These monomers are usually

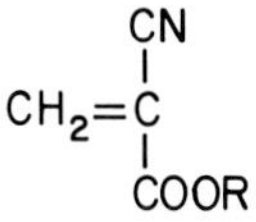

CN
|
CH_2=C
|
COOR

FIG. 1. A. The monomer of alkyl-2-cyanoacrylates are derivatives of ethylene combined with nitride (CN) and alkyloxycarbonyl group (COOR).

synthesized by base-catalyzed condensation of formaldehyde and a cyanoacetate. This condensation produces polycyanoacetate that subsequently can depolymerize to yield a monomer. The monomers are electronegative and, in the presence of anions, rapidly polymerize and convert to a solid, thus becoming adhesive (Fig. 2). The anions needed for polymerization could be an OH of water or an NH_2 group of tissue protein. The process of polymerization takes place in the absence of heat or catalysis. The rate of polymerization depends on how much of the monomer surface is exposed to the substrate and will continue until the depletion of the monomer or the addition of an acid group (H^+). Thus, a thin layer of adhesive will polymerize much faster than a thick layer or a large drop. In the presence of excessive water, polymerization is so fast that the compound will turn white and convert to powder, which does not leave enough time to bring the two surfaces together for adhesion. Since the process of polymerization is reversible, the polymer can degrade and recompose to formaldehyde and cyanoacetate.

DEGRADATION AND TOXICITY

An ideal surgical adhesive should be biodegradable within a reasonable period of time, and its byproduct should be nontoxic. Neither is true of cyanoacrylate polymers. In the presence of water, there is cleavage of carbon-to-carbon of the polymer of cyanoacrylate molecules, leading to formation of formaldehyde and cyanoacetate. Formaldehyde is probably the cause of tissue toxicity of cyanoacrylate adhesives. The rate of degradation of cyanoacrylates is different for each homolog. The rate of toxicity is proportional to the rate of degradation. This rate is generally slower for longer, less toxic alkyl groups, compared to methyl-cyanoacrylates with faster degradation and higher toxicity.

Ocular toxicity of methyl-cyanoacrylates has been evaluated by many investigators (1,5,17,19,53). Its application on an intact cornea causes destruction of epithelial cells, corneal haze, and inflammatory reaction. In the lower cul-de-sac, this agent leads to inflammation and symblepharon. Its injection intracorneally causes limbal hyperemia, severe inflammatory reaction, and

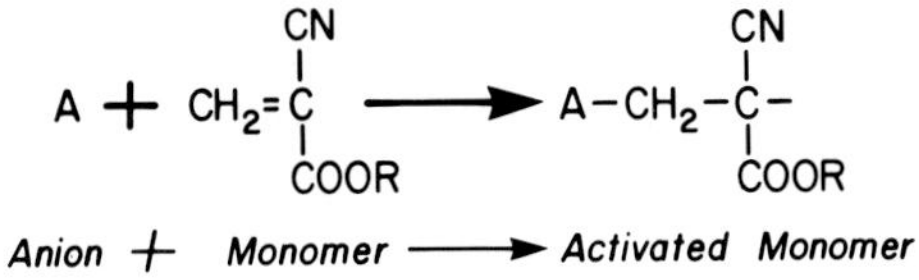

A + CH₂=C(CN)(COOR) → A-CH₂-C(CN)(COOR)

Anion + Monomer → Activated Monomer

FIG. 1. B. In the presence of anion (A^-) the monomer of cyanoacrylates becomes activated and initiates polymerization.

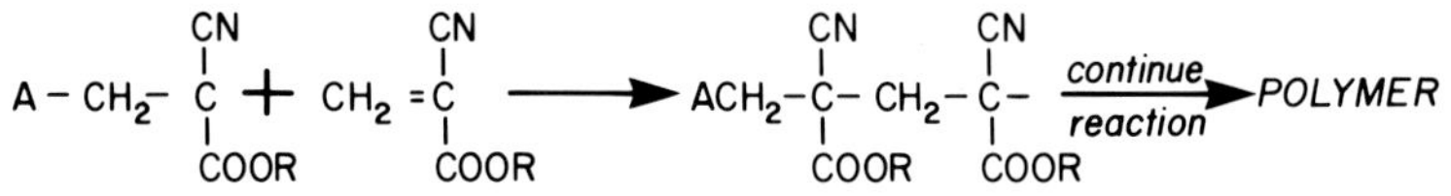

$$A-CH_2-\underset{\underset{COOR}{|}}{\overset{\overset{CN}{|}}{C}} + CH_2=\underset{\underset{COOR}{|}}{\overset{\overset{CN}{|}}{C}} \longrightarrow ACH_2-\underset{\underset{COOR}{|}}{\overset{\overset{CN}{|}}{C}}-CH_2-\underset{\underset{COOR}{|}}{\overset{\overset{CN}{|}}{C}}- \xrightarrow[reaction]{continue} POLYMER$$

FIG. 2. Activated monomer of cyanoacrylate initiates a chain reaction, converting the liquid monomer into a solid polymer.

corneal vascularization. Because of these toxic reactions, methyl-cyanoacrylates have not been recommended in ocular surgery.

The alkyl derivatives of cyanoacrylates are less toxic because of a slower degradation rate. The degradation of n-butyl alpha cyanoacrylates, commonly used for clinical application, is extremely slow. Once implanted subcutaneously, 92% of this agent is retained at 5 months (40). Intracorneal injection of hexyl, octyl, decyl, and isobutyl monomers in experimental animals causes corneal inflammation and vascularization in addition to anterior chamber reaction (1,21). Injection of hexyl and decyl monomers into the anterior chamber leads to a marked reaction, corneal opacification and vascularization. Iris edema, necrosis of pigment epithelium, peripheral anterior synechiae, and inflammatory reaction in the vitreous have been seen on histological examination (21). Injection of similar monomers into the extraocular muscle of rabbits produces an inflammatory response (21). Isobutyl monomers injected into the extraocular muscles cause loss of the muscle nuclei, fibroblastic invasion, and acute inflammatory response, in addition to giant-cell formation around the locus of adhesion (38). Similar agents used topically on the cornea for adhesion of contact lens after removal of epithelium lead to a transient stromal edema and vascularization (19). Favorable results with isobutyl monomers in experimental scleral-buckling procedures with inflammatory reaction limited to the vicinity of adhesion have been reported (56).

The toxic effect of cyanoacrylates has also been evaluated on tissue culture of rabbits and human cells (39). Isobutyl monomers were found to be more toxic than octyl monomers. Marked reduction of toxic effect of the latter after several washings suggests that impurity of the monomer causes toxicity. Fibroblasts used in tissue culture have shown methyl-cyanoacrylates to be more toxic than isobutyl and octyl (12). Exposure of liver tissue culture to various monomers did not show a significant difference between the toxicity of methyl and butyl cyanoacrylates (24).

Refojo and his co-workers (46) have classified the available cyanoacrylates on the basis of toxicity in three groups: the best tolerated (octyl, heptyl, hexyl, butyl, and isobutyl 2-cyanoacrylate), less well tolerated (trifluoroisopropyl 2-cyanoacrylate), and least tolerated (methyl 2-cyanoacrylate). In conclusion, all the existing cyanoacrylates are toxic, and the rate of toxicity depends on the type of monomer, the amount of adhesive use, the mode of application, and the purity of the samples.

AVAILABILITY

Eastman 910 (Krazy Glue®) is methyl-2-cyanoacrylate. It is commercially available but too toxic for clinical use. The medical grade of adhesive (*n*-butyl-2-cyanoacrylates) is manufactured by Braun in West Germany and also by the Tri-Hawk Company in Canada (histacryl glue). It has been colored blue to make it more visible. These agents are not approved by the Food and Drug Administration. Carbohexoxymethyl—2-cyanoacrylate monomer can be obtained from Ethicon (CHC adhesive) in the United States but requires an application for investigation from the company.

BACTERIOTOXICITY AND MITOGENICITY

The effect of cyanoacrylates on bacterial growth is controversial. The bacteriotoxic property of different monomers of cyanoacrylates has been tested by Lehman and his co-workers (32), who concluded that cyanoacrylates are increasingly bacteriotoxic in inverse proportion to the monomers' chain length. Methyl and ethyl cyanoacrylates were equally bacteriotoxic. On the other hand, Matsumoto and his colleagues (36) claimed that methyl, *n*-butyl, and isobutyl polymers possess no bacteriotoxic or bacteriostatic properties. These agents have been tested in dogs, rats, and mice for carcinogenicity with negative results (37).

STRENGTH OF TISSUE ADHESIVES

Several factors influence the bond strength and duration of tissue adhesives. These include technique of application, type of adhesive, nature of surface, and purity of adhesive.

A thin film of adhesive between two dry, smooth, and clean surfaces will polymerize rapidly and form a tight bond. Polymerization is so fast that after the initial contact, no adjustment or realignment is possible. Once the substrate has been exposed to monomers and polymerization has occurred, reapplication of more monomers will fail to provide a strong bond. In the presence of excessive moisture or water, the monomer turns white and becomes powdery. Epithelial surface does not maintain a bond, and for application on the cornea, the epithelium should be removed.

The higher monomer of cyanoacrylate provides the best bond strength in tissue. The tensile strength of various adhesives has been evaluated in experimental ophthalmology for bonding tissue to tissue and tissue to alloplastic material. Refojo et al. (44) have noted the strongest bond with *n*-butyl and isobutyl cyanoacrylates used in gluing corneal stroma to corneal stroma. Adhesives have been used to glue a contact lens (PMMA) to the cornea, and silicone rubber to the sclera. The bond strength of a contact lens to Bowman's membrane decreased by one-half within 1 month (44). Isobutyl and *n*-decyl cyanoacrylate failed to provide adequate bond strength between the muscle and the sclera when used for sutureless muscle surgery (16). Cyanoacrylates used for corneoscleral wounds in experimental animals generally provided greater tensile strength during the early postoperative period compared to suture wounds (6). Beyond 6 days, the suture wound was found to be stronger.

CLINICAL USE OF ADHESIVES

Surgical glue is currently under FDA investigation, requiring an application by the user from Ethicon for investigator status. The patient also must sign a consent form, and the result of treatment must be reported to the company. Despite these limitations, these glues have been enthusiastically used by several investigators, and the results in some instances are encouraging. Surgical glues have been used for sealing corneal perforations or descemetocele, sealing of leaking bleb of glaucoma or leaking wound of cataract surgery, tarsorrhaphy and plastic lid procedures, punctal occlusion, clinical replacement of artificial corneal epithelium and endothelium by alloplastic material, and scleral-buckling procedures for retinal detachment.

Corneal Perforations

One of the most promising uses of adhesives is sealing off perforated corneal ulcers or impending perforations. The glue was first successfully used by Webster and his co-workers (58) in two cases with perforated corneal ulcers in 1968. Since then, several studies have shown its effectiveness for perforated corneal ulcers and impending perforations (8,13,25–27,29,59). It can act as a temporizing procedure or, in some instances, a definitive treatment. Hirst and his co-workers (26), in a prospective trial study, compared the effect of tissue adhesive to other methods of therapy for perforated corneal ulcers at the Wilmer Institute between 1960 and 1980. Thirty-five patients were treated with tissue adhesive and 69 patients were treated initially with other methods, such as conjunctival flaps or keratoplasty. A lower rate of enucleation and better final visual acuity has been claimed in the patients treated by tissue adhesive compared to the control group. More recently, Weiss and his co-workers (59) have reported on 80 patients with either corneal perforation or impending perforation, the largest series to date. Forty-four percent healed with only application of glue. Although 11% of the cases developed complications such as glaucoma and corneal infiltration, 80% achieved a good visual outcome.

Initially, tissue adhesive was recommended for sealing off perforated ulcers of less than 1 mm in diameter without incarceration of intraocular content. However, use of sodium hyaluronate as a spacing agent between the intraocular tissue and the perforated site has enabled sealing off larger perforations in both experimental animals and humans (25).

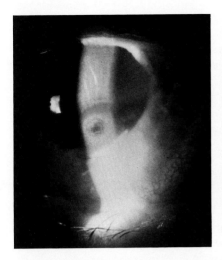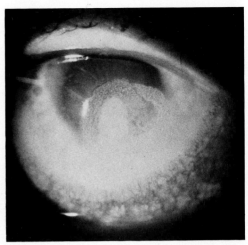

FIG. 3. Left: Perforated corneal ulcer in a 65-year-old female. Note flat anterior chamber and folds in the Descemet's membrane. **Right:** Same as **left** after application of cyanoacetate on the perforation site. The leak was sealed off and anterior chamber formed within 20 min.

The application of tissue adhesives for corneal perforations is simple (Fig. 3). The procedure is performed with topical anesthesia in the emergency room or in the operating room under the microscope. A lid speculum is inserted. The corneal epithelium is debrided from the ulcer site and the surrounding area. Using a "weck" sponge, the surface is dried. A small drop of tissue adhesive on the undersurface of a bent iris spatula or a polyethylene disc is brought into contact with the perforated site. The adhesive also can be applied directly with a thin polyethylene tube or with a 27-gauge needle on a tuberculin syringe. After contact with the tissue, the adhesive polymerizes rapidly and seals the perforation in 5 to 10 min. The anterior chamber will start to re-form under close observation. A continuous-wear soft contact lens is filled, and the patient is kept on prophylactic topical antibiotics.

Tissue adhesives can be retained for a few months, until the ulcer has healed. The healing usually occurs under the adhesive. The tissue adhesive can be removed earlier with a pair of fine forceps if the cornea is vascularized, or before a definitive surgical procedure such as conjunctival flap or corneal transplantation.

Postoperative Leaking Wounds

Although only a few cases of postoperative leaking wounds have been treated with surgical glue, the approach seems promising. Some of these cases are technically difficult with conventional suturing technique. The external fistula of filtering bleb following glaucoma surgery has successfully been sealed with surgical glue by Grady and Forbes (23), and Awan and Spaeth (2). Similarly, the wound dehiscence following keratoplasty, cataract wound, and leaking corneal wounds after repair has successfully been sealed off (26,54). In all of these instances, the technique is similar to that for closure of perforated corneal ulcers. Under topical anesthesia, the area is dried, the glue is applied, and the cornea is covered by a bandage contact lens. The anterior chamber should start to form within a few minutes. The glue either will fall off spontaneously or can be removed after wound healing.

Plastic Lid Procedure and Tarsorrhaphy

Surgical glues seem to be indicated, particularly for temporary tarsorrhaphy, in cases of facial paralysis and exposure keratitis. A technique has been reported by Schimek and Ballou (48) to glue the eyelashes of the upper lid to the skin of the lower lid.

In their series, they used Eastman 910 with good results. Streit and his co-workers (54) applied methyl-2-cyanoacrylate to the eyelashes of upper and lower lids. Immediate closure of the lid resulted in rapid polymerization and temporary tarsorrhaphy that could last for 2 to 3 weeks. An accidental tarsorrhaphy also has been reported in a boy who splashed acrylic adhesive in his left eye (3). Regardless of the technique, extreme care must be exercised to avoid excessive glue in the lid margin or conjunctival contact with the glue because, in either instance, the solid polymerized glue mechanically will erode the corneal tissue (52).

Surgical glue also has been used successfully for sutureless plastic correction of blepharochalasis. In a case reported by Kosko (31), a desired amount of redundant skin of the upper lid was delineated. The base was pressed together by a hemostat. The excessive skin fold was cut off and a line of surgical glue was applied to the cut edge. The wound healed satisfactorily without a bandage, and there was no irritation.

Punctal Occlusion

Tissue adhesives have been used for the occlusion of lacrimal puncta in patients with keratoconjunctivitis sicca. They have been used as a temporary measure prior to permanent occlusion by electrocoagulation in borderline cases and in patients with temporary dry-eye condition. In a technique described by Patten (42), *n*-butyl cyanoacrylate was introduced into the punctum by a thin polyethylene tube after dilation and epithelial debridement with a fine, hand-held electric corneal rust remover. The adhesive was retained an average of 2.5 weeks and could be removed electively at the time of permanent punctal occlusion. No complications were encountered in 15 eyes that had tissue adhesive punctal occlusion.

Retinal Detachment and Sclera

Surgical adhesives can potentially be more applicable for a variety of surgical procedures on the sclera, because the semisolid and relatively avascular sclera provides a suitable surface for application of glue. Several encouraging reports on the use of cyanoacrylates for sutureless scleral surgery in experimental animals have been published (7,9,17,28,35,49). Methyl-cyanoacrylate (Eastman 910) has been used to glue scleral flaps and intrascleral implants (17). Isobutyl cyanoacrylate has been used to glue silicone on the sclera as explant, or to glue a silicone sheet over hydrogels and silicone rubber as implants or explants (35). Encircling silicone has been glued to the sclera or on the silicone sheet (35).

Although the glue has been used enthusiastically for various kinds of scleral and retinal surgery in humans on occasion (18,50,51), it has not as yet been accepted as a replacement for conventional suturing technique. Spitznas and his co-workers (51) have applied the surgical glue in 100 patients with a variety of disorders, such as needle perforation of the sclera and choroid, securing thin sclera with lyophilized dura mater or preserved sclera closure of scleral trapdoor and securing encircling elements. They claimed the adhesive to be nontoxic to the vitreous, with minimal irritation of the choroid and retina. This sutureless approach can reduce the risk of perforation in patients with thin sclera from previous surgical procedure or in patients with staphyloma. The glue has been used to obtain scleral-buckling effect by scleral graft in patients with staphylomatous or necrotic scleral area by Regenbogen and his co-workers (47), who observed mild postoperative reaction lasting not more than 1 week.

Artificial Epithelium (Epikeratoprosthesis) and Artificial Endothelium

For a brief period of time, surgeons were removing the diseased corneal epithelium in corneal edema and attempting to replace it with an alloplast material (4,14,15,30). The entire epithelium was denuded from the cornea and then a hard contact lens was cemented in the Bowman's membrane to provide optically clear interface and relieve the signs and symptoms of epithelial edema. Although the prosthesis did remain in place, in some instances for months, the major complications were regrowth of epithelium, infection, and vascularization. These complications, plus the introduction of gas-permeable soft contact lenses for protection of the corneal surface, led this investigator to abandon the idea of epikeratoprosthesis. Surgical adhesive has also been used to glue the artificial membrane replacing corneal endothelial cells, but the results have been discouraging (15).

ADHESIVES IN EXPERIMENTAL OPHTHALMOLOGY

Since the introduction of cyanoacrylate (surgical glue) in 1960, its substitution in a wide variety of surgical procedures has been attempted in experimental animals. The subject was extensively reviewed by Refojo and his co-workers in 1971 (46). Discussion of all the available literature on this subject is beyond the scope of this text and does not contribute to the surgical pharmacology.

REFERENCES

1. Aronson, S. B., McMaster, P. R. B., Moore, T. E., Jr., and Coon, M. A. (1970): Toxicity of the cyanoacrylates. *Arch. Ophthalmol.*, 84:342–349.
2. Awan, K. J., and Spaeth, P. G. (1974): Use of isobutyl-2-cyanoacrylate tissue adhesive in the repair of conjunctival fistula in filtering procedures for glaucoma. *Ann. Ophthalmol.*, 6:851–853.
3. Balent, A. (1976): An accidental tarsorrhaphy caused by acrylic adhesive. *Am. J. Ophthalmol.*, 82:501.
4. Bloome, M. A., and Piepergerdes, L. G. (1970): Epikeratoprosthesis in rhesus monkeys. *Am. J. Ophthalmol.*, 70:997–1002.
5. Bloomfield, S., Barnert, A. H., and Kanter, P. D. (1963): The use of Eastman 910 monomer as an adhesive in ocular surgery. I. Biologic effects on ocular tissue. *Am. J. Ophthalmol.*, 55:742–748.
6. Bloomfield, S., Barnert, A. H., and Kanter, P. D. (1963): The use of Eastman 910 monomer as an adhesive in ocular surgery. II. Effectiveness in closure of limbal wounds in rabbits. *Am. J. Ophthalmol.*, 55:946–953.
7. Bonnet, M., and Taillanter, N. (1979): Surgical glue in the preparation of lyophilized episcleral implants for retinal detachment surgery. *Bull. Soc. Ophthalmol. Fr.*, 79:661–662.
8. Boruchoff, S. A., Refojo, M., Slansky, H. H., Webster, R. G., Freeman, M. I., and Dohlman, C. H. (1969): Clinical applications of adhesive in corneal surgery. *Trans. Am. Acad. Ophthalmol. Otolaryngol.* 73:499–505.
9. Calabria, G. A., Pruett, R. C., Refojo, M. F., and Schepens, C. L. (1970): Sutureless scleral buckling: An experimental technique. *Arch. Ophthalmol.*, 83:613–618.
10. Carton, C. A., Kessler, L. A., Seidenberg, B., and Hurwitt, E. S. (1960): A plastic adhesive method of small blood vessel surgery. *World Neurol.*, 1:356–362.
11. Coover, H. W., Jr., Joyner, F. B., Shearer, N. H., Jr., and Wicker, T. H. (1959): Chemistry and performance of cyanoacrylate tissue adhesives. *Soc. Plastics Eng. J.*, 15:413–417.
12. deRenzis, F. A., and Aleo, J. J. (1970): An in vitro bioassay of cyanoacrylate cytotoxicity. *Oral Surg.*, 30:803–808.
13. Dohlman, C. H., Boruchoff, S. A., and Sullivan, G. L. (1967): A technique for the repair of perforated corneal ulcers. *Arch. Ophthalmol.*, 77:519–525.
14. Dohlman, C. H., Carrol, J. M., Richards, J., and Refojo, M. F. (1970): Further experience with glued-on contact lenses (artificial epithelium). *Arch. Ophthalmol.*, 83:10–20.
15. Dohlman, C. H., Refojo, M. F., and Rose, J. (1967): Synthetic polymers in corneal surgery. I. Glyceryl methacrylate. *Arch. Ophthalmol.*, 77:252–257.
16. Dunlap, E. A., Dunn, M., and Rossomondo, R. (1969): Adhesives for sutureless muscle surgery. *Arch. Ophthalmol.*, 82:751–755.
17. Ellis, R. A., and Levine, A. M. (1963): Experimental sutureless ocular surgery. *Am. J. Ophthalmol.*, 55:733–741.
18. Faulborn, J. (1976): Treatment of giant retinal tears after perforating injuries with vitrectomy and a cyanoacrylate tissue adhesive. *Adv. Ophthalmol.*, 33:204–207.
19. Gasset, A., Hood, C. I., Ellison, E. D., and Kaufman, H. E. (1970): Ocular tolerance to cyanoacrylate monomer tissue adhesive analogues. *Invest. Ophthalmol. Vis. Sci.*, 9:3–11.
20. Ginsberg, S. P., and Polack, F. M. (1972): Cyanoacrylate tissue adhesive in ocular disease. *Ophthalmic Surg.*, 3:126–132.
21. Girard, L. J., Cobb, S., Reed, T., Williams, B., and Minaya, J. (1969): Surgical adhesives and bonded contact lenses: An experimental study. *Ann. Ophthalmol.*, 1:65–74.
22. Gottlob, R., ed. (1968): *Adhesives in Surgery.* Proceedings of the International Symposium, Vienna Academy of Medicine, Vienna.
23. Grady, F. J., and Forbes, M. (1969): Tissue adhesive for repair of conjunctival buttonhole in glaucoma surgery. *Am. J. Ophthalmol.*, 68:656–658.

24. Hegyeli, A. F. (1973): Use of organ culture to evaluate biodegradation of polymer implant materials. *J. Biomed. Mater. Res.,* 7:205–214.
25. Hirst, L. W., and DeJuan, E., Jr. (1982): Sodium hyaluronate and tissue adhesive in treating corneal perforations. *Ophthalmology,* 89:1250–1253.
26. Hirst, L. W., Smiddy, W. E., and Stark, W. J. (1982): Corneal perforations: changing methods of treatment 1960–1980. *Ophthalmology,* 89:630–634.
27. Hirst, L. W., Stark, W. J., and Jensen, A. D. (1979): Tissue adhesive: New perspectives in corneal perforations. *Ophthalmic Surg.,* 10:58–64.
28. Hung, J. Y., and Hilton, G. F. (1982): Scleral buckling with cyanoacrylate tissue adhesive. *Retina,* 2:179–181.
29. Hyndiuk, R. A., Hull, D. S., and Kinyoun, J. L. (1974): Free tissue patch and cyanoacrylate in corneal perforations. *Ophthalmic Surg.,* 5:50–55.
30. Kaufman, H. E., and Gasset, A. R. (1969): Clinical experience with the epikeratoprosthesis. *Trans. Am. Acad. Ophthalmol. Otolaryngol.* 73:1133–1140.
31. Kosko, P. I. (1981): Upper lid blepharoplasty: Skin closure achieved with butyl-2-cyanoacrylate. *Ophthalmic Surg.,* 12:424–425.
32. Lehman, R. A. W., West, R. L., and Leonard, F. (1966): Toxicity of alkyl-2-cyanoacrylates. II. Bacterial growth. *Arch. Surg.,* 93:447–450.
33. Leonard, F., Kulkarni, R. K., Brandes, G., Nelson, J., and Cameron, J. J. (1966): Synthesis and degradation of poly (alkyl alpha-cyanoacrylates). *J. Appl. Polymer Sci.,* 10:259–272.
34. Levine, A. M. (1964): Sutureless ocular surgery: Results of recent experiments. *EENT Monthly,* 43:55–58.
35. Long, R. S., Mittl, R., and Chuanico, R. (1970): Experimental scleral buckling of the posterior pole using tissue adhesive. *Am. J. Ophthalmol.,* 69:419–422.
36. Matsumoto, T., Dobek, A. S., Pani, K. C., Kovaric, J. J., and Hamit, H. F. (1968): Bacteriological study of cyanoacrylate tissue adhesives. *Arch. Surg.,* 97:527–530.
37. Matsumoto, T., and Heister Kamp, C. A. (1969): Long-term study of aerosol cyanoacrylate tissue adhesive spray: Carcinogenicity and other untoward effects. *Am. Surg.* 35:825–827.
38. Munton, C. G. F. (1971): Tissue adhesive in ocular surgery. A prospective study. *Exp. Eye Res.,* 11:1–6.
39. Nesburn, A. B., and Ziniti, P. (1969): Cell culture toxicity of two cyanoacrylate adhesives. *Invest. Ophthalmol. Vis. Sci.,* 8:648. (Abstract).
40. Pani, K. C., Gladieux, G., Brandes, G., Kulkarni, R. K., and Leonard, F. (1968): The degradation of n-butyl alpha-cyanoacrylate tissue adhesive. *Surgery,* 63:481–489.
41. Parry, T. G. W., and Laszlo, G. C. (1946): Thrombin technique in ophthalmic surgery. *Br. J. Ophthalmol.,* 30:176–178.
42. Patten, J. T. (1976): Punctal occlusion with n-butyl cyanoacrylate tissue adhesive. *Ophthalmic Surg.,* 7:24–26.
43. Price, J. A., Jr., and Wadsworth, J. A. C. (1969): Evaluation of an adhesive in cataract wound closure. *Am. J. Ophthalmol.,* 68:663–668.
44. Refojo, M. F., and Dohlman, C. H. (1969): The tensile strength of adhesive joints between the eye tissues and alloplastic materials. *Am. J. Ophthalmol.,* 68:248–255.
45. Refojo, M. F., Dohlman, C. H., Ahmad, B., Carroll, J. M., and Allen, J. C. (1968): Evaluation of adhesives for corneal surgery. *Arch. Ophthalmol.,* 80:645–656.
46. Refojo, M. F., Dohlman, C. H., and Koliopoulos, J. (1971): Adhesives in ophthalmology: A review. *Surv. Ophthalmol.,* 15:217–236.
47. Regenbogen, L., Romano, A., Zuckerman, M., and Stein, R. (1976): Histocryl tissue adhesive in some types of retinal detachment surgery. *Br. J. Ophthalmol.,* 60:561–564.
48. Schimek, R. A., and Ballou, G. S. (1966): Eastman 910 monomer for plastic lid procedures. *Am. J. Ophthalmol.,* 62:953–955.
49. Seelenfreund, M. H., Refojo, M. F., and Schepens, C. L. (1970): Sealing choroidal perforations with cyanoacrylate. *Arch. Ophthalmol.,* 83:619–625.
50. Spitznas, M., Lossagh, H., Vogel, M., and Joussen, F. (1974): Intraocular use of butyl-2-cyanoacrylate in retinal detachment surgery. A preliminary report. *Mod. Probl. Ophthalmol.,* 12:183–188.
51. Spitznas, M., Lossagh, H., Vogel, M., and Meyer-Schwickerath, G. (1973): Cyanoacrylate in retinal surgery. *Trans. Am. Acad. Ophthalmol. Otolaryngol.,* 77:114–118.

52. Stasior, O. G. (1963): Discussion: Experimental studies employing adhesive compounds in ophthalmic surgery. *Trans. Am. Acad. Ophthalmol. Otolaryngol.,* 67:333–334.
53. Straatsma, B. R., Allen, R. A., Hale, P. N., and Gomez, R. (1963): Experimental studies employing adhesive compounds in ophthalmic surgery. *Trans. Am. Acad. Ophthalmol. Otolaryngol.,* 67:320–333.
54. Streit, S., Ackerman, J., and Kanarek, I. (1981): Cyanoacrylate. *Ann. Ophthalmol.,* 13:315–316.
55. Town, A. E. (1949): The use of fibrin coagulum fixation in intraocular surgery. *Trans. Am. Acad. Ophthalmol. Otolaryngol.,* 54:131–133.
56. Vygantas, M. C., and Kanter, P. J. (1974): Experimental buckling with homologous sclera and cyanoacrylate. *Arch. Ophthalmol.,* 91:126–129.
57. Webster, R. G., Jr., Dohlman, C. H., and Refojo, M. F. (1964): The use of adhesives in anterior segment surgery. *Trans. Pac. Coast Otoophthalmol. Soc. Annu. Meet.* 50:121–135.
58. Webster, R. G., Jr., Slansky, H. H., Refojo, M. F., Boruchoff, S. A., and Dohlman, C. H. (1968): The use of adhesives for the closure of corneal perforations. Report of two cases. *Arch. Ophthalmol.,* 80:705–709.
59. Weiss, J. L., Cot, P. W., Lindstrom, R. L., and Doughman, D. J. (1983): The use of tissue adhesive in corneal perforations. *Ophthalmology,* 90:610–615.

Commentary

Lens Replacement

The loss of refractive power after removal of the crystalline lens must be replaced. For this purpose spectacles, intraocular lenses, contact lenses, or even refractive corneal surgery may be considered. To date about 2 million lens implantations have been performed. Modern intraocular lenses make them feasible for many aphakic patients with a resultant rapid visual rehabilitation. Yet problems with lens design and their chemical composition may still exist. Dr. Tarkkanen has had the opportunity to study an eye, through autopsy, after successful surgery for extracapsular cataract extraction with a J-loop posterior chamber lens 13 months postoperatively. A giant cell inflammatory reaction around the polypropylene loops was still present. One of the loops had eroded deep into the ciliary body. The surrounding fibrovascular tissue may be a source for late vitreous hemorrhage. On the other hand, the tight fixation would allow all physical activities to the patient without fear of luxation. These findings were confirmed by Dr. B. Daicker of Basel, Switzerland, and others. The alternative of capsular fixation has its problems, too. The zonular structure in old age, or, in eyes with the pseudoexfoliation syndrome, may not give the necessary support and posterior subluxation may result.

Dr. Treffers has worked for the next generation of IOLs. In monkeys he has removed the crystalline lens material and filled the bag with a soft gel-like material, hydrogel. This is truly an exciting event. Theoretically it should be possible to restore accommodation as well. Future developments call for close cooperation between the polymer chemist and ophthalmic surgeon.

The Editors

235

Surgical Pharmacology of the Eye,
edited by M. Sears and A. Tarkkanen.
Raven Press, New York © 1985.

Lens Replacement

W. Frits Treffers

Department of Ophthalmology, St. Radboud Hospital, Nijmegen, The Netherlands

SUMMARY: The technique of cataract surgery has changed enormously these last decades, especially since the introduction of the intraocular lens. Over 150 types of intraocular lenses (IOL) are now available. All consist of an optical part and anchoring devices (haptics).

The original IOL were two-plane lenses. Since the introduction of one-plane lenses and viscous surgery, less damage to the intraocular tissues, especially the corneal endothelium, results.

The major problems of the present technique (extracapsular cataract surgery with posterior chamber IOL) remain after cataract, wrinkling of the posterior capsule, and poor visibility of the retinal periphery.

The next generation of IOL made of a soft gel-like material that completely fills the capsular bag should eliminate the above-mentioned complications. Such a gel-like IOL may restore accommodation as well.

Major research has to be done in order to find the right gel material. Cooperation between a polymer specialist and a biomaterial specialist is essential for the ophthalmic research. Technically such a surgical procedure is possible.

Cataract surgery has become an extremely successful and reliable procedure nowadays. Patients who have undergone a removal of their cataract regain a useful visual acuity in more than 90% of the cases. After the extraction of the lens the eye has become aphakic. To compensate for this loss of refractive power, 21.8 diopters (20), we have four options we can choose from: spectacles, contact lenses, intraocular lenses, and refractive corneal surgery. Each option has its pros and cons and will be described briefly.

APHAKIC CORRECTION

Spectacles

This method has been the only way to correct the aphakic patient for a long time and is still widely used; especially when combined with an intracapsular cataract extraction, visual rehabilitation is regained easily. However, sometimes the use of spectacles presents difficulties. The user has a limited peripheral field and a ring-shaped scotoma causing the so-called jack-in-the-box phenomenon. The retinal image is increased by 25%, resulting in acclimatization problems to the new, enlarged outer world, especially in the elderly. Spectacles cannot be applied in case of unilateral cataract, because the difference in retinal images between both eyes causes diplopia, which is not acceptable for the patient. Bilateral aphakic patients have a low visual acuity when the spectacles are not worn. Many patients complain about the poor cosmesis, large eye sizes, of aphakic spectacles.

Contact Lenses

A contact lens is placed directly on the cornea. The aphakic contact lens has the advantage that it can be applied in cases of unilateral cataract, because the increase of the retinal image by 8% of the affected eye hardly causes diplopia.

The aphakic contact lens hardly limits the peripheral field and cosmesis is generally good. A minor disadvantage might be the bad tolerance in dusty environments. On the other hand, the physical disabilities of elderly patients, such as arthritis, paresis, tremor, and dyskinesia, can be or might become a major handicap in the handling of contact lenses. Recurrent infection, dry eyes, cornea defects, recurrent corneal erosions, and lid abnormalities can further restrict the use of contact lenses in the aphakic patient.

There are several types of contact lenses: hard, soft, permanent wear, and extended wear, each with its own advantages and disadvantages. It is not the purpose of this chapter to discuss these items; the reader is referred to the literature.

Intraocular Lens

To eliminate some problems that patients encounter in the unilateral aphakia corrected with contact lenses, Ridley (30) in 1949 implanted an artificial lens in a unilateral traumatic cataract. After an extracapsular cataract extraction Ridley placed the intraocular lens in the posterior chamber. The material the lens was made of was polymethylmethacrylate (PMMA). This material was used for airshields in fighter airplanes in World War II. Some pilots had their eyes perforated by shattered airshield, and it turned out that this material was well tolerated within the eye. So in 1949 Ridley opened a new surgical era in ophthalmology: the intraocular lens.

The patient with an intraocular lens has a full visual field, and the retinal image is about the same size preoperatively. A real aphakia never exists, so the blurred image when such a patient wakes up is eliminated as well. Early complications due to lack of experience and sufficient follow-up prevented general acceptance. A retrospective matched study by Jaffe et al. (13) demonstrated that the surgical results in intracapsular cataract extraction are comparable if the same procedure is combined with intraocular lens implantation.

Today, almost 35 years after Ridley implanted the first intraocular lens, more than 70% of all cataract operations done in the United States in 1982 involved intraocular lens implantation (31). That is almost half a million intraocular lenses annually.

Refractive Corneal Surgery

The purpose of this technique is to increase the total refractive power of the cornea. J. Barraquer can be regarded as a pioneer in this field. In refractive corneal surgery a donor lenticle is frozen, ground so as to correct the aphakia, and implanted into a stromal pocket. McCarey and Andrews (22) inserted a hydrogel implant in the stroma of the cornea for the same purpose. Their short-term results in rabbits proved to be successful. Kaufman (15) described the epikeratophakia technique. In this technique a donor lenticle is sutured on top of the cornea to balance the refractive power deficit created by the removal of the lens.

CATARACT SURGERY

Basically, there are two techniques to remove a cataractous lens, either intracapsular or extracapsular. Anatomically, the lens consists of an elastic capsule, the capsular bag, the lens content, and the lens fibers. The lens is held in place by a suspensory ligament known as the zonule. This is composed of numerous fibrils that insert into the lens capsule and arise from the ciliary body and choroid.

In intracapsular cataract extraction, the entire lens within and without the capsule is taken out. As a consequence, the zonule has to be ruptured. To facilitate this an enzyme, chymotrypsin, is used.

In extracapsular cataract extraction, the lens capsule is opened and sometimes partially removed, depending on the surgeon's preference. The nucleus of the lens is removed by either expression or phacofragmentation. The remaining cortex is taken out through either meticulous rinsing or aspiration in order to clean the capsule. In most procedures one wants to preserve the posterior capsule.

Each technique has its advantages and its disadvantages. Cystoid macular edema, one severe postoperative complication, occurs in a lower incidence if an extracapsular technique has been employed (2,12). Binkhorst (3,4), one of the pioneers of the intraocular lenses, repopularized the extracapsular technique and the fixation of his two-loop lens to both the iris and the capsule. As time progressed, complications such as sphincter erosions, recurrent hemorrhages, subluxation of the intraocular lens, and corneal decompensation showed up. The impossibility of dilating the pupil in the presence of suspected fundus abnormalities led to a different method of fixation of the intraocular lens that permitted mydriasis (34).

A major breakthrough in intraocular lens design has been the development of the so-called one-plane lenses. Implantation of these intraocular lenses is less traumatic compared with the so-called two-plane lenses. The one-plane intraocular lenses are designed for either anterior chamber or posterior chamber use. They represent 97% of the lenses that were implanted in the United States in 1982 (31).

Intraocular Lens

The intraocular lens is composed of an optical part and an anchoring device, called either loops or haptics. The loops and optical part can be made of one piece of material. There are however, many intraocular lenses that have loops made of a different material. The loops have to be attached to the optical part, with the potential risk of loosening as time goes on. At present more than 100 types of intraocular lenses are commercially available. Some are designed for implantation combined with an intracapsular procedure, others for extracapsular procedures.

The ability of the human lens to alter its shape, resulting in a change of refractive power that permits focusing light from a near object and reversing the procedure for a far object, is called accommodation. As the lens ages, its accommodative power is gradually reduced. At the age of 60 or 70 accommodation power is zero. The present generation of intraocular lenses all lack this feature. Future design and research of new intraocular lenses will be devoted to this goal. Some preliminary work in this field has been done already (9,17–19).

Intraocular Lens Material

In most intraocular lenses that are commercially available the optical part is made of a solid polymer, PMMA (29). This material has been in use since World War II and has not shown any evidence of toxicity when implanted in the eye (30).

Although the manufacture of intraocular lenses may require molding, heating, lathing, and drilling, the degree of degrading of the PMMA, resulting in leaching out of potential dangerous monomers, does not appear of clinical importance (8). Recent experiments have shown that leaching of monomers from polymerized PMMA did not harm secondary cultures of rabbit kidney cells (35), nor did it evoke an immune response to secondary PMMA challenge in rabbits (14). However, allergies to monomers of methylmethacrylate have been reported (32). Monomer leaching might be a causal factor in recurrent uveitis in patients who have an intraocular lens (7), although such a response might be attributed to an allergy to protein deposit on the implant (11) as well.

In the human lens potential damage of ultraviolet light is prevented because it is absorbed by the lens during passage. In contrast to the human lens PMMA does not behave like a filter for ultraviolet light (21). Consequently, this potentially dangerous part of the light can reach the retina and cause damage. This has been shown in aphakic monkey eyes (10). Recently, new experimental intraocular lenses that filter the ultraviolet light have been tested in monkeys, with encouraging (27) and effective (28) results.

The loops of an intraocular lens are made of either the same material as the optical part (PMMA) or a different material. The major disadvantage of loops made of PMMA is that the material is rigid at room and body temperature. The actual implantation with this type of loop is harder than with more bendable loops. For this reason many of the intraocular lenses have loops made of different material, polypropylene. This material is resistant to biodegradation and can be regarded as safe for intraocular use (24), although scanning electron microscopy demonstrated surface degradation (6). At one time, the loops were sometimes made of different materials, for example, supramid. Unfortunately, this material turned out to be biodegradable; as a consequence loosening of the loops occurred some years after implantation (Fig. 1). Titanium and platinum have been used as loops. Sphincter erosion and, as a result, a higher incidence of lens dislocation occurred.

Touching the inner lining of the cornea, the endothelium, with the hydrophobic surface of the PMMA of the intraocular lens during the implantation procedure will damage this vulnerable cell layer. The endothelial cells will be torn from the cornea and adhere to the surface of the intraocular lens, as demonstrated with scanning electron microscopy (25). This loss of endothelial cells cannot be compensated for sufficiently, and late corneal decompensation is often the result. Less damage to the endothelium will be done by covering the hydrophobic PMMA surface with a thin hydrophilic layer such as

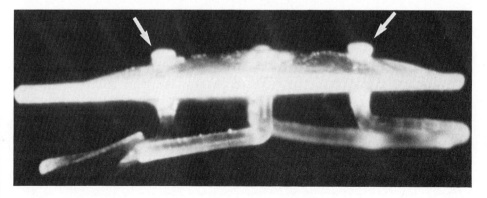

FIG. 1. Removed two-loop lens. Note loosening of the haptic from the optical part (*arrows*).

polyvinylpyrrolidone, methylcellulose, polyvinylalcohol, dextran, and hyaluronic acid.

FUTURE OF INTRAOCULAR LENSES

The ultimate goal of the cataract surgeon is to develop a surgical procedure that not only replaces the cataractous lens but restores its function as well. Although the mechanism of accommodation is not completely understood, it is beyond question that future intraocular lenses have to be developed from a moldable polymer. This type of lens would allow alteration of its shape, thus imitate accommodation.

Polymers are chemical compounds that are composed of many units linked together in a long chain. Polymers that are used for contact lenses can be differentiated into three groups: (a) thermoplastics, (b) synthetic elastomers, and (c) hydrogels.

1. *Thermoplastics.* PMMA is a typical member of this group. The polymer is manufactured under application of heat and pressure. The material is fairly rigid at room temperature. It may show some flexibility but is not elastic at all.
2. *Synthetic elastomers.* Silicon rubber is a member of this group. This group of polymers is flexible and shows a rubber-like behavior. It is possible to change their shape under the influence of force; they return to their original shape as soon as the deforming force is removed.
3. *Hydrogels.* PolyHEMA can be regarded as a typical member of this group. The unit of this polymer is hydroxyethylmethacrylate. The polymer is hydrophilic; it absorbs water and can be described as soft, elastic gel in the hydrated form. The percentage of water absorption of the polymer is dependent on the cross-linking of the polymer chains.

Several aspects that affect the performance of polymers are of importance when they are used as intraocular lenses: density, refractive index, optical transmittance, dimensional stability, mechanical properties, wettability, biocompatibility, toxicity and chemical stability, ease and method of sterilization. Three items will be highlighted because they are of major importance for the development of the new generation of intraocular lenses: mechanical properties, wettability, and biocompatibility.

Mechanical Properties

When a force is exerted on a body—for example, a lens—deformation will occur until an equilibrium is reached. As soon as the deforming force is removed, the lens will return to its original shape with the ideal material. This process is time dependent, but in the ideal material it will be reduced to almost 0 sec. Why is this search for the ideal elastic behavior so important? Imagine that one has been able to manufacture an intraocular lens that meets all the criteria except the ideal elastic behavior. If such an intraocular lens is used and takes 3 or more sec to change focus from far away to a wristwatch, and vice versa, one will not be content with such an intraocular lens. Deformation, back and forth, has to be instantaneous. Both synthetic elastomers and hydrogels have elastic behavior, but there is a relationship between the monomer structure and cross-linkage and the elasticity. Future research has to be devoted to this aspect.

Wettability

The terms hydrophilic and hydrophobic simply mean, respectively, water loving and water hating. When these terms are used in connection with a surface, they have a more specific meaning. *Hydrophilic* means that water will spread spontaneously on the surface of the material, in contrast to *hydrophobic,* which means that a droplet of water on the material will stay a droplet. The angle of the droplet and the material interface determines the wettability of the material tested. In a true hydrophilic surface the angle is zero. Synthetic elastomers exhibit a hydrophobic surface. Hydrogels do not exhibit a hydrophilic surface, as one would expect, but rather a hydrophobic one, as we know from studies with contact lenses. The hydrogels present another potential problem, namely, their tendency to accumulate proteinaceous and other material, such as calcium deposits, on their surface (33), with a risk that transparency will decrease. The behavior of the surface of any material, hydrophilic or not, and the interaction with the tissue the material is implanted into is of major importance for biocompatibility (1).

Biocompatibility

Tissue response to synthetic implants varies from material to material. Both physical and chemical properties are involved in a particular tissue reaction. It is a complicated problem to discover which part is responsible for each of the above-mentioned tissue responses. Tissue response can be understood more easily if one is familiar with the natural wound healing in tissue. If one then compares this with the healing of a similar wound that occurs with an implant, the most striking difference is encapsulation of the implant.

The tissue response, encapsulation, is independent of whether the implant is soft or hard or whether it is biodegradable or not. The only variable seen is the thickness of the capsule (1). For example, if the implant has sharp corners or edges causing mechanical trauma of the surrounding tissue, an increased encapsulation will be the response. A similar tissue response to an intraocular lens has been reported by Wolter (36). On the other hand, the implant surface and its interaction with body fluids (most often blood) represent the chemical part of tissue response to implants. The earliest event is absorption of proteins by the surface of the implant. Depending on the chemistry of the surface, several sorts of proteins will be absorbed, creating either a thrombogenic or a nonthrombogenic response (1). There are indications that the chemical response is related to the wettability of the different implant materials.

It will be understood that both synthetic elastomers and hydrogels are potential candidates for the future intraocular lenses (5). PMMA, although a material that has proved its suitability as a polymer for intraocular lenses, lacks the requested elasticity.

Mehta et al. (23) reported in 1978 a series of 32 patients who underwent implantation of an intraocular lens made of polyHEMA. The lens was pupillary fixated. Their average follow-up time was 3 months. Most eyes seemed to tolerate the polyHEMA polymer quite well. More recently, poly-HEMA has been implanted in rabbit eyes by Packard et al. (26). They found no demonstrable tissue reaction on light microscopy in any of the eyes. They had a follow-up of 3 months.

In an ongoing study by Treffers (*unpublished data*) implantation of a hydrogel intraocular lens in the eye of a monkey was tolerated well. Some promising results were obtained (Fig. 2).

The eye is a unique organ because tissue response can be observed both directly by slit-lamp examination and by histologic examination. This approach gives a more dynamic insight into tissue response. Close cooperation between a biomaterial specialist, a polymer specialist, and the ophthalmic surgeon are essential for the development of the next generation of intraocular lenses.

In a recent study we investigated the ocular response to an intraocular lens made of 55% polyPMMA hydrogel. This hydrogel is commercially available

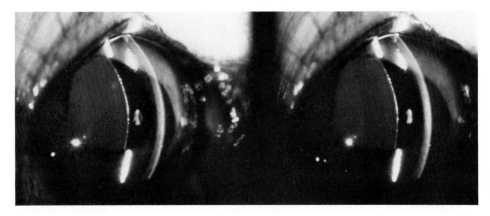

FIG. 2. Monkey eye with hydrogel pseudophakos, 4 weeks postoperative. Stereophotograph.

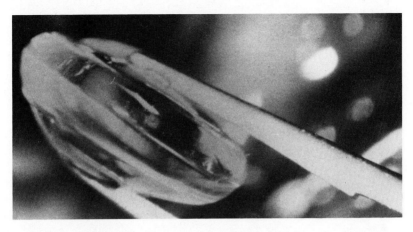

FIG. 3. Prelathed dehydrated hydrogel, 55% polyPMMA intraocular lens. (From ref. 34, with permission.)

and is used normally for contact lenses. The hydrated hydrogel is too rigid to permit accommodation, but the 55% hydrogel has a refractive index comparable with the refractive index of the human lens (33).

Six adult monkeys (10 eyes) were used in this study. The monkeys were operated on under general anesthesia (ketamine, Pavulon®, Ethrane®, N_2O, and O_2); a Zeiss operating microscope was used. In order to obtain optimal visual control, a total iridectomy was done 6 weeks prior to the lens implantation in all but 1 monkey. The technique for a total iridectomy described by Kaufman and Lutjen-Drecoll (16) was used. To immobilize the eye, a suture was placed through the superior rectus muscle. The conjunctiva was opened at the limbus, and the anterior chamber was entered with a superblade and scissors.

The attachment of the zonules on the anterior capsule could be seen easily because of the absence of the iris. The anterior capsule was opened just anterior of the zonules. In all cases, the lens content was removed with an infusion-aspiration technique. A completely empty capsular bag was obtained in all cases. A prelathed hydrated hydrogel intraocular lens was placed within the capsular bag (Fig. 3). The eye was closed with interrupted 10–0 nylon alcon. Chloramphenicol ointment was applied.

The dehydrated polyPMMA absorbs aqueous and fills the capsular bag completely (Figs. 4, 5). In all cases a fibrin-like material in the anterior chamber covering the hydrogel was seen (Fig. 6). In one case the hydrogel lens could not be placed in the capsular bag.

In the remaining 8 cases, the intraocular lens was in the capsular bag. In 4 eyes, the postoperative inflammation was severe, resulting in a fibrosed lens capsule and vascularization. In the other 4 eyes the capsule was clear. In only

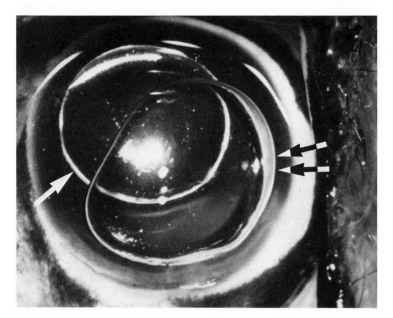

FIG. 4. Hydrogel intraocular lens within the capsular bag (*arrow*), immediately after the lens insertion. The anterior chamber is partly filled with air (*double arrow*). 0 hr. (From ref. 34, with permission.)

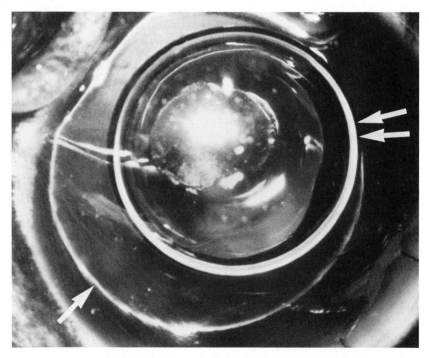

FIG. 5. Hydrogel intraocular lens within the capsular bag (*arrow*). Note the increase in size, due to absorption of aqueous. The anterior chamber is partly filled with air (*double arrow*). 1.5 hr. (From ref. 34, with permission.)

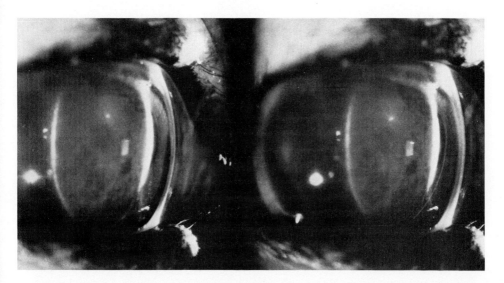

FIG. 6. Hydrogel intraocular lens within capsular bag with fibrin-like material on the surface of the intraocular lens. Four days postoperative. Stereophotograph. (From ref. 34, with permission.)

1 of these 4 eyes did wrinkling of the posterior capsule occur. The hydrogel itself was completely transparent. The follow-up period ranged from 4 to 9 months.

REFERENCES

1. Bagnall, R. D. (1980): Implant biocompatibility. *Biomaterials* 1:97–99.
2. Binkhorst, C. D. (1973): The iridocapsular (two loop) lens and the iris clip (four loop) lens in pseudophakia. *Trans. Am. Acad. Ophthalmol. Otolaryngol.,* 77:589–617.
3. Binkhorst, C. D. (1975): Evaluation of intraocular lens fixation in pseudophakia. *Am. J. Ophthalmol.,* 80:184–191.
4. Binkhorst, C. D., Katz, A., and Leonard, P. A. M. (1972): Extracapsular pseudophakia results in 100 two loop iridocapsular lens implantations. *Am. J. Ophthalmol.,* 73:625–636.
5. Dreifus, M., Wichterle, O., and Lim, D. (1960): Intracameral lenses made of hydrocolloid acrylates. *Cs. Oftalmologie,* 16:154–159.
6. Drews, R. C. (1983): Polypropylene in the human eye. *Am. Intra-Ocular Implant Soc. J.,* 9:137–142.
7. Galin, M. A., Chowchuvech, E., and Turkish, L. (1976): Uveitis and intraocular lenses. *Trans. Ophthalmol. Soc. U.K.,* 96:166–167.
8. Galin, M. A., Turkish, L., and Chowchuvech, E. (1977): Detection, removal and effect of unpolymerized methylmethacrylate in intraocular lenses. *Am. J. Ophthalmol.,* 84:153–159.
9. Gelender, H., Parel, J. M., Treffers, W. F., and Norton, E. W. D. (1985): Phacoersatz: Cataract surgery designed to preserve accommodation. (*Submitted*).
10. Ham, W. T., Mueller, H. A., Ruffolo, J. J., Guerry, D., III, and Guerry, R. K. (1982): Action spectrum for retinal injury from near-ultraviolet radiation in the aphakic monkey. *Am. J. Ophthalmol.,* 93:299–306.
11. Jaffe, N. S. (1976): Postoperative complications early and late. *Trans. Am. Acad. Ophthalmol. Otolaryngol.,* 81:118–119.
12. Jaffe, N. S. (1979): The changing scene of intraocular implant lens surgery. *Am. J. Ophthalmol.,* 88:819–828.

13. Jaffe, N. S., Eichenbaum, D. M., Clayman, H. M., and Light, D. S. (1978): A comparison of 500 Binkhorst implants with 500 routine intracapsular cataract extractions. *Am. J. Ophthalmol.,* 85:24–27.
14. Jennett, J. C., Eifrig, D. E., and Paranjape, Y. B. (1982): The inflammatory response to secondary methylmethacrylate challenge in lens-implanted rabbits. *Am. Intra-Ocular Implant Soc. J.,* 8:35–37.
15. Kaufman, H. E. (1980): The correction of aphakia. XXXVI Edward Jackson Memorial Lecture. *Am. J. Ophthalmol.,* 89:1–10.
16. Kaufman, P. L., and Lutjen-Drecoll, E. (1975): Total iridectomy in the primate in vivo: Surgical technique and postoperative anatomy. *Invest. Ophthalmol. Vis. Sci.,* 14:766–771.
17. Kessler, J. (1964): Experiments in refilling the lens. *Arch. Ophthalmol.,* 71:412–417.
18. Kessler, J. (1966): Refilling the rabbit lens: Further experiments. *Arch. Ophthalmol.,* 76:596–598.
19. Kessler, J. (1975): Lens refilling and regrowth of lens substance in the rabbit eye. *Ann. Ophthalmol.,* 7:1059–1062.
20. LeGrand, Y. (1965): *Optique Physiologique,* 3d ed., p. 70. Editions de la Revue d'Optique, Paris.
21. Mainster, M. A. (1978): Spectral transmittance of intraocular lenses and retinal damage from intense light sources. *Am. J. Ophthalmol.,* 85:167–170.
22. McCarey, B. E., and Andrews, D. M. (1981): Refractive keratoplasty with intrastromal hydrogel lenticular implants. *Invest. Ophthalmol. Vis. Sci.,* 21:107–115.
23. Mehta, K. R., Sathe, S. N., and Karyekar, S. D. (1978): The new soft intraocular lens implant. *Am. Intra-Ocular Implant Soc. J.,* 4:200–205.
24. Mowbray, S. L., Chang, S. H., and Casella, J. F. (1983): Estimation of the useful lifetime of polypropylene fiber in the anterior chamber. *Am. Intra-Ocular Implant Soc. J.,* 9:143–147.
25. Olson, R. J., and Kaufman, H. E. (1982): Ocular tolerance of intraocular lenses in aphakia. In: *Biocompatibility in Clinical Practice,* vol. 2, edited by D. F. Williams, pp. 51–52. CRC Press, Boca Raton, FL.
26. Packard, R. B. S., Gardner, A., and Arnott, E. J. (1981): Poly-HEMA as a material for intraocular lens implantation: a preliminary report. *Br. J. Ophthalmol.,* 65:585–587.
27. Peyman, G. A., Sloan, H. D., and Lim, J. (1982): Ultraviolet light absorbing pseudophakos. *Am. Intra-Ocular Implant Soc. J.,* 8:357–360.
28. Peyman, G. A., Zak, R., and Sloane, H. (1983): Ultraviolet-absorbing pseudophakos: An efficacy study. *Am. Intra-Ocular Implant Soc. J.,* 9:161–170.
29. Refojo, M. F. (1982): Current status of biomaterials in ophthalmology. *Surv. Ophthalmol.,* 26:257–265.
30. Ridley, H. (1952): Intra-ocular acrylic lenses. A recent development in the surgery of cataract. *Br. J. Ophthalmol.,* 36:113–122.
31. Stark, W. J., Leske, M. C., Worthen, D. M., and Murray, G. C. (1983): Trends in cataract surgery and intraocular lenses in the United States. *Am. J. Ophthalmol.,* 96:304–310.
32. Strain, J. C. (1967): Reactions associated with acrylic denture base resins. *J. Prosthet. Dent.,* 18:465–468.
33. Tighe, B. J. (1981): Contact lens materials. In: *Contact Lenses,* vol. 2, edited by J. Stone and A. J. Phillips, pp. 387–389. Butterworths, London.
34. Treffers, W. F. (1980): Intracapsular fixation of extracapsular pseudophakia. *Ophthalmic Surg.,* 11:280–284.
35. Turkish, L., and Galin, M. A. (1980): Methylmethacrylate monomer in intraocular lenses of polymethylmethacrylate. Cellular toxicity. *Arch. Ophthalmol.,* 98:120–121.
36. Wolter, J. R., and Felt, D. P. (1983): Proliferation of fibroplast-like cells on failing intraocular lenses. *Ophthalmic Surg.,* 14:57–64.

Commentary

Induced Hypotony for Cataract Surgery

The presence of a relaxed lens iris diaphragm, indicative of reduced vitreous pressure, is a most desirable feature preparatory to cataract surgery, helping to insure a good result. Ever since Ralph Kirsch made and published his observations about the effect of digital massage on intraocular pressure prior to cataract surgery, all anterior segment surgeons have followed his path. Modifications have been made, and, indeed, mechanical, rather than manual, pressure reduction is currently in style.

Gills (1), Davidson (2), Stark and Maumenee and others have promoted the mechanical method. The Honan reducer (3, 4) is effective in reducing intraocular pressure, and, with it, the chances of vitreous loss for both intracapsular and extracapsular cataract surgery. The gauge on the Honan instrument, however, gives a false sense of security about the safety of the device. Pressure reduction *and* elevation in the eye will depend on the placement of the device (how closely approximated to the eye) and the surrounding orbital tissues. Safety limits have been designated but are not completely accurate. In certain instances of elevated intraocular pressure, the fundus must be examined before and sometimes after application. The response of this "slow" preoperative pressure reduction is only now beginning to be studied. We like to elevate the head slightly before and during cataract surgery (because of possible blood volume increases after release of the Honan) to reduce the pressure on the posterior capsule from the posterior segment.

More needs to be learned about the changes in intraocular pressure, blood flow, and their possible rebounds.

The Editors

REFERENCES

1. Gills, J. P. (1979): Constant mild compression of the eye to produce hypotension. *Am. Intra-Ocular Implant Soc. J.,* 5:52–53.
2. Davidson, B., Kratz, R. P., Mazzocco, T. R., et al. (1979): An evaluation of the Honan intraocular pressure reducer. *Am. Intra-Ocular Implant Soc. J.,* 5:237–238.
3. McDonnell, P. J., Quigley, H. A., Maumenee, A. E., Stark, W. J., and Hutchins, G. M. (1985): The Honan intraocular pressure reducer. *Arch. Ophthal.,* 103:422–425.
4. Jay, W. M., Azia, M. Z., and Green, K. (1985): Effect of Honan pressure reducer on ocular blood flow. *ARVO Abstracts,* 26:105.

Surgical Pharmacology of the Eye,
edited by M. Sears and A. Tarkkanen.
Raven Press, New York © 1985.

Induced Hypotony for Cataract Surgery

Arlo C. Terry and Walter J. Stark

*Wilmer Ophthalmological Institute, The Johns Hopkins Hospital,
Baltimore, Maryland 21205*

Obtaining a soft eye preoperatively is one of the most important aspects of any type of cataract surgery. In extracapsular cataract extraction, a soft eye allows maintenance of the anterior chamber during anterior capsulotomy, aspiration of cortex, and intraocular lens insertion. In intracapsular cataract extraction, delivery of the lens is accomplished in a more controlled fashion in a soft eye. In both types of cataract surgery, there is much less chance of vitreous loss with a soft eye.

We have found the gentle, continuous external compression provided by the Honan monometer to be very effective in inducing hypotony preoperatively. The Honan balloon reduces vitreous volume, decompresses the orbit, and aids in diffusion of the local anesthetic agent. We apply this device for a minimum of 15 min at 30 mmHg immediately prior to proceeding with surgery. Retrobulbar anesthesia itself has been shown to be effective in lowering intraocular pressure, and hyaluronidase enhances this effect (1).

Occasionally we find it necessary to employ a hyperosmotic agent as an adjunct to the Honan balloon in order to induce hypotony. We prefer intravenous mannitol 1½–2 g/kg for this purpose. In patients with poorly controlled diabetes mellitus or cardiovascular compromise, hyperosmotic agents must be used with caution, and we prefer to consult with the patient's internist prior to employing them. We have found preoperative carbonic anhydrase inhibitors to be of no value in inducing hypotony.

General anesthetic agents (except ketamine and possibly trichloroethylene) lower intraocular pressure in proportion to the depth of anesthesia (2,3). The decrease in intraocular pressure is caused by a decrease in the vascular volume in and around the eye, relaxation of the extraocular muscles, depression of central nervous system activity in the diencephalon, and cardiorespiratory effects (2,4). Cardiorespiratory factors that influence intraocular pressure include venous pressure, arterial pressure, and carbon dioxide levels in the blood (2,4,5).

In addition to general anesthetic agents, muscle relaxants may affect the intraocular pressure. Nondepolarizing muscle relaxants such as *d*-tubocurarine and gallamine tend to lower the intraocular pressure, whereas the well-known depolarizing agent succinylcholine produces a transient rise in intraocular pressure lasting for several minutes (2).

A definite relationship between the intraocular pressure and changes in ventilation and inspired P_{CO_2} has been demonstrated in dogs, the intraocular pressure increasing dramatically with increasing percentages of inspired carbon dioxide and decreasing with hyperventilation (6). The same effect has been demonstrated in humans undergoing general anesthesia: an elevated arterial carbon dioxide tension results in increased intraocular pressure, whereas a sudden cessation of CO_2 administration or hyperventilation causes a rapid, simultaneous fall in intraocular pressure to levels below the initial preoperative values (5).

Hvidberg and co-workers (5) have presented evidence suggesting that the drop in intraocular pressure that occurs following hyperventilation is directly related to a decrease in choroidal blood volume, which occurs as the result of a decrease in central venous pressure. These authors further demonstrated that changes in body position (anti-Trendelenburg) may also result in a reduction in the intraocular pressure. They recommend that the PA_{CO_2} be maintained between 25 and 30 mm and that the patient be placed in a 15-degree anti-Trendelenburg position in order to reduce the central venous pressure and thereby avoid an intraoperative elevation in intraocular pressure.

A sudden and dramatic lowering of the intraocular pressure to very low levels occurs when the systolic blood pressure is reduced to 60 mmHg (5,7). This probably occurs as the result of a collapse of the choroidal circulation. Because the uveal vessels possess no precapillary sphincters, there is no compensatory mechanism in the choroid for a decrease in perfusion, and a significant decrease in the systolic blood pressure therefore results in a proportionate decrease in the intraocular pressure (4,5,7). The retinal circulation contributes little to the intraocular pressure because the volume of blood in the retinal circulation is only a fraction of that in the choroidal (7).

In summary, we find the Honan manometer to be the single most effective agent in our preoperative pressure-reducing armamentarium, regardless of whether local or general anesthesia is used. We routinely rely on retrobulbar anesthesia with hyaluronidase to enhance preoperative hypotony and even use it at times in concert with general anesthesia. All of our patients are routinely placed in an anti-Trendelenburg position prior to the beginning of any intraocular procedure. If these measures prove inadequate, we administer intravenous mannitol; and if the patient is under general anesthesia, we request that the anesthesiologist deepen the level of anesthesia, hyperventilate the patient, and/or reduce the patient's blood pressure as appropriate.

REFERENCES

1. Havener, W. H. (1983): *Ocular Pharmacology,* C. V. Mosby, St. Louis.
2. Self, W. G., and Ellis, P. P. (1977): The effect of general anesthetic agents on intraocular pressure. *Surv. Ophthalmol.,* 21:494–500.

3. Crandall, D. C. (1982): Pharmacology of ocular anesthetics. In: *Biomedical Foundations of Ophthalmology,* vol. 3, edited by T. D. Duane and E. A. Jaeger, chap. 35. Harper & Row, Philadelphia.
4. Adams, A. K., and Barnett, K. C. (1966): Anesthesia and intraocular pressure. *Anaesthesia,* 21:202–210.
5. Hvidberg, S. V., Kessing, V., and Fernandes, A. (1981): Effect of changes in P_{CO_2} and body positions on intraocular pressure during general anesthesia. *Acta Ophthalmol. (Copenh.),* 59:465–475.
6. Duncalf, D., and Weitzner, S. W. (1963): The influence of ventilation and hypercapnea on intraocular pressure during anesthesia. *Anesth. Analg.,* 42:232–237.
7. Dias, P. L., Andrew, D. S., and Romanes, G. J. (1982): Effect on the intraocular pressure of hypotensive anaesthesia with intravenous trimetaphan. *Br. J. Ophthalmol.,* 66:721–724.

Commentary

The Pupillary Response to Trauma

Adequate mydriasis is a prerequisite for the execution of a number of commonly performed surgical procedures. The basic laboratory and clinical research about the pupillary reaction to trauma is outlined in this chapter.

Miosis is a phenomenon associated with the nociceptive response to ocular trauma. Miosis is an accompaniment of the vasodilation, breakdown of the blood-aqueous barrier, and the transient intraocular pressure rise after an abrupt influx of plasmoid aqueous. The elements of the response are complex, mediated by neural and/or direct mechanical pathways. Intact sensory nerves can mediate the miotic response to prostaglandins by release of substance P, an undecapeptide and a potent miotic. Direct mechanical stimulation may also release substance P, or, may cause prostaglandin synthesis and secondary release of substance P, and, perhaps other neuropeptides.

In the absence of available specific potent substance P antagonists,[1] the clinical attack to ward off miosis has been: to develop excellent (retrobulbar) sensory anesthesia, to pretreat with inhibitors of prostaglandin synthesis and release (i.e. steroids and/or nonsteroidal agents, especially topical indomethacin), and to employ intraocular direct postsynaptic stimulation of the dilator muscle of the iris, epinephrine, incorporated in ocular perfusion fluids. The value of this armamentarium has not received a randomized clinical trial, but its utility appears reasonable and has been accepted by most ocular surgeons.

Knowledge of the details of this nociceptive response is incomplete, but workable solutions[2] (prophylactic bupivicaine and steroids, and/or topical indomethacin, and "maintenance" perfused pure epinephrine) for a clinical approach to the problem have been found and are improving rapidly.

The Editors

---

[1] See newer developments of potential importance. Stjernschantz, J., von Dickhoff, K., Oksala, O., and Seppä, H. (1985): YAG-laser capsulotomy of rabbit eyes. A study of the acute response. *Invest. Ophthalmol. Vis. Sci. (Suppl.)* 26(8):191.

[2] To this can be added, avoidance of the paracentesis effect by maintenance of the intraocular pressure and a formed anterior chamber. (Salt and/or viscous solutions, extraocular supports, small incisions, and the like).

Surgical Pharmacology of the Eye,
edited by M. Sears and A. Tarkkanen.
Raven Press, New York © 1985.

The Pupillary Response to Trauma

*Joseph Caprioli, **Kanjiro Masuda, and †Johan Stjernschantz

*Department of Ophthalmology, Yale University School of Medicine,
New Haven, Connecticut 06510; †Pharmaceutical Company Oy Star Ab, 33721
Tampere 72, Finland; and **Department of Ophthalmology, School of Medicine,
Tokyo University, Tokyo, Japan

SUMMARY: Atropine-resistant miosis is one of the cardinal responses to ocular irritation. Neither is the response significantly susceptible to blockade of adrenergic, muscarinic, serotonergic, or histaminergic receptors. PGs are synthesized and released into the eye after trauma such as iris stroking, paracentesis, and ocular surgery in animals and humans. Sensory neural blockade or depletion of SP attenuates the response. PGs stimulate receptors on sensory nerve endings, which results in the liberation of SP or related compounds in the eye. PG effects on pupillary constriction are therefore evoked via a mechanism that requires nerve conduction. SP may well represent the final pathway in producing nonmuscarinic miosis caused by ocular trauma. Miosis caused by mechanical stimulation can be achieved by blocking PG synthesis or by blocking SP at the effector postsynaptic level. Perhaps the same mechanism functions in the human eye.

It is well known that the pupil reacts to noxious stimuli by constricting, although the threshold and intensity of miosis may vary in different species. Other components of the ocular irritative response include conjunctival and iridial hyperemia, breakdown of the blood-aqueous barrier, and an increase in intraocular pressure. Traumatic miosis is not mediated by cholinergic receptors; it is prolonged and cannot be blocked by atropine. The irritative response constitutes a logical way of protecting the eye. Pupillary constriction may protect the lens and the posterior pole from penetration by foreign substances. Increased blood flow in the anterior segment, together with increased permeability of the blood-aqueous barrier, makes it possible for phagocytizing cells and immunoglobulins to reach the site of insult rapidly. The price to be paid for this protective system is an increased intraocular pressure (IOP); this is likely secondary to the disruption of the blood-aqueous barrier and in some instances to miosis in eyes with a shallow chamber angle. In rabbits, the increase in IOP after paracentesis is largely due to pupillary block caused by miosis (1). Breakdown of the blood-aqueous barrier in combination with persistent miosis can result in clinically significant posterior synechiae formation.

The pupillary reaction to trauma can cause significant problems during ocular surgery. Miosis can hamper cataract extraction, particularly extracapsular surgery with posterior chamber lens implantation. Preoperative pharmacologic blockade to prevent surgically induced miosis is an important consideration in vitrectomy and procedures for retinal detachment.

MECHANISM OF PUPILLARY REACTION TO TRAUMA

It has been known for at least 150 years that stimulation or cutting of the trigeminal nerve induces miosis. This is true in many mammalian species, and the topic has been reviewed by several authors, including Perkins (43). When trigeminal neurons are depolarized by mechanical or electrical stimuli, the impulses are propagated in all directions of the neuron, including the antidromic direction. Although it is quite clear that stimulation of the trigeminal nerve causes release of neurotransmitter in the iris, it is not clear whether the same transmitter causes the component parts of the ocular irritative response. Observations made by Sears (36,46) and subsequently substantiated (50,52) indicate that there may be separate pathways for the miotic response and the vascular responses.

In the classical experiments by Ambache et al. (4) it was demonstrated that stroking the iris or collapse of the anterior chamber in rabbits causes a release of an active substance, irin, later identified as a prostaglandin E_2 and $F_{2\alpha}$ (3). Thus, pupillary reaction to trauma could be based on at least two mechanisms, one directly nerve-mediated and one prostaglandin-mediated; this dual mechanism has been reviewed (20). A systematic approach to sorting out the dual mechanisms of the ocular reaction to noxious stimuli was undertaken by Jampol et al. (27). Rabbit eyes denervated with retrobulbar injection of alcohol did not react typically to standard external noxious stimuli with nitrogen mustard. However, these eyes still reacted to direct trauma of the iris caused by paracentesis. Stimulation of the trigeminal nerve in rabbits or infusion of formaldehyde into the anterior chamber did not release prostaglandins into the aqueous humor, but direct stroking of the iris did release substantial amounts (18). Later Butler and Hammond (10) showed that the miotic response to intracameral injection of PGE_1, bradykinin, and capsaicin is dependent on intact sensory innervation. The same mechanism has been shown with external irritation of the eye with topical formaldehyde (14) and with laser irradiation of the rabbit iris (13).

Recently, studies by Mandahl and Bill (34,35) have further clarified the role of sensory nerves in the miotic response to autacoids and trauma. Their studies suggested that the miotic response to exogenous PGE_1 and PGE_2 in the rabbit eye requires conductance by sensory nerves. In all likelihood, these autacoids cause miosis by releasing substance P (SP) from nerve terminals, since miosis can be blocked by a specific SP antagonist (D-Arg^1, D-Pro^2, D-Trp^{7,9}, Leu^{11}-SP). Strong irritants such as capsaicin and compound 48/80, when injected into the eye, affect sensory nerve endings directly and have been shown to release substance-P-like immunoreactivity into the aqueous humor of rabbits. It is evident that the miotic response to trauma is largely

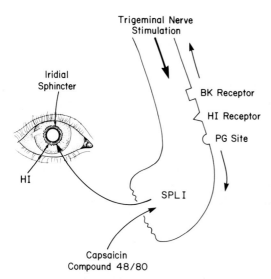

FIG. 1. The hypothetical mechanism of traumatic miosis in the rabbit. Depolarization of trigeminal neurons release SP-like immunoreactivity (SPLI), i.e., SP or a closely related peptide, antidromically in the eye. Autocoids such as bradykinin (BK), histamine (HI), and prostaglandins (PG) release SP-like activity from sensory nerves through a mechanism that requires nerve conduction. Strong irritants such as capsaicin injected into the eye release SPLI activity directly by acting on nerve endings and do not require nerve conduction. SP or a closely related peptide is the final transmitter inducing nonmuscarinic, long-lasting miosis. Some autocoids, e.g., HI, may also act directly on the smooth muscle cells of the sphincter. (Adapted from A. Mandahl, thesis.)

based on the release of SP or related compounds from sensory nerves. Perhaps certain endogenous autacoids, e.g., prostaglandins, bradykinin, and histamine or vasoactive intestinal polypeptide (VIP) (61), may also exert some direct effect on smooth muscle cells of the iridial sphincter. The proposed mechanism of traumatic miosis is schematically represented in Fig. 1.

NEUROPEPTIDES

When evaluating the pathophysiologic roles of various neuropeptides in the iris, it is important to consider their natural distribution in the eye. For example, both oxytocin and vasotocin constrict the rabbit pupil; however, these peptides have not been demonstrated in neural elements of the iris and are unlikely to be involved in the miotic response to irritation. The neuropeptides that have been demonstrated by immunohistochemical and immunoassay techniques to be present in the iris are SP and VIP, which has been found in the choroid (61).

SP

SP has immunohistochemically been identified in the cornea and anterior uvea of many species, including the rat, guinea pig, rabbit, and man (25,57,60). SP-like immunoreactivity is confined to small-caliber nerve fibers, which are abundantly present in the sphincter region of the iris and are thought to convey sensory input. Quantitatively, SP of the anterior uvea varies greatly between species. The rabbit anterior uvea is particularly rich in SP, whereas the primate anterior uvea, including humans, seems to contain much less SP

(Stjernschantz and Sears, *unpublished results*). The concentration of SP in the rabbit anterior uvea measured by immunoassay has been found to be 4.5 − 8.1 pmol × g^{-1} (15,51,64). Sensory denervation of the rabbit eye causes a marked reduction both in the SP that can be measured with radioimmunoassay (12,54) and in the SP that can be detected immunohistochemically (57,59). High-pressure liquid chromatography and immunoassay of SP in the anterior uvea of the rabbit demonstrated that SP-like immunoreactivity corresponds to the undecapeptide of SP (52).

The hypothesis that SP may be released from sensory nerve endings in the eye on irritation or trigeminal nerve stimulation was first published by Bill in 1977. Experiments initiated to test this hypothesis demonstrated that electrical as well as mechanical stimulation of the trigeminal nerve causes a release of SP-like activity into the aqueous humor of rabbits. Intracameral injection of exogenous SP in a dose of 100 ng also induces intense, long-lasting miosis (9). Subsequent studies have verified the potency of SP in the rabbit iridial sphincter muscle (11,34,41,53). Synthetic SP in a dose of 200 to 500 pg (about 10^{-9} M) injected intracamerally caused a marked constriction of the pupil in rabbits (34,53). Intravitreal injection of SP is also effective, but topical application seems to be ineffective, even in high doses (26,53). This is to be expected with a polar and relatively large molecule such as SP, which does not readily penetrate the cornea.

The effects of SP on the iridial sphincter muscle have been studied *in vitro* (17,33,42,47,62). SP in a molar concentration of about 10^{-10} has been shown to cause a measurable contraction of the rabbit iridial sphincter muscle (47). The preparation was about 1,000 times more sensitive to SP than to carbachol (42). The isolated dilator muscle of the rabbit iris was completely insensitive to SP (47). The effect of SP cannot be prevented by adrenergic, cholinergic, serotoninergic, or histaminergic blockade or by blockade of nerve conductance or prostaglandin synthesis. However, (D-Pro^2, D-Trp^{7,9})-SP, an antagonist analog of SP, apparently blocked the response to exogenous SP in the isolated rabbit iris (33). Another SP antagonist, (D-Arg^1, D-Pro^2, D-Trp^{7,9}, Leu^{11})-SP, blocks the contraction of the rabbit sphincter muscle to SP, trigeminal nerve stimulation, capsaicin, PGE$_1$, compound 48/80, and histamine (35). This evidence strengthens the hypothesis that SP is the final transmitter causing miosis during trigeminal nerve depolarization.

At the present time, it is not possible to extrapolate the results from the rabbit to the human eye. However, the finding that there exist many different SP receptors in various tissues (56) and that there seems to be at least some SP-like activity in human irides (Stjernschantz and Sears, *unpublished results*) favors the possibility that a closely related peptide exists in human eyes.

VIP

VIP has been demonstrated by immunohistochemical and radioimmunoassay techniques to be present in the anterior uvea of various species, including guinea pigs, rabbits, and cats. However, VIP seems to be predominantly confined to the choroid and ocular glandular tissue (57,61,64). Stimulation of the facial-intermediate nerve in rabbits causes a marked noncholinergic vasodilation in the choroid and glandular structures; it has been suggested that VIP may be the released neurotransmitter (49). However, in these studies there was no effect on the pupil, and intracameral injections of VIP have not been reported to cause miosis (24,43). *In vitro,* VIP induces relaxation of the rabbit sphincter muscle, which may be linked to an increase in cyclic AMP (23). Currently, there is no evidence that implicates VIP as a mediator in the ocular irritative response.

AUTACOIDS

The autacoids are a group of compounds that include prostaglandins, leukotrienes, histamine, serotonin, bradykinin, and related substances. Evidence to date suggests that prostaglandins, histamine, and bradykinin constrict the pupil by releasing SP from sensory nerve endings through a mechanism that requires nerve conduction (10,34). The antidromic stimulation of the trigeminal nerve liberates SP into the anterior chamber and causes miosis, vasodilation of the iris, breakdown of the blood-aqueous barrier, an increase in the protein content of the aqueous, and a rise in IOP.

Prostaglandins

Ambache (2) demonstrated that the active substance called irin [subsequently identified as prostaglandins E_2 and $F_{2\alpha}$ (3)] is liberated into the aqueous humor after mechanical stimulation of the iris. This provided evidence that prostaglandins (PGs) might mediate ocular irritation caused by antidromic stimulation of the trigeminal nerve. The denervation of the trigeminal nerve abolished the effects of PGE_1 on the pupil and the (IOP). This led to the conclusion that PG-evoked ocular hypertension and miosis is dependent on an intact sensory nerve system (10). Blockade of nerve conduction with tetrodotoxin diminishes the miosis induced by PGE_1 and PGE_2 (34). The degree of miosis produced by PGs depends on the route of drug administration and the species. PGE_2 causes constriction of the isolated sphincter muscle in rabbit eyes and is more potent than acetylcholine (55).

Bhattacherjee et al. (8) demonstrated that epinephrine (which stimulates both α- and β-adrenergic receptors) enhances synthesis of PGs from ^{14}C-arachidonic acid in rabbit ocular tissues. Other investigators suggested that sympathomimetics stimulate ocular PG synthesis via an α-adrenergic mechanism (39,63). Engstrom and Dunham (22) showed that phenylephrine enhances PGE_2 and $PGF_{2\alpha}$ synthesis and release from superfused ^{14}C-arachidonic-acid-labeled iris-ciliary body. Phenoxybenzamine, an α-adrenergic blocker, or indomethacin prevented phenylephrine-induced PG release. Phenoxybenzamine did not inhibit the enzymes involved in PG synthesis. Bradykinin was capable of marked stimulation of PG release from the iris-ciliary body pretreated with phenoxybenzamine.

Leukotrienes

Arachidonic acid is released from the phospholipid pool of almost all cell membranes by mechanical or chemical stimuli and is quickly converted into cyclic endoperoxides (PGG_2 and PGH_2) by cyclooxygenase. Arachidonic acid is also converted into various hydroxyeicosatetraenoic acids (HETEs) and leukotrienes by 12- and 5-lipoxygenase pathways, respectively. Arachidonic acid is first converted by 5-lipoxygenase into unstable compounds, 5-HPETE, which are further converted into the leukotrienes A_4, B_4, C_4, D_4, and E_4. Among these agents, B_4 is found to be a potent chemotactic agent for leukocytes in rabbit eyes (6). A mixture of C_4 and D_4 represents the slow-reacting substance of anaphylaxis and results in smooth muscle contraction. Many lipoxygenase products are synthesized in the anterior uvea and the conjunctiva of several species (7,32); some of these (5-HETE and 12-HETE, 15-HETE and 15-HPETE) have been injected intracamerally in rabbits, and leukotrienes B_4, C_4, and D_4 have been injected intracamerally in guinea pigs, rabbits, and cats (54). Most of the lipoxygenase products showed little activity in the anterior segment of the eye, with three exceptions: leukotriene B_4 caused leukocyte infiltration, and leukotrienes C_4 and D_4 caused nonmuscarinic, prolonged miosis in cats.

Bradykinin

Bradykinin is a potent contractor of smooth muscles. Small doses of bradykinin (0.5×10^{-8} and 1.0×10^{-8} M administered intracamerally into rabbit eyes) result in intense miosis and a sharp increase in IOP. These effects were completely abolished by denervation of the trigeminal nerve. The results indicate that the rise in IOP and intense miosis were dependent on an intact peripheral sensory nervous system. Atropine does not block this miosis. Bradykinin appears to act on the sensory nerve terminals, releasing a mediator that acts directly on the sphincter muscle. Tachyphylaxis develops rapidly by successive applications of bradykinin (66).

PREVENTION OF SURGICAL MIOSIS

The miotic response to intraocular surgery is well known to ophthalmic surgeons and can occasionally prevent adequate exposure for certain surgical maneuvers. This has become increasingly important in recent years with the popularity of extracapsular cataract extraction and intraocular implantation of posterior chamber lenses. Surgically induced, atropine-resistant miosis can complicate the performance of an adequate anterior capsulotomy, the aspiration of peripheral cortical material, and the placement of a posterior chamber lens implant. Miosis caused by ocular surgery appears to be evoked via a pathway of PG synthesis and release followed by the liberation of SP or related substances from the sensory nerve endings. Since SP does not cause miosis via muscarinic receptors, antimuscarinic drugs such as atropine and tropicamide do not inhibit the miosis. Surgical miosis can theoretically be blocked by inhibiting PG synthesis or by blocking the effects of SP directly.

Inhibitors of PG Synthesis

Nonsteroidal anti-inflammatory drugs inhibit the synthesis of prostaglandins and suppress the inflammatory process (65). The route of administration is an issue here. Systemically administered indomethacin does not penetrate well into the human eye as compared to topical application (44). Oral indomethacin showed a mean aqueous humor level below the lower limit of sensitivity of the assay and a mean serum level of 642 ng/ml. Patients receiving the topical 1% aqueous suspension had a mean aqueous level of 198 ng/ml and no detectable serum level. Patients receiving the topical 1% oil suspension had a mean aqueous level of 429 ng/ml, which was significantly higher than that of the aqueous suspension.

Since PGs are released in response to surgical trauma, the use of PG synthesis inhibitors in patients who are about to undergo intraocular surgery was undertaken (37). Indomethacin in oil (0.5%) was used in soft cataract aspiration (45) and in intracapsular extraction of senile cataracts (38). Preoperative instillation of 0.5% indomethacin in oil significantly decreased miosis during soft cataract aspiration, thereby reducing accidental iris aspiration and facilitating total cortical removal. Klug et al. (30) studied the effects of topical indoxole on pupillary constriction induced by trauma to the rabbit iris. Indoxole was found to maintain mydriasis significantly more effectively than topical indomethacin. More recently, the effect of topical indomethacin was studied compared to placebo in preventing miosis during extracapsular cataract extraction (29). Indomethacin significantly reduced the amount of pupillary constriction intraoperatively, simplifying cortical removal and lens implantation.

SP Inhibitor

Direct inhibition of SP at the effector level may block the component of miosis produced by the irritative response. One such compound, (D-Pro^2, D-Trp^{7,9})-SP is a synthetic SP analog, which in small doses inhibits the irritant effects of exogenous SP and reduces the inflammatory response to infrared irradiation of the iris (21). The increase of protein concentration in the aqueous humor caused by SP and PGE$_1$ was significantly reduced after pretreatment with (D-Pro^2, D-Trp^{7,9})-SP. Large doses of (D-Pro^2, D-Trp^{7,9})-

SP, however, cause miosis, breakdown of the blood-aqueous barrier, and a rise in the IOP mimicking SP effects on the eye (35). This drug appears to act as an antagonist of SP, with partial agonist activity that becomes manifest at high doses. Further research in this area may produce more specific compounds that could be instilled in the eye at the time of surgery to prevent traumatic miosis.

REFERENCES

1. Al-Ghadyan, A., Mead, A., and Sears, M. L. (1979): Increased pressure after paracentesis of the rabbit eye is completely accounted for by prostaglandin synthesis and release plus pupillary block. *Invest. Ophthalmol. Vis. Sci.*, 18:361–365.
2. Ambache, N. (1955): Irin, a smooth-muscle-contracting substance present in rabbit iris. *J. Physiol. (Lond.)*, 129:65P–66P.
3. Ambache, N., and Brummer, H. D. (1968): A simple chemical procedure for distinguishing E from F prostaglandins, with application to tissue extracts. *Br. J. Pharmacol. Chemother.*, 33:162–170.
4. Ambache, N., Kavanagh, L., and Whiting, J. (1965): Effect of mechanical stimulation on rabbit's eye: Release of active substance in anterior chamber perfusates. *J. Physiol. (Lond.)*, 176:378–408.
5. Beitch, B. R., and Eakins, K. E. (1969): The effects of prostaglandins on the intraocular pressure of the rabbit. *Br. J. Clin. Pharmacol.*, 37:158–167.
6. Bhattacherjee, P., Hammond, B., Salmon, J. A., Stepney, R., and Eakins, K. E. (1981): Chemotactic response to some arachidonic acid lipoxygenase products in the rabbit eye. *Eur. J. Pharmacol.*, 73:21–28.
7. Bhattacherjee, P., Hammond, B. R., Williams, R. N., and Eakins, K. E. (1980): Arachindonic and lipoxygenase production in ocular tissues and their effect on leukocyte infiltration in vivo. *Proc. Int. Soc. Eye Res.*, 1:32–36.
8. Bhattacherjee, P., Kulkarni, P. S., and Eakins, K. E. (1979): Metabolism of arachidonic acid in rabbit ocular tissues. *Invest. Ophthalmol. Vis. Sci.*, 18:172–178.
9. Bill, A., Stjernschantz, J., Mandahl, A., Brodin, E., and Nilsson, G. (1979): Substance P: Release on trigeminal nerve stimulation, effects in the eye. *Acta Physiol. Scand.*, 106:371–373.
9a.Bito, L. Z., Nicholas, R. R., and Baroody, R. A. (1982): A comparison of the miotic and inflammatory effects of biologically active polypeptide and prostaglandin E_2 on the rabbit eye. *Exp. Eye Res.*, 34:325–337.
10. Butler, J. M., and Hammond, B. R. (1977): Effect of sensory denervation on the response of the rabbit eye to bradykinin and PGE_1. *Trans. Ophthalmol. Soc. U.K.*, 97:668–674.
11. Butler, J. M., and Hammond, B. R. (1980): The effects of sensory denervation on the response of the rabbit eye to prostaglandin E, bradykinin and substance-P. *Br. J. Clin. Pharmacol.*, 69:495–502.
12. Butler, J. M., Powell, D., and Unger, W. G. (1980): Substance-P levels in normal and sensorily denervated rabbit eyes. *Exp. Eye Res.*, 30:311–313.
13. Butler, J. M., Unger, W. G., and Cole, D. F. (1980): Axon reflex in ocular injury: Sensory mediation of the response of the rabbit eye to laser irradiation of the iris. *Q. J. Exp. Physiol.*, 65:1981–1982.
14. Butler, J. M., Unger, W. G., and Hammond, B. R. (1979): Sensory mediation of the ocular response to neutral formaldehyde. *Exp. Eye Res.*, 28:577–589.
15. Camras, C. B., and Bito, L. Z. (1980): The pathophysiological effects of nitrogen mustard on the rabbit eye. II. The inhibition of the initial hypertensive phase by capsaicin and the apparent role of substance-P. *Invest. Ophthalmol. Vis. Sci.*, 19:423–428.
16. Casey, W. J. (1974): The effect of prostaglandin E_2 on the rhesus monkey pupil. *Prostaglandins*, 6:243–251.
17. Cohen, S., Dusman, E., Blumberg, S., and Teichberg, V. I. (1981): In vitro contraction of the pupillary sphincter by substance-P and its stable analogs. *Invest. Ophthalmol. Vis. Sci.*, 20:717–721.

18. Cole, D. F., and Unger, W. G. (1973): Prostaglandins as mediators for the responses of the eye to trauma. *Exp. Eye Res.,* 17:357–368.
19. Eakins, K. E. (1970): Increased intraocular pressure produced by prostaglandins E_1 and E_2 in the cat eye. *Exp. Eye Res.,* 10:87–92.
20. Eakins, K. E. (1977): Prostaglandin and non-prostaglandin mediated breakdown of the blood-aqueous barrier. *Exp. Eye Res.,* 25(Suppl.):438–498.
21. Engberg, G., Svensson, T. H., Rosell, S., and Folkers, K. (1981): A synthetic peptide as antagonist of substance P. *Nature,* 293:222–223.
22. Engstrom, P., and Dunham, E. W. (1982): Alpha-adrenergic stimulation of prostaglandin release from rabbit iris-ciliary body in vitro. *Invest. Ophthalmol. Vis. Sci.,* 22:757–767.
23. Hayashi, K., and Masuda, K. (1982): Effects of vasoactive intestinal polypeptide (VIP) and cyclic AMP of the isolated sphincter pupillae muscles of the albino rabbit. *Jpn. J. Ophthalmol.,* 26:437–442.
24. Hayashi, K., Mochizuki, M., Masuda, K., Nishiyama, A., and Mishima, S. (1982): Die Wirkung des vasoaktiven, intestinalen polypeptids (VIP) auf das Auge. *Klin. Monatsbl. Augenheilk,* 180:82–85.
25. Hokfelt, T., Johansson, O., Kellerth, J-O, Ljungdahl, A., Nilsson, G., Nygards, A., and Pernow, B. (1977): Immunohistochemical distribution of substance-P. In: *Substance-P,* edited by U. S. von Euler and J. Pernow, pp. 117–145. Raven Press, New York.
26. Holmdahl, G., Hakansson, R., Leander, S., Rosell, S., Folkers, K., and Sundler, F. (1981): Substance-P antagonist (D-Pro², D-Trp⁷·⁹)-SP inhibits inflammatory responses in the rabbit's eye. *Science,* 214:1029–1031.
27. Jampol, L. M., Neufeld, A. H., and Sears, M. L. (1975): Pathways for the response of the eye to injury. *Invest. Ophthalmol. Vis. Sci.,* 14:184–189.
28. Kelly, R. G. M., and Starr, M. S. (1971): Effects of prostaglandins and a prostaglandin antagonist on intraocular pressure and protein in the monkey eye. *Can. J. Ophthalmol.,* 6:205–211.
29. Keulen-deVos, J. C. J., Van Rij, G., Renardel de LaVolette, J. C. G., and Jansen, J. T. G. (1983): Effect of indomethacin in preventing surgically induced miosis. *Br. J. Ophthalmol.,* 67:94–96.
30. Klug, R. D., Krohn, D. L., Breitfeller, J. M., and Dieterich, D. (1981): Inhibition of trauma-induced miosis by indoxole. *Ophthalmic Res.,* 13:122–128.
31. Kulkarni, P. S., and Srinivasan, B. (1982): The effects of intravitreal and topical prostaglandins on intraocular inflammation. *Invest. Ophthalmol. Vis. Sci.,* 23:383–392.
32. Kulkarni, P. S., and Srinivasan, B. (1983): Synthesis of slow reacting substance-P-like activity in rabbit conjunctiva and anterior uvea. *Invest. Ophthalmol. Vis. Sci.,* 24:1079–1085.
33. Leander, S., Hakansson, R., Rosell, S., Folkers, K., Sundler, F., and Tornquist, K. (1981): A specific substance-P antagonist blocks smooth muscle contractions by non-cholinergic, non-adrenergic nerve stimulation. *Nature,* 294:467–469.
34. Mandahl, A., and Bill, A. (1981): Ocular responses to antidromic trigeminal stimulation, intracameral prostaglandin E_1 and E_2, capsaicin, and substance-P. *Acta Physiol. Scand.,* 112:331–338.
35. Mandahl, A., and Bill, A. (1983): Effects of the substance-P antagonist (D-Arg¹, D-Pro², D-Trp⁷·⁹, Leu¹¹)-SP on the miotic response to substance-P, antidromic trigeminal nerve stimulation, capsaicin, prostaglandin E, compound 48/80, and histamine. *Acta Physiol. Scand.,* 117:139–144.
36. Maul, E., and Sears, M. L. (1976): Objective evaluation of experimental ocular irritation. *Invest. Ophthalmol. Vis. Sci.,* 15:308–312.
37. Mishima, S., and Masuda, K. (1977): Clinical implication of prostaglandins and synthesis inhibitors. In: *Symposium on Ocular Therapy,* vol. 10, edited by I. H. Leopold and R. P. Burns, pp. 1–19. Wiley, New York.
38. Mochizuki, M., Sawa, M., and Masuda, K. (1977): Topical indomethacin in intracapsular extraction of senile cataract. *Jpn. J. Ophthalmol.,* 21:215–226.
39. Neufeld, A. H., Chavis, R. M., and Sears, M. L. (1973): Degeneration release of norepinephrine causes transient ocular hyperemia mediated by prostaglandins. *Invest. Ophthalmol. Vis. Sci.,* 12:167.
40. Nilsson, S., and Bill, A. (1979): Effect of the vasoactive intestinal polypeptide on the intraocular pressure and regional blood flow. *Acta Physiol. Scand.,* 108:51A.

41. Nishiyama, A., Masuda, K., and Mochizuki, M. (1981): Ocular effects of substance-P. *Jpn. J. Ophthalmol.,* 25:362–369.
42. Nishiyama, A., Mochizuki, M., and Masuda, K. (1982): Effects of substance-P on the isolated iris sphincter muscle of the albino rabbit. *Jpn. J. Ophthalmol.,* 26:29–36.
43. Perkins, E. S. (1957): Influence of the fifth cranial nerve on the intraocular pressure of the rabbit eye. *Br. J. Ophthalmol.,* 41:257–300.
44. Sanders, D. R., Goldsteck, B., Kraff, C., Hutchins, P., Berstein, M. S., and Evans, M. A. (1983): Aqueous penetration of oral and topical indomethacin in humans. *Arch. Ophthalmol.,* 101:1614–1616.
45. Sawa, M., and Masuda, K. (1976): Topical indomethacin in soft cataract aspiration. *Jpn. J. Ophthalmol.,* 20:514–519.
46. Sears, M. L. (1960): Miosis and intraocular pressure changes during manometry. *Arch. Ophthalmol.,* 63:707–714.
47. Soloway, M. R., Stjernschantz, J., and Sears, M. L. (1981): The miotic effect of substance-P on the isolated rabbit iris. *Invest. Ophthalmol. Vis. Sci.,* 20:47–52.
48. Starr, M. (1971): Further studies on the effect of prostaglandins on intraocular pressure in the rabbit. *Exp. Eye Res.,* 11:170–174.
48a.Stern, F. A., and Bito, L. Z. (1982): Comparison of hypotensine and other ocular effects of prostaglandins E_2 and $F_{2\alpha}$ on cat and rhesus monkey eyes. *Invest. Ophthalmol. Vis. Sci.,* 22:588–598.
49. Stjernschantz, J., and Bill, A. (1980): Vasomotor effects of facial nerve stimulation: non-cholinergic vasodilation in the eye. *Acta Physiol. Scand.,* 109:45–50.
50. Stjernschantz, J., Geiser, C., and Bill, A. (1979): Electrical stimulation of the fifth cranial nerve in rabbit: Effects on ocular blood flow, extravascular albumin content and intraocular pressure. *Exp. Eye Res.,* 28:229–238.
51. Stjernschantz, J., Gregerson, D., Bausher, L., and Sears, M. L. (1982): Enzyme-linked immunosorbent assay of substance-P. A study in the eye. *J. Neurochemistry,* 38:1323–1328.
52. Stjernschantz, J., and Sears, M. L. (1982): Identification of substance-P in the anterior uvea and retina of the rabbit. *Exp. Eye Res.,* 35:401–404.
53. Stjernschantz, J., Sears, M. L., and Stjernschantz, L. (1981): Intraocular effects of substance-P in the rabbit. *Invest. Ophthalmol. Vis. Sci.,* 20:53–60.
54. Stjernschantz, J., Sherk, T., Borgeat, P., and Sears, M. L. (1984): Intraocular effects of lipoxygenase pathway products in arachidonic acid metabolism. *Acta Ophthalmol. (Copenh.),* 62:104–111.
55. Takats, I. (1976): Effect of prostaglandin E_2 on the isolated rabbit iris sphincter. *Graefes Arch. Klin. Exp. Ophthalmol.,* 200:257–262.
56. Teichberg, V. W., Cohen, S., and Blumberg, S. (1981): Distinct classes of substance-P receptors revealed by a comparison of the activities of substance-P and some of its segments. *Regul. Pept.,* 1:327–333.
57. Terenghi, G., Polak, J. M., Probert, L., McGregor, G. P., Ferri, G. L., Blank, M. A., Butler, J. M., Unger, W. G., Zhang, S-Q., Cole, D. F., and Bloom, S. R. (1982): Mapping, quantitative distribution, and origin of substance P- and VIP-containing nerves in the uvea of guinea pig eye. *Histochemistry,* 75:399–419.
58. Tervo, K., Eranko, L., Vannas, A., Tervo, T., and Ahonen, R. (1983): Substance-P immuno-reaction and acetylcholinesterase activity in the anterior segment of the human eye. *Invest. Ophthalmol. Vis. Sci.,* 24(Suppl.):261.
59. Tervo, K., Tervo, T., Eranko, L., Eranko, O., and Cuello, A. C. (1981): Immunoreactivity for substance-P in the gasserian ganglion ophthalmic nerve and anterior segment of the rabbit eye. *Histochem. J.,* 13:435–443.
60. Tornquist, K., Mandahl, A., Leander, S., Loren, I., Hakansson, R., and Sundler, F. (1982): Substance-P reactive nerve fibers in the anterior segment of the rabbit eye: Distribution and possible physiological significance. *Cell. Tissue Res.,* 222:467–477.
61. Uddman, R., Alumets, J., Ehinger, B., Hakansson, R., Loren, I., and Sundler, F. (1980): Vasoactive intestinal peptide nerves in ocular and orbital structures of the cat. *Invest. Ophthalmol. Vis. Sci.,* 19:878–885.
62. Ueda, N., Muramatsu, I., Sakakibara, Y., and Fujiwara, M. (1981): Non-cholinergic, non-adrenergic contraction and substance-P in rabbit iris sphincter muscle. *Jpn. J. Pharmacol.,* 31:1071–1079.

63. Unger, W. (1979): Prostaglandin mediated inflammatory changes induced by alpha-adrenoceptor stimulation in the sympathectomised rabbit eye. *Graefes Arch. Klin. Exp. Ophthalmol.,* 211:289–300.
64. Unger, W. G., Butler, J. M., Cole, D. F., Bloom, S. R., and McGregor, G. P. (1981): Substance-P, vasoactive intestinal polypeptide (VIP) and somatostatin levels in ocular tissue in normal and sensorily denervated eyes. *Exp. Eye Res.,* 32:797–801.
65. Vane, J. R. (1971): Inhibition of prostaglandin synthesis as a mechanism of action of aspirin-like drugs. *Nature [New Biology],* 231:232–235.
65a.Waizman, H. B., and King, C. D. (1967): Prostaglandin influence on intraocular pressure and pupil size. *Amer. J. Physiol.,* 212:329–334.
66. Zhang, S. Q., Butler, J. M., Ohara, K., and Cole, D. R. (1982): Sensory neuromechanisms in contraction of the isolated sphincter pupillae: The role of substance-P and the effects of sensory denervation on the response to miotics. *Exp. Eye Res.,* 35:43–54.

Commentary

Intraoperative Mydriasis and Miosis, Hemostasis: Methods, and Useful Enzymes

In the introductory comments to Joaquín Barraquer's marvelous book "*Microsurgery of the Cornea*" Professor José A. Salva Miguel, Professor of Pharmacology at the University of Barcelona said, "Among my pupils, I remember with special affection, Joaquín Barraquer. During his years of medical school the interest he demonstrated for pharmacology led me to believe that he would become the rigorous scientist with a broad base of knowledge." Certainly in these chapters we have the evidence that supports these comments about the great physician-scientist, Professor Joaquín Barraquer.

These sections on enzymes, hemostasis, and pupillary pharmacology must be studied. The editors have a few thoughts to add. Maintenance of ocular hemostasis includes avoidance of venous congestion and sudden decompression. In the former regard, it is important to raise the head of the operating table slightly. With the now common use of scleral incisions it is necessary to examine the sclera carefully to avoid branches of the muscular arteries. Useful intraocular techniques for hemostasis include mechanical compression by an instrument as by forceps, for example, to pinch a vessel; increasing intraocular pressure such as with Healon®, air, or fluid to tamponade the eye; intraocular vasoconstriction by drugs; sometimes even a well placed suture to capture a vessel can be helpful. Corneal incision for blood dyscrasias, and the continued maintenance of intraocular pressure (tamponade) in patients with persistent hypertension are most important considerations.

On the subject of secondary hyphema, it has been well demonstrated that topical anti-inflammatory steroids have antifibrinolytic action. So while epsilon aminocaproic acid has documented antifibrinolytic action, it is a drug that must be given systemically, *and* has mild as well as potentially serious side effects. The same end (antifibrinolysis) can be accomplished by a few topical drops of steroid. Therefore we prefer topical steroid in primary hyphema to prevent blow-out of the clot and the development of secondary bleeding or blackball.

With respect to enzymes, occasional use of α-chymotrypsin in eyes that may require anterior segment reconstruction *sometimes* can be helpful and less traumatic to remove a scar when that scar is contained within the posterior capsule. Fibrous tissue will, of course, not be affected, but often fibrous tissue that does not incorporate the zonular area but is part of the capsule can be removed in this way.

On the subject of the pupil, avoiding direct trauma to the iris, warming the anesthetic injection fluid and perfusion fluid to at least room temperature, before use to reduce nociception, can be helpful. Unsuccessful preoperative attempts to dilate the pupil by pharmacologic means may, in certain instances, be followed by intraocular infusions of epinephrine diluted in BSS plus. Attempts to dilate a miotic pupil have been tried using argon laserplasty, but the fibrinous reaction could be quite undesirable. Recent attempts at mydriasis have been made using argon laser fiber optic probe. In appropriate cases, four clean linear surgical iridotomies may be quite useful for either anterior segment surgery or in aphakic eyes for surgery of the vitreous and/or retina. The vitrector can be used to do sphincterectomy, when necessary.

Additional scholarship and clean surgical maneuvers are beautifully described herein and should be considered in adjunct to the use of preoperative topical and systemic medications (for mydriasis) described in other chapters.

The Editors

Surgical Pharmacology of the Eye,
edited by M. Sears and A. Tarkkanen.
Raven Press, New York © 1985.

Intraoperative Mydriasis and Miosis

Rafael I. Barraquer and Joaquín Barraquer

Instituto Barraquer, Barcelona 21, Spain

SUMMARY: **Mydriasis:**
1. Preoperative mydriasis:
    a. For ICCE: phenylephrine 10% or 2.5%, 1 drop 2 hr preoperatively and (optional) 1 drop 1 hr preoperatively. Cyclopentolate 1% or tropicamide 1%, 1 drop 30 min preoperatively, 1 drop 25 min preoperatively.
    b. For ECCE, retina and vitreous surgery, the same regimen as above plus: Homatropine 5%, 1 drop every 15 min starting 2 hr preoperatively; *or,* scopolamine 1%, 1 drop 1 hr preoperatively, and 1 drop 30 min preoperatively; *and/or,* atropine 1%, 1 drop 72 hr preoperatively, 1 drop 48 hr preoperatively, 1 drop 24 hr preoperatively, and 1 drop 12 hr preoperatively.
2. To avoid undesired intraoperative miosis: Avoid opiates. Avoid trauma to the eye tissues (particularly the iris), both physical (rubbing, turbulent irrigation, ultrasound) and chemical (irrigating solutions, gas, drugs and preservatives). Healon® may be useful to dilate maximally an already mydriatic pupil and to maintain dilation throughout surgery.
3. To redilate an intraoperatively constricted pupil: Parasympatholytics are of little help. Sympathomimetics can be used, watching for local or systemic toxicity: To avoid cardiac complications intracameral epinephrine with halothane anesthesia may be up to 68 μg/kg. Watch for local (intraocular) toxicity of epinephrine solutions, probably caused by preservatives. Do not use commercially available 1:10,000 epinephrine. Best for intraocular use is Parke-Davis 1:1,000 intracardiac epinephrine, diluted to 1:8,000, or into a bottle of 500 ml. of BSS.

Miosis:
1. Preoperative miosis (to protect lens during corneal trephination, to have a tense iris for laser iridotomy or corioplasty, for a very basal and self-repositioning peripheral iridectomy, for best trabecular access in goniotomy or laser trabeculoplasty): Use any kind of topical parasympathomimetic of the muscarinic type, as pilocarpine 1% or 2%, 1 drop 2 hr preoperatively, 1 drop 1 hr preoperatively. Avoid anticholinesterase agents (as echothiophate iodide, isoflurophate, and demecarium) as they may interact with succinylcholine leading to prolonged apnea, and increase the toxicity of local anesthetics of the ester type, which may lead to hypotension and convulsions.
2. Intraoperative miosis (to reposition anterior hyaloid and iris diaphragm after ICCE, to reduce iris prolapse, to perform a basal iridectomy after operating with a maximally dilated pupil): Best intracameral drug for fast, non toxic, intense, short-lasting effect is acetylcholine 0.5 to 1%. When a longer lasting effect is desired (although it may favor postoperative iritis and/or pupillary block), the effect of acetylcholine may be potentiated with eserine, or carbachol 0.01% may be used.

Since the structural division of the eye into anterior and posterior chambers by the iris is a main feature of intraocular topography, the size of the pupil is a determinant factor for most intraocular surgery. The need of a mydriatic or miotic iris is not only different according to the observation and maneuvering requirements of each specific procedure, but usually varies between intraoperative steps and/or postoperative status. However, the surgeon's personal preferences are a common source of variability among these requirements.

FACTORS INFLUENCING INTRAOPERATIVE PUPIL SIZE

Before considering the pharmacological tools the ophthalmic surgeon may use to adapt the pupil size to his preferences, during each step of an intraocular procedure, we should review the physiologic and pharmacologic factors—as anesthesia and response to surgical trauma—whose intraoperative interactions will condition the use of other agents.

Pupil and Anesthesia

Effect of Anesthetic Agents on the Iris

The classical description of Guedel's surgical anesthetic planes includes a progressive dilatation of the pupils with the deepening of anesthesia (43,44). However, these observations were made mainly using ether (diethilic ether), known to be a sympathetic activator (14,82). Most inhaled agents used today for general anesthesia, such as halothane (Fluothane®), enflurane (Ethrane®), or methoxyflurane (Penthrane®), induce a depression of the sympathetic activity and a parasympathetic predominance resulting in miosis and accommodation (19,83). Nitrous oxide, cyclopropane or fluroxene (Fluoromar®) are sympathetic stimulators and would be expected to produce mydriasis, unless this effect is masked by the miosis induced by associated drugs (83).

Barbiturates have been found to exert an antiadrenergic effect on the CNS at the anesthesic doses (52). Barbiturate intoxication usually leads to mydriasis, although miosis is also seen, and hippus is common (64). However, the barbiturates commonly used to start general anesthesia, such as thiopental (Pentothal®), are unlikely to affect pupil size significantly during surgery, due to their ultrashort action. Similarly, the parasympatholytic action of systemic atropine, at the doses given to prevent excessive bronchial secretion or cardiac side effects of anesthetics (0.5 mg., which equals 1 drop of a 1% collyrium), may not be expected to produce significant mydriasis.

Muscle relaxants of both types—competitive or stabilizing, such as *d*-tubocurarine (Mioflex®, Tubarine®), gallamine (Galaflex®, Flaxedil®), or pancuronium (Pavulon®), and noncompetitive or depolarizing, such as succinylcholine (Anectane®, Scoline®) or decamethonium (Syncurine®)—exert their action on the skeletal and extraocular striate neuromuscular junction. Although *d*-tubocurarine has some blocking action on the nicotinic receptors of autonomic ganglia, which would equally inhibit sympathetic and parasympathetic activity, it does not affect the autonomic neuromuscular (adrenergic or muscarinic cholinergic) junctions (35,55). The association of sedative drugs such as benzodiazepines or opiate analgesics such as pentazocine lactate (Fortral®, Talwin®), meperidine chlorhydrate (Petidine®), or fentanyl citrate (Sublimaze®), frequently used to supplement general anesthesia, or particularly the latter in its association with droperidol (Inapsine®) known as Innovar® for neuroleptoanalgesia, will also favor miosis.

Another factor not to be overlooked is the ventilatory status of the anesthetized patient. Whereas correct ventilation or hyperventilation favors the general tendency to miosis, hypoventilation—which might occur during spontaneous ventilation, often preferred for ophthalmic surgery to avoid the risk of anesthetic agent hyperdosage and intraocular pressure (IOP) rise that the intrathoracic pressure inversion may cause during mechanically assisted respiration—will result in a Pa_{CO_2} rise (hypercarbia) and Pa_{O_2} fall (hypoxia) leading to mydriasis. The demand for a supplementary respiratory effort by means of the accessory respiratory muscles, as may happen if the endotracheal intubation is partially obstructed by secretions (which is more likely to happen in children, where the small caliber is a concurrent factor) will also result in sympathetic stimulation and a tendency to mydriasis.

Local anesthetics block the generation and conduction of nerve impulses, probably by interfering with the axon membrane ionic dynamics (Na^+, Ca^{2+}) (26,86). They may also block the ganglionic synapse acting on both the preganglionic terminal and the ganglionic cells. Retrobulbar injection of local anesthetics should be expected to block both the sympathetic and parasympathetic orbital fibers as well as the sensory, not having a significant influence in pupil size unless associated to epinephrine. However, a mechanical dilator tonus predominance may be present, leading to mydriasis.

Although the sensitivity of nerve fibers to local anesthetics depends on their caliber (nonmyelinized fibers, such as the sympathetic, are blocked faster and longer) (40) and type (some delta A myelinized fibers have been found to be blocked before C fibers) (74), a differential blocking effect is expected to occur only during the first minutes after the injection. Absolute differential block was found only when the nerve section exposed to the anesthetic was limited to a few millimeters (36).

Cocaine is the only exception to this rule, due to its ability to block the presynaptic reuptake of catecholamines, resulting in an indirect sympathomimetic effect (it has no effect on denervated structures) and sensitivity to exogenous catecholamines (79). Introduced by Koller in 1884, cocaine was the first drug used successfully as a local anesthetic in ophthalmology (57).

For many years cocaine has been a very popular ophthalmic anesthetic for a wide range of procedures, from superficial manipulations to cataract extraction. The combined anesthetic and sympathomimetic effects, producing hemostasia and mydriasis, together with its simplicity and adequate short-term action, were considered very convenient by many surgeons before new drugs and the more sophisticated techniques of retrobulbar and general anesthesia were introduced. About 15 to 20 min after instillation of cocaine, the pupil begins to dilate, reaching a maximum size within the first hour and returning to normal size within several hours (47). However, the fact that the mydriasis obtained is never maximal and the lack of abolition of parasympathetic reflexes (which may be convenient if miosis is desired at the end of the procedure), together with its toxicity on corneal epithelium and its addicting potential—not to the patient but to the personnel having access to the drug— have greatly limited its use. Although all topical anesthetics are toxic to corneal epithelium, the effect of cocaine is greater, leading to grayish corneal pits and irregularities that may obscure visualization of intraocular structures and to loosening of the epithelium, which may result in large erosions.

Interactions Between Anesthetic and Autonomic Drugs

The intraoperative use of autonomic drugs affecting the pupil size is limited by the possibility of adverse interactions with anesthetics. The most commonly used halogenated inhaled general anesthetics (halothane, enflurane, methoxy-flurane, and trichloroethylene) and cyclopropane sensitize the heart to cate-cholamines, leading to severe ventricular arrhythmias.

According to Kratz and associates (59) the maximum advisable dose of locally injected epinephrine, when these anesthetics are used, is 10 ml of a 1:100,000 solution (100 μg) in any 10-min period, or 30 ml(300 μg)/hr, provided an adequate ventilation is assured. However, Smith and associates (94) concluded that as much as 68 μg/kg, which in an average adult person means almost 5 mg or 5 ml of 1:1,000 solution, could be safely injected into the anterior chamber during halothane anesthesia in patients undergoing cataract extraction by phacoemulsification and aspiration. The rich adrenergic supply of the iris would be able to capture the exogenous epinephrine very rapidly and thus prevent its systemic distribution (94). On the other hand, we must be aware of the fact that systemic absorption speed and rates of drugs administered into the conjunctival sac, and then carried to the nasopharynx via the lacrimal ducts, might be almost half of an intravenous injection, as has been shown with tetracaine (1). External instillation may be safer for intraocular structures but hazardous in relation to systemic side effects.

The safety margin with catecholamines varies for each anesthetic, cyclopro-pane having the least (11). Methoxyflurane would be safer; it does sensitize the ventricles to catecholamines, although to a lesser degree than halothane or enflurane. Fluroxene and isoflurane (Forane®) are halogenated anesthetics believed not to exert a heart sensitizing effect, although they are much less used, the latter having found to be a potential carcinogen (102).

Neuroleptoanalgesia, as obtained with Innovar® (2.5 mg droperidol and

0.05 mg/ml fentanyl), permits a safe association with vasopressors but has a miotic effect due to its opiate component (not depending on parasympathetic activity); a spasmodic diminution of the pupil size, causing difficulties with cataract extraction or posterior segment visualization, and not responding to 1% atropine and 10% phenylephrine (Neo-Synephrine®) has been reported (80).

Local anesthetics, on the contrary, have a reduced toxicity when associated with sympathomimetics (used as vasopressors and to prolong anesthesia, rather than as mydriatics). Cocaine, procaine (Novocain®), tetracaine (Pontocaine®, Prescaina®) and the remaining anesthetics of the ester type are metabolized by blood esterases, and their toxicity (including hypotension and convulsions) will be increased by anticholinesterase agents such as echothiophate iodide (phospholine iodide) or isoflurophate (Floropryl®, DFP). Although these are unlikely to be used as intraoperative miotics, special attention must be given to glaucoma patients chronically using these drugs.

Effect of Surgical Manipulation on the Iris

It is a not infrequent observation that a preoperatively fully dilated pupil becomes progressively miotic during surgery, making difficult posterior segment visualization and any transpupillary maneuver. Various physiologic mechanisms explaining this phenomenon have been postulated, including the photomotor reflex to the intense operating field illumination, the predominating miotic effect of general anesthesia, hypotony, and liberation of local mediators from the injured tissues. Histamine and prostaglandins were the first substances implicated; 25 mg of the antihistamine promethazine (Phenergan®) given 2 hr preoperatively was found to maintain a well-dilated pupil in 12 of 14 cataract extractions (compared to 8 of 13 control eyes) (34).

Lately substance P (SP), a neuropeptide found in various nervous structures including the eye's sensory nerves (21), appears particularly relevant in the miotic aspect of the ocular nociceptive response (65,98,101). As this has been the subject of a previous chapter, we will only mention here that miosis resulting from mechanical (instrumental, irrigation turbulence, or bubble rubbing) or chemical (drugs, gas, irrigating solutions) irritation of ocular structures does not depend on sympathetic nor parasympathetic activity and thus cannot be prevented by parasympatholytic drugs such as atropine or cyclopentolate (Ciclogyl®). Sympathomimetic agents could, however, antagonize this effect, acting postsynaptically on the iris dilator, which appears insensitive to SP (98).

Several experimental facts found in rabbits—such as the requirement of an intact sensory innervation to obtain a miotic reaction to prostaglandin E_1 (PGE) or bradykinin (20) and the ineffectiveness of indomethacin (an inhibitor of the synthesis and release of prostaglandins) pretreatment in blocking the trigeminal antidromic stimulation-induced miosis (25,67), a phenomenon associated with the release of SP into the anterior chamber (15)—permits us to expect a certain degree of intraoperative miosis, in spite of maximum care in avoiding direct trauma to the iris. If this reduction in pupil size depends on an axon-reflex-triggered release of SP, we may expect it from the sole stimulus of corneoscleral incision, although further iris trauma will obviously increase the response.

Capsaicin, a vanillic acid derivative, is known to cause a depletion of SP from sensory nerve fibers (51) and to prevent in rabbits the initial IOP rise after topical application of nitrogen mustard (22). We still do not know, however, whether capsaicin pretreatment could prevent SP-mediated miosis. Although there is evidence suggesting that enkephalins may inhibit the release of SP from sensory nerves, preliminary experiments by Stjernschantz and Sears (100) and by Bill (15) have failed to reveal any significant attenuation of the iris response to trigeminal antidromic stimulation in rabbits.

INTRAOPERATIVE MANAGEMENT OF PUPIL SIZE

Mydriasis

A widely dilated pupil is generally preferred in any procedure requiring visualization and/or maneuvering in the retropupillary area and posterior segment of the eye, including cataract extraction—both intracapsular (ICCE) and particularly extracapsular (ECCE)—conventional retinal detachment surgery, and vitreous surgery. This is usually accomplished preoperatively by topical sympathomimetics alone or combined with parasympatholytics (muscarinic blockers). Agents that act rapidly and do not have an excessively long duration are logically preferred. However, preoperative mydriasis may not be sufficient or the pupil may contract during surgery following the mechanisms noted above. As related to intraoperative trauma, this is more likely to occur during longer and more aggressive procedures requiring extensive intraocular irrigation and prolonged maneuvering with intraocular instruments, as in conventional ECCE or vitreous surgery, and particularly when ultrasound is used. An intraoperative mydriatic approach may be required in these situations.

Although a miotic pupil is preferred at the end of ICCE to obtain a better vitreous anterior face reposition, the instillation of atropine drops is a frequent practice at the end of other procedures. This may be intended to maintain mydriasis postoperatively to allow fundus observation. In other cases it is cycloplegia (ciliary muscle relaxation) rather than mydriasis that is sought, to obtain a retroposition of the lens/zonular plane and a deepening of the anterior chamber in filtering procedures—particularly when the possibility of ciliary block (malignant glaucoma) is feared—to avoid the formation of posterior synechiae or pupillary block in ECCE by tensing the lens posterior capsule, or simply to prevent postoperative pain and iridocyclitis.

Preoperative Methods: Influencing Factors

A single drop of 10% phenylephrine (PHL) 1 to 2 hr prior to the operation frequently results in mydriasis sufficient for ICCE. Although the individual responses may vary widely, maximal mydriasis is not always mandatory, particularly for ICCE. The erysiphake can pass through a relatively small pupil like a button through its buttonhole, and the vacuum grasp of the lens will slightly reduce its equatorial diameter. Moreover, maximal mydriasis may make difficult the practice of a basal peripheral iridectomy.

Other procedures, such as ECCE and vitreous surgery, require maximal dilatation of the pupil and abolition of the light reflexes. A topical combination of 2.5% to 10% PHL and a parasympatholytic agent, such as cyclopentolate, tropicamide (Mydriacyl®), atropine (all three in 0.5% to 1% solutions), or 5% homatropine, will be useful. The specific combination and administration pattern largely varies among ophthalmologists, ranging from single-drop to multiple applications every 5, 10, or 15 min during the 2-hr preoperative period. A number of factors influence the response to mydriatics, including drug concentration, administration vehicle and method, previous treatments and interactions with other drugs, age, and pigmentation of the iris.

According to Haddad and associates (45), the effect of a freshly prepared solution of PHL increases from 0.1% to 5%. Little improvement in mydriasis can be obtained with solutions above 5%. However, the mydriatic effect of the 10% commercial solution was found similar to a 2.25% freshly prepared solution of PHL.

Sympathetic pupillary tone is usually reduced in old age, resulting in a miotic pupil (58). However, a similar dilatation may be obtained in young and old subjects with 10% PHL, and a sufficient mydriatic effect of 1 drop of 2.5% PHL has been found more often in patients over 60 years of age (89). Tachyphylaxis, an effect consisting of decreased response to the drug following repeated use on subsequent days and associated with a tendency to miosis, is more likely to occur in older patients (45). Infant eyes having a poorly developed iris dilator may show a reduced response to mydriatics.

The administration of the drug in the form of a conjunctival pack has been postulated to enhance the mydriatic effect, avoiding the need for repeated instillations (27). To obtain maximal mydriasis throughout a vitreous operation, Michels (72) suggests, apart from the topical treatment, a 0.2 to 0.3 ml subconjunctival injection of a 0.5% PHL and 0.4% homatropine combination with procaine in an isotonic solution. The use of such methods should be cautiously evaluated in relation to possible systemic side effects (38). Moreover, there is evidence suggesting that intraocular penetration of subconjunctivally administered drugs is actually insignificant compared to the topical transcorneal route (28).

Highly pigmented irises are resistant to mydriatics of both types, requiring higher doses or repeated applications. Melanin metabolites such as dihydroxyphenylalanine (DOPA) have been found to inactivate epinephrine (4). Atropine, cyclopentolate, and related drugs (among others) are bound by melanin, which may lead to a slow onset and prolonged duration of cycloplegia (77).

Cocaine sensitizes the iris dilator to catecholamines, allowing a response to lesser amounts of exogenous epinephrine or PHL. However, it actually decreases the strength of contraction of the muscle (88), its association to catecholamines not being of any real value. Epinephrine associated to retrobulbar anesthesia will enhance the action of dilating drops and may have a mydriatic effect by itself. Chronic users of miotic drops (and some older patients) may have a fibrotic small pupil that will not react to mydriatics, even if the miotic therapy has been discontinued several weeks before surgery. Intraoperative pupil dilatation in these patients will be feasible only by mechanical methods.

Local Toxicity

It is a common observation that PHL enhances the drying changes of the corneal epithelium, and it has been reported to induce epithelial sloughing (75). The cytotoxicity of PHL has been assessed in rabbit corneas, where 2.5% and 10% drops were found to induce edema, and vacuolation within keratocytes and endothelial cells when the epithelium had been removed (but not when it was intact). This was considered the result of an increase in intracellular osmolarity (30). Although the low pH of the commercial drug vehicle (47) and the presence of benzalkonium chloride as a preservative had been previously implied (78), 2.7% PHL prepared to isotonicity in distilled water produced the same degree of edema and vacuolization, ruling out the vehicle factor (30). These effects would therefore be related to the drug itself or possibly to metabolites or breakdown products, such as 1,2,3,4-tetrahydro-4,6-dihydroxy-2-methylisoquinoline and a 4,8-dihydroxy analog, both found in buffered PHL (73) and capable of acting osmotically within the cornea to increase its thickness. Similar effects would be expected when PHL is injected intracamerally.

Systemic Toxicity

Although PHL is an α-adrenergic agent whose vasopressor effects are well recognized when used parenterally, conjunctival instillation rarely produces systemic side effects. Classical papers following its introduction in ophthalmology showed no effect or only a slight increase in blood pressure after topical use of one drop of 10% PHL (48). Even among hypertensive patients, only 6% developed elevations of blood pressure, all of them less than 10 mmHg (70). Other studies, using repeated applications, found 10 to 40 mmHg increases in both systolic and diastolic pressures in normal and hypertensive patients (90), or no increase 90 min after the last drop (95).

However, adverse reactions including severe hypertension with occipital headache, subarachnoid hemorrhage, and ventricular arrhythmia have been occasionally reported since 1956 (61,70,97,101,105). By 1978, about 50 cases could be gathered. Fraunfelder and Scafaldi (38) reviewed 32 systemic reactions attributable to 10% PHL from the United States National Registry of Drug-Induced Ocular Side Effects. Eleven of 15 patients with myocardial infarctions died. Seven others required cardiopulmonary resuscitation for arrhythmia or arrest. The rest had a marked rise in blood pressure, tachycardia, or reflex bradycardia. This most commonly occurred 20 min after the last application. Seven patients had been treated with a cotton pledget, subconjunctival injection, or by irrigation of the lacrimal sac. The authors conclude that these methods and repeated applications should be avoided. Only 1 drop per eye per hour is allowable.

Although the controlled hypotension obtained in general anesthesia may be protective against the vasopressor effect of PHL, 2 patients in the above-mentioned series were under general anesthesia. One had a cardiac arrest 1 to 2 min after a subconjunctival injection of 0.1 ml 10% PHL; the other had severe postoperative hypertension (240/160) lasting 8 hr.

Although the upper safety limit for intravenous PHL is only 1.5 mg in young healthy adults (10 mg subcutaneously) (53), a single drop of 10% PHL contains 3.3 (97) to 6.7 (61) mg of the drug. As the mucosal (particularly the nasopharyngeal) absorption of drugs may be almost as fast as intravenously (101), the sparsity of overdoses may be due to the fact that commercial 10% solutions have an actual activity equivalent to a 2.25% freshly prepared solution of PHL (45).

The 2.5% solution is preferred for infants and the elderly, since topical use of 10% PHL in neonates has been documented to cause marked increase in blood pressure (17), and no significant adverse effects have been reported with the use of the 2.5% solution. However, a transient blood pressure rise (both systolic and diastolic) averaging 24% and lasting 30 min has been observed in preterm infants, 8 min after 1 drop of 2.5% PHL and 0.5% tropicamide (62).

Patients with heart disease, aneurysm, advanced arteriosclerosis, and hypertension should be cautiously treated, particularly if they are receiving reserpine or guanethidine. Formal contraindications include patients using antidepressants of both types, tricyclic or monoamine oxidase inhibitors, even up to 21 days after cessation of the latter. Atropinized patients may show a potentiation of the pressor effect of PHL and tachycardia (53).

The previous instillation of a drop of anesthetic (0.5% proparacaine) increased the pupillary dilatation after a single drop of 2.5% PHL combined with either 0.5% cyclopentolate or 0.5% tropicamide (5). The toxic effect of local anesthetics on corneal epithelium could cause an increase in corneal permeability. Although this would allow mydriasis without the need of repeated instillations and diminish the risk of systemic side effects, it would also increase the risk of endothelial damage.

Using three applications of 0.005-ml microdrops of a 5% PHL and 0.5% tropicamide combination, Brown and Hanna (18) obtained the same mydriasis and cycloplegia as with regular (0.05 to 0.07 ml) (37) drops of 10% PHL with 1% tropicamide. Although the technical difficulties in instillating such minute quantities may make this method rather unpractical, it is interesting that the lacrimation and lid squeezing that follows the irritation caused by regular drops dilutes or evacuates part of the drug, reducing the intraocular penetration and favoring its lacrimal drainage and systemic absorption through the nasal mucosa. Fortunately, most of these tears are lost!

We should also mention the possible systemic adverse effects of the parasympatholytics used for preoperative mydriasis, although more infrequent than reactions to PHL. A single drop of 1% atropine contains 0.5 (47) to 0.75 mg (41) of drug. The lethal dose is about 100 mg for adults and 10 mg for children. However, it is unlikely that preoperative use of these agents by qualified personnel results in atropinic intoxication.

Small doses of atropine (49), homatropine (104), scopolamine (39), and particularly 2% cyclopentolate drops have shown CNS toxicity (especially in children), including dysarthria, disorientation, hallucinations, psychotic reactions and convulsions (6,13,16,66,81,93). Although the incidence of these reactions is reduced with the 1% cyclopentolate solution, they are generally considered as idiosyncratic responses to the drug (16). Even tropicamide drops have been reported to produce in a 5-year-old child generalized muscle rigidity, opisthotonos, pallor, and cyanosis (103).

Intraoperative Methods

If preoperative mydriasis is not sufficient or the pupil constricts during the operation despite all precautions (minimal contact of the instruments with the iris, avoidance of hypotony, use of the least toxic irrigating solution, avoiding unnecessary extensive irrigation and turbulent flux close to the iris, use of air or gas restricted to the end of the procedure, etc.), an intraoperative mydriatic method is indicated. Three alternatives are apparent: instillation with external drops, intraocular instillation, and mechanical methods.

Since intraoperative miosis seems to have little dependence on parasympathetic activity (see Effect of Surgical Manipulation on the Iris, above), cycloplegic drugs are not a suitable approach (at least alone); only an active enhancer of iris dilator contraction (α-adrenergic) may have a valuable effect.

Repeated external instillation of PHL increases the risk of systemic toxicity and local toxicity on corneal epithelium, which may lead to loosening and opacities that make visualization difficult, particularly of the posterior segment structures. If the epithelium has already been removed or has lost its integrity, which is more likely to happen in diabetics, there will be an increased toxicity on corneal endothelium and risk of postoperative decompensation and permanent corneal edema. This is obviously not the best approach.

Michels (72) proposes the application of a small cotton pledget or cellulose sponge soaked with PHL to a localized peripheral area of the cornea where the epithelium has been removed. A redilatation of the pupil would be obtained in 5 to 15 min following this method, which combines increased transcorneal penetration and localization of possible endothelial damage.

Intraocular instillation of mydriatics, including PHL and epinephrine, are definitely effective, causing prompt mydriasis in seconds. Their use is limited, however, because of their toxicity and interaction with anesthetics, and special care should be taken with the solutions employed (31).

The transcorneal toxic effects of PHL on the endothelium should be expected to be amplified when the drug is introduced directly into the anterior chamber. Lang and Hassard (60) performed endothelial cell counts in patients after ICCE and found higher cell loss when 10% PHL had been added to other anterior chamber reconstituents (balanced salt solution, Miochol®, air) during the operation, as compared to air or Miochol® alone. The final dilution of PHL is not precise, but the results (mean loss at 20 days 11.7% to 19.4% in the different combinations with PHL against 7.8% with Miochol® alone and 8.9% with air alone) seem rather optimistic, considering the high concentration of PHL used and the fact that some cell loss always occurs after ICCE (60).

The intraocular use of commercial epinephrine in cataract surgery has been reported to cause corneal edema (33). Experimental studies showed that 1:1,000 commercial epinephrine was clearly damaging to corneal endothelium (50). However, sodium bisulfite preservative produced similar damage, used in concentrations present in commercial epinephrine solutions. Endothelial damage could be prevented by diluting commercial epinephrine (with preservative) to 1:5,000, or using preservative-free 1:1,000 epinephrine (92). Concentrations of 1:10,000 or even less may be effective for mydriasis when injected in the anterior chamber (72). Pigment epithelium toxicity manifested as epinephrine maculopathy (56) is a possibility to be kept in mind.

The systemic side effects of epinephrine combine the pressor activity of its α-adrenergic aspect (similar to PHL) with the β-adrenergic, particularly in the heart. The risk of severe ventricular arrhythmia following the use of halogenated anesthetics that sensitize the heart to catecholamines (see Interactions Between Anesthetic and Autonomic Drugs, above), although responding to extremely complex mechanisms, is more likely to occur with β-adrenergic compounds as epinephrine or isoproterenol. Pure α-adrenergic agents such as PHL or norepinephrine do not have direct action on the myocardium (cardiac side effects would be a consequence of a vagal response following stimulation of the baroreceptors by the increase in blood pressure). This would allow safe use of PHL with halothane anesthesia (96). Moreover, the rich adrenergic supply of the iris, being able to capture rapidly the exogenous catecholamines injected into the anterior chamber, makes this way of administration safer than topical or subconjunctival (in relation to systemic toxicity). The maximal safe dose for epinephrine here would be as much as 68 μg/kg (94).

The last possible approach is the mechanical. Although this goes beyond our pharmacologic subject, it may be the actual approach many surgeons follow to manage a nondilating or reconstricting pupil. Among the various methods used we may note:

1. Instrumental dilatation of the pupil. A relatively small but elastic pupil will allow dilatation with a small iris speculum or with the erysiphake and then further "passive mydriasis" as the lens is removed through it and attached to the cryoprobe or erysiphake, or by means of Smith's technique.

2. Iris sections and resections. Although this is an aggressive approach, it may be the only possibility in the case of a small, fixed, or fibrotic pupil. Attempted instrumental dilatation of such pupils might result in sphincter tears and pupil distortion. Methods include single or double radial iridotomies—either complete or just sphincterotomies—and sector iridectomy, or the sectorialization of a peripheral iridectomy by means of a radial iridotomy toward its vertex. These procedures allow an anatomic restitution, if desired, by simple iris sutures (10–0 nylon or Prolene) at the end of the operation. In vitreous surgery portions of the pupillary margin and sphincter are occasionally excised to obtain a permanently wider pupil (71).

3. Viscous mydriasis. The intracameral injection of a high-viscosity solution such as 2% sodium hyaluronate (Healon®) may result in a more complete mydriasis. A subtotally dilated pupil will enlarge as the iris is compressed backward and peripherally by the hyaluronate "drop" filling the anterior chamber. This will facilitate surgical maneuvers, protect intraocular tissues from trauma, and help in maintaining the iris in its dilated position; it has particular value in ECCE.

Miosis

The intraoperative need for a miotic iris includes procedures in which a deeper anterior chamber and lens protection is desired, especially in the reposition of the iris and anterior vitreous face after ICCE. Specific steps such as peripheral iridectomy require miosis after a procedure has been performed with a dilated pupil, as in ECCE. Furthermore, most anterior segment laser procedures (iridotomy, iridoplasty, trabeculoplasty) require a tense, miotic iris.

Preoperative Methods

When miosis is preferred during the whole operation (from its beginning), as in penetrating corneal grafts, goniotomy, and peripheral iridectomy (in the management and prophylaxis of angle-closure glaucoma), this is commonly obtained by preoperative topical parasympathomimetic drugs such as pilocarpine, when the patient is not already being treated with miotics.

Acetylcholine (ACH) (Miochol®) and methacholine (Mecholyl®) cannot be used externally, because of their high water solubility (which causes a very poor transcorneal absorption unless iontophoresis is used) and short life—they are destroyed (ACH particularly rapidly) by cholinesterase. When anticholinesterase miotics are used—particularly long-acting ones such as echothiophate, isoflurophate, or demecarium—special attention should be paid to the enhancement of local anesthetics toxicity (see Interactions Between Anesthetic and Autonomic Drugs, above), as well as to the danger of prolonged apnea resulting from the use of succinylcholine for endotracheal intubation (42,76).

Intraoperative Methods

Intraoperative miosis is useful in all situations in which there is danger of vitreous prolapse and vitreous loss. Immediately after, and even during, the cataract removal from the posterior chamber, open-sky instillation of 0.5% to 1% ACH promptly results in reduction of the pupil to 2-mm diameter. This may help in completing the separation of the lens from the anterior hyaloid and prevent anterior vitreous bulging, reducing the possibility of hyaloid rupture, vitreous loss, and vitreous incarceration in the corneoscleral incision. It will also prevent iris prolapse, facilitate the placement of sutures, and avoid the formation of anterior synechiae or iris incarcerations.

ACH-induced miosis, together with the filling of the anterior chamber with an air bubble, also has diagnostic value, since a previously inadverted vitreous strand will become apparent by the distortion of the bubble and the displacement of the pupil in its attempt to contract. The air bubble will also have a "synergistic" effect with ACH when a vitreous *champignon* is present, bulging into the anterior chamber and opposing mechanical resistance to miosis; in spite of ACH instillation the pupil may not reduce. Once the vitreous has been pushed backward by the air, miosis can be attained.

Although the main application of intraoperative miosis is at the end of ICCE, it may be a valuable help in repositioning the prolapsing iris after a peripheral iridectomy or an anterior chamber lavage (as for hyphema) has been performed. Other uses include various situations involving risk of vitreous presentation, as in capsulectomy, open-sky intraocular foreign body, and retina and vitreous surgery.

ACH was first synthesized by Baeyer in 1867 (8). Its pharmacologic actions were studied by Dale, Loewi, and Navratil. The two latter demonstrated in 1924 its role as a neurotransmitter (54). ACH is the chemical mediator of the nerve impulse for a variety of synapses, including the autonomic ganglia (nicotinic), muscarinic autonomic effectors (such as the iris sphincter), striate neuromuscular junctions, and several locations in the CNS and retina.

Amsler and Verry (3) first recognized in 1949 its miotic effect and the potential clinical value of its intracameral injection. José Ignacio Barraquer introduced its use in cataract surgery, which was first published in 1952 (9). Several reports afterward confirmed its value in ICCE and other intraocular procedures (10,23,46,84,87,91).

Although as little as 1:5,000 ACH elicits a certain degree of miosis when instilled close to the iris, optimal response is obtained with the 1% freshly prepared solution (10). Physostigmine (eserine) (1 μg/ml), as a reversible cholinesterase inhibitor, potentiates the action of ACH by 100 times (88), not only causing the response to minute quantities of ACH (10^{-6} mg/ml) but also, in contrast to the sensitization of cocaine to epinephrine, enhancing the strength of muscle contraction (2). Intraoperative ACH-induced miosis takes place in spite of previous mydriatic treatment. Concurrent factors such as general anesthesia and iris response to trauma play a favorable role here.

ACH is destroyed rapidly by cholinesterase, which is in accordance with the physiologic mechanism that allows the successive repolarization of neuromuscular end plates in order to become receptive to the next impulse (63). This is the cause of the short miotic action of ACH and also of its lack of toxicity. However, a systemic reaction after the intracameral injection of 20 mg ACH (which would be 40 ml of the 0.5% solution!) after cataract extraction (7) has been reported, consisting of an immediate drop in blood pressure to 75 mmHg systolic and bradycardia (48 beats/min), both lasting 20 min without further consequences.

Carbamylcholine or carbachol (Carcholin®) has been advocated since 1965 as an alternative to ACH (85). When injected into the anterior chamber, it is a very powerful, apparently nontoxic (69) miotic, 100 times more effective than ACH—this difference increases to 4,800 times in the isolated bovine iris strip model (106)—and much longer lasting, since it is not attacked by cholinesterase (it cannot be potentiated by anticholinesterases as eserine). In rabbits 0.01% carbachol produced greater miosis than 1% ACH (68) and was found as effective for prompt miosis after cataract surgery (12,29) but with a much longer effect, lasting up to 15 hr.

When a prolonged miosis is desired, other muscarinic drugs (e.g., pilocarpine) or anticholinesterases (e.g., eserine) may be used with ACH. However, strong miosis is associated with postoperative pain and may cause iridocyclitis, posterior synechiae, and pupillary block. Pilocarpine has also been advocated as an intraoperative miotic (32). However, it has been found to have a dose-related toxicity on rabbit corneal endothelium, producing ultrastructural changes, such as the margination of nuclear heterochromatin and cytoplasmic vacuolation. Although these toxic effects are less likely to occur when given externally, we have a quite different situation in the intracameral application, which allows the direct contact of a high concentration of the drug with the corneal endothelium (25).

ACKNOWLEDGMENTS

We thank Dr. Ignacio Zabal and Dr. Antoni Monsó for their advice regarding anesthesia influences on the pupil. Dr. Joaquín Rutllán helped us in the bibliographic search. We also thank Miss Montserrat Veses for typing the manuscript.

REFERENCES

1. Adriani, J., and Campbell, D. (1956): Fatalities following topical application of local anesthetics to mucous membranes. *J.A.M.A.,* 162:1527–1528.
2. Alphen, Van G. W. H. M., Robinette, S. L., and Macri, F. J. (1962): Drug effects on ciliary muscle and choroid preparations in vitro. *Arch. Ophthalmol.,* 68:81–93.
3. Amsler, M., and Verrey, F. (1949): Mydriase et myose directes et instantanées par les médiateurs chimiques. *Ann. Oculist. (Paris),* 182:936–937.
4. Angenent, W. (1953): Destruction of epinephrine by the dopa-oxidase system of ocular tissue. *Science,* 116:543–544.
5. Apt, L., and Henrick, A. (1980): Pupillary dilatation with single eyedrop mydriatic combinations. *Am. J. Ophthalmol.,* 89:553–559.
6. Awan, K. J. (1976): Systemic toxicity of cyclopentolate hydrochloride in adults following topical ocular instillation. *Ann. Ophthalmol.,* 8:803–806.
7. Babinski, M., Smith, R. B., and Wickerham, E. P. (1976): Hypotension and bradycardia following intraocular acetylcholine injection. *Arch. Ophthalmol.,* 94:675–676.
8. Baeyer, A. (1867): Ueber das Neurin. *Justus Liebigs Annln. Chem.,* 142:322–326.
9. Barraquer, J. I. (1952): Novedades y estado actual de la cirugía de la catarata y su terapéutica actual. *Aggior. di Ter. Oftal.,* 4:1–24.
10. Barraquer, J. I. (1964): Acetylcholine as a miotic agent for use in surgery. *Am. J. Ophthalmol.,* 57:406–408.
11. Barton, D. (1971): Side reactions of drugs in anesthesia. *Int. Ophthalmol. Clin.,* 11:185–200.
12. Beasley, H. (1972): Miotics in cataract surgery. *Arch. Ophthalmol.,* 88:49–51.
13. Beswick, J. A. (1962): Psychosis from cyclopentolate. *Am. J. Ophthalmol.,* 53:879.
14. Bhatia, B. B., and Burn, J. H. (1933): The action of ether on the sympathetic system. *J. Physiol. (Lond.),* 78:257–270.
15. Bill, A., Stjernschantz, J., Mandahl, A., Brodin, E., and Nilsson, G. (1979): Substance P: Release on trigeminal nerve stimulation, effects in the eye. *Acta Physiol. Scand.,* 106:371–373.
16. Binkhorst, R. D., Weinstein, G. W., Baretz, R. M., and Clahane, A. C. (1963): Psychotic reaction induced by cyclopentolate (Cyclogyl). Results of a pilot study and a double-blind study. *Am. J. Ophthalmol.,* 55:1243–1245.
17. Borromeo-McGrail, V., Bordiuk, J. M., and Shennan, A. T. (1973): Systemic hypertension following ocular administration of 10% phenylephrine in the neonate. *J. Pediatr.,* 51:1032–1033.
18. Brown, C., and Hanna, C. (1978): Use of dilute drug solutions for routine cycloplegia and mydriasis. *Am. J. Ophthalmol.,* 86:820–824.
19. Burch, P. G. (1969): Accommodation during general anesthesia. *Arch. Ophthalmol.,* 81:202–206.
20. Butler, J. M., and Hammond, B. (1977): Neurogenic responses of the eye to injury. Effect of sensory denervation on the response of the rabbit eye to bradykinin and prostaglandin E_1. *Trans. Ophthalmol. Soc. U.K.,* 97:668–674.
21. Butler, J. M., Powell, D., and Unger, W. G. (1980): Substance P levels in normal and sensorily denervated rabbit eyes. *Exp. Eye Res.,* 30:311–313.
22. Camras, C. B., and Bito, L. Z. (1980): The pathophysiological effects of nitrogen mustard on the rabbit eye. 2. The inhibition of the initial hypertensive phase by capsaicin and the apparent role of substance P. *Invest. Ophthalmol. Vis. Sci.,* 19:423–428.
23. Catford, G. V., and Millis, E. (1967): Clinical experience in the intraocular use of acetylcholine. *Br. J. Ophthalmol.,* 51:183–187.
24. Cole, D. F., and Unger, W. G. (1973): Prostaglandins as mediators for the responses of the eye to trauma. *Exp. Eye Res.,* 17:357–368.
25. Coles, W. H. (1975): Pilocarpine toxicity. Effects on the rabbit corneal endothelium. *Arch. Ophthalmol.,* 93:36–41.
26. De Jong, R. H. (1970): *Physiology and Pharmacology of Local Anesthesia,* Charles C Thomas, Springfield, IL.
27. De Ocampo, G., and Lim-Catipon, P. (1968): Phenylephrine pack for flat anterior chamber following cataract extraction. *Am. J. Ophthalmol.,* 66:881–883.
28. Doane, M. G., Jensen, A. D., and Dohlman, C. H. (1978): Penetration routes of topically applied eye medications. *Am. J. Ophthalmol.,* 85:383–386.

29. Douglas, G. R. (1973): A comparison of acetylcholine and carbachol following cataract extraction. *Can. J. Ophthalmol.,* 8:75–77.
30. Edelhauser, H. F., Hine, J. E., Pederson, H., Van Horn, D. L., and Schultz, R. O. (1979): The effect of phenylephrine on the cornea. *Arch. Ophthalmol.,* 97:937–947.
31. Edelhauser, H. F., Van Horn, D. L., Hyndiuk, R. A., and Schultz, R. O. (1975): Intraocular irrigating solutions: Their effect on the corneal endothelium. *Arch. Ophthalmol.,* 93:638–657.
32. El-Guindi, N. M. (1966): Pilocarpine irrigation of anterior chamber after cataract extraction. *Bull. Ophthalmol. Soc. Egypt,* 59(Suppl. 63):173–179.
33. Emery, J. M., Landis, D. J., and Benolken, R. M. (1974): Phacoemulsification. II. The phacoemulsifier: An evaluation of performance safety margins. In: *Current Concepts in Cataract Surgery: Selected Proceedings of the Third Biennial Cataract Surgical Congress,* edited by J. M. Emery and D. Paton, pp. 208–222. C. V. Mosby, St. Louis.
34. File, T. M. (1961): Studies on the use of antihistamines in cataract surgery. *Am. J. Ophthalmol.,* 51:1240–1243.
35. Foldes, F. F., ed. (1966): *Muscle Relaxants.* F. A. Davis, Philadelphia.
36. Franz, D. N., and Perry, R. S. (1974): Mechanisms for differential block among single myelinated and non-myelinated axons by procaine. *J. Physiol. (Lond.),* 236:193–210.
37. Fraunfelder, F. T., and Hanna, C. (1977): Trends in topical ocular medication. In: *Symposium of Ocular Therapy,* edited by I. H. Leopold and R. P. Burns, vol. 10, p. 85. John Wiley, Baltimore.
38. Fraunfelder, F. T., and Scafaldi, A. F. (1978): Possible adverse effects from topical ocular 10% phenylephrine. *Am. J. Ophthalmol.,* 85:447–453.
39. Freund, M., and Merin, S. (1970): Toxic effects of scopolamine eye drops. *Am. J. Ophthalmol.,* 70:637–639.
40. Gasser, H. S., and Erlanger, J. (1929): The role of fiber size in the establishment of a nerve block by pressure or cocaine. *Am. J. Physiol.,* 88:581–591.
41. German, E., and Siddiqui, N. (1970): Atropine toxicity from eyedrops. *N. Engl. J. Med.,* 282:689.
42. Gesztes, T. (1966): Prolonged apnea after suxamethonium injection associated with eye drops containing an anticholinesterase agent. *Br. J. Anesth.,* 38:408–409.
43. Gillespie, N. A. (1943): The signs of anesthesia. *Curr. Res. Anesth. Analg.,* 22:275–282.
44. Guedel, A. E. (1951): *Inhalation Anesthesia: A Fundamental Guide,* 2nd ed. Macmillan, New York.
45. Haddad, N. J., Moyer, N. J., and Riley, F. C. (1970): Mydriatic effect of phenylephrine hydrochloride. *Am. J. Ophthalmol.,* 70:729–733.
46. Harley, R. D., and Mishler, J. E. (1966): Acetylcholine in cataract surgery. *Br. J. Ophthalmol.,* 50:429–433.
47. Havener, W. H. (1978): *Ocular Pharmacology,* 4th ed., pp. 75–76, 242, 248. C. V. Mosby, St. Louis.
48. Heath, P., and Geiter, C. W. (1949): Use of phenylephrine hydrochloride (Neo-Synephrine Hydrochloride) in ophthalmology. *Arch. Ophthalmol.,* 41:172–174.
49. Hoefnagel, D. (1961): Toxic effects of atropine and homatropine eyedrops in children. *N. Engl. J. Med.,* 264:168.
50. Hull, D. S., Chemotti, M. T., Edelhauser, H. F., Van Horn, D. L., and Hyndiuk, R. A. (1975): Effect of epinephrine on corneal endothelium. *Am. J. Ophthalmol.,* 79:245–250.
51. Jessel, T. M., Iversen, L. L., and Cuello, A. C. (1978): Capsaicin-induced depletion of substance P from primary sensory neurones. *Brain Res.,* 152:183–188.
52. Johnson, E. S., Roberts, M. H. T., and Straughn, D. W. (1969): The responses of cortical neurones to monoamines under different anesthetic conditions. *J. Physiol. (Lond.),* 203:261–280.
53. Keys, A., and Violante, A. (1942): The cardiocirculatory effects in man of Neo-Synephrine. *J. Clin. Invest.,* 21:1–5.
54. Koelle, G. B. (1975): Neurohumoral transmission and autonomous nervous system. In: *The Pharmacologic Basis of Therapeutics,* 5th ed., edited by L. S. Goodman and A. Gilman, Ch. 21. Macmillan, New York.
55. Koelle, G. B. (1975): Neuromuscular blocking agents. In: *The Pharmacologic Basis of Therapeutics,* 5th ed., edited by L. S. Goodman and A. Gilman, Ch. 28. Macmillan, New York.

56. Kolker, A. E., and Becker, B. (1968): Epinephrine maculopathy. *Arch. Ophthalmol.,* 79:552–562.
57. Koller, K. (1884): Uber die Verwendung des Cocain zur Anästhesierung am Auge. *Wien. Med. Bl.* 7:1352–1357.
58. Korczyn, A. D., Laor, N., and Nemet, P. (1976): Sympathetic pupillary tone in old age. *Arch. Ophthalmol.,* 94:1905–1906.
59. Kratz, R. L., and Epstein, R. A. (1968): The interaction of anesthetic agents and adrenergic drugs to produce cardiac arrhythmias. *Anesthesiology,* 29:763–784.
60. Lang, R. M., and Hassard, D. T. R. (1981): Effects on the corneal endothelium of anterior chamber reconstituents instilled during intracapsular cataract extraction. *Can. J. Ophthalmol.,* 16:70–72.
61. Lansche, R. K. (1966): Systemic reactions to topical epinephrine and phenylephrine. *Am. J. Ophthalmol.,* 61:95–98.
62. Lees, B. J., and Cabal, L. A. (1981): Increased blood pressure following pupillary dilatation with 2.5% phenylephrine hydrochloride in preterm infants. *Pediatrics,* 68:231–234.
63. Leopold, I. H. (1966): Cholinesterases and the effects and side-effects of drugs affecting cholinergic systems. *Am. J. Ophthalmol.,* 62:771–777.
64. Lubeck, M. J. (1971): Effects of drugs on ocular muscles. *Int. Ophthalmol. Clin.,* 11:35–62.
65. Mandahl, A., and Bill, A. (1980): Effects of substance P, PGE$_2$, and capsaicin on the pupillary sphincter, modification by tetrodotoxin. *Acta Physiol. Scand.,* 109:26A.
66. Mark, H. H. (1963): Psychotogenic properties of cyclopentolate. *J.A.M.A.,* 430:214.
67. Maul, E., and Sears, M. L. (1976): The contralateral effect of antidromic stimulation of the trigeminal nerve on the rabbit eye. *Invest. Ophthalmol. Vis. Sci.,* 15:564–566.
68. McDonald, T. O., Beasley, C., Borgmann, A., and Roberts, D. (1969): Intraocular administration of carbamylcholine chloride. *Ann. Ophthalmol.,* 1:232–239.
69. McDonald, T. O., Roberts, M. D., and Borgmann, A. R. (1970): Intraocular safety of carbamylcholine chloride (carbachol) in rabbit eyes. *Ann. Ophthalmol.,* 2:878–883.
70. McReynolds, W. U., Havener, W. H., and Henderson, J. W. (1956): Hazards of the use of sympathomimetic drugs in ophthalmology. *Arch. Ophthalmol.,* 56:176–179.
71. Michels, R. G. (1979): Vitrectomy techniques in retinal reattachment surgery. *Ophthalmology,* 86:556–585.
72. Michels, R. G. (1981): *Vitreous Surgery,* pp. 140, 391. C. V. Mosby, St. Louis.
73. Millard, B. J., Priaulx, D. J., and Shatton, E. (1973): The stability of aqueous solutions of phenylephrine at elevated temperatures: Identification of the decomposition products. *J. Pharm. Pharmacol.,* 25(Suppl.):24–31.
74. Nathan, P. W., and Sears, T. A. (1961): Some factors concerned in differential nerve block by local anesthetics. *J. Physiol. (Lond.),* 157:565–580.
75. *National Drug Registry of Drug-Induced Ocular Side Effects.* (1978): Case reports. University of Arkansas for Medical Sciences, Little Rock.
76. Pantuck, E. J. (1966): Echothiophate iodide eye drops and prolonged response to suxamethonium. *Br. J. Anesth.,* 38:406–407.
77. Patil, P. N. (1974): Iris pigmentation and atropine mydriasis. *Pharmacologist,* 16:311–312.
78. Pfister, R. R., and Burstein, N. (1976): Effects of ophthalmic drugs, vehicles and preservatives on corneal epithelial surface: Scanning electron microscope study. *Invest. Ophthalmol. Vis. Sci.,* 15:246–259.
79. Philpot, F. J. (1940): The inhibition of adrenalin oxidation by local anesthetics. *J. Physiol. (Lond.),* 97:301–314.
80. Pontinen, P. J., Mietinen, P., and Reinikainen, M. (1966): Neuroleptoanalgesia in cataract surgery. *Acta Ophthalmol. (Copenh.),* 80(Suppl.):1–36.
81. Praeger, D. L., and Miller, S. N. (1964): Toxic effects of cyclopentolate. Report of a case. *Am. J. Ophthalmol.,* 58:1060–1061.
82. Price, H. L. (1957): Circulating adrenaline and noradrenaline during diethyl ether anesthesia in man. *Clin. Sci.,* 16:377–387.
83. Price, H. L. (1975): General anesthetics. In: *The Pharmacological Basis of Therapeutics,* 5th ed., edited by L. S. Goodman and A. Gilman, chs. 6, 7. Macmillan, New York.
84. Ray, R. R. (1968): The use of acetylcholine in peripheral iridectomy. *An. Inst. Barraquer,* 8:117–122.
85. Reed, H. (1965): Use of carbamylcholine chloride. *Am. J. Ophthalmol.,* 59:955–956.

86. Ritchie, J. M. (1971): The mechanism of action of local anesthetics. In: *Local Anesthetics,* vol. 1, *International Encyclopedia of Pharmacology and Therapeutics,* sect. 8, edited by P. Lechat, pp. 136–166. Pergamon Press, Oxford.

87. Rizzuti, A. B. (1967): Acetylcholine in surgery of the lens, iris and cornea. *Am. J. Ophthalmol.,* 63:484–487.

88. Sachs, E., and Heath, P. (1940): The pharmacological behavior of the intraocular muscles. *Am. J. Ophthalmol.,* 23:1376–1380.

89. Salminen, L., Aaltonen, H., and Jäntti, V. (1980): Mydriatic effect of low-dose phenylephrine. *Ophthalmic Res.,* 12:235–239.

90. Samantary, S., and Thomas, A. (1975): Systemic effects of topical phenylephrine. *Indian J. Ophthalmol.,* 23:16–17.

91. Schimek, R. A. (1961): The use of intraocular acetylcholine in anterior segment surgery. *An. Inst. Barraquer,* 2:687–688.

92. Schulz, R. O., Edelhauser, H. F., Van Horn, D. L., and Hyndiuk, R. A. (1976): Hazards of intraocular irrigating solutions and epinephrine in cataract surgery. In: *Current Concepts in Cataract Surgery,* edited by J. M. Emery, pp. 269–276. C. V. Mosby, St. Louis.

93. Simcoe, C. W. (1962): Cyclopentolate (Cyclogyl) toxicity. Report of a case. *Arch. Ophthalmol.,* 67:406–408.

94. Smith, R. B., Douglas, H. N., Petruscak, J., and Breslin, P. (1972): Safety of intraocular Adrenaline with halothane anesthesia. *Br. J. Anesth.,* 44:1314–1317.

95. Smith, R. B., Read, S., and Oczypok, P. M. (1976): Mydriatic effect of phenylephrine. *Ear Nose Throat J.,* 55:36–48.

96. Snow, J. C. (1982): *Anesthesia in Otolaryngology and Ophthalmology,* 2nd ed., pp. 220–225. Appleton-Century-Crofts, New York.

97. Solosko, D., and Smith, R. B. (1972): Hypertension following 10 percent phenylephrine ophthalmic. *Anesthesiology,* 36:187–189.

98. Soloway, M. R., Stjernschantz, J., and Sears, M. (1981): The miotic effect of substance P on the isolated rabbit iris. *Invest. Ophthalmol. Vis. Sci.,* 20:47–52.

99. Stjernschantz, J. (1981): Neuropeptides in the eye. In: *New Directions in Ophthalmic Research,* edited by M. L. Sears, pp. 327–358. Yale University Press, New Haven and London.

100. Stjernschantz, J., Sears, M., and Stjernschantz, L. (1981): Intraocular effects of substance P in the rabbit. *Invest. Ophthalmol. Vis. Sci.,* 20:53–60.

101. Vaughan, R. W. (1973): Ventricular arrhythmias after topical vasoconstrictors. *Anesth. Analg.,* 52:161–163.

102. Vitcha, J. F. (1971): A history of Forane. *Anesthesiology,* 35:4–7.

103. Wahl, J. W. (1969): Systemic reaction to tropicamide. *Arch. Ophthalmol.,* 82:320–321.

104. Walsh, F. B., and Hoyt, W. F. (1969): *Clinical Neuro-Ophthalmology,* 3rd ed., vol. 3, p. 2661. Williams & Wilkins, Baltimore.

105. Wilensky, J. T., and Woodward, H. J. (1973): Acute systemic hypertension after conjunctival instillation of phenylephrine hydrochloride. *Am. J. Ophthalmol.,* 76:156–157.

106. Yamauchi, D. N., De Santis, L., and Patil, P. N. (1973): Relative potency of cholinomimetic drugs on the bovine iris sphincter strips. *Invest. Ophthalmol. Vis. Sci.,* 12:80–82.

Surgical Pharmacology of the Eye,
edited by M. Sears and A. Tarkkanen.
Raven Press, New York © 1985.

Hemostasis: Methods

Rafael I. Barraquer and Joaquín Barraquer

Instituto Barraquer, Barcelona 21, Spain

SUMMARY: Intraocular surgery is commonly a fairly hemostatic surgery: Several intraocular tissues are normally avascular (cornea, lens, vitreous). There are few "great" vessels. The uvea is, however, a highly vascularized tissue. Although it shows little bleeding tendency in some instances (iridectomy), it occasionally leads to disaster (expulsive hemorrhage).

Physiological hemostasis should always be assessed preoperatively (by clinical history, laboratory tests) and corrected if necessary.

Vitamin K_1 (10 mg every 12 hr, intravenous, three times, repeating tests after 48 hr) is only indicated when there is a true hypovitaminosis K situation. No hemostatic improvement can be expected from giving vitamin K to a patient with adequate ingestion and absorption. Only a little improvement can be found when a faulty liver function is the cause, since vitamin K cannot be expected to improve the factor production of non-functioning hepatocytes, and only compensate the decreased vitamin K absorption due to the cholestatic component of the liver disfunction.

Although there is no definite clinical evidence of their usefulness in preventing surgical bleeding, agents that improve platelet function, as calcium dobesilate (Doxium®) and antifibrinolytics as EACA or tranexamic acid might theoretically improve hemostasis. There is some clinical evidence of the usefulness of the last in the prevention of traumatic secondary hyphema, which theoretically could be applied to the prevention of precocious postoperative hyphema too.

Intraoperative hemostatic methods do not act directly on physiological mechanisms for hemostasis, but consist of a series of measures directed to prevent or stop bleeding by attention to circulatory parameters: reducing arterial pressure, venous pressure and ocular congestion). Local factors: avoidance of sudden ocular decompression, ensuring preoperative ocular hypotony). Ocular vessels: use of local vasoconstrictors; mechanical compression with instruments, air bubble, saline or viscous solutions; and, if necessary, coagulation with heat, electrodiathermy, or laser).

SURGICAL HEMOSTASIS VERSUS PHYSIOLOGICAL HEMOSTASIS

Analgesia and anesthesia, antisepsis and asepsis, are classically considered the fundamentals of modern surgery. The role of hemostasis, although it actually is a better landmark between "ancient" and "medical" surgery, has been often overlooked, perhaps because its principles have developed since the time of Ambroise Paré more than 400 years ago and have become an almost unnoticed aspect of our daily practice.

Advances in the knowledge of the physiologic mechanisms of hemostasis and the development of pharmacologic agents and therapeutic methods capable of interfering with them permit us today to obtain purposely a status of decreased coagulation (anticoagulant drugs, inhibitors of the platelet aggregation), destroy formed blood clots (fibrinolytic agents), or correct certain conditions in which the hemostasis mechanisms are insufficient. However, we still have no way of improving the efficiency of physiologic hemostasis *when it is not pathologically altered.* Since hemostasis may be considered the result of a complex equilibrium between opposing mechanisms, it is difficult to think of improving that equilibrium when already present, particularly since most therapeutic actions will alter it in either direction.

Physiologic hemostasis may be defined as the ensemble of mechanisms intended to prevent or limit the loss of blood elements after a disruption of the vascular walls and to restore normal circulation. We may consider four phases:

1. Reflex vasoconstriction (active and transient contraction of the smooth muscle cells of the vessel wall).
2. Adhesion and aggregation of platelets ("primary" hemostasis, or plug formation).
3. Formation and apposition of fibrin ("secondary" hemostasis, or production of the fibrin clot by the coagulation system).
4. Fibrinolysis (simultaneously activated to prevent excessive clotting and assure the reestablishment of normal circulation).

Although all these mechanisms may take place everywhere in the circulatory apparatus and in the tissues where the blood has exited the vessels, their main physiologic function (particularly the platelet plug formation) is limited to the microcirculation (arteriole/capillary bed/venule), as they have little effect in preventing bleeding from a ruptured large vessel.

Surgical hemostasis might be called "therapeutic," as opposed to "prophylactic" physiologic hemostasis. It mainly consists of a series of measures dealing with vascular and circulatory—not properly "hemostatic"—factors: reduction of the blood effluence (controlled hypotension, local vasoconstriction), minimization of tissular congestion (avoidance of rises in venous pressure), and of course the multiple and commonly *physical* methods of obturating the bleeding vessels (mechanical compression, cold irrigation, thermal, electrodiathermal, and photothermal cauterization).

These measures can be applied independently of the hemostatic status of the patient and are actually used in case physiologic hemostasis cannot be expected to stop the bleeding by itself (e.g., a large vessel). However, defective coagulation or platelet function will obviously be a risk factor for intraoperative or postoperative bleeding and thus require maximal use of surgical hemostatic methods in spite of the preoperative diagnosis and medical hemostatic therapy.

PREOPERATIVE EVALUATION OF HEMOSTATIC COMPETENCE

Although intraoperative hemostatic methods do not act directly on the physiologic mechanisms of hemostasis, the preoperative assessment of hemostatic competence serves the role of screening high-risk patients. It should be done 48 hr (at least) prior to surgery, to allow additional laboratory tests, reevaluation, and the possible correction of the important problems in time (86). This is particularly useful in those cases having a minor (and thus previously undetected) hemostasis disorder, not causing hemorrhagic manifestations but possibly leading to intraoperative or postoperative bleeding complications.

A scrupulous clinical history and complete physical examination are essential; they are considered more important than laboratory tests (48). The questioning should be oriented to (a) antecedent hemorrhages (prolonged bleeding after banal trauma such as shaving or domestic cuts, after a dental extraction, unexplained hematuria, epistaxis or bruises, delayed rebleeding at the site of venous punctures, etc.); (b) general diseases favoring surgical bleeding (diabetes, hypertension, obesity, and "bull neck"); and (c) the use of drugs interfering with hemostasis—particularly aspirin (20) and other nonsteroidal anti-inflammatory drugs such as indomethacin, whose inhibitory effect on platelet aggregation will be commonly ignored by the patient (who is more likely to be aware of being on heparin or oral anticoagulant treatment). Since several hemostasis disorders are genetically inherited, it is also valuable to inquire about familial antecedents.

However, history and physical exam are frequently negative, and a laboratory study is necessary. Among the multiple hemostatic tests we must select a few for routine screening. The platelet count is the best indicator for "primary" hemostasis (plug formation). It may be considered pathologic under 150,000/μl (thrombocytopenia) and over 500,000/μl (thrombocytosis). The bleeding time (Duke's method) (31) has the advantage of detecting not only defects in the number of platelets but in their function (thrombocytopathy), as occurs in several infrequent primary diseases (such as von Willebrand's and Glanzmann's thromboasthenia) and also secondary to more frequent conditions (such as cirrhosis, uremia, and platelet antiaggregant therapy) (3,44). Bleeding time is, however, a rather unprecise method.

"Secondary" hemostasis, or the formation of the fibrin clot by the cascade reactions of the coagulation system, is best explored by the activated partial thromboplastine time (PTT), normally between 22 and 46 sec (it varies according to the technique used, but a difference of 8 to 10 sec as related to a control plasma is considered pathologic). It does not detect variations in platelet factor III and may be normal, with a fibrinogen value as low as <100 mg/100 ml (normal 200 to 400 mg/100 ml), which could lead to intraoperative bleeding. To have additional information on the "extrinsic" coagulation pathway and factor VII (not explored by PTT), prothrombin time (PT, Quick's time) is done. Although its systematic use is contested, PT is mandatory when PTT is abnormal. PT is a better indicator for liver-synthesized coagulation factors (V, VII, IX, X, prothrombin).

When clinical history, physical exam, platelet count, and PT are normal but PTT is altered, specific evaluation of "intrinsic" pathway factors are indicated. A very long PTT (more than double normal value) suggests a lack in activating factors (XI, XII, Fletcher, or Fitzgerald), among which XI is the most significant for surgery. This may be confirmed if PTT decreases when repeated after prolonged incubation with contact factor. A milder increase in PTT may indicate a deficient VIII or IX factor (A and B hemophilia, respectively). If these are found normal, the interaction of an abnormal protein—as in myeloma, macroglobulinemia, or systemic lupus—with the coagulation factors should be considered (86).

When both PTT and PT are altered (and the rest is normal), a hypovitaminosis K situation (oral anticoagulants, inadequate ingestion, intestinal or pancreas disease causing malabsorption, alteration of the intestinal flora by broad-spectrum antibiotics, cholestasis caused by liver, pancreas or bile duct disorder), defective liver function, presence of inhibitors of coagulation factors, or disseminated intravascular coagulation (DIC), and hyperfibrinolysis are suggested (9,44).

Those patients having history of probable abnormal hemorrhage but normal platelet count and PTT should be carefully explored for vasculopathic bleeding diseases (capillary telangiectasia or Rendu-Osler-Weber disease, Ehlers-Danlos syndrome, Marfan's syndrome, Schönlein-Henoch's purpura and other vasculitis, disglobulinemic purpura), thrombocytopathic diseases (prolonged bleeding time), lack of factor XIII (fibrin stabilizer) ("clot solubility in urea" test positive), or fibrinogen disfunction.

PREOPERATIVE MANAGEMENT OF DEFECTIVE HEMOSTASIS

When a high-risk patient is detected, the indication of preoperative corrective therapy will depend on the degree of severity of the defect and the kind of surgery to be performed. The therapeutic methods vary according to the specific hemostatic deficiency. None of the multiple drugs advocated to reduce "vascular fragility" have clearly proved useful.

Defective Primary Hemostasis

Although any platelet count under 150,000/μl may be considered pathologic, over 30,000/μl is considered relatively safe for minor surgery, which in ophthalmology may extend to keratoplasty. Both thrombocytopenia and thrombocytopathy may be managed with the three following approaches. A specific or etiologic treatment will require further examinations, such as a bone marrow aspiration or biopsy and antiplatelet antibody determination.

Substitutive Therapy: Platelet Transfusion

Although this is undoubtedly an effective method, it has some inconveniences, such as availability, technical complexity, and the risk of hepatitis transmission; we still have no way of detecting and avoiding the non-A, non-B virus (28). Other transfusion-transmitted infections include cytomegalovirus and mononucleosis (42). It is indicated in patients with symptomatic hemorrhage due to platelet defect or dysfunction, except in the case of an immune thrombocytopenia.

The survival time after the transfusion may be expected to be about 4 days, if the patient has never received platelets previously, only washed erythrocytes. It is therefore adequate to give platelets 24 hr prior to surgery and to repeat the bleeding time test just before the operation. Better maintenance is obtained afterward with frequent small transfusions rather than larger and less frequent doses.

The usual goal of platelet transfusion is to obtain a preoperative count of $100,000/\mu l$. A 7×10^{10} platelet unit is necessary for each $10,000/\mu l$ increment desired in a 70-kg sensitized patient with anti-HLA antibodies, using platelets from a single HLA-compatible donor and supposing 65% of the given platelets are actually recovered (80,91).

Enhancers of the Platelet Function

Benzosulfonated agents such as calcium dobesilate (Doxium®) have been found to improve platelet aggregation and may be useful, particularly in thrombocytopathic conditions but also in thrombocytopenia.

Antifibrinolytic Agents

Epsilon-aminocaproic acid (EACA) and tranexamic acid are inhibitors of fibrinolysis and thus indirectly enhance the efficiency of thromboplastic mechanisms. These are the only drugs that can be useful in any kind of defective hemostasis, primary or secondary.

Specific (Etiologic) Therapy

Certain cases may be treated with a specific approach. A bone marrow aspiration or biopsy will be helpful to differentiate hypoplastic thrombocytopenia due to reduced formation of platelets (lack of megacariocytes or myelofibrosis) from those cases with excessive destruction but normal production of platelets, as in immune thrombocytopenia, thrombotic thrombocytopenia (Moschcowitz's purpura), and DIC (73).

Determination of a platelet-bound IgG rise will indicate an immune thrombocytopenia. This can be induced by transfusion or drugs. In this case, suppression of the drug and waiting 1 to 3 weeks is commonly sufficient. When the cause is idiopathic or autoimmune (Werlhof's disease), a remission may be expected in 80% of the acute-type patients after 1 to 6 months. If surgery is urgent, it can be treated with prednisone (1.5 mg/kg/day). If this fails, splenectomy is indicated (39). Even 30% of the splenectomized patients relapse. Repeated steroid treatment or immunosuppressors such as vincristine (1.2 mg/m^2 body surface/week) or cyclophosphamide (2.5 mg/kg/day) over 1 to 2 months can be successful (13). Although vincristine may induce some increase in the platelet number in hypoplastic thrombocytopenia (1), such patients commonly need a platelet transfusion. Since this condition may be due to a large number of possible ambient toxins and drugs, it is difficult to identify the actual inducer; all candidate drugs used during the past 12 months should be investigated (73).

Other situations may paradoxically require anticoagulant (heparin) or platelet antiaggregate therapy (aspirin, dipyridamole). The first is true for DIC, although the cause of this condition should be investigated and treated, and substitutive therapy will also be necessary. The second may be useful in thrombotic thrombocytopenia, together with steroids, plasmapheresis, and splenectomy (30).

Defective Secondary Hemostasis

The defects in coagulation factors mainly produce high risk of hemorrhage postoperatively. Their management includes, other than substitutive therapy, vitamin K and also the above-mentioned antifibrinolytic agents.

Substitutive Therapy

Inherited defects in coagulation factors are commonly isolated (factor VIII in A hemophilia, factor IX in B hemophilia). When indicated, its correction can only be done with transfusions. We have already commented on the risks of this treatment, which is higher when concentrates coming from multiple donors are used, compared to fresh or frozen-fresh plasma or cryoprecipitates. The detection of the specific defect and correction methods are widely described in the literature (14,33,65,92).

Although patients with von Willebrand's disease show a defective platelet adhesivity that may cause postoperative hemorrhage, it is actually a defect in a factor associated with factor VIII and will be corrected with plasma cryoprecipitates (0.6 bag/kg every 8 hr for 4 days preoperatively and every 24 hr for 6 days postoperatively) (16).

Vitamin K

Multifactorial defects commonly relate to liver-synthesized factors (I, II, V, VII, IX, X) associated with prolonged PT. Other possible situations include DIC and the collapse syndrome following massive bleeding and transfusion (47). Vitamin K_1 therapy—10 mg/12 hr, i.v., three times, repeating tests after 48 hr—is indicated only when there is a true hypovitaminosis K. No hemostatic improvement can be expected from giving vitamin K_1 to a patient with an already adequate ingestion and absorption. When faulty liver function is the cause, vitamin K_1 may not be expected to improve the factor production of nonfunctioning hepatocytes. A certain improvement can, however, be found with vitamin K_1; the decreased absorption of vitamin K due to the cholestatic component of the liver dysfunction could account for this improvement. Substitutive therapy may be required in any case, since lack of platelets and other factors, such as fibrinogen, are frequent findings (86).

Management of the Patient on Anticoagulant Therapy

The preoperative suppression of anticoagulants depends on whether the therapy must be resumed after surgery. The coagulation tests must be repeated prior to the operation to assess its normalization. The short half-life of sodium heparin usually makes its suppression 4 to 6 hr preoperatively sufficient. When urgent, the antidote protamine sulfate (1 mg, i.v., for each $50 \times T$ heparin units, "T" being the number of hours elapsed since the last dose), can be used (86). The waiting time after subcutaneous calcium heparin is longer and less predictable, requiring repeated tests.

If heparin has to be resumed after surgery, intraoperative hemostasis must be particularly careful. A half-dose should be given during the first 4 postoperative days.

Patients using oral anticoagulants (antivitamin K) may be given intravenous vitamin K_1 (10 mg/12 hr). If this does not attain a PT normalization or the surgeon cannot wait, plasma (20 ml/kg) can be administered. When the treatment must be resumed postoperatively, it is better not to use vitamin K_1. We may simply suppress antivitamins several days before surgery, waiting for PTT and PT to be normalized, or preoperatively shift to heparin therapy and suppress it as noted above. Antivitamins may be resumed at the usual doses 24 hr after the operation. When urgent, small (0.5-mg), repeated doses of vitamin K_1, or complete vitamin K_1 doses together with calcium heparin, may be used (56).

Inhibitors of platelet aggregation, such as aspirin, dipyridamole, or indomethacin have to be suppressed several days before surgery, if the bleeding time is dangerously prolonged, since these drugs act through the whole lifetime of platelets. In case of urgency, a platelet transfusion might be required.

Fibrinolysins, such as streptokinase, urokinase, or human activated plasminogen (fibrinolysin) have a few hours half-life, and their activity may be counteracted by EACA, but a fibrinogen restitution may be needed (47).

SURGICAL HEMOSTASIS IN THE EYE: THE LOCAL FACTORS

The particular anatomic and physiologic features of the eye represent several advantages and disadvantages regarding surgical hemostasis. Fortunately, the normal tissues most commonly manipulated during intraocular surgery have little tendency to important bleeding, since some of them are avascular (cornea, lens, vitreous), or sparsely vascularized (sclera). Even a more vascularized part (such as the iris), provided it is not pathologically altered, shows surprisingly little tendency to bleed when it is cut and resected. Moreover, ocular surgery (as microsurgery) benefits from the fact that it does not deal with large-caliber vessels.

On the other hand, the richly vascular uveal tissue—although it is most commonly entered through its less vascularized zone, the pars plana—may be the source of important bleeding, as in the most feared hemorrhagic complication of intraocular surgery, expulsive hemorrhage. The pathogenesis of this disastrous accident is not fully understood, but it appears clearly unrelated to a direct surgical trauma to the choroid.

The chambers of the eye are actually transcellular (avascular) spaces whose fluid-exchange dynamics—particularly that of the aqueous humor as indicated by its most apparent parameter, intraocular pressure (IOP)—are essential in the maintenance of the organ's homeostasis, but they obviously differ from the intravascular space or the interstitial spaces of other tissues. This must be carefully considered, since the coagulation and fibrinolytic mechanisms (in the case of an intraocular hemorrhage) will depend on the specific thromboplastic and fibrinolytic activities of the intraocular tissues involved, in addition to the hemostasis factors that will enter the globe within the hemorrhage itself. Moreover, the presence of blood inside the eye will interfere with the aqueous humor dynamics, which may lead to increased IOP, as in the glaucoma secondary to large hyphema and ghost cell glaucoma (12,61).

According to Pandolfi (57,58), the thromboplastic and fibrinolytic activities of the normal cornea are weak. However, the reaction of corneal epithelium and endothelium to trauma includes the finding of plasminogen activators, which would be intended to oppose the formation of fibrin deposits on the corneal surfaces in these situations. The thromboplastic and fibrinolytic activities of the lens are also very low. On the contrary, uveal tissues have an important fibrinolytic activity, which probably would be responsible for the lower activity found in the ocular fluids and the resorption of blood clots and fibrin deposits in the anterior chamber (in contact with the iris). On the other hand, this would also make hemostasis difficult in the case of a choroidal hemorrhage. The retina is also strongly fibrinolytic, but this is balanced by its thromboplastic activity, one of the strongest in the organism, together with the brain.

The pathologic changes in the chronically diseased eye should also be considered. Myopia, diabetes, glaucoma, hypertension, and arteriosclerosis, among other conditions, are associated with increased vascular fragility and intraoperative bleeding. The last three particularly are commonly postulated as etiologic factors in expulsive hemorrhage.

Neovascularization consists of fragile vessels whose walls are composed of only endothelial cells, having a great tendency to bleed. This might represent a serious source of complications in both anterior segment (corneal vascularization, rubeosis iridis) and posterior segment (retinal and vitreous neovascularization) surgery. Furthermore, neovessels will not respond to vasoconstrictors and thus will require physical management in the case of bleeding. Regarding this, several anatomic features of the eye may be noted:

1. It is a closed cavitary structure. This allows the manipulation of IOP as a hemostatic tool. A surgically controlled IOP rise will have a compressive effect on all intraocular vessels.
2. It has a series of transparent media. This permits the use of light as a cautery (argon and carbonic laser endophotocoagulator and photocautery).
3. As a neural structure, it can be damaged by the high-frequency currents of electrodiathermy, particularly the optic nerve, although the risk is minimized by the use of the bipolar diathermy.

INTRAOPERATIVE HEMOSTASIS: METHODS

Once the physiologic hemostatic status of the patient has been assessed, and corrected if defective, we face surgery knowing that our intervention will nevertheless produce some bleeding. It is clear that several risk factors, such as chronic conditions increasing the vascular fragility (myopia, arteriosclerosis, glaucoma) or the presence of neovascularization, cannot be corrected preoperatively. A hemostasis defect might be only partially corrected but surgery still indicated by urgency or other reasons. These situations oblige the maximal use of intraoperative hemostasis.

Intraoperative methods do not act on physiologic hemostasis (platelet aggregation, fibrin deposition) but consist of a series of measures directed to physically prevent or stop bleeding. We may consider the following factors:

1. Physical prevention of bleeding by (a) reduction of blood arterial pressure, which may be systemic (controlled hypotension by anesthesia and hypotensors) or local (vasoconstrictors); (b) avoidance of venous congestion by postural control of cephalic venous pressure (anti-Trendelenburg position) or adequate ventilation, avoiding positive intrathoracic pressure; (c) avoidance of sudden ocular decompression by preoperative hypotony (urea, mannitol, massage) and progressive decompression of high-risk eyes (paracentesis); and (d) management of vascularized tissue by minimization of surgical trauma, blunt dissection and scissors instead of knife cut and tearing, and preventive coagulation.

2. Physical arrest of bleeding by (a) mechanical compression, which may be instrumental (forceps, sponge, marten-hair brush) or hydrostatic, viscous, and tensioactive (infusion-controlled intraocular hyperpressure, air bubble, sodium hyaluronate); (b) local vasoconstriction through cold irrigation or sympathomimetics (epinephrine, phenylephrine, naphazoline) and (c) coagulation of the bleeding vessels by thermal cautery (heated glass rod, electric resistor or galvanocautery), electric high-frequency AC diathermy (unipolar, bimanual, coaxial, and forceps bipolar), or photothermal coagulation (xenon and laser endophotocoagulation and photocautery).

Most of these methods are obviously not pharmacologic. Anesthetics and vasoconstrictors are almost the sole drugs used in surgical hemostasis. Vasoconstrictors are actually seldom used in intraocular surgery, apart from retrobulbar anesthesia.

Anesthesia and Hemostasis

General Anesthesia

A certain degree of blood hypotension, leading to less tendency to bleed, is a common feature in general anesthesia. Most halogenated inhaled anesthetics, such as halothane (Fluothane®), enflurane (Ethrane®), and to a lesser extent methoxyflurane (Penthrane®), depress cardiac output and produce vasodilatation (64). On the other hand, they sensitize the myocardium to catecholamines, leading to severe ventricular arrhythmia, which limits the association with local vasoconstrictors (see Interactions Between Anesthetic and Autonomic Drugs, previous chapter).

Barbiturates have also a peripheral vasodilatation activity, but having ultrashort effect [e.g., thiopental (Pentothal®)], their use as inductors of anesthesia produces little modification of blood pressure. Other general anesthetics, such as gamma-hydroxybutyric acid (GABA) and ketamine (Ketalar®) are vasoconstrictors; they increase blood pressure and may cause intraoperative bleeding. Nitrous oxide (N_2O) and cyclopropane combine a sympathetic vascular effect with cardiac depression, having no important net action on blood pressure (64).

Correct ventilation favors hypotension and tends to reduce bleeding. The halogenated general anesthetics, particularly methoxyflurane, induce respiratory depression and should be used with pure O_2 as vehicle. Assisted respiration assures good ventilation, but positive intrathoracic pressure elevates central venous pressure and leads to cephalic congestion and increased risk of hemorrhage. It also increases the risk of anesthetic overdosage. Spontaneous respiration is preferred, although it may lead to hypercarbia and hypoxia, which induces sympathetic stimulation, blood pressure rise, and increased bleeding. However, many ophthalmologists and anesthesiologists prefer sufficient spontaneous ventilation.

An incorrect intubation or one partially obstructed by secretions will produce an increment in the respiratory effort, causing both arterial and central venous pressures rise. Correct suppression of the tracheal irritative reflexes is essential, since they may cause straining, bucking, coughing, or vomiting. This is particularly critical at the time of extubation and during the recovery from anesthesia. Since marked rises in venous pressure and IOP may result, leading to severe complications in the operated eye (including hemorrhage), this should be avoided by maintaining a deep level of anesthesia until the extubation, and the use of antiemetic drugs such as promethazine (Phenergan®).

A greater reduction of intraoperative bleeding is obtained with controlled hypotension. Halogenated anesthetics alone are hypotensors, but an effort to decrease blood pressure could lead to overdosage. Potent hypotensive agents with short effect combined with anesthetics are preferable. This includes ganglionic (nicotinic) blockers, such as hexamethonium (C6), or trimethaphan (Arfonad®) 2 to 4 mg/min in 5% dextrose intravenous infusion, and direct-acting strong vasodilators such as sodium nitroprusside (Nipride®) 0.5 to 8 μg/kg/min or nitroglycerine infusion, starting at 1 μg/kg/min. Details on the technique are widely described in the literature (41,69,75).

An 80 mmHg systolic pressure is well tolerated by young, healthy patients, provided adequate ventilation, blood volume and tissular perfusion are guaranteed. However, severe complications—including heart failure and coronary, cerebral, or central retinal artery thrombosis, hepatic or renal failure with oliguria or anuria, reactional bleeding, etc.—may occur in the elderly or in patients with antecedent heart failure, hypertension, arteriosclerosis, hepatic or renal failure, cerebrovascular disease, or marked anemia. Some of these dangers may be reduced with the use of induced hypothermia—32°C to 30°C—during anesthesia (75).

Local Anesthesia

Although local anesthetics do not have a specific autonomic effect—they block all nervous fibers depending on their caliber and type—they usually lead to vasodilatation and increased local bleeding, particularly lidocaine (Xylocaine®) (35). Cocaine is the only local anesthetic having a clear sympathomimetic (vasoconstrictor) activity, due to its ability to block the catecholamine reuptake by the presynaptic adrenergic terminal (62). As mentioned previously, its use is very limited today due to its addicting potential (see Effect of Anesthetic Agents on the Iris, previous chapter). Mepivacaine (Carbocaine®) is also said to potentiate the action of norepinephrine on nerve fibers and produce mild peripheral vasoconstriction (36).

On the other hand, all local anesthetics except cocaine may be safely associated with epinephrine diluted from 1:50,000 to 1:400,000, resulting in vasoconstriction and a bloodless operating field. This is particularly useful in extraocular surgery—dacryocystorhinostomy, lid, and orbit surgery. Epinephrine reduces the absorption speed of local anesthetics and thus prolongs their action and reduces their potential toxicity. However, the association of lidocaine and epinephrine may lead to a spasm of the ophthalmic artery (40). Side effects of the injection of epinephrine include transient nervousness, tremor, tachycardia and palpitations, pallor, and apprehension that may cause undesired reactions—such as vomiting during surgery—particularly if the patient has not been previously warned. It is recommended that the surgeon wait for these transient effects to subside before starting the operation. They should not be confused with the initial symptoms of local anesthetic intoxication, which, unlike epinephrine, is associated with hypotension and causes true disorientation, twitching, and convulsions (32).

The use of retrobulbar epinephrine should be avoided in patients with myocardial or coronary disease or in the presence of α-adrenergic modifying drugs, including reserpine, guanethidine, L-DOPA, cocaine, and both types of antidepressants—tricyclics and monoamine oxidase inhibitors. The latter in particular may induce hypertensive crises and should be discontinued several weeks before elective surgery. Interactions with epinephrine may be managed with intravenous β-blocking agents, such as tolazoline chlorhydrate (Priscoline®) or phentolamine mesylate (Regitine Mesylate®) (50).

Ophthalmologists who prefer local anesthesia argue its simplicity, lesser incidence of systemic complications, safer associations with vasopressors, and minimization of the likelihood of postoperative nausea and vomiting, thus lessening the likelihood of intraocular bleeding. However, mastery of ophthalmic general anesthesia may overcome most problems (e.g., with the use of antiemetics), permit more complex techniques, and enhance local safety—a more hypotonic eye, prevention of sudden movement of the patient, etc. Retrobulbar anesthesia has specific hemorrhagic risks, such as intraocular bleeding after scleral transfixion (32) and retrobulbar hemorrhage. When this occurs, the operation has to be stopped or postponed, the patient observed closely, and a drainage performed if necessary. This complication produces orbital hypertension, which may lead to oculocardiac reflex and optic nerve ischemia.

Intraoperative Hemostatic Pharmacologic Agents

Vasoconstrictors

Catecholamines may be applied directly into the eye during surgery to reduce or stop bleeding, due to their constrictor effect on the vascular smooth-muscle cells, provided they exist in the bleeding vessel wall and respond to α-adrenergic stimulation. However, the intraocular hemostatic use of both epinephrine and phenylephrine is not very extended, probably due to the local toxicity shown by these drugs or their commercial vehicles, particularly on the corneal endothelium, and the possibility of systemic adverse reactions and interactions with anesthetics (see preceding chapter). On the other hand, the systemic absorption of intraocular catecholamines might be greatly limited by the local reuptake effect of the rich adrenergic iris innervation. This would allow the safe use of doses much higher than that permitted for retrobulbar injection—up to 68 μg/kg (74), instead of maximum 300 μg/hr for injected epinephrine (38).

It has to be kept in mind that newly formed vessels absolutely lack muscle cells and will not respond to vasoconstrictors. Normal retinal vessels are believed not to have adrenergic innervation.

Apart from catecholamines, other very strong vasoconstrictors might be used. These include several peptides, such as angiotensin II (Hypertensin®), normally occurring in the human blood as the active short-life agent of the blood pressure/volume homeostasis renin-angiotensin system. Agiotensin II has been clinically used to reestablish blood pressure, not having a tendency to induce arrhythmia and being safely used with halogenated anesthetics and cyclopropane (21). Alitesin and bombesin are other remarkable vasopressor peptides found in amphibia (23). We have no knowledge of the surgical hemostatic use of these substances, although we think that they might be useful if they prove nontoxic to the eye structures; a very localized action can be expected, as they are rapidly destroyed by peptidases, thus avoiding systemic side effects. Thromboxane A_2 (TXA_2) might also be a useful hemostatic agent. It is released by activated platelets to start platelet aggregation, and it is the strongest vasoconstrictor known to date.

Hyperosmolar Agents

Hyperosmolar agents causing preoperative dehydration of the vitreous and ocular hypotony may help in prevention of bleeding, particularly in the congestive glaucomatous eyes. A previously lowered IOP will minimize the sudden ocular decompression caused by the incision, which otherwise induces venous congestion and might be one of the mechanisms leading to choroidal (expulsive) hemorrhage.

However, hyperosmolar agents cause a rapid expansion of intravascular volume, as they dehydrate intracellular and transcellular spaces, resulting in increased blood pressure (up to 300/176) (34). This might lead not only to increased surgical bleeding but to the known acute hypertensive systemic complications. Since mannitol produces a more abrupt effect than urea, it is more likely to induce such undesired reactions. As an alternative, mechanical pressure or massage may be used to preoperatively soften the eye.

Other Hemostatic Substances

Some materials have a combined hemostatic effect: mechanical tamponade and creating a matrix that favors platelet aggregation. This would be the case with microfibrillar collagen hemostat (MCH), a fluffy, fibrous, off-white

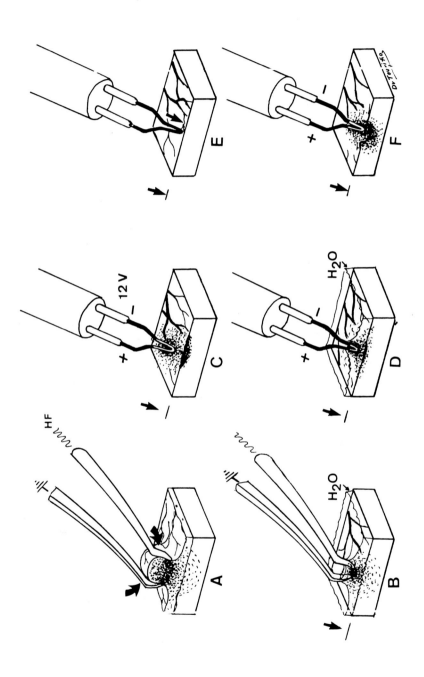

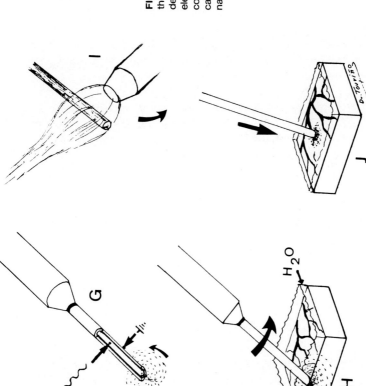

FIG. 1. Different types and modalities of the use of cauteries. **A, B:** Forceps-delivered bipolar diathermy; **C, D, E, F:** electric (low voltage DC) cautery; **G, H:** coaxial bipolar probe; **I, J:** glass rod cautery. See the text for further explanation. (**A** to **F** modified from ref. 76).

material prepared from bovine corium collagen, efficiently used in various fields of surgery. Its use in ophthalmology has been proposed only for extraocular (orbital or oculoplastic) surgery (2). The hemostatic effect seen with sodium hyaluronate (Healon®) appears not always related to the sole viscous hydrostatic compression and might be due to a similar mechanism.

Intraoperative Use of Physical Hemostatic Methods

To most ophthalmic surgeons, hemostasis means mechanical maneuvers and the use of cautery. The classical compression methods, using forceps, silicone sponges, marten-hair brush—or simply waiting for physiologic hemostasis—is often successful when bleeding comes from small vessels. The closed chambers of the eye permit the use of an increase in the hydrostatic pressure to restrain bleeding. This is commonly used in vitreous surgery where we can control the infusion of irrigating solutions. Similar effect may be obtained with viscous solutions such as sodium hyaluronate and air bubbles in the anterior chamber. A cold irrigation may favor vasoconstriction. The coagulation of the bleeding vessels is, however, the most reliable hemostatic method.

The effect of cauteries varies according to their type and mode of application. Galvanocautery—an electric resistor heated by a low voltage (6 to 12 V) DC— is convenient for a superficial cauterization when applied already heated (Fig. 1C) and particularly soft in a wet field (Fig. 1D). Its effect is deeper when turned on after it has touched the tissue (Fig. 1E,F). The use of a flame-heated glass rod, as suggested by José Ignacio Barraquer, would have the advantages of simplicity, soft and diffuse effect, and the possibility of seeing the coagulating vessels through it (Fig. 1I,J). However, electrical cauteries have the advantage of being regulable in their intensity, according to the effects seen in tissues.

Electric diathermy induces tissue heating and coagulation by the flow of high-frequency AC radiation through the tissue. In the unipolar mode, current flows from the probe tip to a grounded plaque placed at the back of the patient. The pathway followed by the current through the patient is not controlled by the surgeon; it depends on the specific conductivity of tissues. This implies the risk of optic nerve damage when unipolar diathermy is used in the vitreous chamber.

In the various bipolar diathermy devices (15,49,52), the current jumps between two electrodes placed in the same operating field. Its effect, apart from intensity regulation, is better controlled by the surgeon. When the electrodes are connected to two different instruments or to the arms of a forceps, the radiation field is ellipsoidal between the two tips. The effect is deeper if the tissue is grasped (Fig. 1A). When a superficial burn is desired, the current is allowed to jump between the tips in a wet field without touching the tissue, which will be affected by a lesser density of contiguous radiation (Fig. 1B).

In the coaxial bipolar probe, the current flows from a central or axial electrode to a surrounding outer, or coaxial diameter electrode (59), producing a localized, spheroidal, high-radiation-density field around its tip (Fig. 1G,H). The electrodes are insulated by a silicone sheet. The distance (radius) between the electrodes is critical, since the probe becomes unipolar when the radius becomes infinitely large. Coaxial diathermy may be particularly useful in posterior segment surgery. However, the bimanual technique (51)—each electrode connected to a different instrument—has the advantage in intraocular use (particularly in the vitreous) of not requiring the removal of instruments and replacing for the coagulator, which may save precious seconds when there is a bleeding vessel.

The photothermal effect is another possible approach to hemostatic coagulation. The potential risks of intraocular diathermy have favored the development of endophotocoagulation devices, and their application as photocautery in the case of the carbon dioxide laser. Xenon light and argon laser (24) are transmitted by intraocular transparent media and can be delivered at a distance from the target. However, they depend on pigment absorption and are less effective as vessel coagulators. Since infrared radiation is poorly transmitted by intraocular fluids, CO_2 laser has to be used following an air-tissue interface technique, or very close to the tissue within a wet field by means of an endoocular probe (53,54). It does not depend on pigment absorption. A similar approach might be followed using a neodymium-YAG laser in the continuous running mode, with the advantage of transmission by intraocular fluids.

Surgical Hemostasis During the Specific Intraocular Procedures

Although all surgical intraocular procedures have common aspects, we may group them, for practical reasons, into anterior and posterior segment surgery.

Anterior Segment Surgery

Apparently innocent maneuvers, such as the passing of a traction suture under the superior rectus muscle, may lead to the formation of a hematoma. This is rarely a serious complication, but if it reaches a large size, it may compress the globe, causing an IOP rise and leading to complications if inadverted, or forcing postponement of the intervention. Inadequate grasping of the presumed rectus muscle may lead (particularly in high myopes) to the perforation of the globe, retinal detachment, and intraocular hemorrhage.

The dissection of the conjunctival flap is a common source of minor bleeding; since it is external, it ceases partly spontaneously and is easily cauterized. Careful coagulation of episcleral vessels is particularly necessary in glaucoma filtering procedures and pterygium surgery. Both the presence of a hemorrhage in the scleroconjunctival interface or an exuberant healing reaction due to excessive cauterization may lead to the failure of the operation. A Desmarres scarifier is useful in cleaning the scleral surface of redundant episcleral tissue. The precise localization of the bleeding sources is facilitated by gentle irrigation of the field. A superficial coagulation of scleral tissue by means of bipolar diathermy is useful to prevent bleeding from the cut edges of the trabeculectomy scleral trapdoor, as well as from the path of scleral sutures.

The corneoscleral incision is the common origin of most significant bleeding in cataract surgery. Several factors should be balanced in order to decide its best placement. Although a corneal incision is obviously hemostatic, it certainly induces more postoperative astigmatism. Furthermore, for a given sectorial amplitude (i.e., 180° incision), the more we go into the cornea, the smaller the resulting opening, forcing a greater folding of the cornea and endothelial trauma—apart from the increased risk of touching the endothelium with instruments.

The *ab interno* technique with the Graefe knife permits the obtention of a two-plane (corneoscleral and conjunctival) incision with a single maneuver, although it commonly leads to greater bleeding than the less elegant *ab externo* technique. The shearing effect of scissors is somehow hemostatic, since it compresses the tissue while cutting. Special care must be taken at the 3- and 9-hr meridians, where thicker scleral branches of the posterior long ciliary arteries approach the limbus. It is advisable to cornealize the corresponding segments of the incision. A hemostatic single-maneuver, two-plane corneo-scleroconjunctival incision can be obtained following the Riquelme's modification of the José Ignacio Barraquer *ab externo* keratome-and-straight-scissors technique: To obtain a suitable-size limbus-based conjunctival flap, the perilimbic conjunctiva is pulled toward the cornea while the corneoscleral and conjunctival planes are cut simultaneously with the scissors (66).

The cauterization of the limbic incision vessels can be easily performed with galvanocautery. Excessive coagulation may lead to defective coaptation of the wound and postoperative astigmatism. The main intraoperative intention of limbic hemostasis is to prevent the entrance of blood into the anterior chamber. This may also be achieved, in spite of bleeding, by the previous filling of the chamber with sodium hyaluronate. This is particularly useful in the case of bleeding from the trephination edge of a vascularized cornea during penetrating keratoplasty. It is better to wait for the spontaneous hemostasis of these vessels, since cauterization would induce astigmatism and impair graft adaptation. The immediate placement and suturing of the graft also helps in stopping that bleeding. The simple apposition of tissue by suture placement is hemostatic. The same principle applies when a limbic vessel bleeds during suturing. Here, an air bubble in the anterior chamber will prevent the entrance of blood and maintain the shape of the cornea while the sutures are adjusted.

In spite of its rich vascularization, the iris shows little tendency to bleed when an iridectomy is performed. This is believed to be a consequence of the elastic conditions of iris tissue and particularly iris vessels, not a greater content of elastic fibers (6). Apart from the obvious risk of rubeosis, a fibrotic or inflamed iris will show increased tendency to bleed. Serious bleeding after iridectomy is commonly the result of inadequate technique: tearing of the iris root, iridodialysis, or lesion of the ciliary body. This is also avoided during trabeculectomy by an adequate selection of the area to be resected. A relatively anterior (corneal) trabeculectomy, including the corneoscleral trabeculum, is safer. A too posterior resection may lead to bleeding of the ciliary body or deep scleral vessel and does not improve the filtering effect of the procedure.

In the case of hemorrhage coming from the iris, ciliary body, or vascularized tissue in the retropupillary space (vascularized secondary cataract, persistent hyperplastic primary vitreous, cyclitic membrane), bipolar diathermy is preferable, since simple cautery may be ineffective in the wet field. However, mechanical methods (instrumental compression, air bubble, sodium hyaluronate) may be tried before using diathermy.

Special procedures involving the ciliary body—iridocyclectomy for small melanoma of the iris-ciliary body and antiglaucomatous cyclectomy—require special prophylactic hemostasis, such as preventive transcleral diathermy, direct ciliary body coagulation, and the subscleral application of naphazoline- or epinephrine-soaked sponges.

Posterior Segment Surgery

The classical retinal detachment procedures present similar problems, as described above, regarding conjunctival and episcleral hemostasis. In the case of a reoperation, the dissection is more laborious due to the presence of adhesions, and there will be increased tendency to bleed from scar tissue. Blunt dissection is always more hemostatic than cutting or tearing. Attention should be given to the presence of scleral thinning or ectasia, in high myopes or secondary to a previous too tight indentation procedure, which could lead to perforation and choroidal hemorrhage.

The diathermal coagulations and cryoapplications for retinopexy purposes should not be excessive. Transillumination may be useful to avoid the vortex veins and the long posterior ciliary arteries. In the case of a bleeding vortex it is preferable not to attempt coagulation, since this could lead to a choroidal hemorrhage.

The practice of an evacuation puncture is more safely done with a diathermy needle. A coaxial bipolar probe will give a more constant effect in a wet field.

Bleeding from the pars plana sclerotomy in vitrectomy is prevented by superficial cauterization of the sclera and preventive diathermy of the underlying uvea prior to penetration with the knife.

The hemostasis inside the vitreous chamber may be attained by simply raising the IOP by means of an increment in the infusion. A decrease in IOP down to 5 mmHg may be useful to assess the effectiveness of hemostasis after a bleeding vessel has been coagulated (51).

Bipolar diathermy is particularly useful in the vitreous cavity, since it is a wet field where thermal cauteries would be ineffective, and unipolar diathermy has greater risk of damaging the optic nerve or retina. Even with bipolar diathermy there is some electrical hazard that could be ruled out with the use of photocautery. The coagulation of a fibrovascular pedicle inside the cavity is obviously safer than acting on the retinal surface. In the first situation the tissue may be touched or grasped between the two electrodes, and the intensity increased until the desired effect is observed. Adhesion between coagulated tissue and instruments should be avoided. When the retina has to be coagulated, it is preferable to avoid proximity to the optic nerve and macula. To obtain a superficial effect it is recommended that the current flow between the two tips without directly touching the retina with the instruments (51). Although a coaxial bipolar probe gives a very uniform and circumscribed field (rather "recurrent" from the tip to a more proximal zone of the external electrode) the bimanual technique has the advantage of using the instruments already inside the vitreous cavity and not needing to replace them, as well as the possibility of holding the tissue between the electrodes.

Prevention and Management of Expulsive Hemorrhage

Expulsive hemorrhage (EH) is the most feared complication of intraocular surgery. Its natural course when the globe is opened consists of iris bulging with anterior chamber collapse, followed by spontaneous exit of the lens, iris, and vitreous, then retina and choroid, and finally blood. Even if this autoevisceration of the globe is avoided by rapid closure of the wound, the final result is frequently the loss of the eye.

Fortunately, EH is an infrequent accident. Its incidence [reviewed by Taylor (79)], ranges between 0.05% and 0.40%, with an average of 0.2%. This is low enough so that many ophthalmologists have not experienced EH, and it explains our ignorance of its precise pathophysiology.

EH is classically associated with cataract surgery, although it has also occurred during glaucoma (85) and other open-globe procedures (26), and even during retina-detachment surgery (90). It may happen during the operation or postoperatively. In the Pau (60) review of 59 cases, only one-third occurred during surgery, another one-third during the 3 to 6 postoperative hr, and the remaining one-third up to 9 days later. Lately EHs have been reported on the 14th (72) and 16th (5) postoperative days. When the sutures are strong enough to hold, or in the case of closed-globe surgery, we may talk about "nonexpulsive choroidal hemorrhage" (68).

Pathophysiology of EH

Multiple risk factors have been advocated with EH. Almost any ophthalmologist would agree that glaucoma, hypertension, arteriosclerosis, myopia, diabetes, obesity, "bull neck," and cephalic congestion may be considered dangerous. However, the low incidence of EH has not permitted a precise evaluation of the risk involved in each of these factors or in their association.

Although glaucoma (46,88) and arterial hypertension are probably the most significant risk factors, EH has been also found in nonglaucomatous and normotensive patients (27). Hematologic disorders are another possible etiology. EH has been reported as the first manifestation of an acute leukemia in a bilateral case (71). EH has also occurred in children and young patients.

Nontraumatic spontaneous massive choroidal hemorrhages (11) probably have a pathophysiology similar to EH; they are particularly similar to the nonexpulsive surgical cases. They actually can become expulsive if the globe was perforated by a corneal ulcer (88,89), or to induce hemophthalmos (29), or even in the spontaneous rupture of the eye seen in glaucoma patients (63). They may be confused with melanomas (4,18) and may actually happen in association with melanomas (84). Surgical EH from a previously undiagnosed melanoma has also been reported (83).

There are few pathologic studies on EH, possibly due to the fact that many such eyes are treated by evisceration rather than enucleation [for review see Manschot (45,46)]. The most accepted mechanism is the rupture of a short or long posterior ciliary artery. This is also suggested by the bright red appearance of the blood when a posterior sclerectomy is done after EH. In the case of a melanoma, the bleeding would come from a necrotic area of the tumor (84) or from a tear in choroidal vessels following the displacement of a nonnecrotic tumor after the opening of the globe (83).

The cause of the arterial rupture would be the necrosis of its wall, at the level of its penetration into the suprachoroidal space or in the choroid, always after leaving the scleral canal (46). In glaucomatous eyes the nutrition of the arterial wall would be defective, due to the resistance created by the high IOP against the diffusion of nutrients from the vascular lumen, leading to necrosis. The degenerative changes caused by hypertension and arteriosclerosis or associated with high myopia and diabetes would be additional causes. Apart from the pathologic fragility of the vessel, hemodynamic factors should be considered.

The choroid is a fundamentally vascular tissue in a very lax connective matrix. Its vascular content may vary widely, depending on

1. The *perfusion pressure,* which itself depends on
   a. the blood pressure in posterior ciliary arteries;
   b. the resistance of the capillary beds; and
   c. the venous pressure in the vortexes.
2. The *resistance of the tissue* against distention
   a. the elastic resistance of the choroidal tissue, and
   b. the intraocular pressure.

Moreover, IOP and choroidal perfusion certainly interact, but the involved mechanisms are still unclear. The uveal vessels have both sympathetic and parasympathetic innervation, which regulate their circulatory conditions and may subsequently influence the formation of aqueous humor. On the other hand, an increase in IOP will tend to collapse the uveal vascular beds or at least increase the resistance to perfusion. When IOP suddenly drops after the eye is opened, these interactions are abruptly altered. Although adaptation may be expected to follow, the initial reaction may include choroidal congestion or even choroidal effusion *ex vacuo.* This could also be the origin of an arterial rupture, at a fragile or necrotic section, and EH. However, the *ex vacuo* hypothesis cannot be applied easily to the postoperative and nonexpulsive cases. Arterial and venous pressure should also be considered.

When the iris/lens diaphragm starts to bulge after the corneoscleral incision has been done (Fig. 2A), the surgeon may consider the following: (a) the IOP has not been sufficiently decreased preoperatively, particularly if the eye was glaucomatous; (b) there is not enough muscle relaxation; (c) there is an increasing choroidal congestion. Since the IOP factor has become almost a constant (zero) after the opening of the globe, choroidal engorging depends only on vascular factors.

Arterial hypertension can be accounted for as follows:

1. A hypertensive patient whose blood pressure has not been corrected preoperatively. General anesthesia is not deep enough, or a controlled hypotension technique is required.
2. There is a sudden rise in blood pressure, secondary to a shallowing of the anesthesia, or a sympathetic stimulation due to
   a. lack of abolition of the endotracheal reflexes—the "anxiety" of the intubated patient;
   b. insufficient ventilation, causing hypoxia and hypercarbia; or
   c. systemic side effects of local epinephrine or phenylephrine.

Venous hypertension may be due to one of the following:

1. A patient with chronic obstructive bronchopneumopathy not corrected preoperatively.
2. An increase of the respiratory effort due to bronchoconstriction during anesthesia, an incorrect location of the endotracheal tube, or partial obstruction by excessive secretions.
3. Positive intrathoracic pressure due to assisted respiration.
4. Sudden Valsava effect caused by coughing, bucking, straining, or vomiting.
5. Increase in vortex pressure secondary to orbital hypertension:
   a. excessive or inadequately distributed retrobulbar injection, or
   b. retrobulbar hemorrhage.

If the choroidal congestion progresses, it may lead to simple vitreous loss after the lens extraction (Fig. 2B). Since the sclera has little or no distensibility, any increase in choroidal thickness results in reduction of the vitreous cavity. A sudden choroidal engorgement may be associated with transudation. Since choroidal interstitial fluid cannot diffuse to the retina, due to the pigment epithelium continuous intercellular-junction barrier, this is likely to result in a

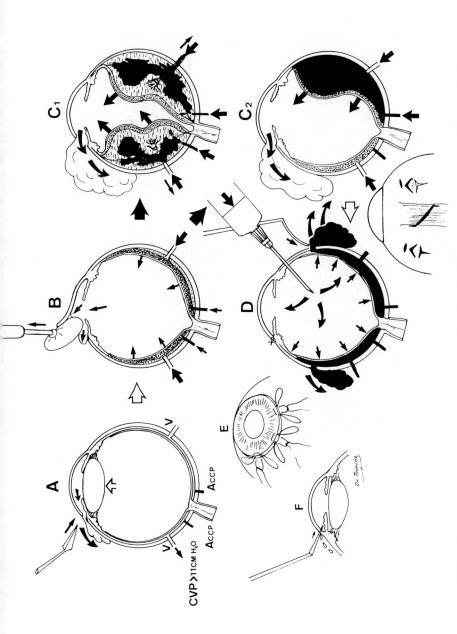

FIG. 2. Pathophysiology, prevention, and management of expulsive hemorrhage. **A:** Iris/lens diaphragm bulging after eye decompression; **B:** choroidal congestion and effusion causing vitreous loss after cataract extraction; **C1, C2:** proposed mechanisms of expulsive hemorrhage; **D:** various measures in the preoperative management of expulsive hemorrhage; **E:** prophylactic multiple preplaced sutures; **F:** progressive decompression of the eye. (See text for details.)

suprachoroidal fluid collection, a *choroidal effusion*. As the suprachoroidal virtual space becomes real, the actual dissecting forces may result in large-vessel tearing and massive hemorrhage, provided the effusion is sudden enough or the vessel wall is already weak or necrotic. (Fig. 2C1). Once EH has begun, progressive tearing of all large vessels can be expected, as the choroid is pushed away from the sclera. This fact should be kept in mind regarding the extreme urgency in stopping EH, to avoid the total lysis of the choroidal circulation.

The importance of venous hypertension in pathogenesis of both the vitreous losses and EH has been emphasized by Roveda and Roveda (67). However, the pathologic evidence of arterial necrosis cannot be overlooked. The simple ocular decompression could lead to the rupture of a necrotic ciliary artery, particularly if the blood pressure is high, without the intermediate stage of choroidal congestion and effusion (Fig. 2C2). The results will be similar.

Prevention of EH

The prophylaxis of EH consists of a series of measures whose efficiency is very difficult to assess. Although some cases have been reported associated to hematologic disease (11,71), the fact that bleeding comes from a ruptured, relatively large vessel indicates that the physiologic hemostatic status is a minor factor.

Anesthesia has a certain value in the prevention of EH and its cause. Whether local or general anesthesia is safer remains, however, unestablished. In a poll improvised by Welsh, Girard, and Jaffe (22), one-sixth of the ophthalmologists present using general anesthesia admitted to having experienced EH. When asking the local anesthesia users, who were the majority of the audience, "many hands" were raised.

General anesthesia permits a better control of blood pressure, particularly if a controlled hypotension technique is used, and lowers IOP too. However, general anesthetics such as halothane, cyclopropane, and ketamine actually increase the cerebral blood flow, which includes that of the eye. Although tracheal intubation causes reflex release of catecholamines and blood pressure rise, this is inhibited by a sufficiently deep general anesthesia. The same applies to coughing and straining. The use of systemic atropine avoids excessive bronchial secretion or constriction.

It has been said that general anesthesia leads to postoperative vomiting, with greater risk of EH. In a series of seven postoperative EHs (25), six were associated with vomiting, but five had been operated on with local anesthesia. The venous congestive factor can be reduced by simply positioning the patient in anti-Trendelenburg (67).

A preoperatively hypotonic eye is essential to minimize the decompression effect. This can be achieved by using inhibitors of carbonic anhydrase (acetazolamide) or hyperosmotic agents (see Hyperosmolar Agents, above) together with deep general anesthesia and muscle relaxants. When compressive maneuvers are used, a sudden decompression should also be avoided.

Local anesthesia avoids ventilatory problems, if not already present, and permits a safe association with local catecholamines. Nevertheless, it is questionable whether a reduction in blood flow is an improvement in the case of an ischemic or necrotic arterial wall. Retrobulbar anesthesia may cause orbital hypertension, thus raising IOP and impairing venous drainage of the choroid.

In regard to surgical maneuvers, little can be done to prevent EH, provided the techniques are correct and carefully performed. Special security measures can be taken in high-risk patients, such as progressive decompression of the globe by paracentesis, letting successive minute quantities of aqueous humor escape over time intervals (Fig. 2F), or preplacing multiple security sutures (Fig. 2E).

Prophylaxis of EH includes postoperative procedures. Vomiting and trauma could be the cause of postoperative EH. From a series of 1,607 "missionary" cataract extractions performed during 2 months—all bilateral and using local anesthesia—Goren (27) reported seven EHs, all postoperative, one bilateral. He associated that high incidence of 0.435% with a rather primitive method of transporting the patient from the operating table to a stretcher and from there to the bed—in the arms of a lone attendant. The simple improvement of this method resulted in only 1 case of EH in a subsequent 1,300-cataract-extraction series.

Management of EH

EH may occur despite all preventive measures. The prognosis is always poor. Old texts (70,81) recommended immediate enucleation. Verhoeff (85) in 1915 was the first to report a successful conservative treatment multiple posterior evacuating sclerotomies, in a case of EH during a filtering procedure. In 1938, Vail (82) followed a similar technique in a case of EH after a cataract extraction. The eye regained a vision of 20/25. However, the number of successfully treated eyes reported is small, and frequently the eye becomes extremely hard and painful, forcing secondary enucleation or evisceration, or undergoes fast phthisis changes in spite of sclerotomy treatment. Sometimes the globe is not lost, but no vision is retained. The causes of the fatal outcome, in cases in which primary expulsion has been overcome, can be related to the following:

1. *Massive ischemia of the choroid*—and therefore of the photoreceptors and ciliary processes—leading to phthisis bulbi. It is apparent that if the "progressive rupture of choroidal vessels" hypothesis is correct, prognosis depends on rapidity in initiating intraoperative treatment.
2. *Ischemia of internal retinal layers and optic nerve head,* due to compression and collapse of the central retinal artery system. The maintenance of a very high IOP in the postoperative period also darkens prognosis.

The intraoperative management of EH can be resumed in two ways (Fig. 2D):

1. *External decompression.* The posterior sclerotomy, to externally drain the hemorrhage may be simple or multiple. Most authors do not specify its precise location, although it is advisable to practice it as posteriorly as possible without losing time, since the source of bleeding is believed to be very posterior indeed. It is also advisable to maintain the exit opened by means of twisting the knife inside the sclerotomy, introducing a cyclodialysis spatula or a polyethylene aspirating tube, cauterizing the sclerotomy edges, enlarging the sclerotomy to a *V* or *T* shape, or doing a triangular sclerectomy. Bordeianu (8) advocates the practice of a large, very posterior *Z* incision, 4 × 10 to 15 mm, under a rectus muscle (to avoid vorticose veins) to be left unsutured.

2. *Internal recompression or tamponade.* To overcome the expulsion of the ocular content, the wound has to be closed as fast as possible with a number of sutures strong enough to resist the subsequent IOP rise. To counteract the buildup of the suprachoroidal blood collection, several internal tamponade maneuvers have been proposed using saline (7) and air (37) injections. This would help in the external emptying of the hemorrhage through the sclerotomy and in repositioning the retina and choroid, preventing the progressive tearing of vessels. The central retinal artery pulse should be monitored. Other possibilities would be the injection, through the corneoscleral wound or through a pars plana puncture, of a viscous solution (such as sodium hyaluronate), silicone, or an inflatable device similar to the balloon proposed for the management of giant retinal tears (17).

Prevention of Postoperative Hemorrhage

Postoperative bleeding includes hyphema and vitreous hemorrhage. A small amount of blood in the anterior chamber has little importance, since the high fibrinolytic activity of the iris will promote its fast reabsorption. Secondary bleeding may lead to a more serious postoperative hemorrhage, which could be the cause of secondary glaucoma and corneal staining.

The preoperative normalization of hemostasis plays a significant role in preventing these complications. However, surgical maneuvers and intraoperative hemostasis are also factors to be considered.

A postoperative hyphema may result from iridectomy or corneoscleral wound bleeding, or from anterior displacement of a posterior-segment hemorrhage. An altered iris is, as already mentioned, more prone to bleed. A lesion in the iris root or ciliary body, or iridodialysis during the practice of iridectomy may lead to intraoperative or postoperative hemorrhage.

Wound bleeding may be precocious, occurring during the days following the operation, or as late as several years postoperatively (77,78,87). It may be related to one or more of the following:

1. *A too scleral lesion,* particularly if deep vessels are affected. We have already commented the advantages and disadvantages of the different locations of the corneoscleral incision (see Anterior Segment Surgery, above).
2. *A defect in sutures.* A loose or gaping incision, or the use of thicker and more irritating sutures, will promote a more important healing reaction. The newly formed vessels in the scar tissue easily bleed following minimal trauma. The recovery of normal IOP after surgery or a transient postoperative hypertension may reopen a defective sutured wound and produce hyphema.
3. *Postoperative trauma.* Even a well-sutured wound may bleed if trauma is strong enough to partially reopen it. Special care should be taken in postoperative handling of the eye (tonometry, removal of sutures, etc.).
4. *Wound neovascularization.* This is the advocated cause of late hyphema after surgery (78,87). It usually occurs several years postoperatively and may be recurrent. It has been reported even in the case of a corneal incision.

Multiple, least irritating, and subconjunctival sutures are preferable to avoid wound gaping, excessive healing reaction with neovascularization, and postoperative knot-induced conjunctival irritation, which could lead to lid spasms and wound reopening. The removal of sutures should be very careful, preferably late and under operating room conditions. Subconjunctival sutures may not be removed unless they spontaneously perforate the conjunctiva.

The final sequence of the hemostatic process includes an activation of the fibrinolytic system. This is the postulated mechanism of secondary bleeding 2 to 6 days following an ocular contusion (10) and could also apply to surgical trauma. Antifibrinolytic agents as EACA (19) and tranexamic acid (55) have been reported to cause a statistically significant reduction in the incidence of traumatic secondary hyphema. This might be also useful in preventing precocious bleeding after surgery. However, late hyphema due to wound neovascularization is probably related to the fragility of new vessels rather than to fibrinolytic activation. The postoperative use of drugs interfering with platelet aggregation—including aspirin and ethanol—should be avoided (32).

Apart from the antifibrinolytic approach, none of the proposed preventive or conservative treatments of secondary hyphema, including mydriatics, miotics, and estrogens, or prolonged bed rest, binocular patching, and restricted activity have proved significantly useful (32).

ACKNOWLEDGMENTS

We thank Dr. Emilio Iglesias-Touriño, who is the author of the drawings and collaborated in their conception. Dr. Pedro Borrat advised us regarding hematologic aspects and medical hemostatic therapy, as Drs. Ignacio Zabal and Antoni Monsó did regarding anesthesia influences on hemostasis. We also thank Miss Montserrat Veses for typing the manuscript.

REFERENCES

1. Ahn, Y. S., Harrington, W. J., Seelman, R. C., et al. (1974): Vincristine therapy of idiopathic and secondary thrombocytopenia. *N. Engl. J. Med.,* 291:376–380.
2. Allavie, J. J., and Kalina, R. E. (1981): Microfibrillar collagen hemostat in ophthalmic surgery. *Ophthalmology,* 88:443–444.
3. Arkel, Y. S. (1976): Evaluation of platelet aggregation and disorders of hemostasis. *Med. Clin. North Am.,* 60:881–911.
4. Auw-Yang Sien (1948): A case of choroidal apoplexy diagnosed as a sarcoma of the choroid. *Ophthalmologica,* 11:1–10.
5. Awan, K. J. (1975): Expulsive choroidal hemorrhage. *Can. J. Ophthalmol.,* 10:427–432.
6. Babel, J. (1962): L'iridectomie sous l'angle de l'anatomie, de la physiologie, et de la pathologie. *An. Inst. Barraquer,* 3:137–145.
7. Bair, H. L. (1966): Expulsive hemorrhage at cataract operation. *Am. J. Ophthalmol.,* 61:992–994.
8. Bordeianu, C. D. (1982): L'hemorragie expulsive: Accident insurmontable? Discussion d'une possibilité de traitement. *J. Fr. Ophtalmol.,* 5:257–261.
9. Bowie, E. J. W., and Owen, C. A., Jr. (1974): Symposium on the intravascular coagulation-fibrinolysin system. *Mayo Clin. Proc.,* 49:676–679.
10. Bramsen, T. (1979): Fibrinolysis and traumatic hyphema. *Acta Ophthalmol. (Copenh.),* 57:447–454.
11. Cahn, P. H., and Havener, W. H. (1963): Spontaneous massive choroidal hemorrhage, with preservation of the eye by sclerotomy. *Am. J. Ophthalmol.,* 56:568–571.
12. Campbell, D. G., and Essigmann, E. M. (1979): Hemolytic ghost cell glaucoma. Further studies. *Arch. Ophthalmol.,* 97:2141–2146.
13. Caplan, S. N., and Berkman, E. M. (1976): Immunosuppressive therapy of idiopathic thrombocytopenic purpura. *Med. Clin. North Am.,* 60:971–986.
14. Cardamone, J. M., and Reese, E. P., Jr. (1976): Ocular enucleation in a patient with severe classic hemophilia A. *Am. J. Ophthalmol.,* 82:767–769.
15. Charles, S., White, J., Dennison, C., and Eichenbaum, D. (1976): Bimanual polar intraocular diathermy. *Am. J. Ophthalmol.,* 81:101–102.
16. Chediak, J. R., Telfer, M. C., and Gren, D. (1977): Platelet function and immunologic parameters in von Willebrand's disease following cryoprecipitate and factor VIII concentrate infusion. *Am. J. Med.,* 62:369–376.
17. Couvillon, G. C., Freeman, H. M., and Schepens, C. L. (1970): Vitreous surgery. III. Intraocular balloon: Instrument report. *Arch. Ophthalmol.,* 83:713–714.
18. Crigler, L. W. (1932): Subchoroidal hemorrhage diagnosed as sarcoma of the choroid. *Arch. Ophthalmol.,* 8:690–694.
19. Crouch, E. R., and Frenkel, M. (1976): Aminocaproic acid in the treatment of traumatic hyphema. *Am. J. Ophthalmol.,* 81:355–360.
20. Davis, D. W., and Steward, D. T. (1977): Unexplained excessive bleeding during operation: Role of acetyl salicylic acid. *Can. Anesth. J.,* 24:452–458.
21. Douglas, W. W. (1975): Polypeptides, angiotensin, plasma cynines, and other vasoactive agents. Prostaglandins. In: *The Pharmacological Basis of Therapeutics,* 5th ed., edited by L. S. Goodman and A. Gilman, ch. 30. Macmillan, New York.
22. Emery, J. M. (1976): *Current Concepts in Cataract Surgery,* p. 28. C. V. Mosby, St. Louis.
23. Ersparmer, V. (1971): Biogenic amines and active polypeptides of the amphibian skin. *Pharmacol. Rev.,* 11:327–350.
24. Fleischman, J. A., Swartz, M., and Dixon, J. A. (1981): Argon laser endophotocoagulation. An intraoperative trans-pars plana technique. *Arch. Ophthalmol.,* 99:1610–1612.
25. François, J., Wannebroucq, Ch., and G. Legrand (1966): Les hémorragies expulsives. A propos de 6 cas. *Bull. Soc. Ophtal., Fr.,* 66:579–585.
26. Girard, L. J., Spak, K. E., Hawkins, R. S., and Caldwell, D. (1973): Expulsive hemorrhage during intraocular surgery. *Trans. Am. Acad. Ophthalmol. and Otolaryngol.,* 77:109–115.
27. Goren, S. B. (1966): Expulsive subchoroidal hemorrhage following cataract surgery. *Am. J. Ophthalmol.,* 62:536–537.

28. Gradey, C. F. (1978): Transfusion and hepatitis update in 78. (Editorial.) *N. Engl. J. Med.,* 298:1413–1415.
29. Grafenberg, E. (1907): Hoemophthalmus bei Glaukom. *Arch. Augenheilkd.,* 56:38–52.
30. Grundlach, W. J., and Tarnasky, R. (1979): TTP and antiplatelet therapy. (Correspondence.) *Blood,* 53:798.
31. Harker, L. A., and Slichter, S. J. (1972): The bleeding time as a screening test for evaluation of platelet function. *N. Engl. J. Med.,* 287:155–159.
32. Havener, W. H. (1978): *Ocular Pharmacology,* 4th ed., pp. 81, 109, 702–719. C. V. Mosby, St. Louis.
33. Hilgartner, M. W., and Sergis, E. (1977): Current therapy for hemophiliacs: Home care and therapeutic complications. *Mt. Sinai J. Med. (NY),* 44:316–331.
34. Jaffe, N. S. (1976): Discussion: Ophthalmic anesthesia. In: *Current Concepts in Cataract Surgery,* edited by J. M. Emery, p. 29. C. V. Mosby, St. Louis.
35. de Jong, R. H. (1970): *Physiology and Pharmacology of Local Anesthesia.* Charles C Thomas, Springfield, IL.
36. Jorfeldt, L., Löfström, B., Prenow, B., and Whren, J. (1970): The effect of mepivacaine and lidocaine on forearm resistance and capacitance vessels in man. *Acta Anaesthesiol. Scand.,* 14:183–189.
37. Krasnov, M. M. (1960): The method of forced blood evacuation from the subchoroidal space in the treatment of expulsive hemorrhage. *Am. J. Ophthalmol.,* 49:402–403. (Abstract.)
38. Kratz, R. L., and Epstein, R. A. (1968): The interaction of anesthetic agents and adrenergic drugs to produce cardiac arrythmias. *Anesthesiology,* 29:763–784.
39. Lacey, J. V., and Penner, J. A. (1977): Management of idiopathic thrombocytopenic purpura in the adult. *Semin. Thromb. Hemost.,* 3:160–174.
40. Laroche, L. (1983): Les hémorragies en chirurgie oculaire. *Clinique Ophtalmologique* (Lab. Martinet), 2:111–123.
41. Leigh, J. M., Millar, R. A., eds. (1975): Symposium on deliberate hypotension in anesthesia. *Br. J. Anaesth.,* 47:743.
42. Lerner, P. I., and Sampliner, J. E. (1977): Transfusion-associated cytomegalovirus mononucleosis. *Ann. Surg.,* 185:406–410.
43. Lerner, R. G. (1977): The difibrination syndrome. *Med. Clin. North Am.,* 60:871–880.
44. Lusher, J. M., and Barnhart, M. I. (1977): Congenital disorders affecting platelets. *Semin. Thromb. Hemost.,* 4:123–186.
45. Manschot, W. A. (1942): Expulsive hemorrhage. *Acta Ophthalmol. (Copenh.),* 19:237–246.
46. Manschot, W. A. (1955): The pathology of expulsive hemorrhage. *Am. J. Ophthalmol.,* 40:15–24.
47. Marder, V. J. (1979): The use of thrombolytic agents: Choice of patient, drug administration and laboratory monitoring. *Ann. Intern. Med.,* 90:802–808.
48. Marengo-Rowe, A. J., and Leveson, J. E. (1977): Evaluation of the bleeding patient. *Postgrad. Med. J.,* 62:171–177.
49. Mehta, R. F., and Bankes, J. L. K. (1977): Haemostasis in cataract surgery. The Downs bipolar coagulator. *Trans. Ophthalmol. Soc. U.K.,* 97:112–113.
50. Meyers, E. F. (1980): Anesthetic complications in ophthalmological patients. In: *Complications in Ophthalmic Surgery,* edited by S. R. Waltman and T. Krupin, pp. 1–27. J. B. Lippincott, Philadelphia.
51. Michels, R. G. (1980): *Vitreous Surgery,* p. 173. C. V. Mosby, St. Louis.
52. Michels, R. G., and Rice, T. A. (1977): Bimanual bipolar diathermy for treatment of bleeding from the anterior chamber. *Am. J. Ophthalmol.,* 84:873–874.
53. Miller, J. B., Smith, M. R., and Boyer, D. S. (1979): Intraocular carbon dioxide laser photocautery. II. Preliminary report of clinical trials. *Arch. Ophthalmol.,* 97:2123–2127.
54. Miller, J. B., Smith, M. R., Pincus, F., and Stockert, M. (1979): Intraocular carbon dioxide laser photocautery. I. Animal experimentation. *Arch. Ophthalmol.,* 97:2157–2162.
55. Nortensen, K. K., and Sjölie, K. (1978): Secondary hemorrhage following traumatic hyphema. A comparative study of conservative and tranexamic acid treatment. *Acta Ophthalmol. (Copenh.),* 56:763–768.
56. Nussbaum, M., and Moschos, C. B. (1976): Anticoagulants and anticoagulation. *Med. Clin. North Am.,* 60:855–869.

57. Pandolfi, M. (1978): Intraocular hemorrhages: A hemostatic therapeutic approach. *Surv. Ophthalmol.,* 22:322–324.
58. Pandolfi, M. (1979): *Hemorrhages in Ophthalmology.* Georg Theme, Stuttgart.
59. Pao, D. S. (1979): Coaxial bipolar probe. *Arch. Ophthalmol.,* 97:1351–1352.
60. Pau, H. (1958): Der Zeitfaktor bei der expulsiven Blutung. *Klin. Monatsbl. Augenheilkd.,* 132:865–869.
61. Phelps, C. D., and Watzke, R. C. (1975): Hemolytic glaucoma. *Am. J. Ophthalmol.,* 80:690–694.
62. Philpot, F. J. (1940): The inhibition on adrenalin oxidation by local anesthetics. *J. Physiol. (Lond.),* 97:301–314.
63. Pietruschka, G., and Schill, H. (1964): Ueber die Spontane Bulbusrupstur. *Klin. Monatsbl. Augenheilkd.,* 145:167–174.
64. Price, H. L. (1975): General anesthetics. In: *The Pharmacological Basis of Therapeutics,* 5th ed., edited by L. S. Goodman and A. Gilman, Ch. 6, 7. Macmillan, New York.
65. Richards, R. D., and Spurtling, C. L. (1973): Elective ocular surgery in haemophilia. *AMA Arch. Ophthalmol.,* 89:167–168.
66. Riquelme, J. L. (1983): Incisión conjuntivo-esclero-corneal simplificada para la extracción de la catarata. *Rev. d'Or de Oftalmología,* 2:41–44.
67. Roveda, J. M., and Roveda, C. E. (1979): Pression veineuse dans les hémorragies expulsives et les pertes de vitré. *J. Fr. Ophthalmol.,* 2:343–348.
68. Samuels, B. (1931): Postoperative non-expulsive subchoroidal hemorrhage. *AMA Arch. Ophthalmol.,* 6:840–851.
69. Schettini, A., Freund, H. R., and Owre, E. S. (1967): Deliberate hypotension with halothane/oxygen anesthesia in head and neck surgery. *Am. J. Surg.,* 114:543–547.
70. de Schweinitz, G. E. (1921): *Diseases of the Eye.* 9th ed., p. 739. W. B. Saunders, Philadelphia.
71. Secheyron, P., Poitevin, B., and Deodati, F. (1978): Hémorragie expulsive bilatérale du vitré: Première manifestation d'une leucemie aiguë. *Bull. Soc. Ophtalmol. Fr.,* 78:489–490.
72. Shaffer, R. N. (1966): Posterior sclerotomy with scleral cautery in the treatment of expulsive hemorrhage. *Am. J. Ophthalmol.,* 61:1307–1309.
73. Simpson, M. B. (1978): Platelet function and transfusion therapy in the surgical patient. In: *Platelet Physiology and Transfusion,* edited by C. J. Schiffer, pp. 51–68. American Association of Blood Banks, Washington, DC.
74. Smith, R. B., Douglas, H. N., Petruscak, J., and Breslin, P. (1972). Safety of intraocular adrenaline with halothane anesthesia. *Br. J. Anaesth.,* 44:1314–1317.
75. Snow, J. C. (1982): *Anesthesia in Otolaryngology and Ophthalmology,* 2nd ed., pp. 225–230. Appleton-Century-Crofts, New York.
76. Spaeth, G. L. (1982): Instrumentation and sutures. In: *Ophthalmic Surgery,* edited by G. L. Spaeth, p. 78. W. B. Saunders, Philadelphia.
77. Speakman, J. S. (1975): Recurrent hyphema after surgery. *Can. J. Ophthalmol.,* 10:299–304.
78. Swan, K. C. (1976): Late hyphema due to wound vascularization. *Trans. Am. Acad. Ophthalmol. Otolaryngol.,* 81:138–144.
79. Taylor, D. M. (1974): Expulsive hemorrhage. *Am. J. Ophthalmol.,* 78:961–966.
80. Tomasulo, P. A. (1978): Management of the alloimmunized patient with HLA-matched platelets. In: *Platelet Physiology and Transfusion,* edited by C. J. Schiffer, pp. 69–92. American Association of Blood Banks, Washington, DC.
81. Torok, E. V., and Grout, G. H. (1913): *Surgery of the Eye,* pp. 187, 270, 420. Lea & Febiger, Philadelphia.
82. Vail, D. T. (1938): Posterior sclerotomy as a form of treatment in subchoroidal expulsive hemorrhage. *Am. J. Ophthalmol.,* 21:256–259.
83. Varela, H. (1964): Expulsive hemorrhage at cataract surgery. Unsuspected choroidal melanoma. *Arch. Ophthalmol.,* 71:209–210.
84. Verhoeff, F. H. (1904): Sarcoma of the choroid with destructive hemorrhage. *Arch. Ophthalmol.,* 33:241–249.
85. Verhoeff, F. H. (1915): Scleral puncture for expulsive sub-choroidal hemorrhage following sclerostomy-scleral puncture for post-operative separation of the choroid. *Ophth. Rec.,* 24:55–59.
86. Watson-Williams, E. J. (1979): Hematological and hemostatic considerations before surgery.

In: *Symposium on the Medical Evaluation of the Preoperative Patient. Med. Clin. North Am.,* 63:1157–1181.

87. Watzke, R. C. (1980): Intraocular hemorrhage from vascularization of the cataract incision. *Ophthalmology,* 87:19–23.
88. Williams, K., and Rentries, P. K. (1970): Spontaneous expulsive choroidal hemorrhage. *Arch. Ophthalmol.,* 83:191–194.
89. Winslow, R. J., Stevenson, W., and Yanoff, M. (1974): Spontaneous expulsive choroidal hemorrhage. *Arch. Ophthalmol.,* 92:33–36.
90. Wolter, J. R. (1961): Expulsive hemorrhage during retinal detachment surgery. A case with survival of the eye after Verhoeff sclerotomy. *Am. J. Ophthalmol.,* 51:264–266.
91. Yankee, R. A., Grumet, F. C., and Rogentine, G. N. (1969): Platelet transfusion therapy: The selection of compatible platelet donors for refractory patients by lymphocyte HL-A typing. *N. Engl. J. Med.,* 281:1208–1212.
92. Zauber, N. P., and Levin, J. (1977): Factor IX levels in patients with hemophilia B (Christmas disease) following transfusion with concentrates of factor IX or fresh frozen plasma (FFP). *Medicine (Baltimore),* 56:213–224.

Surgical Pharmacology of the Eye,
edited by M. Sears and A. Tarkkanen.
Raven Press, New York © 1985.

Useful Enzymes

Rafael I. Barraquer and Joaquín Barraquer

Instituto Barraquer, Barcelona 21, Spain

SUMMARY: α-Chymotrypsin: Enzymatic zonulolysis is usually accomplished two minutes after irrigation of the posterior chamber with 1 ml of 1:5,000 solution. α-Chymotrypsin is useful for ICCE at any age over 30. Although it may not be necessary in patients over 60 with mature cataracts, it will always reduce the need of traction and thus the risk of intraoperative traction-induced retinal detachment. It will also reduce the risk of capsule rupture in cases of hypermature and intumescent cataracts. Zonular detritus may induce a transient postoperative rise in ocular pressure. Wash the anterior chamber with irrigating solution after enzymatic zonulolysis has been accomplished to avoid this possible occurrence.

Urokinase: Management of vitreous hemorrhage: Although its usefulness has not been clearly established, the intravitreal injection of 5,000 to 55,000 P.U. of urokinase in 0.2 to 0.3 ml distilled water is a less aggressive alternative that can be tried before vitrectomy in patients who fail to respond to conservative therapy. Best results have been obtained in traumatic cases. Management of traumatic hyphema: In cases of large or total, generally secondary, hyphema (with risk of corneal blood staining, fibrous membrane formation, and persistent secondary glaucoma) that fails to reabsorb with conservative therapy or anterior chamber saline lavage, urokinase might be useful. Five 0.3 ml. doses from 5,000 P.U. dissolved in 2 ml distilled water, each left in the anterior chamber for 3 minutes, are recommended.

ALPHA-CHYMOTRYPSIN

Ophthalmic surgery has pioneered the intraoperative use of enzymes since enzymatic zonulolysis (EZ) (167,168) was discovered in 1957. However, alpha-chymotrypsin (α-CT) has remained almost the only enzymatic tool ophthalmologists use during surgery. Management of intraocular hemorrhages by means of the injection of a fibrinolytic agent such as urokinase, although not intraoperative may nevertheless be considered a surgical procedure.

The increased danger of vitreous loss, the large incision required, and the fragility of the lens capsule associated with the resistance of the zonules were the main classical intraoperative problems of phacoerysis, or intracapsular cataract extraction (ICCE). During the first half of the century, some of the former problems were solved by the introduction of corneoscleral sutures and improvement in lens-grasping devices—the erysiphake by Ignacio Barraquer in 1917 (13), the development of several new capsule forceps, and lately, the introduction of the cryoprobe by Tadeusz Krwawicz in 1961 (104). The resistance of the zonules remained, however, an unsolved problem. Techniques such as Kirby's mechanical zonulotomy were indeed complicated and not exempt from risk (99).

On May 27, 1957, Joaquín Barraquer injected a solution of α-CT 1:500 into the vitreous of an almost blind eye with a massive vitreous hemorrhage that had not resorbed after 1 year of conservative treatment. Next day he observed that although the hemorrhage was still present, the lens had disappeared from its normal location in the retropupillary space and was luxated into the vitreous cavity. After several experiments in animals and donor eyes, followed by clinical trials, the technique of EZ was disclosed before the Royal Academy of Medicine and Surgery of Barcelona in April 1958 (14).

EZ consists of the destruction or weakening of the Zinn's zonules by the action of a solution of α-CT. It makes ICCE easier by elimination of its major obstacle: the need for mechanical liberation of the lens from its attachment to the ciliary zone, which was the source of many complications, such as capsule rupture, vitreous loss, pupil distortion, corneal and iris posterior epithelial trauma, and possibly retinal detachment, among others.

The history of its discovery is another example of the role of exploited chance in scientific advances. A measure of its fast, widespread diffusion is the fact that during the year following its introduction more than 100 papers referring to it had been published throughout the world (166). In 1959 a report to the American Academy of Ophthalmology and Otolaryngology (AAOO) by a committee on the use of α-CT, chaired by Derrick T. Vail, included the experience of 151 institutions and more than 200 ophthalmologists (191). The EZ technique has remained the same with few variations and has been almost routinely used for ICCE during the last quarter of a century.

EZ introduces a radical change in cataract surgery. Whereas in classical ICCE methods the separation of the lens from the zonules and its delivery are done almost simultaneously, EZ makes possible the atraumatic separation of these structures and the division of that surgical step into two phases: (a) the *liberation* of the lens from its attachment, and (b) the *extraction* of the lens from the posterior chamber of the eye. The separation of these two phases means a structural improvement in the security of surgical maneuvers.

Biochemistry of Chymotrypsin

α-CT is a proteolytic enzyme liberated by the pancreas. It was first isolated in a crystalline form by Kunitz and Northrop in 1933 (105). It belongs, together with trypsin (TPS), to the endopeptidase group of hydrolases: the enzymes capable of breaking the peptidic bonds, not only terminally but also centrally located in protein chains.

Its precursor, chymotrypsinogen, an enzymatically inactive protein secreted by the pancreas, consists of a single chain of 254 amino acids, transversely joined by 5 disulfide links. Its original molecular weight of 23,240 is slightly reduced during activation to α-CT due to the elimination of four amino acids. The conversion process takes place under the action of TPS, and maybe the same α-CT also, following three steps (28,45):

1. The chymotrypsinogen chain is divided between the 15 and 16 positions, producing pi-chymotrypsin (π-CT), proteolytically active but unstable.
2. The dipeptide Ser (14)-Arg (15) is separated, producing delta-chymotrypsin (δ-CT), which is more active than α-CT.
3. The dipeptide Thr (147)-Asn (148) is finally cut and eliminated to produce α-CT. The original single chain maintains its five disulfide links, but has been split into three peptidic chains containing 13, 131, and 97 amino acids (Fig. 1).

When this process takes place through a "slow pathway" as a consequence of low TPS concentration, α-CT may produce further forms such as beta-chymotrypsin (β-CT) and gamma-chymotrypsin (γ-CT), both active (175).

The catalytic locus of α-CT is probably composed of the 57 (His), 195 (Ser), and possibly also 102 (Asp) residues (29,45). Although they may appear distant

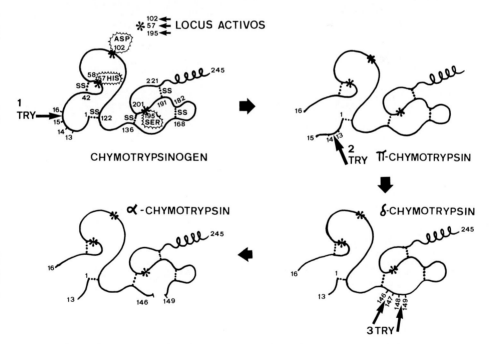

FIG. 1. Conversion process of chymotrypsinogen into α-chymotrypsin, under the action of trypsin. See text for details. TRY, trypsin. (From refs. 28 and 45).

to each other according to their position in the chain, X-ray analysis of the tertiary (tridimensional) structure of the enzyme has shown (with a 2-Å resolution) that they actually are very close (181).

α-CT has endopeptidase and also some exopeptidase (aminopeptidase) activity. It specifically hydrolyzes the peptidic bonds whose carbonyl group is produced by an aromatic ring carrying amino acid (tyrosine, tryptophan, or phenylalanine) and also, but less effectively, leucine and threonine. Apart from the peptidic, it is also capable of attacking the bonds of amides, esters, hydrazides, hydroxyamides, and even carbon-carbon bonds (174) (Fig. 2).

Whether any specific bond hydrolysis is involved in EZ remains to be determined. A histochemical study on the effect of α-CT in rabbit and cat zonules failed to detect changes in protein-bound NH_2, tryptophan, or tyrosine. Only a negativization of the PAS reaction was seen in cat zonules treated for 2 to 4 min in a 1:10,000 to 1:5,000 α-CT solution (68). In regard to substrate specificity, α-CT and TPS are believed to supplement each other.

The activity and stability of α-CT is increased by calcium (94,199). The desirability of using a high-calcium solution with α-CT is questionable, since

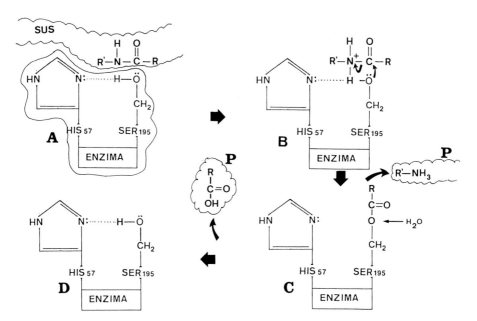

FIG. 2. Proposed mechanism of action of chymotrypsin. **A:** Free enzyme approaching substrate (SUS). The hydroxyl from Ser 195 and the imidazole from His 57 are linked by a hydrogen bond. **B:** The imidazole group from His 57 is now linked by a hydrogen bond with the substrate amine group, which results in orientation of the carbonyl group carbon in such a way that it can be attacked by the hydroxylic oxygen of Ser 195. **C:** The substrate acyl group is transferred to the Ser 195 hydroxyl. Acyl-chymotrypsin is formed and the amine-end peptide product (P) is released. **D:** The acyl-end peptide product (P) is finally released by means of the acceptance of an H_2O molecule, and free chymotrypsin is regenerated. Enzima, enzyme. (From refs. 28 and 45.)

this might extend the activity of the enzyme beyond the optimum for EZ and damage other ocular tissues.

Inhibitors of α-CT could be used to eliminate further activity of the enzyme once EZ has been accomplished. There are two kinds of inhibitors. Competitive antagonists, such as β-phenyl-propionic acid (BPPA) and chloramphenicol (21,90), combine in a reversible way with the catalytic locus of the enzyme and compete for it with the substrate. The degree of inhibition depends on the substrate/inhibitor concentration ratio. Noncompetitive antagonists such as di-isopropyl-fluorophosphate (DFP) (21) inactivate the enzyme, probably by binding to a different locus that is not affected by the concentration of the substrate. One percent epinephrine (but not 0.1%) was found to inactivate α-CT after 1 hr (46). Aqueous humor also has some inhibitory effects on α-CT (24,171).

Histology of EZ

Zinn's zonules, or suspensory ligament of the lens, is a vitreous-related structure corresponding to the embryonic tertiary vitreous and consisting of a series of fibers radially stretched between the equatorial zone of the lens capsule and the vitreal surface of the ciliary zone, including the pars plicata valleys and the pars plana.

According to its termination, anterior or posterior to the lens equator, two sheets of fibers can be described. However, these layers fuse together as the fibers pass backward through the ciliary valleys and to the pars plana. Some of them appear to arise from the vitreous base and anterior retina (44,87,120,198).

The size and shape of the fibers vary considerably, depending on the number of fibrils aggregated and the fixation and preparation method employed, their diameter ranging from 1 to 40 μm. Their ultrastructure shows a longitudinal array of fine fibrils, 60 to 75 (109) or 80 to 120 Å (87,158) thick in humans and monkeys, separated by less osmophilic ground substance (Fig. 3A). The ruthenium red staining found in monkey and rabbit suggests an acid glycosaminoglycan covering (183), but the composition of fibrils is still not determined. Evidence against the classical idea of a collagen composition is based on their resistance to collagenase (148), a different amino acid composition lacking hydroxyproline, and a low glycine content; cystine is present in significant amounts (198). Their birefringence is not inverted by phenol (10,172). The small diameter and lack of periodicity or banding (109)—or a short periodicity (110 to 180 Å) similar to vitreous fibrils (87) [490 Å banding in whole bundles of tightly packed fibrils (158)]—and their tritiated-glucose and amino acid uptake rate (studied in the developing mouse) (75) suggest a sort of procollagen. Other studies relate them to elastic fiber microfibrils (183,184).

The anchoring of zonules to the lens capsule and the internal limiting layer (ILM) of the ciliary zone is believed not to involve the underlying epithelial

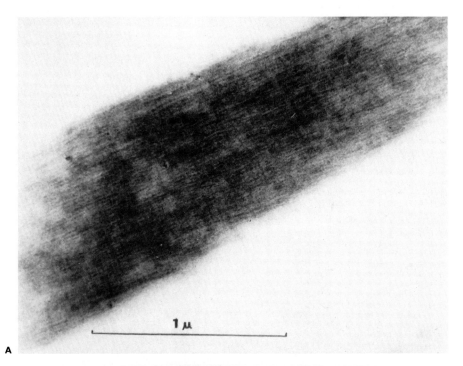

1 μ

A

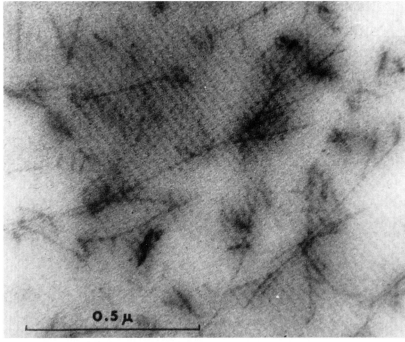

0.5 μ

B

FIG. 3. Transmission electron microscopic evidence of enzymatic fragmentation of zonular fibrils. **A:** Longitudinal section through an isolated human zonular fiber, showing its oriented fibrillar structure. Original magnification × 60,000. **B:** Isolated human zonular fiber after 5 min in 1:5,000 α-CT. Note the regularity of fibril fragmentation. Original magnification × 100,000. (From ref. 110 with permission.)

cells (87), although some fibrils have been traced to the intercellular spaces of both layers of the ciliary epithelium, where they may connect with the plasma membranes, and to the space between the basement membrane of the pigmented layer and the elastic tissue of Bruch's membrane (158,163,164). As the fibers approach the lens, they split into finer ones in a fan-vault arrangement [also found in their pars plana end (44)] before attaching to the equatorial lens capsule, that is crenated in this zone and covered by a pericapsular membrane or zonular lamella not present in the polar faces of the lens. This structure may be considered a part of the zonular attachment apparatus, having a fibrillar structure similar to zonular fibers (87,109).

The destructive effect of α-CT on human and monkey zonules has been demonstrated at the concentrations used in surgery (1:10,000 to 1:5,000, without difference between them), using optic (108), transmission (109), and surface (44) electron microscopy, and also by microcinematography (107).

Rupture of the zonules may be considered as following three steps:

1. Thinning and stretching of zonular fibers and dilatation of the ciliary ring (Fig. 4A). This increase in diameter, observed in human eyes *in vitro* and in monkey eyes *in vivo,* (108) may be responsible, together with the spheroidalization of the loosened lens, for the "coming forward" effect seen as a result of EZ. A "coagulation" effect on fiber attachments to lens capsule and on the zonular lamella may be seen by surface electron microscope (SEM) (44) (Fig. 5).

2. Rupture of the fibers takes place randomly and without detaching from the lens capsule or the ILM (Fig. 4B). Fibrils are fragmented to segments approximately 1,000 Å long (109). The uniformity of these fragments suggests a regular occurrence in the fibril protein of a peptide bond attacked by α-CT (Fig. 3B). The low-power appearance is that of a progressive loosening and rarefaction of the fibers, with the appearance of whitish corpuscles adhering to the remaining fibers or floating in the aqueous humor (107). They probably represent aggregates of fibril fragments.

3. In the late stages, the rupture and fragmentation process eventually leads to total disintegration of the zonules. However, the pars plana portion of the fibers may be relatively spared (44), and a few floppy fragments may remain attached to the lens or ciliary zone (Figs. 4C, 6).

No alterations of the vitreous anterior face, ciliary epithelium, ILM, or lens capsule have been observed (14,82,109) even after prolonged exposure to α-CT at the concentration mentioned. Only the zonular lamella over the equatorial lens capsule, whose structure resembles zonular fibers, is fragmented in a similar way. The hyalocapsular ligament of Wieger, commonly present in monkeys and younger humans, is not affected by α-CT (109).

Studies in other mammals (rabbit, sheep, cow, pig) (23,25,41,74,169) have also found facilitated ICCE after 1:5,000 α-CT. Dog zonules seem resistant to the enzyme (P. Amalric, personal communication). Rabbit zonules are composed of fibers 333 to 666 nm in diameter (average 470) (200), and fibrils

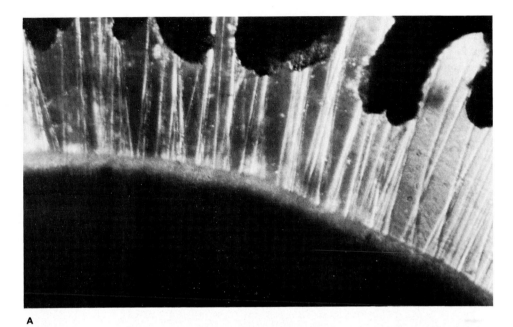

A

B

FIG. 4. Enzymatic zonulolysis in a human eye, after 0.5 ml 1:5,000 α-chymotrypsin in the posterior chamber, *in vitro*. Original magnification × 80. **A:** Before the instillation of the enzyme. **B:** One minute after the instillation. Note the "fluffy" appearance of the zonular fibers.

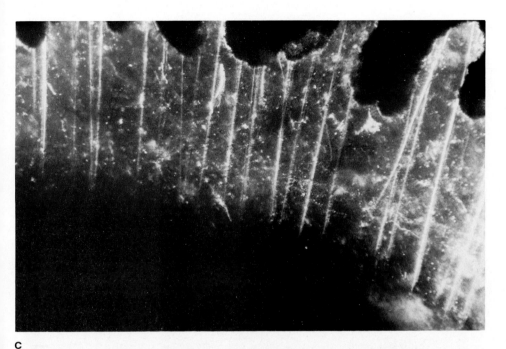

C

D

FIG. 4. Cont. C: One and a half minutes after the instillation. A few very thin fibers remain. Floating zonular detritus can be seen as bright particles. **D:** Two minutes after the instillation. Zonules have been completely dissolved by the enzyme.

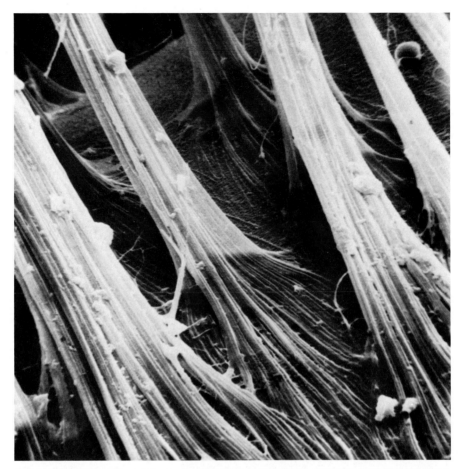

FIG. 5. Effect of α-CT on the zonular attachments to the lens equator. **A:** Surface electron-microscopic (SEM) close-up view of the lens equatorial ending of zonules. Note the overlapping of fibril endings, circumferential crinkling of zonular lamella, and polymorphous deposits.

similar to those found in humans (80 to 120 Å) (143), whereas cattle zonular fibers measure 400 to 666 nm in diameter (average 515) (200). Atypical 700-Å banded collagen-like fibrils are shown in a paper (84) as coming from bovine zonules. These fibers were *in vitro* (not under the normal physiologic tension) little affected by several proteolytic enzymes, including α-CT, TPS, elastase, and other proteases.

Although optic microscopic evidence of fiber rupture (rabbit) (169) and even spontaneous luxation and separation of the lens (rabbit, cow, sheep, 1:2,000 to 1:1,000 α-CT) (41) have been reported, several investigators denied the fiber fragmentation in these animals (23,25). The ultrastructure of rabbit zonules appeared unaffected by α-CT, collagenase, or hyaluronidase (184).

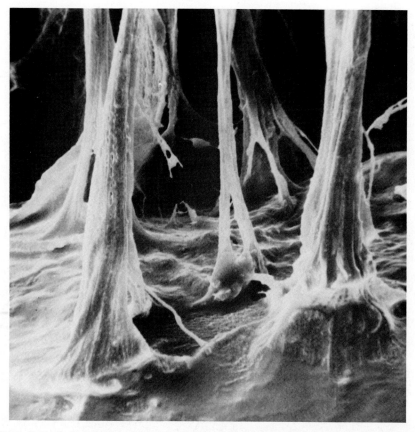

FIG. 5. Cont. B: Footplate appearance of coagulated zonular bundles as they lift away with the zonular lamella from the lens capsule, after α-CT treatment. (*Macaca fascicularis*). Original magnification × 1,400. (From ref. 44 with permission.)

The enzymatic facilitation of ICCE in this case would be explained as the consequence of a weakening effect in the fibers not manifested in morphologic changes.

Indications for EZ

The cataract extraction method should be selected according to type of cataract, the condition of the eye and the patient, the indication for surgery, and also the surgeon's personal preference. The following indication pattern will thus be personal, although a reasoned one.

EZ is the method of choice for ICCE. In congenital and juvenile cataracts (under 20 years) ICCE is contraindicated by several facts (low scleral rigidity, presence of Wieger's ligament, tendency to pupillary block, etc.) that produce

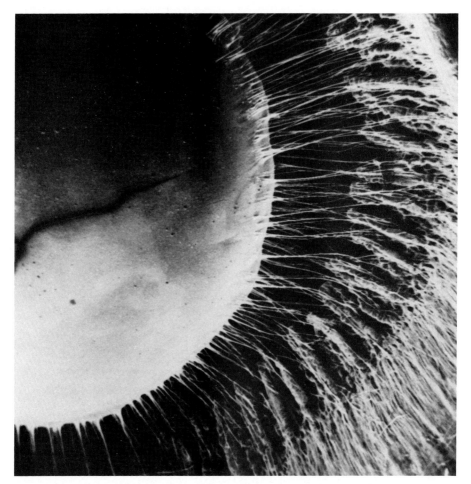

FIG. 6. Surface electron-microscopic (SEM) evidence of enzymatic zonulolysis. **A:** Posterior view of a 70-year-old human zonular system. Original magnification × 25.

a high risk of massive vitreous loss and other complications, and this cannot be obviated by the use of α-CT. EZ is particularly indicated for (a) young adults, (b) high myopia, (c) antecedent retinal detachment (in the same or fellow eye), and (d) intumescent cataract.

The advantages of EZ are evident in patients whose zonules are more resistant than in older ones. In high myopia and antecedent retinal detachment the minimization of retinal traction during ICCE is largely preferred in spite of a possible noxious effect of the enzyme on a weakened retina. The higher risk of capsule rupture in intumescent cataract is minimized by the EZ obviation of traction maneuvers. There are no truly absolute contraindications for EZ, although some of the following conditions might limit its use:

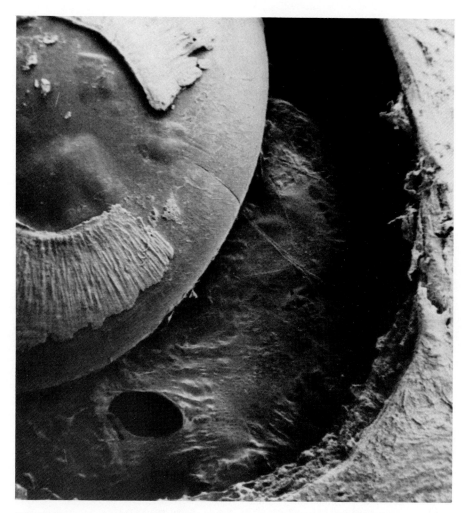

FIG. 6. Cont. B: Complete dissolution of the zonular system by α-CT. Bare lens equator, anterior hyaloid face (holed in the 5 o'clock meridian), and ciliary processes coated with coagulated material are exposed. (*Macaca fascicularis*). Original magnification × 30. (From ref. 44 with permission.)

1. *Allergic hypersensitivity to α-CT.* Although this is a most uncommon condition, patients who have previously had systemic α-CT (or in the fellow eye) could be sensitized. Allergy to systemic α-CT has been reported to consist of urticarial reactions and anaphylactic shock (177,194). However, intraocular injections of α-CT failed to elicit any local reactions in systemically sensitized guinea pigs (169). We have never seen such reactions in our practice, and in a patient operated on elsewhere and having secondary glaucoma in the second operated eye—which had been considered the consequence of an allergic

reaction to α-CT after its use in the first eye operation—we verified that it was actually due to a vitreous pupillary block.

2. *Vitreous in the anterior chamber.* This condition means a lack of integrity in the zonules, but the rest may be resistant. When the vitreous is fluid and easily fills the whole chamber, it will probably coat the zonules also and have an inhibitory effect on α-CT (16). Whether this is due to enzymatic antagonism or to simply avoiding the contact between the enzyme and its substrate is still to be determined. The lack of anterior hyaloid membrane and the fluidity of the vitreous would, however, facilitate the posterior penetration of the enzyme and increase the risk of retinal damage. Consistent vitreous may enter the anterior chamber through a restricted zonular defect, either preexisting or resulting from surgical manipulation. If the zonules still show a high resistance during lens extraction, which is most infrequent, α-CT may be carefully applied to the intact sector of the zonules.

3. *Corneal endothelial dystrophy.* The existence of *cornea guttata,* Fuchs's dystrophy, or other posterior corneal dystrophies has been considered a contraindication for EZ. In 1962, J. McLean (123) reported an unfortunate course of endothelial dystrophy in one eye after EZ-ICCE. Since we know that ICCE alone or any intraocular (particularly anterior segment) surgical procedure (apart from EZ) may produce a decrease in the endothelial cell population and thus decompensate a dystrophic cornea, it seems difficult to specifically blame α-CT for that complication.

Experimental work in rabbits showed an increase in endothelium mitotic rate (which is a reaction to noxious stimulus in that animal) after the injection of 1:5,000 α-CT into the anterior chamber, subsequently rinsed with a 0.9% NaCl solution, 3 min later. One-third of the animals developed transient corneal edema. However, *the injection of the saline solution alone produced almost the same results* (169), as has been proved lately (50). As we mentioned in previous chapters, irrigating solutions and drug vehicles are of primary importance in evaluating side effects attributed to intraocularly applied drugs.

Our personal experience with EZ in cases of compensated cornea guttata and posterior polymorphous corneal dystrophy has been the absence of any adverse reaction attributable to α-CT. On the contrary, EZ combined with the Smith's or cryoprobe sliding methods for lens delivery reduces endothelial trauma to its minimum. For additional protection, the endothelium can be previously coated with a thin layer of sodium hyaluronate (Healon®). No progression of corneal endothelial dystrophy following EZ has been observed by other authors (83).

4. *Lack of a conjunctival flap.* α-CT has been reported to induce a delay in wound healing (15,20,38,125,189,195) and thus increase the risk of postoperative hypotony and flat chamber. No experimental work has confirmed that clinical impression (18,23,33,54), and other authors deny this effect (30,161). A number of surgeons use EZ successfully with corneal incisions. Even crediting the delayed-healing hypothesis, the double-plane incision (corneoscleral plus

conjunctival flap) gives us security in the event of a filtering wound. However, when a corneal incision without a conjunctival flap is indicated—e.g., when a filtering bleb is to be spared or when a too corneal incision has been performed accidentally—it might be better not to use the enzyme.

Technique of Enzymatic Zonulolysis

We should consider three steps (16):

Preparation of the α-CT Solution

The apparent zonular specificity of α-CT is not only a consequence of the biochemical aspects of its activity but also depends on its *concentration* at the site of action and the length of *time* it acts before it is inhibited, destroyed, or washed away. The optimum concentration is around 1:5,000. Greater dilutions may be ineffective. Greater concentrations do not improve EZ, and they increase the danger of damaging other ocular structures. The duration of action may be controlled by simply irrigating the ocular chambers. The use of an enzymatic inhibitor might not be exempt from danger to intraocular structures and is not necessary, since aqueous humor has α-CT-inhibitory activity (24,171), and washing the chamber eliminates the residual enzyme and zonular debris.

Another factor in enzyme activity is *temperature*. The optimum for α-CT would be 37°C, but room temperature is, for practical purposes, almost as good.

Special attention must be given to intraocular irrigating solutions, which are the vehicles for intraocular intraoperative drugs such as acetylcholine and α-CT. Sterile isotonic physiologic saline (0.9% NaCl) has been shown to cause endothelial degenerative changes and swelling in rabbit and monkey corneas. Improved solutions containing pH buffers and other physiologic cations (K^+, Ca^{2+}) such as lactated Ringer's or balanced salt solution (BSS) may still produce corneal changes if continuously perfused for periods of time longer than 1 hr. The addition of 0.5 μM adenosine and 0.3 μM reduced glutathione (GSH), as in BSS-Plus or glutathione bicarbonated Ringer's (GBR), prevented stromal swelling and ultrastructural endothelial changes throughout a 5-hr perfusion time (50).

Our experience with *artificial aqueous humor* (HAA), a commercial solution similar to BSS, is clinically excellent, although in EZ-ICCE the corneal endothelium is exposed to a small amount of it and for a short period of time. A fresh solution must be used, since the enzyme loses its activity within a few hours after being dissolved (46). The calcium content of the dissolving solution is a factor that must be considered since we know that

1. Calcium is an α-CT enzymatic activity enhancer (94). Whether this is desirable, depending on its influence in both EZ efficiency and the risk of

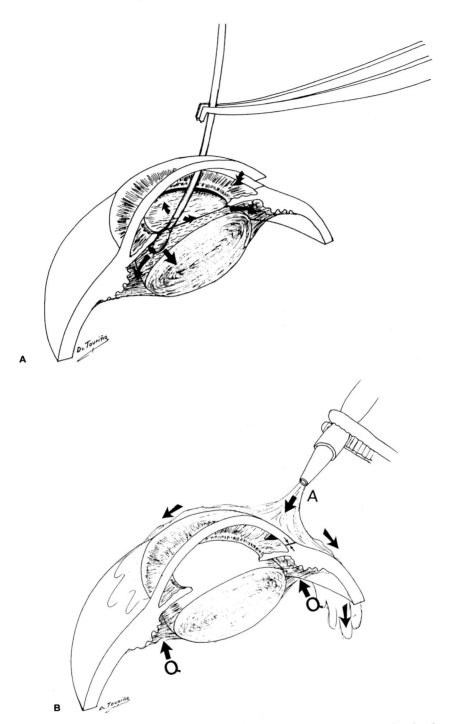

FIG. 7. Enzymatic zonulolysis technique. **A:** Instillation of the enzyme into the posterior chamber of the eye. The cannula is secured by the forceps, and the lens is slightly depressed to avoid trauma to the posterior epithelium of the iris. **B:** External irrigation (A) immediately follows the introduction of the enzyme (Q), to minimize its effect on the corneoscleral wound.

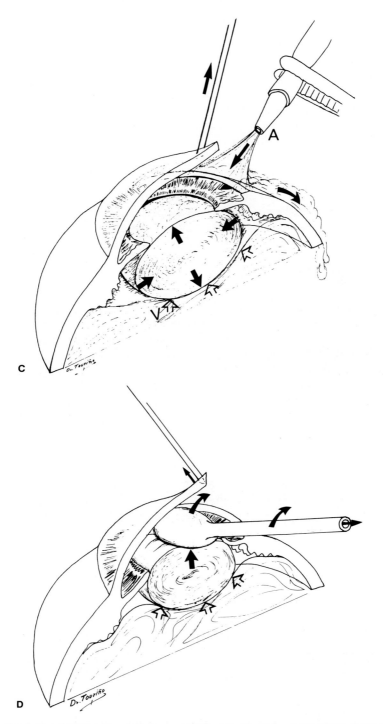

FIG. 7. Cont. C: Internal washout of the remaining enzyme and zonular debris follows the accomplishment of zonulolysis, which may be indicated by a "coming forward" tendency and spheroidalization of the lens. V, anterior vitreous face. **D:** Open-sky extraction with the erisiphake tumbling maneuver. This technique allows a progressive separation of the lens capsule from the anterior vitreous face, and lens diameter is slightly reduced as some anterior cortex prolapses into the erisiphake vault.

damaging other ocular structures, has not been determined. The calcium content of aqueous humor, HAA, or BSS is negligible at this point.

2. Calcium stabilizes the α-CT solution and thus extends the time of maintained activity of the dissolved enzyme (199).

3. Calcium-free medium has been shown to produce corneal changes similar to those obtained with physiologic saline (0.9% NaCl) perfusion over 1 hr (50,98).

The syringe and cannula must be clean, thoroughly rinsed with distilled water (since traces of detergents or alcohol may inactivate the enzyme and damage intraocular structures), and autoclave sterilized. External sterilization of the α-CT vials should be avoided because the enzyme might be inactivated by the accidental penetration of some of the sterilizing agents into the vial.

Application of the α-CT Solution

The introduction of the enzyme must be carried out precisely, as close as possible to the zonula (directly into the posterior chamber), and in the operatory time preceding the lens extraction. After the incision, iridectomy, and hemostasis have been completed, the anterior chamber must be free of blood; if present, it should be expelled by irrigation, or with a marten-hair brush in the case of adherent clots.

The syringe is held in one hand, and the base of the attached cannula is steadied with a forceps held in the other hand. To avoid trauma to the iris and dispersion of pigment, an olive-tipped cannula is preferred, and a slight depression of the lens is made while injecting (Fig. 7A). The danger of luxating the lens is minimal, since this maneuver requires less pressure than grasping the lens with a capsule forceps. Only 0.5 ml of the enzyme solution is required. For uniform action, injection should be slow and directed to each quadrant; for best reaching the upper quadrants it is convenient to pass the cannula through the peripheral iridectomy. Contact of the cannula with the corneal endothelium is prevented by having an assistant raise the cornea slightly, or by the prelocation of a sodium hyaluronate retrocorneal cushion.

Irrigation of the Incision and the Anterior Chamber

Immediately after the injection of the enzyme solution, the incision is irrigated with HAA or BSS to prevent prolonged contact of the wound edges with α-CT. If EZ is used with a corneal incision without a conjunctival flap, the incision should be irrigated simultaneously with the injection of the enzyme solution into the posterior chamber. Contact of the corneal wound edges with the enzyme is thus reduced to a minimum (Fig. 7B).

The duration of action of α-CT is varied according to the case and degrees of zonulolysis desired. In standard cases *2 min* is sufficient. When an intumescent cataract is present, this time may be doubled to minimize the need of traction. The lens can be seen assuming a spherical shape and coming forward as the zonulolysis becomes complete. However, these signs are often masked by hypotony, particularly under general anesthesia conditions. Once the α-CT action time has elapsed, the anterior chamber is irrigated (with HAA or BSS) in order to remove the remaining enzyme (Fig. 7C). This washing effect is completed after the lens removal (Fig. 7D) by the intracameral irrigation with acetylcholine.

Side Effects and Complications Attributed to EZ

Since EZ is only part of a surgical procedure (ICCE), the complications observed in EZ-ICCE must be compared to non-EZ ICCE in order to estimate the risks specifically attributable to EZ. Among these, we must differentiate between three possible agents involved: (a) the enzymatic activity of α-CT; (b) the toxicity of the solution components (50,180); and (c) the mechanical hazards related to the instillating media (the cannula, the turbulence created by the solution).

From the literature that has appeared following the introduction of EZ (167,168) and from the experience accumulated during the past 25 years, we may conclude that *the use of α-CT following the described EZ technique does not increase significantly the rate of intraoperative and postoperative complications of ICCE,* and *actually diminishes* the appearance of some of them. However, there have been a number of side effects, such as the following:

1. Damage to ocular tissues, including corneal changes (endothelial degeneration, swelling); iris pigment dispersion and atrophy; heterochromia; intraoperative miosis and paralytic mydriasis; lens capsule rupture; anterior hyaloid membrane rupture and vitreous loss; retinal degeneration and retinal detachment.
2. Decreased hemostasis and postoperative hyphema.
3. Delayed wound healing and related complications, such as postoperative hypotony and subconjunctival filtration; delayed re-formation and loss of anterior chamber; iris prolapse and anterior synechiae; reopening of the wound.
4. Secondary glaucoma (transient enzymatic glaucoma).

Effect of EZ on Ocular Tissues

Most experimental studies on the effect of α-CT on ocular tissues have failed to find any significant undesirable histopathologic change attributable to the EZ use of the enzyme (82,92,109,135). We have already discussed the influence of the irrigating solutions and mechanical trauma (including contact with the cannula) in the described corneal changes, whereas α-CT seems to produce little harm to the endothelium by itself. However, according to its protease activity, the enzyme can be expected to attack stromal protein if exposed to it, as has been shown in rabbits, by intracorneal injections of α-CT (6).

Iris changes such as intraoperative miosis (20) are most probably attributable to mechanical irritation (rubbing) and reflex endogenous release of miotic agents such as substance P and prostaglandins and not to a specific effect of α-CT. *In vitro* exposure of the iris to the enzyme over 20 hr produced relaxation of the sphincter (82), which would be in agreement with the observation by Joaquín Barraquer of an immediate and permanent paralytic mydriasis after the application of 1:500 α-CT in a previously blind eye, during the trial series presented in his first communication on EZ (14). However, M. J. Roper-Hall (165) reported in 1963 a series of 17 cases accidentally operated on with 1:100 α-CT. No significant increase in the number of complications was observed (as compared to a 1:5,000 α-CT group). None developed paralytic mydriasis (165).

Iris pigment dispersion (20) and atrophy, or postoperative partial heterochromia are also due mainly to mechanical trauma: rubbing of the cannula or other instruments against the posterior epithelium of the iris, or the turbulence created by injecting the solution too fast. *In vitro* exposure of the iris to α-CT had variable results, and depigmentation was found only after a very long immersion time (20 hr) (82).

Although F. Clement (41) found in 1959 a 10-fold increase in sheep and cow lens capsule fragility to vacuum suction (twofold in rabbit) after treatment with 1:2,000 to 1:1,000 α-CT, histologic and ultrastructural studies have failed to demonstrate any enzyme-induced lens capsule changes (23,109). Our clinical experience indicates that EZ has no effect on the capsule itself, and on the contrary, the elimination of traction maneuvers reduces risk of mechanical rupture of the capsule. In fact, the reduction of incidence of accidental extracapsular extraction was the most statistically significant advantage of EZ found by the AAOO Committee on the use of α-CT (190), apart from the facilitation of cataract extraction (174).

A similar argument could apply to hyaloid integrity and vitreous loss (20,55,134,189). Although some authors reported an increased incidence of vitreous loss after EZ-ICCE during the years immediately following its introduction, histologic studies (109) and long-term experience have shown that α-CT does not affect the anterior hyaloid membrane, even after long periods of exposure. Again, the obviation of pressure and traction maneuvers minimizes the danger of mechanical hyaloid rupture and therefore of vitreous loss.

The effect of α-CT on the retina was experimentally studied by A. E. Maumenee (119) in 1959 and also by several European authors (85,156). Maumenee found that "a very tangential injection" of 0.5 ml 1:5,000 α-CT through the sclera, choroid, and retina into the rabbit vitreous body produced, after 5 to 15 days, various degrees of retinal degeneration and atrophy—

mainly related to the supporting structures of the retina, with relative sparing of the neural elements—"limited to one side of the eye" (presumably the side of the injection), whereas the opposite side retained its normal architecture. Introduction of fresh human retinas in 1:500 α-CT solution for 20 min failed to elicit any pathologic change.

It is understandable that the local application of a proteolytic enzyme close to a tissue results in damage to the tissue's proteins. In this chapter, three facts must be pointed out: (a) only the rabbit retina was affected, (b) the exposure period was extremely long compared to EZ, and (c) only the area of the retina surrounding the injection site was damaged, suggesting that the vitreous might be a barrier against the diffusion of the enzyme, in accordance with our impression that vitreous coating the zonules may inhibit EZ (16). Considering all this, together with our clinical experience, we may conclude that it is very unlikely that the use of α-CT following the described EZ technique affects the retina in the majority of the cases. On the contrary, EZ diminishes the risk of retinal detachment secondary to intraoperative tractions on the ora serrata, vitreous base, or retina.

Effect of α-CT on Hemostasis

Systemic (intravenous) administration of α-CT to several animals has produced a shock syndrome that has been associated with hemorrhagic pathologic changes and a prolongation in bleeding time, probably due to a depletory action on blood fibrinogen. Using fast intravenous injection, the median lethal dose (LD_{50}) ranges from 24,000 U/kg in the rabbit to 85,000 U/kg in the mouse (80,182). Attempts at human systemic use of α-CT have never been very encouraging (177,194).

In his first series of about 1,000 EZ-ICCEs, José Ignacio Barraquer (20) in 1961 commented on his impression (not statistically proved) of a higher incidence of postoperative hyphema in the older patient group, and also cases of retinal hemorrhages "opposite to the irrigation point." These complications were then attributed to the initial use of too high a concentration of the enzyme and did not reappear in subsequent series, nor in the Joaquín Barraquer series. In the AAOO Committee series the number of hyphemas (6% in 107, 4% in 481) and intraoperative hemorrhage (2% in 107, 1% in 481) were relatively higher in the first (younger) group, but the total was considered not significantly larger than expected for non-EZ ICCE (190). Subsequent clinical experience has confirmed that α-CT as used in EZ does not cause hemorrhagic complications.

EZ and Delayed Wound Healing

The first postoperative complications that consistently seemed to implicate α-CT was a delay in wound closure following EZ-ICCE, as manifested through different accidents such as reopening of the wound, subconjunctival filtration or "edema", hypotony, delayed re-formation and loss of the anterior chamber, formation of anterior synechiae, and iris prolapse (15,20,38,125,189,195). Further clinical studies specifically oriented to determine the role of α-CT in these complications failed to find a conclusive implication of the enzyme (30,161,187). On the other hand, all experimental work failed to demonstrate an α-CT-induced delayed-cicatrization mechanism (18,23,33,54). It was also noted that most of the reopening cases lacked a complete conjunctival flap.

Improvements in the surgical techniques were recommended (15), stressing the necessity of obtaining a good conjunctival flap—even having somehow to scleralize the incision—irrigating the wound just after the injection of α-CT, and making the incision closing as waterproof as possible (without inducing corneal astigmatism), generalizing the use of the operating microscope, increasing the number of corneoscleral stitches (7 to 9 instead of 3), and using the double-step closure with the conjunctival flap. These modifications of the techniques have almost ruled out this kind of complication, dependent or not on EZ.

Secondary Glaucoma After EZ

In 1964, R. E. Kirsch (100) first described a transient hypertension in the early postoperative course of EZ-ICCE patients. This would later be called "transient enzymatic glaucoma" (71). Controversy followed, since other authors failed to find that hypertension (17) and actually found a more frequent postoperative hypotension (72). This could be due to the different techniques used in the application of the enzyme, the subsequent irrigation of the anterior chamber, and the wound closure.

In 1971, D. Anderson (5) showed in monkeys (*Aotus*) the transient occlusion of the trabeculum by an important apposition of microspherules, presumed to be aggregates of fragmented zonular material, after the closed posterior chamber injection of 1:100 α-CT, not followed by lens extraction nor anterior chamber perfusion. Previous histologic reports have failed to find trabecular damage due to the enzyme. Lately, D. Pita-Salorio (150) showed that the apposition of these spherules was loose and easily prevented by irrigating the anterior chamber following EZ.

In May 1977, J. L. Ruiz Bulumar (166) reported a revision of 833 cases of ICCE performed at our institution from June 1974 to February 1977. All cases presenting ocular hypertension previous to surgery had been excluded from the study. The postoperative intraocular pressure, averaged for each eye in three mean values for the periods covering (a) the first 3 postoperative days, (b) days 4 to 10, and (c) day 15 were compared for α-CT (92.6%) and classical ICCE (7.4%) groups. The percentage of cases with hypertension was similar in both groups for each period, and the decreasing rate throughout the three periods was rapid and almost parallel (hypertension in α-CT patients: (a) 35%,

(b) 16%, and (c) 4.4%; hypertension in non-α-CT patients: (a) 23%, (b) 15%, and (c) 4.9%) (166).

We may conclude that transient postoperative ocular hypertension is present in both groups. The hermeticity of microsurgical wound closure is certainly a pathogenetic factor in this benign and transient complication of ICCE. The possible pathogenetic influence of EZ can be minimized by proper irrigation of the chamber after zonulolysis, as described in the original technique. This possible iatrogenic effect of α-CT can be overlooked in view of its proved advantages.

Alternative Enzymes

Following the introduction of α-CT/EZ, several papers on the relative efficiency of various enzymes on the zonules were published. R. M. Fasanella (53) presented to the Third International Course of Ophthalmology of the Instituto Barraquer (Barcelona, 1961) his experimental work. Comparing the action of lysozime (muramidase), hyaluronidase, *Bacillus subtilis* protease, 0.2% heparin, and TPS on the rabbit zonules, only TPS was effective in zonulolysis (as effective or better than α-CT). *Bacillus subtilis* protease 1:1,000 was effective on bovine zonules but in rabbits only produced corneal damage (53).

In another study (53) carried out in rhesus monkeys (*Macaca mulatta*), different brands of α-CT (Chymotrase®, Chymenon®) and δ-CT were found equally effective. Other agents, such as 20% EDTA (Endrate Disodium®, Versenate®), 1:5,000 fibrinolysin plus desoxyrribonuclease (Elase®), collagenase, and pepsin, produced complete zonulolysis in times ranging from 2.5 to 26.5 min but produced total vitreous loss or vitreous presentation in several cases. Effects of desoxyribonuclease alone oscillated between none and the total exit of the lens with the vitreous, a response that could also be obtained in the saline controls. Hyaluronidase (Wydase®) and Adolph's Meat Tenderizer™ had no effect. TPS was not tested. Finally, ficin, a strong proteinase extracted from *Ficus,* widely used in industry, was able to produce complete zonulolysis in monkeys in 50 to 70 sec when used in a 1:5,000 solution and in 14 sec when used in a 1:1,000 solution. Effects on the cornea could not be assessed (53).

Several authors proposed the clinical use of TPS and claimed superiority of this enzyme over α-CT (34,52,86,89). However, it is questionable whether a stronger activity is an advantage or may lead to greater incidence of adverse side effects (155). Unfortunately, very little work on TPS has been done since. In a more recent paper, brinolase, a fibrinolytic enzyme, was found more effective than α-CT for EZ in young monkeys (154).

UROKINASE

Management of spontaneously unresolving intraocular hemorrhages, a relatively common cause of blindness—particularly vitreous hemorrhages, whose incidence in general population was calculated in 0.05% to 0.35% in developed countries (58)—classically consisted of a great variety of conservative treatments having in common their poor results. Although surgical removal of opaque vitreous was performed as early as 1890 (56), only a few surgeons entered this field (19,122,137) until the introduction of micromechanized pars plana vitrectomy (116). Today, vitreous hemorrhage is one of the main indications for vitrectomy. However, this is a complex and difficult technique, not free of complications and danger to eye structures (69,124,128,133). The use of fibrinolytic enzymes such as urokinase (UKN) appears as a biochemical alternative to the mechanical approach to these hemorrhages.

Basic Aspects

The dynamics of blood clot formation and resolution greatly depend on the tissue in which they take place. According to radioisotope studies (160), resolution of a vitreous hemorrhage after the clot is formed takes place in four stages: (a) lysis of fibrin; (b) free diffusion of red blood cells within the vitreous; (c) phagocytosis of red blood cells and hemolysis; and (d) reabsorption of red cell breakdown products.

Fibrinolysis, which is the first step, is normally the final consequence of the activation, by a humoral or tissue factor (plasminogen activator), of the plasminogen-plasmin (profibrinolysin-fibrinolysin) system (7). Plasmin is a proteolytic enzyme, able to digest cross-linked fibrin by attacking peptide bonds involving lysine. It is also active against several humoral coagulation factors, including prothrombin, fibrinogen, and factors V, VIII, and XII. Its effectiveness against a formed fibrin clot (as in a tissue medium) seems to be much higher than in circulating plasma (102).

Hemorrhages in fluid vitreous (retrovitreal or retrohyaloid space) usually resorb more readily than those occurring in formed vitreous gel. This could be due to the dilution blood undergoes before clotting in the first situation (140), whereas the blood trapped in vitreous gel will clot faster and without dilution. Moreover, the presence of a collagen fibril matrix in the vitreous gel may initiate platelet aggregation and membrane formation independently from fibrin deposition (43).

Although a vitreous plasminogen activator (VPA) has been demonstrated (66) in normal human vitreous, its fibrinolytic activity is much lower than the retina's. This fact could also explain the faster resolution of retrovitreal space hemorrhages in contact with, or close to the retinal activator (141).

Experimental work on methods for spontaneous resolution of vitreous hemorrhage have included physical [diathermy (57,67,192), ultrasound (22), X-rays (91), laser (27)], chemical or pharmacologic [surfactants such as saponin or phenylhydrazine, urea (31), ACTH, cortisone (173)] and enzymatic—EZ was discovered as the accidental result of an experiment on the fibrinolytic use of α-CT agents [TPS (31,36,130), hyaluronidase (147,151,173), collagenase

(31,149), streptokinase (STKN) (31,114,173)]. Only STKN-activated plasminogen (114) showed any promising results. Since unresolving vitreous hemorrhage may be due to defective VPA activity, it appears reasonable to use an alternative plasminogen activator. However, STKN produced severe chorioretinitis and retinal necrosis when injected into the rabbit vitreous (31,173), and it is also known to be antigenic to man.

UKN is a naturally occurring direct plasminogen activator present in human urine. MacFarlane and Pilling (115) first recognized in 1947 the fibrinolytic activity of normal urine, which was then related to its ability to activate the plasmin system (196), due to the presence of a specific activator (UKN) (8).

UKN was seen to concentrate 100-fold in urine foam, which made it possible to prepare it in pharmacologic quantities (35). It is chemically characterized as a colorless, water-soluble protein that, when pure, is fairly stable within a large temperature and pH range (152). It is a nonhomogeneous proteolytic enzyme; under certain conditions it can be separated into four different components. Its molecular weight is relatively low (53,000), and according to its activity it can be measured in Ploug units (P.U.) or CTA units (CTA U.)—1 P.U. approximately equals 1.43 CTA U. As a human-species-specific protein, it is not antigenic to man, nor is it toxic or pyrogenic (4).

UKN's ability to dissolve blood clots is by direct (first-order kinetics) activation of plasminogen into plasmin, probably by splitting lysine and arginine bonds. It has greater affinity for gel-phase plasminogen within a thrombus than for soluble plasma plasminogen. UKN cannot attack plasminogen-free fibrin except at very high concentration, possibly due to an unspecific proteolytic activity (101).

Animal studies of the ocular toxicity of UKN showed that 12,500 to 25,000 P.U. may induce degenerative changes in monkey (103) and rabbit retina (142). The antigenicity of human UKN to these animals can explain the uveitic reaction and subsequent retinal changes as an immune reaction to xenogenic antigen, which is not to be expected in man. However, early postoperative hypopyon and uveitis, without retinal involvement, is a common feature after clinical intravitreal use of this enzyme (37,88,136). Plasmin itself and fibrin degradation products (121,179) are known to be able to activate complement-mediated chemotaxis (193) or directly activate leukocytes (131); this partially explains UKN-induced uveitis in man. Furthermore, leukocyte lysosomal protease may attack fibrin and help in clot lysis (Fig. 8), apart from the phagocytic role of these cells in clot resolution.

Injection of autologous whole blood into the rabbit vitreous (known to have an extremely low fibrinolytic activity) was followed by a mild macrophage reaction, and very few polymorphs were found (77). The hemorrhagic vitreous would thus be not only defective in VPA activity (61) but also in the cellular elements that participate in further phases of clot resolution. Red blood cells may remain intact in the vitreous gel after fibrin has been degraded unless they are removed by macrophage endocytosis (59).

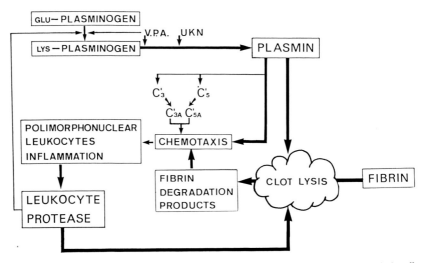

FIG. 8. Mechanism of urokinase-induced clot lysis. Flow chart of possible synergistic effects between plasminogen activator and leukocytic activity in promoting clot lysis. (Modified from ref. 65).

UKN may have a double effect in the vitreous, both leading to clot lysis: plasmin activation and inflammation (chemotaxis). According to Forrester and Williamson (65), UKN-accelerated clearance of vitreous clots, as assessed in rabbits, would be explained by a synergistic action of both effects; whereas in human vitreous hemorrhages, where the presence of fibrin is presumed but seldom detected (60,88), the inflammatory (chemotactic) effect in clot lysis would be more important than fibrinolysis itself.

On the other hand, the increasing presence of the various cellular types involved in inflammation might be a factor in clot fibrous organization. It has been shown that intravitreal injection of leukocytes (106), lymphocytes (126), or platelets (43) (each alone), or whole blood (77), can produce the formation of cellular or acellular membranes. However, the fibrous component of these hematogenous vitreous membranes appears to be the result of cortical vitreous collagen fibril displacement, rather than newly formed collagen (77). True fibrous membrane formation requires the presence of fibroblasts in the vitreous, which is unlikely to occur unless a clearly severe injury or chronic retinal disease is present, a less reproducible feature in animal models but frequent in human vitreous hemorrhage.

Clinical Aspects

UKN was first clinically tried as a fibrinolytic agent in management of hyphema (145), pulmonary (188) and cerebral (113) embolism, and a retinal vascular occlusion (1,3,73,111,129). Williamson and Forrester (197), and shortly afterward, Dugmore and Raichand (49), first reported in 1972 its favorable effect in a case of a diabetic vitreous hemorrhage previously unresolved for more than 4 years. After the intravitreal injection of 5,000 P.U. of UKN in 1.5 ml distilled water, vision ultimately restored from light perception to 6/12 (62).

Use of UKN in the Management of Vitreous Hemorrhages

Following the first experiences noted above, UKN was tested in several centers around the world (37,63,96,118,136,162) and subsequently claimed to be at least as successful or better than vitrectomy in management of vitreous hemorrhages. It would also have a lower rate of (milder) complications. Its only disadvantage would be the high cost of the purified enzyme, although neither vitrectomy can be considered economic.

The visual results reported to date are summarized in Table 1. Almost two-thirds of the eyes (99 out of 160) had improved vision, although only 68 eyes (42.5%) had an objective improvement, consisting of two or more Snellen lines. Improvement of only one Snellen line or its equivalent (i.e., from light perception to hand movement, or from that to finger counting) was considered

TABLE 1. Visual results from published UKN series

Study	Eyes	Improved		Unchanged	Worse
		Objective	Subjective		
USA					
Burnley, 1973 (49)	3	3	—	—	—
UK					
Glasgow, 1974 (62)	11	10	—	1	—
1976[a]	11	8	—	3	—
1982 (65)	10	8	2	—	—
London, 1974 (40)	15	2	—	11	2
1974 (88)	18	2	1	15	—
Spain					
Oviedo, 1975 (96)	5	5	—	—	—
Barcelona, 1984 (118)	33	12	16	5	—
Australia					
Melbourne, 1977 (37)	32[b]	10	9	10[c]	3[c]
Denmark					
Aarhus, 1978 (32)	13	1	2	10[d]	—
Japan, 1980 (136)	9	7	1	1	—
Totals	160	68 (42.5%)	31 (19.4%)	46 (28.8%)	5 (3.1%)

[a] J. Williamson, personal communication to G. Crock.
[b] Two additional cases were lost to follow-up.
[c] In a further report (44) one of the "unchanged" eyes developed a cataract and worsened vision (prior to its extraction).
[d] In six eyes the vision prior to UKN was reduced to light perception with bad light projection. Maximum follow-up time was 5 months.

only subjective. Furthermore, several authors report a certain degree of vitreous clearing, even in cases in which visual acuity did not improve. Although "subjective improvement" is difficult to quantify, it may have a noticeable influence in a patient's quality of life (44).

As a less aggressive alternative to vitrectomy, UKN "should become the first line of attack in vitreous haemorrhages, vitrectomy reserved for those patients who fail to respond," Chapman-Smith and Crock (37) concluded. However, other studies reported unfavorable results—mainly consisting of no improvement rather than worsening—and suggested "that this use of UKN is not indicated in the management of long-standing vitreous haemorrhage" (40), and that "in most cases in which an improvement in vision has been reported, the improvement is due to the aspiration of this debris and not to any specific action of UKN" (88). This discrepancy, based on the results obtained, might be due to (a) different patient selection criteria, including etiology, nature of the hemorrhage, and other conditions that affect final visual acuity, such as the functional status of the retina and the presence of vitreous membranes, or neo-vascularization; (b) differences in the technique employed; (c) different follow-up and subsequent treatment.

The distribution of treated patients according to etiology follows a pattern similar to the general distribution of massive vitreous hemorrhage etiology (26,93,132), diabetes being the main cause. As summarized in Table 2, best results are seen in traumatic hemorrhages, followed by hypertensive hemorrhages or those secondary to retinal vein occlusion; diabetes and Eales' disease have the lowest improvement rate. However, the etiological distribution does not vary significantly between the "good" and "bad" result reports (Table 3).

Other conditions that affect visual prognosis, such as retina function or membrane formation, are difficult to assess preoperatively unless specific exploration is done. When electrophysiologic tests are not available, evaluation of light projection may be a valuable guide. Several cases among the reported "negative" (unchanged) actually had preoperatively only light perception with bad light projection (32,88).

TABLE 2. *Vitreous hemorrhage etiology and UKN visual improvement*

Eyes	Diagnoses	Total improved[a]	Subjective[a]	<0.5	≥0.5
61	Diabetes	28 (45.9%)	14 (50%)	10 (35.7%)	4 (14.2%)
20	Hypertension and retinal vein occlusion	13 (65%)	2 (15.4%)	4 (30.8%)	7 (53.8%)
12	Trauma	10 (83.3%)	—	2 (20%)	8 (80%)[b]
8	Eales' disease	3 (37.5%)	1 (33.3%)	2 (66.7%)	—

[a] The 9 "subjective improvement" cases in the 1977 Melbourne series were reported without specifying their etiology.
[b] Three of these eyes reached a 6/6 vision.
From refs. 37, 40, 64, 88, 96, 119.

TABLE 3. *Etiology distribution in published UKN series*

Study	Cases	Diabetes[a]	HT-RVO[a]	Trauma[a]	Eales'[a]	Other
Glasgow, 1974 (64)	7	2 (2)	4 (4)	1 (1)	—	—
London, 1974 (40)	15	12 (1)	1 (0)	1 (0)	1 (1)	—
1974 (88)	18	10 (1)	5 (0)	—	1 (0)	1 retinal detachment (0) 1 unknown (1)
Oviedo, 1975 (96)	5	1 (1)	2 (2)	2 (2)	—	—
Melbourne, 1977 (37)	27	15 (6)[b]	5 (3)[b]	2 (1)[b]	3[b]	2 overanticoagulated[b]
Aarhus, 1978 (32)	13	8 (3)	—	4 (0)	1 (0)	—
Barcelona, 1984 (118)	33	27 (17)	3 (3)	6 (6)	3 (2)	—

[a] Numbers in brackets indicate improved vision cases.
[b] "Subjective improvement" cases with etiology not reported.
HT-RVO, Hypertension–retinal vein occlusion.

Intravitreal persistence of blood may lead to permanent retinal damage through iron intoxication of photoreceptors (9,39). Electroretinogram (ERG) and electro-oculogram (EOG) changes may be detected as soon as 6 weeks after bleeding (96,97). Membrane formation and secondary retinal detachment—another cause of somber prognosis—are unpredictable. These facts should encourage early use of UKN, whereas most cases reported were operated on after at least 6 months of evolution. Ultrasonography including B-scan should be performed routinely to detect previous retinal detachment or vitreous fibrosis. Since UKN will not attack *true* fibrous membranes, these patients are direct candidates for vitrectomy, although other less invasive methods recently proposed, such as high-intensity focused ultrasound (42) and intravitreal corticosteroids (185,186), may be promising alternative approaches.

The simplicity and safety of the UKN technique is one of its advantages over vitrectomy. It commonly includes local anesthesia, a small conjunctival flap, and a 2-mm sclerotomy over the temporal pars plana, with a preplaced mattress suture. Diathermy may be used for a safer penetration (118). The amount of UKN used ranges from 2,500 (40) to 55,000 P.U. (37). Although in the first report the enzyme was dissolved in 1.5 ml distilled water (197), up to 25,000 P.U. can be dissolved in 0.2 to 0.3 ml (88). However, even such a small quantity can produce a severe IOP rise when injected. Preoperative hypotensors such as intravenous acetazolamide (64) or osmotic agents (96) have been recommended. Most surgeons first perform an anterior chamber paracentesis and aqueous humor extraction. The speed of injection is also a factor to be considered. When possible, papillar vessels should be monitored for vascular embarrassment (37). The preplaced suture should be adjusted while the cannula is withdrawn to avoid regurgitation or vitreous presentation.

Holmes-Sellors and associates (88) reported that vitreous aspiration and saline injection allowed fundus visualization in one eye but without any improvement in visual acuity. However, following the technique described above, it is unlikely that "aspiration of debris" or mechanical disruption of the vitreous is the cause of improvement.

Follow-up time is an important parameter when comparing results. Although immediate vitreous clearing and "clot explosion" is a feature seen occasionally since the first intravenous fibrinolysin trials (F. Lithgow, *personal communication*), it is advisable to wait at least 3 months before evaluating the outcome of UKN treatment. Sometimes visual recovery takes place very late after UKN. One of the hypertensive patients in our series (118) who had improved only from hand movements to 0.04 vision during the first 3 months following UKN, reached a 0.9 vision 1 year later. However, it is difficult to determine whether this is a late effect of the enzyme or due to the natural evolution of the hemorrhage, which is rather unpredictable.

Although a number of clinical factors (age, size of the hemorrhage, location, etiology, recurrence) (12,65,93) have a certain value, we still know too little about the natural mechanism of vitreous blood reabsorption to be confident in our prognosis. Many vitreous hemorrhages will resolve spontaneously, some within days and without lasting visual impairment, others gradually and incompletely over a longer period (weeks to months) and leaving some visual reduction. Resolution may start after a long period of unchanged appearance. However, in other cases reabsorption does not take place, leaving an almost blind eye (11).

To overcome this difficulty, a controlled prospective clinical trial was started by J. V. Forrester and J. Williamson (65), comparing UKN with conservative treatment. Their preliminary report confirms the clearing effect of UKN on vitreous opacity, although this is a slow process. Statistically significant difference was found only after 3 months, compared to untreated eyes, which showed little opacity change after 1 year. Some visual acuity improvement was found in 9 out of 10 UKN-treated eyes by 3 months, whereas only 4 out of 11 controls improved. This improvement did not completely parallel opacity reduction, since it also depends on retinal and optic nerve function, but gained further in the treated group by 1 year (65).

Indications for any specific procedures should be evaluated according to their ability to resolve the pathologic condition to which they are applied, and to restore the normal physiologic function, along with difficulty of use, cost, and complications that can follow—all in comparison to alternative methods. In the case of vitreous hemorrhage, there is evidence that UKN provides better management than simple expected or conservative methods. Mechanical removal of hemorrhagic vitreous by a vitrectomy technique is clearly a successful approach from the anatomic point of view, although it is a much more complicated and aggressive procedure with a more than negligible rate of severe complications (cataract, retinal tear or detachment, secondary glaucoma, corneal problems, lost vision, hypotony, and pthisis bulbi) and often a deceptive visual outcome.

TABLE 4. *Complications of intravitreal UKN*

Study	Eyes	Transient hypertensive uveitis	Hypopyon	Cataract	Late glaucoma
London, 1974 (40, 88)	33	—	16	—	1
Glasgow, 1974 (62)	11	2	2	—	—
1982 (65)	10	10	4	2	1
Melbourne, 1977 (37)	34	Several	22	3	1[a]
Japan, 1980 (136)	9	1	7	—	—
Barcelona, 1984 (118)	33	1	1	—	—
Totals	130	14	52	5	3

[a] Associated with cataract.

The main complications observed after UKN treatment, as summarized in Table 4, include a mild uveitis frequently associated to IOP rise (up to 36 mmHg) (37), but it was usually transient, responding well to medical therapy. Hypopyon was a common feature but also transient. As previously discussed, these inflammatory features may have a role in clot lysis. A similar uveitis (hemophthalmitis) has also been described in spontaneously resolving vitreous hemorrhage (26).

The only long-standing complications were a few cases of cataract development (most of the "worse" group), also seen in control group (65), and occasional long-standing secondary glaucoma, medically controllable (37,65,88).

Although a β-wave amplitude drop in the ERG for UKN-treated eyes has been reported, no serious long-term effects on retinal function have been associated with UKN (40). The only histopathologic report of an UKN-treated eye, from a diabetic patient who died 6 days after the intravitreal injection of 25,000 P.U., showed only "red cell debris and macrophages in and on a retinal surface membrane, having the appearance in places of the internal limiting membrane of the retina" (37). This contrasts with animal studies in which similar doses produced a localized whitish reaction on the retinal surface, which was considered a toxic effect (103). Since UKN is a human protein, the subsequent immune reaction seen in animals cannot be expected in man.

A slight increase in corneal thickness after intravitreal UKN has also been reported (32). Since this hardly can be a result of surgical trauma—as vitrectomy-associated corneal edema actually is—it has been suggested that the fibrinolytic system has an influence on the corneal-thickness regulation. Inhibition of this effect by tranexamic acid, an antifibrinolytic agent, would support this hypothesis.

A reevaluation of several reports on vitrectomy results (117,144) permitted Chapman-Smith and Crock to compare UKN favorably with vitrectomy in the management of vitreous hemorrhage on a visual basis (37), as well as being a clearly simpler and safer technique that can be repeated or followed by vitrectomy in case it fails.

Use of UKN in the Management of Hyphema

The prognosis of traumatic hyphema depends on its size, persistence, and effect on IOP (79,146,159). Primary hyphema are frequently small (less than half the anterior chamber volume), do not affect IOP, and resorb spontaneously without leaving sequelae (51,157,196). However, a number of cases will later develop secondary bleeding, which often results in large or total hyphema (black ball hemorrhage) (176), usually associated with IOP rise and a tendency to persist, clot, and leave complications (such as corneal blood staining, fibrous membrane formation, and persistent secondary glaucoma) that obscure visual outcome (47,138,178).

Since conservative treatment often fails in clearing total hyphema, and medical therapy has been found unable to control subsequent IOP rise (76,81), management of this problem has been controversial. Classical as well as micromechanical (48,127,176) surgical approaches have been proposed but may be technically difficult. The use of fibrinolysins is a compromise (78,112,145,157).

UKN was first clinically tried in the management of hyphema (145), and found to be effective in cases of persistent, clotted, total hyphema in which conservative therapy had failed. In a series of 157 eyes with large traumatic hyphema (157), 20 out of 57 saline anterior chamber washouts failed to remove the clots and received a 5,000-P.U.-UKN second washout (always through a small incision) that was effective in all cases. The enzyme was dissolved in 2 ml distilled water and injected in 5 0.3-ml doses, each left in the anterior chamber for 3 min and the last left at the end of the procedure if any residual clot was present. IOP normalized and blood completely reabsorbed 20% immediately, 40% the first day, 65% within 3 days, and 90% after 1 week. Only two eyes needed a third 10,000-P.U. washout, which was finally successful. Although simple saline irrigation may sometimes be enough, reduction of corneal staining, clotting, and rise in IOP rates were more marked in the UKN group. Fibrous membrane formation was reduced only where UKN was used. Although final visual acuity was equally poor in all groups, this can be attributed to associated ocular injuries, including vitreous hemorrhage in almost half of the cases.

Other fibrinolytic agents, such as human activated plasminogen (fibrinolysin) have also been effective in management of total hyphema, although no comparative studies have been done (79,138,153,170). Its only advantage over UKN would be lower cost and the possibility of a more abundant washout (250-ml solution per bottle) (79)—which actually implies a greater mechanical washout effect, with subsequent higher danger of traumatizing intraocular structures. Experimental and clinical STKN trials had various results (70,95,139), frequently resulting in severe corneal damage due to the antigenic properties or STKN or its lack of purity, being associated with other enzymes (streptodornase, hyaluronidase) known to be toxic to intraocular structures (2,147,151).

The main advantage of fibrinolytic management in resolving total hyphema, apart from its effectiveness, is that the technique is less invasive, requiring neither a large corneoscleral incision, maneuvering with instruments inside the anterior chamber, nor extensive turbulent-flux irrigation. No complications attributable to the use of UKN or plasmin in anterior chamber have been reported. A question still unsettled is how long to wait before surgery. The lower aggressivity of enzymatic techniques allows a safer approach.

ACKNOWLEDGMENTS

We thank Dr. Emilio Iglesias-Touriño, who is the artist of all drawings and collaborated in their conception. Dr. Joaquín Rutllán was an inestimable help in the literature search regarding zonulolysis, as Dr. Pedro Borrat was regarding general medical aspects and literature on fibrinolysis, a subject on which Dr. Francisco Mateus and Dr. Federico Lithgow gave us valuable advice based on their long-standing clinical experience. We also thank Miss Montserrat Veses for typing the manuscript, and Mr. Andrés Maeso and the Department of Photography for their efforts in preparing the graphic materials.

REFERENCES

1. Albalad, E., Olivan, J. M., Lopez De C, A., Rabinal, F., and Honrubia, F. M. (1977): La uroquinasa en el tratamiento de las oclusiones vasculares retinianas. *Arch. Soc. Esp. Oftal.,* 37:1075–1082.
2. Alfano, J. E., and Clampitt, J. (1965): Injection of hyaluronidase into the anterior chamber of the rabbit. *Am. J. Ophthalmol.,* 39:198–202.
3. Algan, B. (1973): Les possibilités actuelles du traitement médical des tromboses veineuses rétiniennes. *Ann. Oculist. (Paris),* 206:797–834.
4. Alkjaersig, N., Fletcher, A. P., and Sherry, S. (cited by Forrester, J. V. et al., 1974). (1958): *J. Biol. Chem.,* 233:86.
5. Anderson, D. (1971): Experimental alpha-chymotrypsin glaucoma studied by scanning electron microscopy. *Am. J. Ophthalmol.,* 71:470–476.
6. Appelmans, M., Michiels, J., De Backer, P., and Alaerts, R. (1958): Action de l'alpha-chymotrypsine sur la cornée du lapin. Le D.F.P. est-il un antidote? *Bull. Soc. Belge Ophthalmol.,* 120:543–570.
7. Astrup, T. (1954): In: *Proceedings of I International Conference on Thrombosis and Embolism, Basel,* edited by T. Koller and W. R. Merz. Schwabe, Basel.
8. Astrup, T., and Sterndorff, I. (cited by Konttinen, Y. P.). (1952): An activator of plasminogen in normal urine. *Proc. Soc. Exp. Biol. Med.,* 81:675.
9. Babel, J. (1964): L'action toxique de l'hémosidérine sur les tissus oculaires. *Arch. Ophtal. (Paris),* 24:405–416.
10. Bairati, A. (1946): Studi sulla natura e sulla minuta struttura delle fibre della zonula dello Zinn. *Bull. Sci. Med. (Bologna),* 118:1.
11. Ballantyne, A. J., and Michaelson, I. C. (1970): *Textbook of the Fundus of the Eye.* Livingstone, Edinburgh.

12. Balmer, F. (1964): Zur prognose der Blutungen in der Glaskörper. *Ophthalmologica,* 147:425–447.
13. Barraquer, I. (1917): Extracción ideal de la catarata. *Ann. Real Acad. Med. y Cir. Barcelona,* 2:57–60.
14. Barraquer, J. (1958): Zonulolisis enzimática. Contribución a la cirugía del cristalino. *Ann. Real Acad. Med. y Cir. Barcelona,* 38:255–266.
15. Barraquer, J., and Rutllan, J. (1960): Crítica de la zonulolisis enzimática basada en nuestra experiancia. *Arch. Soc. Oftal. H.A.,* 20:850–863.
16. Barraquer, J., and Rutllan, J. (1964): *Cirugía del Segmento Anterior del Ojo Vol. I: Generalidades. Extracción Intracapsular del Cristalino.* Instituto Barraquer, Barcelona.
17. Barraquer, J., and Rutllan, J. (1967): Enzymatic zonulolysis and postoperative hypertension. *Am. J. Ophthalmol.,* 63:159.
18. Barraquer, J., and Rutllan, J. (1968): Influencia de la quimotripsina sobre la cicatrización de las incisiones esclero-corneales. *An. Inst. Barraquer,* 8:181–187.
19. Barraquer, J. I. (1957): La evacuación total del cuerpo vítreo para el tratamiento de sus opacidades graves no evolutivas. *Rev. Esp. Oto-Neuro-Oftal. y Neurol.,* 14:193–197.
20. Barraquer, J. I. (1962): Complicaciones por el uso de la alfa-quimotripsina. Su profilaxis. *An. Inst. Barraquer,* 3:249–253.
21. Bart, P., and Seblaek, B. (1955): Protein interactions. IV. Inhibition of alpha-chymotrypsin by D.F.P. and chloramphenicol. *Chem. Listy.,* 49:1617–1620.
22. Baum, G. (1957): The effect of ultrasonic radiation upon the rate of absorption of blood from the vitreous. *Am. J. Ophthalmol.,* 44:150–158.
23. Bedrossian, R. H. (1959): Alpha-chymotrypsin. Its effect on the rabbit zonule, lens capsule and corneal wound healing. *Arch. Ophthalmol.,* 62:216–222.
24. Bedrossian, R. H., and Weimar, V. (1963): Inhibitory effects of aqueous humor on alpha-chymotrypsin. *Trans. Am. Acad. Ophthalmol. Otolaryngol.,* 67:822–828.
25. Begue, H., and Waksmann, J. (1959): Action de l'alpha-chymotrypsine sur l'insertion cristallinienne de la zonule chez l'animal. *Bull. Soc. Ophtalmol. Fr.,* 3:235–237.
26. Benson, W. E., and Spalter, H. F. (1971): Vitreous haemorrhage: A review of experimental and clinical investigations. *Surv. Ophthalmol.,* 15:297–311.
27. Bernardczykowa, A., and Kaluzny, J. (1970): [The influence of laser energy on experimental vitreous hemorrhages in the rabbit]. *Klin. Oczna.,* 40:163–166 (in Polish).
28. Bernhard, S. (1968): *The Structure and Function of Enzymes.* W. A. Benjamin, New York.
29. Blow, D. M., Birktoft, J. J., and Hartley, B. S. (1968): Role of a burred aid group in the mechanism of action of chymotrypsin. *Nature,* 221:337–340.
30. Boberg-Ans, J. (1962): No complications due to the use of alpha-chymotrypsin in 107 consecutive cases of intracapsular lens extraction. *An. Inst. Barraquer,* 3:227–248.
31. Boyer, K. H., Suran, A. A., Hogan, M. J., and McEwen, W. K. (1958): Studies on simulated vitreous haemorrhages. II. The effects of lytic enzymes, surface-active agents, and urea. *Arch. Ophthalmol.,* 59:333–336.
32. Bramsen, T. (1978): The effect of urokinase on central corneal thickness and vitreous haemorrhage. *Acta Ophthalmol.,* 56:1006–1012.
33. Brini, A., and Meyer, A. (1960): La chymotripsine exert-elle une influence sur la cicatrisation de la cornée? *Bull. Soc. Ophtalmol. Fr.,* 4:9–10.
34. Castren, J. (1960): Trypsin and alpha-chymotripsin in cataract surgery. *Acta Ophthalmol.,* 38:247–253.
35. Celander, D. R., Langlinais, R. P., and Guest, M. M. (cited by Konttinen, Y. P.) (1955): Application of foam technique to the partial purification of a urine activator of plasma profibrinolysin. *Arch. Biochem. Biophys.,* 55:286.
36. Chandler, M. R., and Rosenthal, E. (1958): The effect of intramuscularly administered trypsin in blood injected into the vitreous of rabbits. *Arch. Ophthalmol.,* 59:706–711.
37. Chapman-Smith, J. S., and Crock, G. W. (1977): Urokinase in the management of vitreous haemorrhage. *Br. J. Ophthalmol.,* 61:500–505.
38. Charamis, J., Aruga, H. et al. (1961): Table ronde sur l'alpha-chymotrypsine. Premier Congrès de la Societé Européenne d'Ophtalmologie, Athens, 1960. *An. Inst. Barraquer,* 2:319–343.
39. Cibis, P. A., and Yamashita, T. (1959): Experimental aspects of ocular siderosis and hemosiderosis. *Am. J. Ophthalmol.,* 48:465–480.
40. Cleary, P. E., Davies, E. W. G., Shilling, J. S., and Hamilton, A. M. (1974): Intravitreal

urokinase in the treatment of vitreous haemorrhage. *Trans. Ophthalmol. Soc. U.K.,* 94:587–590.
41. Clement, F. (1958): Estudio experimental de la zonulólisis enzimática de Barraquer. *IV Reun. Nac. Esp. Cienc. Fisiol. Granada; An. Inst. Barraquer,* 1:18–22.
42. Coleman, D. J., Lizzi, F. L., El-Mofty, A. A. M., Driller, J., and Francen, L. A. (1980): Ultrasonically accelerated resorption of vitreous membranes. *Am. J. Ophthalmol.,* 89:131–136.
43. Constable, I. J., Aguri, M., Chesney, C. M., Swann, D. A., and Colman, R. W. (1973): Platelet induced vitreous membrane formation. *Invest. Ophthalmol. Vis. Sci.,* 12:680–685.
44. Crock, G. (1978): The fifth generation of surgery. Opening lecture of the VIIth International Course of Ophthalmology of the Instituto Barraquer. *An. Inst. Barraquer,* 14:17–30, 35–91.
45. Cunningham, L. (1965): The structure and mechanisms of action of proteolitic enzymes. In: *Comprehensive Biochemistry,* edited by M. Florkin and E. H. Stotz. vol. 16, pp. 85–188. Academic Press, New York.
46. Damaskus, C. W. (1960): Various laboratory aspects of alpha-chymotrypsin. *Am. J. Ophthalmol.,* 49:31–35.
47. Darr, J. L., and Passmore, J. W. (1967): Management of traumatic hyphaema. *Am. J. Ophthalmol.,* 63:134–136.
48. Diddle, K. R., Dinsmore, S., and Murphree, I. L. (1981): Total hyphaema evacuation by vitrectomy instruments. *Ophthalmology,* 88:917–921.
49. Dugmore, W. M., and Raichand, M. (1972): Intravitreal urokinase in the treatment of vitreous haemorrhage. *Lancet,* 2:660.
50. Edelhauser, H. F., Van Horn, D. L., Hyndiuk, R. A., and Schulz, R. O. (1975): Intraocular irrigating solutions. Their effect on the corneal endothelium. *Arch. Ophthalmol.,* 93:648–657.
51. Edwards, W. C., and Layden, W. E. (1973): Traumatic hyphaema. *Am. J. Ophthalmol.,* 75:110–116.
52. Escariz, B. H. (1959): Nuevos aportes al empleo de la tripsina en la operación de catarata. *Sem. Med.* (Buenos Aires), 114:398–403.
53. Fasanella, R. M. (1962): Experimental work in enzymatic zonulolysis. *An. Inst. Barraquer,* 3:183–193.
54. Fink, A. I., Bernstein, H. N., and Binkhorst, R. (1960): Effect of alpha-chymotrypsin on corneal wound healing. *Arch. Ophthalmol.,* 64:104–107.
55. Flom, L. (1960): Alpha-chymotrypsin and ruptured hyaloid. *Am. J. Ophthalmol.,* 49:357–358.
56. Ford, V. (1890): Proposed surgical treatment of opaque vitreous. *Lancet,* 1:462.
57. Forgacs, J. (1962): La résoption spontanée et consecutive à la diathermocoagulation superficielle de l'hemorragie experimentelle du corps vitré. *Ann. Oculist. (Paris),* 195:743–760.
58. Forrester, J. V. (1980): M.D. thesis., University of Glasgow.
59. Forrester, J. V., Edgar, W., Prentice, C. R. M., Forbes, C. D., and Williamson, J. (1977): The effect of fibrinolytic inhibition in the resolution of experimental vitreous haemorrhage. *Am. J. Ophthalmol.,* 84:810–814.
60. Forrester, J. V., and Lee, W. R. (1981): Cellular composition of post-haemorrhagic opacities in the human vitreous. *Albrecht v. Graefés Arch. Klin. Exp. Ophthalmol.,* 215:279–296.
61. Forrester, J. V., Prentice, C. R. M., Williamson, J., and Forbes, C. D. (1974): Fibrinolytic activity of the vitreous body. *Invest. Ophthalmol. Vis. Sci.,* 13:875–879.
62. Forrester, J. V., and Williamson, J. (1973): Resolution of intravitreal clots by urokinase. *Lancet,* 2:179–181.
63. Forrester, J. V., and Williamson, J. (1974): Lytic therapy in vitreous haemorrhage. *Trans Ophthalmol. Soc. U.K.,* 94:583–586.
64. Forrester, J. V., and Williamson, J. (1974): Total vitreous haemorrhage. A method of treatment. *Trans. Ophthalmol. Soc. U.K.,* 94:992–999.
65. Forrester, J. V., and Williamson, J. (1982): Urokinase in vitreous haemorrhage: A prospective clinical trial. In: *Urokinase: Basic & Clinical Aspects,* Serono Symposium No. 48, edited by P. M. Mannuci and A. D'Angelo. Academic Press, London and New York.
66. Forrester, J. V., Williamson, J., and Prentice, C. R. M. (1978): In: *IIIrd Mackenzie Memorial Symposium on Vision and Circulation, Glasgow,* edited by J. S. Cant. Kimpton, London.
67. Franceschetti, A., and Forni, S. (1954): Surgical treatment (surface diathermo-coagulation) of Eales' disease. *XVI Congr. Ophth. Acta,* 1:215–223.

68. Franklin, S. H. (1974): Histochemical inquiry concerning the site and nature of alpha-chymotryptic activity in enzymatic zonulolysis. *An. Inst. Barraquer,* 5:124–138.
69. Freeman, H. M., Hirose, T., and Schepens, C. L., eds. (1977): *Vitreous Surgery and Advances in Fundus Diagnosis and Treatment.* Appleton-Century-Crofts, New York.
70. Friedman, M. W. (1952): Streptokinase in ophthalmology. *Am. J. Ophthalmol.,* 35:1184–1187.
71. Galin, M. A., Barasch, K. R., and Harris, L. S. (1966): Enzymatic zonulolysis and intraocular pressure. *Am. J. Ophthalmol.,* 61:690–696.
72. Garcia-Sanchez, J., and Sanchez-Salorio, M. (1969): Influencia de la alfaquimotripsina sobre la tensión en el ojo operado de cataratas. *An. Inst. Barraquer,* 9:187–197.
73. Gastaldi, G. M., and Diotti, G. (1969): L'impiego di un attivatore del plasminogeno (urochinasi) in alcune affezioni emorragiche e tromboemboliche dell'occhio. *Minerv. Oftalmol.,* 11:82–84.
74. Geraits, W., Chan, G., and Guerry, D. (1960): The effect of alpha-chymotrypsin on zonular and anterior hyaloid membrane: Experiments on eyes in the human, the rabbit and the dog. *South. Med. J.,* 53:82–85.
75. Gloor, B. P. (1974): Zur Entwicklung des Glaskörpers und der zonula. VI. Autoradiographische Untersuchungen zur Entwicklung der Zonula der Maus mit 3H-markierten Aminosäuren und 3H-glucose. *Albrecht v. Graefe's Arch. Klin. Exp. Ophthalmol.,* 189:105–124.
76. Gregersen, E. (1962): Traumatic hyphaema. I. Report of 200 successive cases. II. Prognostic significance of admission practice. *Acta Ophthalmol. (Copenh.),* 40:192–201.
77. Grierson, I., and Forrester, J. V. (1980): Vitreous haemorrhage and vitreal membranes. *Trans Ophthalmol. Soc. U.K.,* 100:140–147.
78. Heath, W. (1966): Experience with urokinase in secondary traumatic hyphaema. *Trans Ophthalmol. Soc. U.K.,* 86:843–845.
79. Heinze, J. (1975): The surgical management of total hyphaema. *Aust. J. Ophthalmol.,* 3:20–23.
80. Hendley, C. D. et al. (1956): Studies on proteolytic enzymes. I. Toxicology of crystalline trypsin and chymotrypsin. *Arch. Int. Pharmacodyn. Ther.,* 106:164–177.
81. Henry, M. M. (1960): Nonperforating eye injuries with hyphaema. *Am. J. Ophthalmol.,* 49:1298–1300.
82. Hervouet, F. (1962): Nouvelles précisions histologiques sur l'action de l'alpha-chymotripsine sur les tissus oculaires. *An. Inst. Barraquer,* 3:194–198.
83. Hill, H. F. (cited by McLean, J.). (1962): In: Discussion of Zonulolysis. *An. Inst. Barraquer,* 3:274.
84. Hofmann, H. (1960): Versuche über den Wirkkungsmechanismus zonulolytischer fermente. *Albrecht v. Graefe's Arch. Klin. Exp. Ophthalmol.,* 162:111–119.
85. Hofmann, H. (1962): In: Discusión sobre zonulolisis enzimática. *An. Inst. Barraquer,* 3:264–268.
86. Hofmann, H., and Lembeck, F. (1959): Vergleich der zonulolytischen Wirkung von Alpha-Chymotrypsin und Trypsin. *Klin. Mbl. Augen-heilk.,* 134:316–322.
87. Hogan, M. J., Alvarado, J. A., and Weddell, J. E. (1971): *Histology of the Human Eye.* W. B. Saunders, Philadelphia.
88. Holmes-Sellors, P. J., Kanski, J. J., and Watson, D. M. (1974): Intravitreal urokinase in the management of vitreous haemorrhage. *Trans. Ophthalmol. Soc. U.K.,* 94:591–598.
89. Hruby, K. (1959): Die Expression der Katarakt nach Zonulolyse mittels Trypsins. *Klin. Mbl. Augenheilk.,* 134:527–531.
90. Huang, H. T., and Nieman, C. (1951): The reaction of cloramphenicol (cloromycetin) with alpha-chymotrypsin. *J. Am. Chem. Soc.,* 73:4039–4040.
91. Hufford, C., Curtlwiler, F., and Roberts, J. (1952): Roentgen therapy in vitreous haemorrhages and haemorrhagic glaucoma. *Radiology,* 59:161–166.
92. Iserle, J., Anton, M., Riebel, O. (1960): Histological picture of the human eye operated upon by fermentative zonulolysis. *Ophthalmologica,* 140:251–258.
93. Jaffe, N. S. (1969): *The Vitreous in Clinical Ophthalmology.* C. V. Mosby, St. Louis.
94. Jennings, R. R., Kerr, R. J., and Niemann, C. (1958): The effect of calcium chloride on several alpha-chymotrypsin-catalyzed hydrolyses. *Biochim. Biophys. Acta,* 28:144–147.
95. Jukofsky, J. L. (1951): A new technique in the treatment of hyphaema. *Am. J. Ophthalmol.,* 34:1692–1696.

96. Junceda-Avello, J., Suarez-Antuña, S., and Muro Sanchez, I. (1975): Tratamiento actual de las hemorragias en vítreo. *Arch. Soc. Esp. Oftal.*, 35:915–920.
97. Karpe, G. (1969): Early diagnosis of siderosis retinae by the use of electroretinography. *Doc. Ophthalmol.*, 2:277–296.
98. Kaye, G. I., Mishima, S., Cole, J. D., et al. (1968): Studies on the cornea. VII. Effects of perfusion with a Ca^{++}-free medium on the corneal endothelium. *Invest. Ophthalmol. Vis. Sci.*, 7:53–66.
99. Kirby, D. B. (1950): *Surgery of Cataract.* J. B. Lippincott, Philadelphia.
100. Kirsch, R. E. (1964): Glaucoma following cataract extraction associated with the use of alpha-chymotrypsin. *Arch. Ophthalmol.*, 72:612–620.
101. Kjeldgaard, N. O., and Ploug, J. (1957): Urokinase: An activator of plasminogen from human urine. II. Mechanism of plasminogen activation. *Biochim. Biophys. Acta*, 24:283–289.
102. Konttinen, Y. P. (1968): *Fibrinolysis: Chemistry, Physiology and Clinics.* Star, Tampere, Finland.
103. Koziol, J., Peyman, G. A., Sanders, D. R., Vichek, J., and Goldberg, M. F. (1975): Urokinase in experimental vitreous haemorrhage. *Ophthalmic Surg.*, 6:79–82.
104. Krwawicz, T. (1961): Intracapsular extraction of intumescent cataract by application of low temperature. *Br. J. Ophthalmol.*, 45:279–283.
105. Kunitz, M., and Northrop, J. H. (1933): Isolation of a crystalline protein from the pancreas, and its conversion into a new crystalline proteolytic enzyme by trypsin. *Science*, 78:558–559.
106. Lam, K. W., Ashrafzadeh, T., and Lee, C. B. (1972): Vitreous membranes: Induction in rabbits by intravitreous leukocyte injections. *Arch. Ophthalmol.*, 88:655–658.
107. Legrand, J., Hervouet, F., Baron, A., and Lenoir, A. (1960): La zonulolyse par action de l'alpha-chymotrypsine. In: *Zonulólisis enzimática. Edición conmemorativa*, film edited by J. Barraquer. Presented to the Tertium Forum Ophthalmologicum, Bogotá, March, 1980.
108. Ley, A. P., Holmberg, A., and Yamashita, T. (1959): Histology of zonulolysis with alpha-chymotrypsin. *Am. J. Ophthalmol.*, 47:876–877.
109. Ley, A. P., Holmberg, A., and Yamashita, T. (1960): Histology of zonulolysis with alpha-chymotrypsin employing light and electron microscopy. *Am. J. Ophthalmol.*, 49:67–80.
110. Ley, A. P., Holmberg, A., and Yamashita, T. (1960): *An. Inst. Barraquer*, 1:451–468.
111. Limon, S., and Coscas, G. (1975): Les thrombolytiques dans le traitement des oblitérations vasculaires rétiniennes. *Gazet Med. France*, 82:4165–4175.
112. Linn, J. G., Jr., and Ozment, T. L. (1950): Effects of injection of hyaluronidase into anterior chamber. *Am. J. Ophthalmol.*, 33:33–44.
113. Lithgow, F. (1968): Un caso de trombosis cerebral tratado con fibronolysin. *An. Inst. Barraquer*, 8:301–306.
114. Maberly, A. C., and Chisholm, L. D. J. (1970): The effect of fibrinolytic agent on vitreous haemorrhage in rabbits. *Can. J. Ophthalmol.*, 5:55–69.
115. MacFarlane, R. G., and Pilling, J. (cited by Konttinen, Y. P.). (1947): Fibrinolytic activity of normal urine. *Nature*, 159:779.
116. Machemer, R., Parel, J-M., and Buettner, H. (1972): A new concept for vitreous surgery. I. Instrumentation. *Am. J. Ophthalmol.*, 73:1–7.
117. Mandelcorn, M. S., Blankenship, G., and Machemer, R. (1976): Pars plana vitrectomy for the management of severe diabetic retinopathy. *Am. J. Ophthalmol.*, 81:561–570.
118. Mateus, F., and Barraquer, R. I. (1984): Tratamiento de las hemorragias intraoculares mediante la inyección en la cámara vítrea de urokinasa. *An. Inst. Barraquer* (*in press*).
119. Maumenee, E. A. (1960): Effect of alpha-chymotrypsin on the retina. *Trans. Am. Acad. Ophthalmol. Otolaryngol.*, 64:33–36.
120. McCulloch, C. M. (1954): The Zonule of Zinn: Its origin, course, and insertion, and its relation to neighboring structures. *Trans. Am. Ophthalmol. Soc.*, 52:525–585.
121. McKenzie, R., Pepper, D. S., and Kay, A. B. (cited by Forrester, J. V. et al., 1979). (1975): The generation of chemotactic activity for human leukocytes by the action of plasmin on human fibrinogen. *Thromb. Res.*, 6:1.
122. McKinney, J. W. (1964): Vitreous replacement for massive vitreous haemorrhage. *Am. J. Ophthalmol.*, 57:790–793.
123. McLean, J. (1962): Alpha-chymotrypsin extraction in corneal dystrophy. *An. Inst. Barraquer*, 3:224–226.

124. McPherson, A., ed. (1977): *New and Controversial Aspects of Vitreoretinal Surgery.* C. V. Mosby, St. Louis.
125. McWilliam, R. J. (1961): Impairment of wound healing after zonulolysis. *Trans. Ophthalmol. Soc. U.K.,* 81:105–111.
126. Megusar, M. A., Lam, K.-W., Tolentino, F. L., and Liu, H. S. (1975): Lymphocyte induced vitreous membranes: A comparative study with leukocyte and platelet-induced vitreous membranes. *Invest. Ophthalmol. Vis. Sci.,* 14:240–243.
127. Michels, R. G. (1978): Anterior segment application of vitrectomy techniques. *Trans. Ophthalmol. Soc. U.K.,* 98:458–465.
128. Michels, R. G. (1981): *Vitreous Surgery,* 212–237, 384–336. C. V. Mosby Co., St. Louis.
129. Mikuni, M., Kimura, S. (1965): Clinical application of urokinase to ocular diseases. *Jpn. J. Clin. Ophthalmol. (Rinsho Ganka),* 19:1155–1163.
130. Montauffier, R. J., and De la Bernardie-et-Camo, R. (1957): La trypsine dans les hémorragies du vitré. *Bull. Soc. Ophtalmol. Fr.,* 57:380–384.
131. Moroz, L. (cited by Forrester, J. V., et al., 1982). (1974): *N. Engl. J. Med.,* 301–310.
132. Morse, P. H., Aminlari, A., and Scheie, H. G. (1974): Spontaneous vitreous haemorrhage. *Arch. Ophthalmol.,* 92:297–298.
133. Muiños, A., Bonafonte, S., and Iglesias-Touriño, E. (1982): *Cirugía del Vítreo,* pp. 176–180, 196, 226, 322–347. Editorial Jims, Barcelona.
134. Murray, R. G., and Drance, S. M. (1960): The use of alpha-chymotrypsin in cataract surgery. *Arch. Ophthalmol.,* 63:910–917.
135. Offret, G., Haye, C., and Campinchi, R. (1959): Examen histologique d'un globe opéré de catarate avex zonulolyse enzymatique. *Bull. Soc. Ophtalmol. Fr.,* 72:135–146.
136. Okisaka, S., Sugimachi, Y., Ishida, N., Momose, T., Taketani, P., and Hiwatari, S. (1980): Intravitreal urokinase in the treatment of vitreous haemorrhage. *Jpn. J. Clin. Ophthalmol. (Rinsho Ganka),* 37:1025–1030.
137. O'Malley, C. C. (1952): Vitreous withdrawal as a therapeutic procedure. *Trans. Ophthalmol. Soc. U.K.,* 71:773–778.
138. Oosterhuis, J. A. (1968): Fibrinolysin irrigation in traumatic secondary hyphaema. *Ophthalmologica,* 155:357–378.
139. O'Rourke, J. F. (1955): An evaluation of intraocular streptokinase. *Am. J. Ophthalmol.,* 39:119–136.
140. Pandolfi, M. (1978): Intraocular haemorrhages: A hemostatic therapeutic approach. *Surv. Ophthalmol.,* 22:322–334.
141. Pandolfi, M., Coccheri, S., and Astrup, T. (1962): Thromboplastic and fibrinolytic activities in tissues of the eye. *Proc. Soc. Exp. Biol. Med.,* 109:159–161.
142. Pandolfi, M. (cited by Forrester, J. V., et al., 1982). (1979): Bibliotheca Anatomica 18:292.
143. Pappas, G. S., and Smelser, G. K. (1958): Studies on the ciliary epithelium and the zonule. I. Electron microscope observation on change induced by alternation of normal aqueous humor formation in the rabbit. *Am. J. Ophthalmol.,* 46:299–315.
144. Peyman, G. A., Huamonte, F. U., and Goldberg, M. F. (1976): One hundred consecutive pars plana vitrectomies using the Vitrophage. *Am. J. Ophthalmol.,* 81:263–271.
145. Pierse, D., and Legrice, H. (1963): Urokinase in ophthalmology. *Lancet,* 2:1143–1144.
146. Pilger, I. S. (1975): Medical treatment of traumatic hyphaema. *Surv. Ophthalmol.,* 20:28–34.
147. Pirie, A. (1949): Effect of hyaluronidase injection on vitreous humor of rabbit. *Br. J. Ophthalmol.,* 33:678–684.
148. Pirie, A., and van Heyningen, R. (1956): *Biochemistry of the Eye.* Blackwell Scientific Publications, Oxford.
149. Pirie, A., Schmidt, G., and Waters, J. W. (1948): Ox vitreous humor. I. The residual protein. *Br. J. Ophthalmol.,* 32:321–329.
150. Pita Salorio, D. (1980): Personal communication. In: La aportación de Barraquer a la cirugía de la catarata. *Arch. Soc. Amer. Oftal. Optom.,* 14:258–260.
151. Planten, J. T., and Hoppenbrouwers, R. E. (1954): Experiments on intraocular hyaluronidase administration. *Ophthalmologica,* 127:117–121.
152. Ploug, J., and Kjeldgaard, N. O. (1957): Urokinase: An activator of plasminogen from human urine. I. Isolation and properties. *Biochim. Biophys. Acta,* 24:278–283.
153. Polychronakos, D., and Triantatylou, G. (1977): Behandlung des traumatischen postoperativen totalen Hyphäma. *Klin. Mbl. Augenheilk,* 170:736–738.

154. Prompitak, A., Corey, P. N., and Chisholm, L. D. J. (1973): A comparison of brinolase and alpha-chymotrypsin on the facility of lens extraction in cynomolgus monkeys (*Macaca fascicularis*). *Am. J. Ophthalmol.*, 76:1018 (Abstract).
155. Radian, A. B., and Radian, A. L. (1963): [Complications of enzymatic zonulolysis with trypsin in cataract extraction]. *Oftalmologica (Buc.)*, 7:165–172 (in Rumanian).
156. Radnot, M., and Pajor, R. (1960): Histological investigations on the effect exerted by alpha-chymotrypsin on the retina. *Acta Ophthalmol. (Copenh.)*, 38:583–585.
157. Rakusin, W. (1971): Urokinase in the management of traumatic hyphaema. *Br. J. Ophthalmol.*, 55:826–832.
158. Raviola, G. (1971): The fine structure of the ciliary zonule and ciliary epithelium with special regard to the organisation and insertion of the zonular fibrils. *Invest. Ophthalmol.*, 10:851–869.
159. Read, J. (1975): Traumatic hyphaema: Surgical and medical management. *Ann. Ophthalmol.*, 7:659–670.
160. Regnault, F. R. (1970): Vitreous haemorrhage: An experimental study. I. A macroscopic and isotopic study of the evolution of whole blood and hemoglobin. *Arch. Ophthalmol.*, 83:458–465.
161. Remky, H. (1962): La cicatrisation après zonulolyse enzymatique. Observations personnelles au sujet de 851 opérations. *An. Inst. Barraquer*, 3:209–215.
162. Ribeiro, P., and Ribeiro, R. (1980): A urokinasa no tratamento das hemorragias vítreas. *Rev. Soc. Port. Oftalmol.*, 6:39–43.
163. Roll, P., Reich, M., and Hofmann, H. (1975): Der Verlauf der Zonulafaser im Bereich der Pars plicata corporis ciliaris, Pars lana, Ora serrata, und der Retina. Electronenoptische Studie. *Albrecht v. Graefes. Arch. Klin. Exp. Ophthalmol.*, 194:109–123.
164. Roll, P., Reich, M., Hofmann, H., and Scher, A. (1975): Der Verlauf der Zonulafasern. Eine weitere electronoptische Studie. *Albrecht v. Graefes Arch. Klin. Exp. Ophthalmol.*, 195:41–47.
165. Roper-Hall, M. J. (1963): Accidental use of alpha-chymotrypsin in 50× recommended strength. *An. Inst. Barraquer*, 4:321–323.
166. Ruiz-Bulumar, J. L. (1983): El empleo de alfa-quimotripsina para la extracción de la catarata y glaucoma enzimático. Presented to the VIIth International Course of the Instituto Barraquer, Barcelona, May 1977. *Revista D'Or de Oftalmología*, 2:59–62.
167. Rutllan, J. (1963): Bibliografía sobre zonulólisis enzimática. *An. Inst. Barraquer*, 4:198–212.
168. Rutllan, J. (1968): II. Bibliografía sobre zonulólisis enzimática *An. Inst. Barraquer*, 8:175–180.
169. Sallmann, L. von (1960): Experimental studies of some ocular effects of alpha-chymotrypsin. *Trans. Am. Acad. Ophthalmol. Otolaryngol.*, 64:25–32.
170. Scheie, H. G., Ashley, B. J., Jr., and Weiner, A. (1961): The treatment of total hyphaema with fibrinolysin (plasmin). *Arch. Ophthalmol.*, 66:226.
171. Scheie, H. G., Yanoff, M., and Tsou, K. C. (1965): Inhibition of alpha-chymotrypsin by aqueous humor. *Arch. Ophthalmol.*, 73:399–401.
172. Scheuner, G., and Häntzchel, H. (1967): Submikroscopische Unterschungen an der Zonula ciliaris, gleichzeitig ein Beitrag zur polarisationsoptischen Bestimmung gerichtet angeordneter saurer Gruppen. *Histochemistry*, 8:9.
173. Schimek, R. A., and Steffensen, E. H. (1955): Vitreous haemorrhage absorption. Experimental study on rabbit eyes of the effects of intravitreal hyaluronidase and streptokinase-streptodornase and the influence of ACTH and cortisone. *Am. J. Ophthalmol.*, 39:677–683.
174. Schwartz, B., Corwin, M., and Israel, A. (1960): A double-blind therapeutic trial of the effect of alpha-chymotrypsin on the facility of cataract extraction. *Trans. Am. Acad. Ophthalmol. Otolaryngol.*, 64:46–54.
175. Schwartz, B., and Schwartz, J. B. (1960): A review of the biochemistry and pharmacology of alpha-chymotrypsin. *Trans. Am. Acad. Ophthalmol. Otolaryngol.*, 64:17–24.
176. Sears, M. L. (1970): Surgical management of black ball hyphaema. *Trans. Am. Acad. Ophthalmol. Otolaryngol.*, 74:820–827.
177. Shimkin, M. B., and Bierman, H. R. (1949): Chymotrypsin in cancer. *Proc. Soc. Exp. Biol. Med.*, 71:250–252.
178. Spaeth, G. L., and Levy, P. M. (1966): Traumatic hyphaema: Its clinical characteristics and failure of estrogens to alter its course. *Am. J. Ophthalmol.*, 62:1098–1106.

179. Stecher, V. J., and Sorkin, E. (cited by Forrester, J. V., et al., 1979). (1972): The chemotactic activity of fibrinolysis products. *Int. Arch. Allergy Appl. Immunol.*, 43:879.

180. Strampelli, B. (1962): L'importance de la pureté de l'alpha-chymotrypsine pour éviter les effets sécondaires. *An. Inst. Barraquer*, 3:203–205.

181. Stryer, C. (1968): Implications of X-ray crystallographic studies of protein structure. *Annu. Rev. Biochem.*, 37:25–50.

182. Tagnon, H. J., Weinglass, A. R., and Goodpastor, W. E. (1945): The nature and mechanism of shock produced by the intravenous injection of chymotrypsin. *Am. J. Physiol.*, 143:644–655.

183. Takei, Y., and Ozanics, V. (1975): Electron microscopic studies on the zonule. I. Fine structure of normal and ruthenium red stained zonular fibrils in the rabbit and monkey. *Jpn. J. Ophthalmol.*, 19:69–93.

184. Takei, Y., and Smelser, G. K. (1975): Electron microscopic studies on zonular fibers. II. Changes of the zonular fibers after treatment with collagenase, alpha-chymotrypsin and hyaluronidase. *Albrecht v. Graefes Arch. Klin. Exp. Ophthalmol.*, 194:153–173.

185. Tano, Y., Chandler, D., and Machemer, R. (1980): Treatment of intraocular proliferation with intravitreal injection of triamcinolone acetonide. *Am. J. Ophthalmol.*, 90:810–816.

186. Tano, Y., Sugita, G., Abrams, G., and Machemer, R. (1980): Inhibition of intraocular proliferations with intravitreal corticosteroids. *Am. J. Ophthalmol.*, 89:131–136.

187. Thorpe, H. E. (1962): Gonioscopy after cataract extraction. *An. Inst. Barraquer*, 3:254.

188. Tow, D. E., Wagner, H. N., Jr., and Holmes, R. A. (1967): Urokinase in pulmonary embolism. *N. Engl. J. Med.*, 277:1161–1167.

189. Townes, C. D. (1960): Unfavorable effects of alpha-chymotrypsin in cataract surgery. *Arch. Ophthalmol.*, 64:108–113.

190. Troutman, R. C. (1960): National survey on the facility of cataract extraction, operative and immediate postoperative complications. *Trans. Am. Acad. Ophthalmol. Otolaryngol.*, 64:37–45.

191. Vail, D. T. (1960): Report of the committee on use of alpha-chymotrypsin in ophthalmology. *Trans. Am. Acad. Ophthalmol. Otolaryngol.*, 64:16–17, 54–57.

192. Verhoeff, F. H. (1948): Successful diathermy treatment of recurring retinal haemorrhages and retinitis proliferans. *Albrecht v. Graefe's Arch. Klin. Exp. Ophthalmol.*, 40:239–244.

193. Ward, P. A. (cited by Forrester, J. V., et al., 1982). (1967): *J. Exp. Med.*, 126:189.

194. West, P. M. (1949): Ineffectiveness of chymotrypsin in malignancy. *Proc. Soc. Exp. Biol. Med.*, 71:252–253.

195. Weekers, R., Lavergne, G., and Stassart-Hourlay, C. (1958): Avantages et inconvenients de la zonulolyse enzimatique par l'alpha-chymotrypsine au cours de l'extraction cristalinienne (etude clinique). *Bull. Soc. Belge. Ophtalmol.*, 120:539–543.

196. Williams, J. R. B. (cited by Konttinen, Y. P.). (1951): The fibrinolytic activity of urine. *Br. J. Exp. Pathol.*, 32:530.

197. Williamson, J., and Forrester, J. V. (1972): Urokinase in the treatment of vitreous haemorrhage. *Lancet*, 2:488.

198. Wollensak, J. von (1965): Zonula Zinii. Histologische und chemische Unterschungen, insbesondere über Zonulolysis enzymatica und Syndroma Marfan. In: *Advances in Ophthalmology*, Vol. 16, pp. 240–335. S. Karger, Basel.

199. Wu, F. C., and Laskowski, M. (1956): The effect of calcium on chymotrypsins A and B. *Biochim. Biophys. Acta*, 19:110–115.

200. Yoshida, T. (1959): Morphological studies by electron microscopy on the ciliary zonule. *Jpn. J. Ophthalmol.*, 3:177–195.

Commentary

Irrigating and Viscous Solutions

Dr. Edelhauser and his team have made important contributions to the surgeon's arsenal. Solutions that maintain ocular integrity are required in extracapsular cataract extraction with or without intraocular lens implantation, penetrating keratoplasty, vitrectomy, and in anterior segment reconstruction after trauma. In some surgical procedures very large volumes of irrigating fluid may be used. Volumes up to one liter have been reported. In this excellent and comprehensive paper the authors have shown the deleterious effects of saline, Plasma-Lyte 148, and lactated Ringer's solution on the corneal endothelium. BSS Plus, which has the ionic and nutrient constituents of aqueous humor (bicarbonate and glutathione are essential) proved to be superior in maintaining the integrity of corneal endothelium. Viscous aqueous substitutes are discussed: 1% sodium hyaluronate, chondroitin sulphate, and 0.5% methylcellulose seem to offer protection of the corneal endothelium that is very similiar. Consideration is given to post-operative ocular hypertension, which may be produced by these agents. It has been shown that the turnover of sodium hyaluronate in the rabbit anterior chamber is about 3 μg/24 hr (1). Perhaps the best way to prevent hypertension would be to remove most of the viscous solution at the close of surgery.

The Editors

REFERENCE

1. Laurent, U. B. G., and Fraser, J. R. E. (1983): *Exp. Eye Res.* 36:493–504.

Surgical Pharmacology of the Eye,
edited by M. Sears and A. Tarkkanen.
Raven Press, New York © 1985.

Irrigating and Viscous Solutions

*Henry F. Edelhauser and **Scott M. Mac Rae

*Medical College of Wisconsin, Milwaukee, Wisconsin 53226;
and **University of Oregon, Portland, Oregon 97201*

INTRAOCULAR IRRIGATING SOLUTIONS

Open-system surgery of the eye first began in the early 1900s. It is not reported what solutions were used at that time to replace aqueous humor. However, it was probably distilled water, tap water, or a Ringer's solution that contained a variety of electrolytes and microscopic particulate matter. The early surgeons probably observed very quickly that distilled water (a solution with no tonicity or osmotic pressure) injected into the eye was disastrous and that it resulted in immediate and permanent clouding of the cornea due to massive and irreversible swelling of the corneal endothelium. Moistening of the corneal epithelium with distilled water during surgery can also cause a reversible form of corneal edema for similar reasons. The hydration properties of the cornea were first studied in 1942 by Kinsey and Cogan (53,54), who showed that corneal swelling in distilled water was more rapid than in various Ringer's solutions. Normal saline, readily available to all surgeons, had been used for years as an intraocular irrigating solution for those procedures of short duration requiring only small amounts of fluid replacement to the eye. Ophthalmic surgeons were concerned, however, with the corneal stria and edema that occurred after intraocular surgery.

It was not until the *in vitro* studies by Harper and Pomerat (35) and Merrill et al. (60) on rabbit corneal explants of epithelium, endothelium, human conjunctiva, and iris that it was reported that saline did not adequately maintain ocular tissues. Saline was shown to be toxic; it had a pH of 6.8 and lacked the necessary ions to maintain the intraocular tissues. From these studies Merrill et al. (60) developed a balanced salt solution (BSS) which was later made commercially as 15 ml BSS (Table 1). This solution has a pH of 7.4 to 8.2 and contains—in addition to sodium chloride—potassium chloride, calcium chloride, and magnesium chloride, and it is buffered with sodium acetate and citrate.

With the extent of the surgical procedures carried on in the late 1950s and early 1960s, 15 ml BSS for ophthalmic use was all that was necessary. This solution was marketed in a squeeze bottle, which facilitated its use during cataract surgery. In 1961 Struve et al. (82) conducted a double-blind study

TABLE 1. Composition of various intraocular irrigating solutions (all concentrations expressed in mM/l of solution

Ingredient	Normal saline[a] 0.9% NaCl	Lactated Ringer's[a]	Plasma-Lyte 148[a]	BSS[a,b] 15 ml	BSS[a,b] 500 ml and 15 ml[c]	BSS Plus[a,b]	GBR[d]	SMA_2[e]	HEPES buffered Ringer's[f]
Sodium chloride	154	102	86	84.8	110	122.2	111.6	112.9	120.5
Potassium chloride		4	5	10.1	10	5.08	4.8	4.8	4.0
Calcium chloride		3	—	4.3	3	1.05	1.1	1.2	2.54
Magnesium chloride		—	1.5	1.5	1.5	0.98	0.78	1.2	—
Magnesium sulfate		—	—	—	—	—	—	—	1.0
Sodium lactate		28	—	—	—	—	—	—	—
Sodium acetate			27	28.6	29	—	—	4.4	—
Sodium gluconate			23	—	—	—	—	—	—
Sodium citrate				5.78	6	—	—	3.4	—
Sodium acid phosphate						3.0	—	—	—
Disodium phosphate						—	0.86	—	1.0
Sodium bicarbonate						25.0	29.2	25.0	—
HEPES						—	—	—	20.0
Dextrose						5.11	5.01	8.3	4.45
Glutathione (reduced)						—	0.30	—	—
Glutathione (oxidized)						0.30	—	—	—
Adenosine						—	0.50	—	—
pH	4.5–7.2	6.0–7.2	7.4	7.4	7.4	7.4	7.4	7.3	7.2
Osmolality (mOsm)	290	277	299	280	305	305	274	290	268

[a] Commercially available.
[b] Alcon Laboratories, Inc., Fort Worth, Texas.
[c] BSS 15 ml (1984) similar to 500 ml.
[d] pH adjusted by bubbling with 5% CO_2/95% air (glutathione bicarbonate Ringer's).
[e] Senju Pharmaceutical Co. Ltd., Osaka, Japan.
[f] University Hospital of Wales, Health Park, Cardiff, Wales.

and compared saline versus 15 ml BSS following intraocular surgery. These investigators performed 50 consecutive cataract extractions with either saline or BSS. They clinically noted the incidence of striate keratitis. Their data showed that it took an average of 4.1 ± 2.0 days with saline and 3.4 ± 1.6 days with BSS for the cornea to clear. They concluded that there was no marked difference in the cornea following the use of saline instead of BSS for cataract extraction. The apparent lack of observed corneal changes could be related to the volume and length of time the irrigating solution was used during cataract surgery.

The newer intraocular surgical procedures (such as intracapsular cataract extraction with implantation of an intraocular lens, extracapsular cataract extraction with implantation of an intraocular lens, Kelman phacoemulsification with or without an intraocular lens, anterior segment reconstruction, penetrating keratoplasty with its variants, and pars plana vitrectomy and lensectomy) required solutions that were able to maintain the cellular metabolism, function, structure, and integrity of the corneal endothelium, lens, and retina.

The first major instrument-type surgery that required a large volume solution was phacoemulsification. At the time, the irrigating solution of choice was Plasma-Lyte 148, apparently based on a stable pH of 7.4. However, many of the ophthalmic surgeons noticed that corneal stria and edema developed after surgery. When one observes the ingredients of Plasma-Lyte 148, it is apparent that corneal edema could occur from the lack of calcium in this solution. As instrumentation developed for vitrectomy, there was also a need for a large-volume irrigating solution to be commercially available.

It was first shown in 1972 by Dikstein and Maurice (17) that the corneal endothelium of an isolated perfused rabbit cornea could maintain the corneal thickness and aid in temperature reversal if a Krebs-Henseleit bicarbonate Ringer's, with the addition of adenosine and reduced glutathione, was used as the perfusate. Similar studies in the laboratory by McCarey et al. (58) correlated the functional and structural changes of the corneal endothelium to the perfusion media composition. These studies showed that a bicarbonate Ringer's solution containing glucose, adenosine, and glutathione prevented the cornea from swelling and maintained the cellular endothelial integrity. It was also the first time that the corneal swelling rate was compared to the specular microscopic endothelial cell pattern. In these studies the corneas that swelled up to 30 μm/hr maintained a normal cellular endothelial pattern, and corneas that swelled above 40 μm/hr showed loss of the endothelial pattern. From these studies it was apparent that the best intraocular irrigating solution should contain concentrations of inorganic and organic constituents similar to aqueous humor (8,12,13). Based on the studies of Dikstein and Maurice (17) and McCarey et al. (58), a glutathione bicarbonate Ringer's (GBR) solution was formulated to maintain the corneal endothelium (Table 1). This solution contained—in addition to the basic salts—sodium bicarbonate, glucose, glutathione, and adenosine. It was maintained at a pH of 7.4 and had an osmolality of 274—slightly hypotonic to human endothelial tissue but isotonic to rabbit tissue.

Past studies in our laboratory have established that normal saline (0.9% NaCl) (21), Plasma-Lyte 148 (23), and lactated Ringer's (18) are damaging to the corneal endothelium. Table 1 lists the composition of the various irrigating solutions. BSS (15 ml), formulated early for routine cataract surgery (60), did protect the corneal endothelium, but over 3 hr the corneas swelled (18). Based on laboratory studies and the difficulty that ophthalmic surgeons were having with extended surgical procedures during which a large-volume irrigating solution was necessary, GBR solution was prepared in a number of hospital pharmacies.

In a clinical study Waltman et al. (83) compared GBR to lactated Ringer's in patients undergoing vitrectomy. The results of this study showed that GBR solution resulted in significantly fewer corneal complications and less endothelial damage when compared to lactated Ringer's. Because of the difficulty of preparing GBR, Christiansen et al. (11) reported that D-5W and sodium bicarbonate could be added to Ringer's injection solution, resulting in a formula similar to GBR. This solution could be prepared aseptically in the operating room by injecting 18 ml commercial 5% dextrose and water and 20 ml sodium bicarbonate solution (available in 50-ml ampules containing 50 mEq sodium bicarbonate) into a 1,000-ml bottle of Ringer's injection or Ringer's lactate. Their studies showed that rhesus monkey lenses remained clear for extended periods of *in vitro* incubation at 37°C; however, it was not as effective as GBR solution. This solution combination was used for a short period in the United States because no better solution was available. However, problems arose because both Ringer's injection solution and lactated Ringer's solution varied in pH. Therefore, with the addition of bicarbonate ion to a solution of a variable pH, precipitation of the calcium occurred and the medium occasionally turned cloudy. To further confirm the importance of the composition of the intraocular irrigating solutions, Wiederholt and Koch (85) showed that the endothelial cell potential in human and rabbit corneas was maintained for 3 to 5 hr with both GBR and BSS (15 ml). However, their results demonstrated the advantage of GBR as an intraocular irrigating solution compared with 0.9% NaCl and BSS.

During the period of years that BSS Plus was being clinically evaluated in double-masked surgical trials, BSS 500 ml became available for large-volume intraocular surgery. The tonicity of this solution was increased over the 15-ml BSS (Table 1) and provided the ophthalmologist with a large-volume irrigating solution. Later GBR solution was approved by the FDA and became commercially available as BSS Plus. Table 1 compares the composition of BSS Plus to GBR. BSS Plus is similar to GBR except that oxidized glutathione is used in place of reduced glutathione, and adenosine is lacking from the media. Such a formula was necessary in order to develop a solution that was stable with a long shelf life. Table 2 compares BSS Plus to the ionic makeup of

TABLE 2. *Chemical composition of primate aqueous and BSS Plus (all concentrations expressed in mM/l or mEq/l of solution)*

Ingredient	Rhesus[a] monkey aqueous humor	Other[b] monkeys aqueous humor	Human[b,c] aqueous humor	BSS Plus
Sodium	152.0		162.9	160.0
Potassium	3.9	3.59	2.2–3.9[e]	5.0
Calcium	1.3	2.54	1.8[f]	1.0
Magnesium	0.8	1.17	1.1[f]	1.0
Chloride	125.0	122.0	131.6	130.0
Bicarbonate	28.0		20.15	25.0
Phosphate	0.4		0.62	3.0
Lactate	4.7		2.5	—
Urea	6.1		—	—
Glucose	2.9		2.7–3.7	5.0
Ascorbate	1.2		1.06	—
Glutathione	0.0001	0.006[d]	0.0019[d]	0.3
Amino acids	2.1		—	—
Protein	4×10^{-4}		—	—
pH	7.49		7.38	7.4
Osmolality[g] (mOsm)	301			305

[a] Gaasterland et al. (27).
[b] Cole (13).
[c] Cole (12).
[d] Riley et al. (75).
[e] Bessiere et al. (8).
[f] Alcon Laboratories data file.
[g] Measured by freezing point.

monkey aqueous humor and human aqueous humor, and it shows that BSS Plus is similar to the ionic and nutrient constituents of aqueous humor. Of importance is the addition of the bicarbonate ion and glutathione. The specific benefit of each one of these ingredients will be addressed later in this chapter.

The Effect of Irrigating Solutions on Rabbit and Human Corneal Endothelium

Figure 1 compares the swelling of rabbit cornea perfused with BSS Plus, lactated Ringer's, and Plasma-Lyte 148. It can be observed in Table 3 that the BSS Plus was able to maintain the corneal endothelium of the rabbit and prevented the cornea from swelling during the 3-hr period. Figure 2 shows that the endothelial morphology was maintained as shown by both scanning and transmission electron microscopy. By comparison, rabbit corneas perfused with Plasma-Lyte 148 swelled at a rate of 84 μm/hr, and over the 2-hr period the junctions between the cells were lost. The endothelial cells balled, and Descemet's membrane was directly exposed to the perfusion medium (Fig. 3). In this case, all barrier function of the corneal endothelium was lost. Lactated Ringer's, though it contained the necessary ions, did cause the cornea of the rabbit to swell at 32 μm/hr, and there was associated damage to the corneal

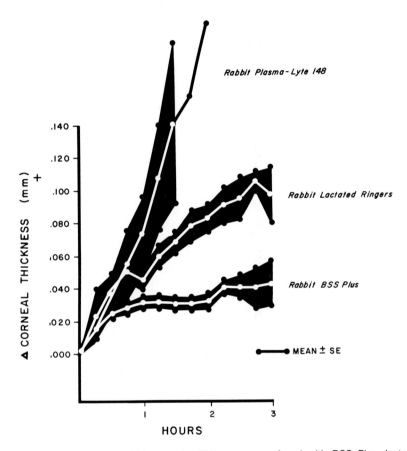

FIG. 1. Changes in corneal thickness of rabbit corneas perfused with BSS Plus, lactated Ringer's, and Plasma-Lyte 148. The white dots and line are the mean change in corneal thickness at each 15-min interval with the shaded range reflecting the standard error of the mean.

TABLE 3. *Corneal swelling rates[a] following endothelial perfusion*
μm/hr (mean ± SEM)

	Rabbit	Human
BSS Plus	0.001 ± 0.01 (N = 11)	−24.6 ± 4.5 (N = 9)
Lactated Ringer's	32.7 ± 3.1 (N = 6)	−5.17 ± 2.67 (N = 4)
Plasma-Lyte 148	84.6 ± 23 (N = 5)	10.06 ± 11.3 (N = 5)

[a] Calculated by regression analysis.

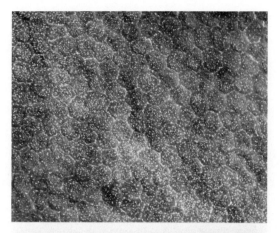

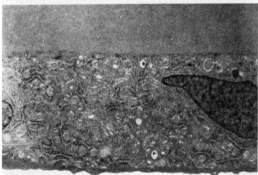

FIG. 2. Top: SEM of rabbit cornea endothelium perfused with BSS Plus for 3 hr. The normal mosaic-like pattern of the endothelial cells is present. ×1,000. **Bottom:** TEM of the same cornea. The posterior surface is smooth and the sub-cellular organelles are normal. ×14,500.

endothelium (Fig. 4). Blebs appeared on the endothelial cells, and associated cellular edema within the endothelial cells was present.

When BSS Plus was perfused to the human corneal endothelium, there was a de-swelling of the cornea of approximately 24 μm/hr (Fig. 5). Both scanning and transmission electron microscopy show that the endothelial cell morphology was maintained for a 3-hr period (the upper length of time that this solution would be used inside the eye during vitrectomy) (Fig. 6). By comparison, when Plasma-Lyte 148 was perfused to the human corneal endothelium, the junctions between the endothelial cells disrupted, and there was a marked degree of swelling (Fig. 7). Lactated Ringer's did maintain the endothelial cells for an extended period of time, but it caused damage as illustrated in Fig. 8 (upper figure shows the paired cornea perfused with BSS Plus; lower figure shows the paired cornea perfused with lactated Ringer's). In this case there is cellular swelling and edema within the endothelial cells. This pair of corneas from a 59-year-old would be expected to show greater stress with a perfusion solution. Figure 9 compares the endothelial cells of a human cornea at age

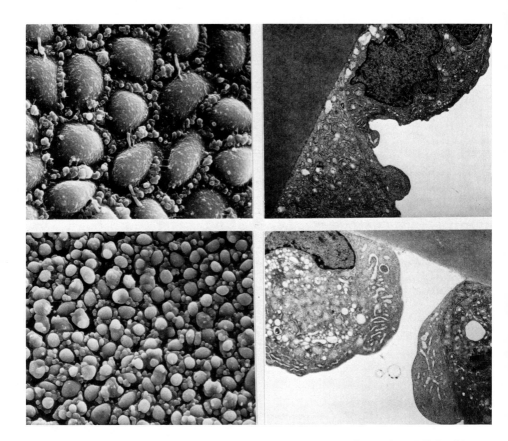

FIG. 3. Top left: SEM of rabbit corneal endothelium perfused with Plasma-Lyte 148 for 2 hr. The endothelial cells are swollen and the junctions between cells have become disruptive. Original magnification ×2,000. **Top right:** TEM of the same cornea. The junction between cells is broken, cytoplasmic vacuoles are present, and mitochondria are condensed. Original magnification ×9,700. **Bottom left:** SEM of rabbit cornea endothelium perfused with Plasma-Lyte 148 for 2 hr. The junctions between cells have completely disrupted, and the endothelial cells have become balled on Descemet's membrane. This is associated with marked corneal swelling. Original magnification ×1,000. **Bottom right:** TEM of the same cornea. Complete junctional breakdown has occurred, the endothelial cells are round with dilated endoplasmic reticulum and mitochondrial condensation. Original magnification ×9,700.

21, and in this case the BSS Plus maintained the endothelial cells, as observed with both scanning and transmission electron microscopy. The lactated Ringer's also maintained the endothelial cells, and there was some swelling of the nucleus. Nevertheless, this younger tissue was able to withstand the stress of the lactated Ringer's, whereas the older tissue could not. It should be pointed out that most of the intraocular surgery performed is in the older population of individuals, and it is these corneas that manifest the greatest degree of postsurgical edema.

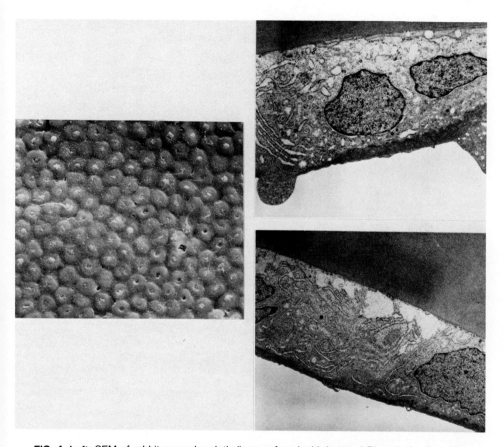

FIG. 4. Left: SEM of rabbit corneal endothelium perfused with lactated Ringer's for 3 hr. The endothelial cells are swollen, cytoplasmic blebbing has occurred, and there are areas of junctional breakdown and cell loss. Original magnification ×1,000. **Top right:** TEM of the same cornea perfused with lactated Ringer's for 3 hr. Note the cytoplasmic blebbing, dilation of the endoplasmic reticulum, and areas of clarified cytoplasm. Original magnification ×12,000. **Bottom right:** TEM of the same cornea illustrating the area of clarified cytoplasm adjacent to Descemet's membrane. Original magnification ×9,600.

The clinical results reported by Benson et al. (7) with BSS Plus have shown that, in a prospective randomized double-blind study, a glutathione-bicarbonate-Ringer's solution (BSS Plus) causes significantly less corneal swelling on the first postoperative day following pars plana vitrectomy than does lactated Ringer's solution. By the seventh postoperative day no difference could be observed between the two solutions. Burke et al. (10), in an open-labeled study, showed that BSS Plus was also safe for pediatric ophthalmic surgery. Recently, de Jong et al. (14), in a prospective double-blind study, compared the effect of GBR to Ringer's solution in a follow-up of 1 week to 28 months,

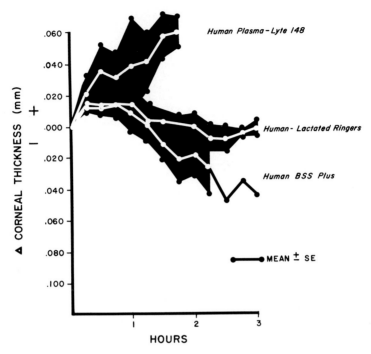

FIG. 5. Changes in corneal thickness of human corneas perfused with BSS Plus, lactated Ringer's, and Plasma-Lyte 148. The white dots and line are the mean change in corneal thickness at each 15-min interval with the shaded range reflecting the standard error of the mean.

and they could find no difference between the two solutions. If a beneficial effect of an irrigating solution is to manifest itself, it would occur within 24 hr. Thereafter the intraocular fluid within the eye would be replaced with newly secreted aqueous humor, and the intraocular effect of the irrigating solution would be minimized.

Other Irrigating Solutions

Other investigators have tried to simplify the GBR solution by removing glutathione (59). Their studies emphasize the importance of bicarbonate as an essential ingredient that should not be omitted from an intraocular irrigating solution. Further studies by this group (73) have suggested that T. C. Earles solution with dextran as an osmotic agent may be beneficial in preventing postsurgical corneal edema. It should be realized from these studies that dextran is not a natural constituent of aqueous humor. Using the basic formulation of GBR, the Japanese formulation SMA_2 (Table 1) has been

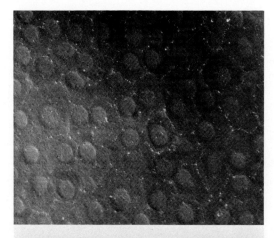

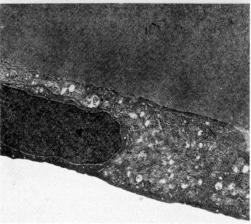

FIG. 6. Top: SEM of human corneal endothelium (51 years old) perfused with BSS Plus for 1.5 hr. The normal mosaic-like pattern of the endothelial cells is present, and their posterior surface is smooth. ×1,000. **Bottom:** TEM of the same cornea. The posterior surface is smooth, and the subcellular organelles are normal. ×5,200.

investigated in rabbits and shown to protect the corneal endothelium and prevent corneal edema (68,69) when perfused to the endothelium for extended periods of time. GBR and SMA$_2$ were also found to support the electroretinogram (ERG) amplitude in isolated rabbit eye cups (66) and to prevent corneal complications after pars plana vitrectomy (57). The essential ingredients of the irrigating solutions were bicarbonate ion and glucose (66). The difference between SMA$_2$ and GBR is the lack of glutathione and the addition of sodium acetate and sodium citrate as the buffers that maintain the solution pH in SMA$_2$. Since acetate and citrate are unnatural buffers to the intraocular tissues, they may not support cellular metabolism as well as a solution without acetate and citrate. There is even the possibility that, with the low calcium concentration of SMA$_2$, the citrate may chelate the solution calcium.

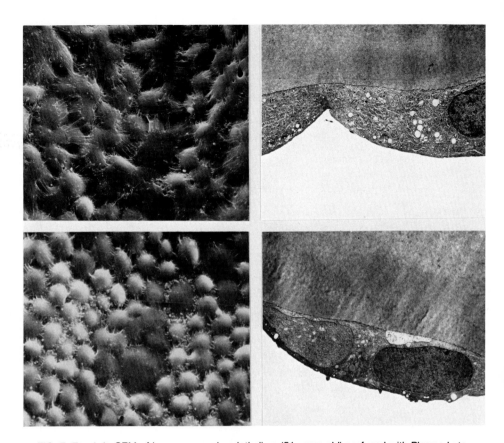

FIG. 7. Top left: SEM of human corneal endothelium (51 years old) perfused with Plasma-Lyte 148 for 1.5 hr. The endothelial cells are separating at their junctions, and the cells are becoming round. Original magnification ×1,000. **Top right:** TEM of the same cornea. The cells have rounded and become vacuolated, and the mitochondria are condensed. Original magnification ×4,400. **Bottom left:** SEM of a human corneal endothelium (97 years old) perfused with Plasma-Lyte 148 for 1.75 hr. The cells are separating at their junctions and becoming round. Original magnification ×1,000. **Bottom right:** TEM of the same cornea illustrating junctional breakdown, rounding of the nucleus, and some cytoplasmic vacuolization. Original magnification ×3,600.

Because of the nature of the bicarbonate buffer solution and the continual loss of CO_2 to the atmosphere, stability can only be achieved in a closed system. Therefore, other buffer systems have been suggested for addition to or replacement of bicarbonate. HEPES, an organic buffer used for tissue culture, has been proposed as an intraocular irrigating and replacement buffer (Table 1) (31). Although a HEPES-buffered irrigating solution will maintain pH and protect the corneal endothelium, there is a loss of the electrical resistance and short circuit current by the endothelium when HEPES is used. However, these

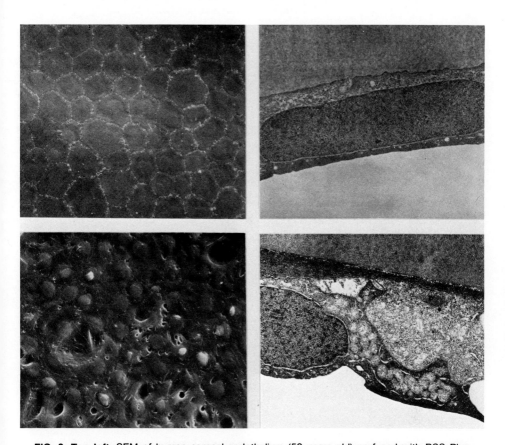

FIG. 8. Top left: SEM of human corneal endothelium (59 years old) perfused with BSS Plus for 3 hr. The endothelium is smooth and junctions are intact. Original magnification ×1,000. **Top right:** TEM of the same cornea illustrating a normal cell ultrastructure after 3 hr of perfusion with BSS Plus. Original magnification ×9,100. **Bottom left:** SEM of the paired human cornea perfused with lactated Ringer's for 3 hr. The endothelial mosaic pattern is present, but the nuclei are prominent and there are breaks in the junctions between cells. Original magnification ×1,000. **Bottom right:** TEM of the same cornea. The outer plasma membrane is irregular due to cytoplasmic vacuolization and swelling of the nucleus, cytoplasm, and mitochondria. Original magnification ×6,100.

parameters are recoverable when the HEPES is replaced with a HCO_3^--buffered irrigating solution. The authors propose that an irrigating solution with HEPES would be used only for a short time period; therefore, minimal endothelial effects would manifest. More recent studies by Geroski et al. (29) have shown that a HEPES-buffered irrigating solution can decrease the Na^+,K^+-ATPase activity of the corneal endothelium over an HCO_3^--buffered solution. It should be noted that HEPES buffer, although one of the most stable buffers to maintain pH of a solution, is not a natural constituent of aqueous humor.

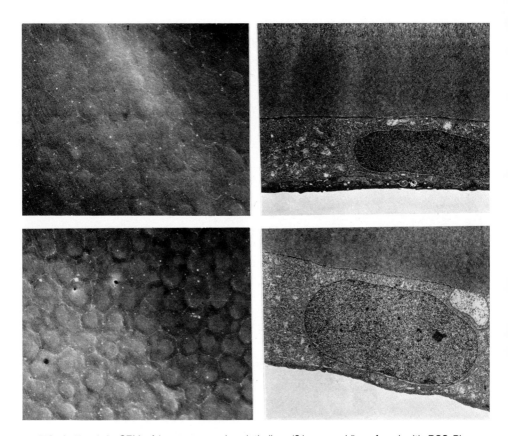

FIG. 9. Top left: SEM of human corneal endothelium (21 years old) perfused with BSS Plus for 2.5 hr. The endothelium is smooth, and the junctions are intact. Original magnification ×1,000. **Top right:** TEM of the same cornea illustrating a normal cell ultrastructure. Original magnification ×5,200. **Bottom left:** SEM of the paired cornea perfused with lactated Ringer's for 2.5 hr. This cornea maintained its thickness. The normal mosaic-like pattern is present, and the endothelium is intact. Original magnification ×1,000. **Bottom right:** TEM of the same cornea. The posterior surface is wavy, the intercellular junctions are intact, and the subcellular organelles are normal. Original magnification ×5,200.

Because of the many intraocular irrigating solutions that are available for ophthalmic use, it is important to review the clinical importance of the various ingredients necessary for the ocular tissues to maintain their normal function.

Sodium, Potassium, and Magnesium

Sodium is the major extracellular ion of plasma and aqueous humor (Table 2) and is essential to maintain cellular tonicity. Sodium is also the major ion transported by cells for cell volume regulation, and it is necessary for the metabolic pump (75) to function within the corneal endothelium.

Potassium is the major intracellular ion of cells and is the ion that is actively transported across the cell membrane to maintain the intracellular potential. The inward transport of K^+ is coupled with the outward transport of Na^+ by the enzyme Na^+,K^+-ATPase. Therefore, the potassium ion at a low concentration (3 to 6 mM/liter) is essential for an intraocular irrigating solution.

Magnesium is an essential element for all cells. It is a cofactor for some ATPases and for many cellular biochemical reactions. Therefore, it should be included in an intraocular irrigating solution in a concentration similar to aqueous humor (Table 2).

Calcium

Calcium ion is essential to the corneal endothelium for maintenance of the barrier function and control of the apical junctional complexes (51). The ultrastructural integrity of the apical junctional complex is dependent on the availability of intracellular and extracellular Ca^{++} (81). An irrigating solution that lacks calcium will cause endothelial junctional breakdown and result in corneal edema (23). Calcium is also an essential ion for the retina in order to regulate the visual cycle (55) and should be included as an ingredient for an irrigating solution that also bathes the retina.

Bicarbonate

The natural extracellular buffer for human tissues is bicarbonate and proteins (blood). For those tissues bathed by special body fluids where protein is lacking (cerebrospinal fluid and aqueous humor) bicarbonate is the major buffer. It is also a major constituent of aqueous humor (Table 2) and should be included as the most important buffer system of an intraocular irrigating solution. There is a great deal of scientific evidence that supports the use of HCO_3^- by the intraocular tissues.

It was first reported by Hodson (37,38) that corneal thickness could be maintained in the rabbit if the concentration of sodium bicarbonate in an endothelial perfusion medium was maintained at 24 mM. Later, Hodson and Miller (39) and Hull et al. (46) provided evidence that an active transport of HCO_3^- across the corneal endothelium contributes to the endothelial pump function. Wiederholt and Koch (85) and Hodson et al. (41) showed that the bicarbonate concentration of GBR was able to maintain the human corneal endothelial potential for extended periods of time.

Bicarbonate has similarly been shown to support retinal function. Winkler et al. (87) and Moorhead et al. (64) reported the beneficial effects on the ERG of an intravitreal bicarbonate buffered Ringer's used for irrigation during vitrectomy. Also, Negi et al. (65,66) concluded that bicarbonate and glucose are essential for maintaining retinal function during intraocular irrigation. All of these reports support the need for an intraocular irrigating solution to contain HCO_3^-, and intraocular irrigating solutions not containing HCO_3^- (Table 1) do not adequately support or maintain the intraocular tissues during the extended periods of time required in certain intraocular surgical procedures.

Dextrose

All cells metabolize glucose for the production of energy necessary for normal function. The ocular tissues use glucose for the production of ATP and the maintenance of cornea, lens transparency, and retinal function. Thus, dextrose is a necessary ingredient for an intraocular irrigating solution used over extended periods of time.

The corneal endothelium has a comparatively high percentage of aerobic glycolysis, as suggested from the pentose shunt studies of Geroski et al. (28). They concluded that 63% of all glucose oxidized to CO_2 occurs by aerobic glycolysis in the endothelium, compared to 34% in the epithelium. In both cases the remaining CO_2 is formed via the pentose shunt. Endothelial cells can be inferred to have a high rate of aerobic glycolysis by their numerous mitochondria, more than any other ocular cell type except retinal photoreceptors (43). The endothelium receives both glucose and oxygen directly from the aqueous, which bathes the apical cellular membranes. Gaasterland et al. (27) reported an average value of 2.94 mM of glucose in the aqueous of fasting rhesus monkeys. Endothelial cells are especially vulnerable to interruptions in their source of nourishment for the control of corneal hydration and clarity. Accordingly, these cells can be affected by the nature of an intraocular irrigating solution used in the course of anterior segment surgery (23).

Glutathione

Glutathione, an important tripeptide with a reactive sulfhydryl group, is found in aqueous humor (Table 2). Its concentration in primates and dogs ranges from 1 to 10 μM and in rabbits from 10 to 30 μM (77). Although the blood contains a high concentration of glutathione, it is mainly present within erythrocytes, and the plasma has only a low concentration of 5 μM or less. While aqueous glutathione may be derived by diffusion from the blood or by an active transport system in the ciliary epithelium analogous to that of the lens, it is probable that it also diffuses from the lens and cornea.

The fluid transport in the isolated cornea was first shown to be influenced by the presence of glutathione by Dikstein and Maurice (17). Anderson et al. (1) found that GSH (the reduced form), when added to a medium deficient in both glucose and adenosine, protected the endothelium from a depletion of ATP. However, later studies by Anderson et al. (2) showed that the addition of glucose alone was equal to GSH in maintaining ATP levels and that adenosine alone was superior. The most important role is indicated by the improved corneal de-swelling and survival time that GSH has over both glucose and adenosine. This effect on the physiologic parameters could be brought about equally well by 240 μM GSH or 20 μM GSSG (the oxidized form), and since such levels of GSSG were always found in solutions of GSH as a result of auto-oxidation, it was suggested that oxidized GSSG was the active one (2). Anderson et al. (2) suggested that membrane thiol groups might interact with the disulfide, resulting in a conformational change that would reduce membrane permeability, thus increasing net fluid transport.

Such a role of the GSSG could be proposed since Riley et al. (77) found 15% oxidized glutathione in aqueous humor. However, Edelhauser et al. (22) found that, when the intracellular endothelial cell glutathione was completely oxidized, endothelial cells lost their barrier functions and the apical junctions became disrupted. When the endothelial cellular concentrations of GSH and GSSG were measured after perfusion of corneas with media of varying glutathione content (67,86), it was found that endothelial fluid transport was disrupted only when the total intracellular glutathione fell below one-third of the *in vivo* value.

These studies also showed that, with the addition of both GSH and GSSG to an irrigating solution, corneal swelling was prevented and the intracellular level of glutathione was maintained. Similarly, Hodson and Wigham (40) and Hodson et al. (41) showed that the transendothelial potential across the human corneal endothelium is stabilized and maintained for up to 6 hr in the presence of 0.5 mM reduced glutathione, whereas a simple salt solution could not maintain this potential.

The role of glutathione is unclear, but there appears to be a critical level required within the endothelial cells and a need for a fraction in both the oxidized and reduced states, suggesting that it might function as a redox buffer system to combat the effects of free radicals. Therefore, a continuous supply of glutathione in the aqueous humor or an irrigating solution could effectively detoxify any injurious radicals produced in the anterior segment or vitreous humor (75,76) during intraocular surgery.

pH and Osmolality

It has been shown that the cornea can tolerate irrigation with physiologic solutions within an osmolality range of 200 to 400 mOsm (22) and within a pH range of 6.8 to 8.2 (26,30). However, an ideal irrigating solution should be iso-osmotic with the intraocular tissues (i.e., 305 mOsm) and contain the essential ingredients to prevent corneal swelling and cellular destruction. Table 1 shows the pH variability of the irrigating solutions. Both 0.9% NaCl and lactated Ringer's can fall below the pH tolerance of the intraocular tissues. The pH of the irrigating solutions can also be changed (buffer capacity) if antibiotics or epinephrine (20) are added. Therefore, the ophthalmic surgeon should be cautious of the additions to an irrigating solution used during intraocular surgery.

Since an individual with an abnormal endothelium can predispose toward bullous keratoplasty after intraocular surgery, it is essential that the most complete intraocular irrigating solution be used: one that contains the essential salts, is buffered with HCO_3^- to pH 7.4, has an osmolality of 305 mOsm, and contains nutrients to support cellular metabolism.

A different surgical problem that occurs with pars plana vitrectomy is the development of a posterior subcapsular lens opacification in diabetic patients. The opacification blocks the appearance of both vitreous cavity and retina, and a lensectomy may double the risk of postoperative neovascular glaucoma. An investigation by Haimann et al. (34) demonstrated that a long-term intraocular irrigating solution was not able to protect against cataract formation in diabetic rabbits. It was found, however, that glucose fortification of BSS Plus to 335 mOsm prevented cataract formation during perfusion in vitrectomies on rabbits. The vitrectomies and perfusions were performed for 2 hr. The increased osmolality acts to guard against the osmotic stress that occurs with solutions of normal osmolality. The reason for this is that the diabetic lenses have polyols trapped within their cells that can cause osmotic stress (49,52). Posterior subcapsular lens opacity does not occur normally because of the higher aqueous glucose content of the diabetic. In a randomized prospective double-blind trial, Haimann and Abrams (33) have shown that glucose fortification of BSS Plus significantly reduces intraoperative lens opacification during diabetic vitrectomy. The important point of this study is that, with a complete intraocular irrigating solution, slight additions can be made to accommodate the surgical need.

VISCOUS AQUEOUS SUBSTITUTES

With the development of intraocular lens implantation after cataract surgery, a problem associated with polymethylmethacrylate implants was the high endothelial cell loss (64%) after surgery (44). Kaufman and Katz (50) demonstrated that direct contact between a polymethylmethacrylate intraocular lens and the corneal endothelium results in a shearing of the endothelial cell membrane or even complete local removal of an area of endothelial cells from Descemet's membrane. Because of the mechanical endothelial cell loss from the intraocular lens, a variety of viscous substances have been used to prevent mechanical trauma to the endothelium. The viscous substances include sodium hyaluronate, chondroitin sulfate, and methylcellulose. A review of each substance is helpful in elucidating its potential intraocular usefulness.

In 1934 Meyer and Palmer (61) isolated hyaluronic acid from the vitreous humor. Based on an extensive laboratory investigation of the biochemical properties of hyaluronic acid, Balazs (4) suggested injecting hyaluronic acid into the vitreous humor for the treatment of retinal detachment; hyaluronic acid replacement of vitreous had been performed by Widder (84) and Hruby

(45). It was not until 1972 that Balazs and Freemen (5) reported on the use of hyaluronic acid in the replacement of both vitreous and aqueous humor.

Miller et al. (62) reported the experimental use of 1% sodium hyaluronate (Healon®) for endothelial protection in rabbits, and in 1981 its use in humans was first described (63). Because of the difficulty in obtaining sodium hyaluronate, Fechner (24) proposed the use of 1% methylcellulose as an inexpensive viscous aqueous substitute for lens implantation that also protected the endothelium when injected into the anterior chamber. Chondroitin sulfate, another natural intraocular substance with greater wettability than sodium hyaluronate, also affords endothelial protection when a 20% concentration is used during intraocular lens implantation (79).

One percent sodium hyaluronate is a naturally occurring glycosaminoglycan consisting of repeating disaccharide units of alternating glucuronic acid and N-acylglycosamine (56,78). It has a molecular weight of greater than $1.1–1.8 \times 10^6$ containing less than 1% protein. Its viscosity ranges between 30,000 and 100,000 centistokes (44,56). Chondroitin sulfate is also a glycosaminoglycan containing alternating disaccharide units of glucuronic acid and galactosamine (78). The molecular weight and viscosity of chondroitin sulfate depend on its formulation. Twenty percent chondroitin sulfate (120 centistokes), however, is considerably less viscous than 1% sodium hyaluronate (56).

Methylcellulose 0.5% and 2% have been used for many years in ophthalmology as wetting agents for the treatment of keratitis sicca. The surgical-grade methylcellulose is hydroxypropyl methylcellulose (25). It consists of two molecules of glucose that bind to form cellobiose, a molecule that humans are unable to break down. The process by which methylcellulose is cleared from the body is at present unknown (25).

Graue et al. (32) reported that sodium hyaluronate had a protective effect on the corneal endothelium as well as being well tolerated in the anterior chamber. Sodium hyaluronate has also been reported by Miller and Stegman (63) to be effective in reducing endothelial cell loss from 54% to 18% in intraocular lens implant surgery. More recently, however, with greater implant experience and uniplanar intraocular lenses, the percentage of endothelial cell loss has been reduced even without the use of a viscous molecule to coat the implant. Hoffer (42) found no significant difference in the amount of endothelial cell loss comparing air to 1% sodium hyaluronate. Many surgeons continue to use 1% sodium hyaluronate, however, because it is difficult to predict which patients will have inadvertent endothelial trauma at the time of lens implantation. Many corneal surgeons use 1% sodium hyaluronate to avoid contact between the iris lens diaphragm and the corneal endothelium as well as to re-form the anterior chamber during corneal transplantation (63,70,74,80). Polack et al. (74) have shown lower postoperative corneal thicknesses following anterior vitrectomy and penetrating keratoplasty using 1% sodium hyaluronate.

In 1980 Denlinger (15,16) reported that sodium hyaluronate was nontoxic when injected into the liquid vitreous of monkeys; however, Hultsch (47) noted that the intraocular inflammatory potential of hyaluronic acid varies with the batch used. This observation may account for the sporadic cases of idiopathic postoperative corneal edema reported to the National Registry of Drug-Induced Ocular Side Effects in Portland, Oregon. Methylcellulose and chondroitin sulfate have not been associated with any significant inflammatory reaction when properly formulated, although their clinical use has been limited (24,25,36,79).

As more experience is gained with viscous aqueous substitutes, clinicians have become aware of the potential for intraocular pressure (IOP) rises with 1% sodium hyaluronate. Binkhorst (9) first reported an increase in IOP (mean 30 mm Hg) the first postoperative day compared with controls (mean 15 mm Hg). Even sharper increases in IOP (mean 38 mm Hg) were noted by Pape and Balazs (70) on the first postoperative day without irrigating the 1% sodium hyaluronate out of the anterior chamber. However, if the 1% sodium hyaluronate was washed out of the anterior chamber with BSS, the IOP rise was lower (mean 19 mm Hg) than in the nonirrigated group.

Passo and Ernest (72) have also documented an increase in IOP (34 mm Hg) at 14.9 hr following use of 0.1 cc of 1% sodium hyaluronate during cataract surgery (control IOP, 14 mm Hg). This pressure increase was minimally affected by medical treatment with acetazolamide. The increase in IOP following intraocular use of sodium hyaluronate causes a decrease in aqueous outflow in monkey (48) and in enucleated human eyes (6). In a laboratory study to document the reported IOP rise, Mac Rae et al. (56) showed that intracameral injection of sodium hyaluronate caused the IOP to increase to 67 mm Hg; and when 20% chondroitin sulfate was used, the pressure increased to 55 mm Hg. The marked increase in IOP occurred at 1 to 6 hr postinjection into the anterior chamber in both rabbits and monkeys. The IOP returned to normal by 24 hr (Fig. 10). When the viscous substances were irrigated from the anterior chamber, or when the viscosity of the substances was decreased (i.e., 0.4% methylcellulose or 10% chondroitin sulfate), IOP was considerably lower (36 mm Hg). Therefore, when any of the viscous substances was used, the IOP was always higher than the IOP following intracameral BSS. Pape (71) also showed that anterior chamber washout was helpful in minimizing the IOP rise after cataract surgery. In enucleated human eyes, however, extensive irrigation was not able to increase the outflow once sodium hyaluronate was used (6).

After intracameral use with 2% methylcellulose, a similar viscosity-induced ocular hypertension occurs that resolves by 24 hr in rabbits (Fig. 11). Fechner (24) noted an increase in IOP (45 mm Hg) with 1% methylcellulose on the first postoperative day in patients who underwent intracapsular cataract extraction with intraocular lens implantation. In a later study, Fechner (25) showed moderate pressure rises in the low 30s on the first postoperative day

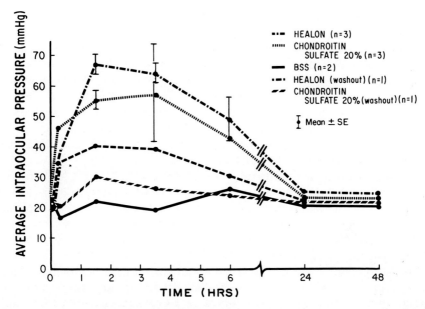

FIG. 10. Intraocular pressure in monkeys after anterior chamber injection (0.15 cc) of sodium hyaluronate (Healon®), 20% chondroitin sulfate with and without washout, and balanced salt solution (BSS, 0.15 ml). (From ref. 56, with permission.)

with both 1% and 2% methylcellulose with and without irrigation to remove the methylcellulose from the anterior chamber. However, Aron-Rosa et al. (3) did not note an elevated IOP when 1% methylcellulose was used for extracapsular cataract extraction although the methylcellulose was irrigated from the eye after lens implantation.

The efficacy of viscous agents in protecting the corneal endothelium from the mechanical trauma of an intraocular lens implant is, nevertheless, a critical

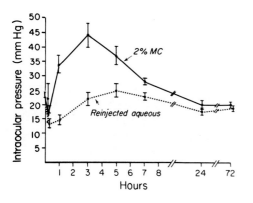

FIG. 11. Intraocular pressure in rabbits after anterior chamber injection of 0.15 cc of 2% methylcellulose (MC). Reinjected aqueous in the paired eye served as a control.

point. It appears that 1% sodium hyaluronate provides excellent corneal endothelial protection. Harrison et al. (36) found the protective properties of 20% chondroitin sulfate to be superior to 1% sodium hyaluronate *in vitro.* However, in subsequent studies 20% chondroitin sulfate was found to be hyperosmolar (656 mOsm) and caused subtle corneal endothelial microvillous changes in rabbits and moderate anterior subcapsular lens vesicles in monkeys (56). The osmotic tolerance of the corneal endothelium has been reported to be between 200 and 450 mOsm (19). Therefore, chondroitin sulfate should be formulated to be in that physiologic range in order to be safe and efficacious for intraocular use.

Another possible alternative may be the combination of a chondroitin sulfate and sodium hyaluronate, since chondroitin sulfate has superior coating properties on intraocular lens implants and sodium hyaluronate provides better support in maintaining the structure of the anterior chamber. For these reasons a combination of the two substances may be beneficial, although clinical data are currently not available.

Methylcellulose has been shown to protect the corneal endothelium from implant damage. In extracapsular cataract extraction and intraocular lens implantation, Aron-Rosa et al. (3) found an endothelial cell loss of 8% using 1% methylcellulose (compared with 25% using air) during implantation. Thus, methylcellulose may prove to be an excellent, inexpensive alternative as a viscous aqueous substitute to protect the endothelium during intraocular surgery.

In summary, the use of the newer intraocular irrigating solutions and an endothelial protective viscous substance have been helpful to the ophthalmic surgeon in reducing postoperative corneal edema following intraocular surgery.

ACKNOWLEDGMENTS

This work was supported in part by grants EY-00933 and EY-07016 from the National Eye Institute. Dr. Edelhauser is a Research to Prevent Blindness, Inc. Olga K. Weiss Research Scholar.

REFERENCES

1. Anderson, E. I., Fischbarg, J., and Spector, A. (1973): Fluid transport, ATP level and ATPase activities in isolated rabbit corneal endothelium. *Biochim. Biophys. Acta,* 307:557–562.
2. Anderson, E. I., Fischbarg, J., and Spector, A. (1974): Disulfide stimulation of fluid transport and effect on ATP level in rabbit corneal endothelium. *Exp. Eye Res.,* 19:1–10.
3. Aron-Rosa, D., Cohen, H., Aron, J. J., and Bouquety, C. (1983): Methylcellulose instead of Healon in extracapsular surgery with intraocular lens implantation. *Ophthalmology,* 90:1235–1238.
4. Balazs, E. A. (1969): The physiology of the vitreous body. In: *Importance of the Vitreous Body in Retina Surgery with Special Emphasis on Reoperations,* edited by C. S. Schepens, pp. 29–48. C. V. Mosby, St. Louis.

5. Balazs, E. A., Freeman, M. I., Kloti, R., Meyer-Schwickerath, G., Regnault, F., and Sweeney, D. B. (1972): Hyaluronic acid and replacement of vitreous and aqueous humor. *Mod. Probl. Ophthalmol.,* 10:3–21.

6. Benson, F. G., Patterson, M. M., and Epstein, D. L. (1983): Obstruction of aqueous outflow by sodium hyaluronate in enucleated human eyes. *Am. J. Ophthalmol.,* 95:668–672.

7. Benson, W. E., Diamond, J. G., and Tasman, W. (1981): Intraocular irrigating solutions for pars plana vitrectomy. *Arch. Ophthalmol.,* 99:1013–1015.

8. Bessiere, E. D., Crockett, R., LeRebeller, M. J., Maurain, C., and Grenie, D. (1973): Methodes chimiques de dosage de l'humeur aqueuse normale. *Albrecht V. Graefes Arch. Klin. Exp. Ophth.,* 187:273–288.

9. Binkhorst, C. D. (1980): Inflammation and intraocular pressure after the use of Healon in intraocular surgery. *Am. Intraocular Implant Soc. J.,* 6:340–341.

10. Burke, M. J., Parks, M. M., Calhoun, J. H., Diamond, J. G., and deFaller, J. M. (1981): Safety evaluation of BSS Plus in pediatric intraocular surgery. *J. Pediatr. Ophthalmol. Strabismus,* 18:45–59.

11. Christiansen, J. M., Kollarits, C. R., Fukui, H., Fishman, M. L., Michels, R. G., and Mikuni, I. (1976): Intraocular irrigating solutions and lens clarity. *Am. J. Ophthalmol.,* 82:594–597.

12. Cole, D. F. (1970): Aqueous and ciliary body. In: *Biochemistry of the Eye,* edited by C. N. Graymore, pp. 105–181. Academic Press, New York.

13. Cole, D. F. (1974): Comparative aspects of the intraocular fluids. In: *The Eye,* vol. 5, *Comparative Physiology,* edited by H. Davson and L. T. Graham, Jr., pp. 71–161. Academic Press, New York.

14. de Jong, P. T. V. M., Strous, C., and Filedt Kok, J. P. (1983): Glutathione bicarbonate Ringers' intraocular irrigating fluid: Prospective double blind study. *Ophthalmologica,* 186:35–40.

15. Denlinger, J. L., and Balazs, E. A. (1980): Replacement of the liquid vitreous with sodium hyaluronate in monkeys. I. Short-term evaluation. *Exp. Eye Res.,* 31:81–99.

16. Denlinger, J. L., El-Mofty, A. A. M., and Balazs, E. A. (1980): Replacement of the liquid vitreous with sodium hyaluronate in monkeys. II. Long-term evaluation. *Exp. Eye Res.,* 31:101–117.

17. Dikstein, S., and Maurice, D. M. (1972): The metabolic basis to the fluid pump in the cornea. *J. Physiol. (Lond.),* 221:29–41.

18. Edelhauser, H. F., Gonnering, R., and Van Horn, D. L. (1978): Intraocular irrigating solutions: A comparative study of BSS Plus and lactated Ringers' solution. *Arch. Ophthalmol.,* 96:516–520.

19. Edelhauser, H. F., Hanneken, A. M., Pederson, H. J., and Van Horn, D. L. (1981): Osmotic tolerance of rabbit and human corneal endothelium. *Arch. Ophthalmol.,* 99:1281–1287.

20. Edelhauser, H. F., Hyndiuk, R. A., Zeeb, A., and Schultz, R. O. (1982): Corneal edema and the intraocular use of epinephrine. *Am. J. Ophthalmol.,* 93:327–333.

21. Edelhauser, H. F., Van Horn, D. L., Hyndiuk, R. A., and Schultz, R. O. (1975): Intraocular irrigating solutions: Their effect on the corneal endothelium. *Arch. Ophthalmol.,* 93:648–657.

22. Edelhauser, H. F., Van Horn, D. L., Miller, P., and Pederson, H. J. (1976): Effect of thiol-oxidation of glutathione with diamide on corneal endothelial function, junctional complexes, and microfilaments. *J. Cell Biol.,* 68:567–578.

23. Edelhauser, H. F., Van Horn, D. L., Schultz, R. O., and Hyndiuk, R. A. (1976): Comparative toxicity of intraocular irrigating solutions on the corneal endothelium. *Am. J. Ophthalmol.,* 81:473–481.

24. Fechner, P. U. (1977): Methylcellulose in lens implantation. *Am. Intraocular Implant Soc. J.,* 3:180–181.

25. Fechner, P. U., and Fechner, M. V. (1983): Methylcellulose and lens implantation. *Br. J. Ophthalmol.,* 67:259–263.

26. Fischbarg, J., and Lim, J. J. (1974): Role of cations, anions and carbonic anhydrase in fluid transport across rabbit corneal endothelium. *J. Physiol. (Lond.),* 241:647–675.

27. Gaasterland, D. E., Pederson, J. E., MacLellan, H. M., and Reddy, V. N. (1979): Rhesus monkey aqueous humor composition and a primate ocular perfusate. *Invest. Ophthalmol. Vis. Sci.,* 18:1139–1150.

28. Geroski, D. H., Edelhauser, H. F., and O'Brien, W. J. (1978): Hexose-monophosphate shunt response to diamide in the component layers of the cornea. *Exp. Eye Res.,* 26:611–619.

29. Geroski, D. H., Grosserode, R. S., and Edelhauser, H. F. (1983): A comparison of HEPES and bicarbonate buffered intraocular irrigating solutions: Effects on endothelial function in human and rabbit corneas. *J. Toxicol.—Cut. & Ocular Toxicol.,* 1:299–309.
30. Gonnering, R., Edelhauser, H. F., Van Horn, D. L., and Durant, W. (1979): The pH tolerance of rabbit and human corneal endothelium. *Invest. Ophthalmol. Vis. Sci.,* 18:373–390.
31. Graham, M. V., and Hodson, S. (1980): Intraocular irrigating and replacement fluid. *Trans. Ophthalmol. Soc., U. K.,* 100:282–285.
32. Graue, E. L., Polack, F. M., and Balazs, E. A. (1980): The protective effect of Na-hyaluronate to corneal endothelium. *Exp. Eye Res.,* 31:119–127.
33. Haimann, M. H., and Abrams, G. W. (1984): Prevention of lens opacification during diabetic vitrectomy. *Ophthalmology,* 91:116–121.
34. Haimann, M. H., Abrams, G. W., Edelhauser, H. F., and Hatchell, D. L. (1982): The effect of intraocular irrigating solutions on lens clarity in normal and diabetic rabbits. *Am. J. Ophthalmol.,* 94:594–605.
35. Harper, J. Y., and Pomerat, C. M. (1958): In vitro observations on the behavior of conjunctival and corneal cells in relation to electrolytes. *Am. J. Ophthalmol.,* 46:269–276.
36. Harrison, S. E., Soll, D. E., Shayegan, M., and Clinch, T. (1982): Chondroitin sulfate, a new and effective agent for intraocular lens insertion. *Ophthalmology,* 89:1254–1260.
37. Hodson, S. (1971): Evidence for a bicarbonate-dependent sodium pump in corneal endothelium. *Exp. Eye Res.,* 11:20–29.
38. Hodson, S. (1974): The regulation of corneal hydration by a salt pump requiring the presence of sodium and bicarbonate ion. *J. Physiol. (Lond.),* 236:271–302.
39. Hodson, S., and Miller, F. (1976): The bicarbonate ion pump in the endothelium which regulates the hydration of rabbit cornea. *J. Physiol. (Lond.),* 263:563–577.
40. Hodson, S. A., and Wigham, C. G. (1980): Effect of glutathione on human corneal transendothelial potential difference. *J. Physiol.,* 301:34–35.
41. Hodson, S., Wigham, C., Williams, L., Mayer, K. R., and Graham, M. V. (1981): Observations on the human cornea in vitro. *Exp. Eye Res.,* 32:353–360.
42. Hoffer, K. J. (1982): Effects of extracapsular implant techniques on endothelial cell density. *Arch. Ophthalmol.,* 100:791–792.
43. Hogan, M. J., Alvarado, J. A., and Weddell, J. E. (1971): *Histology of the Human Eye.* W. B. Saunders Co., Philadelphia.
44. Hoopes, P. C. (1982): Sodium hyaluronate (Healon) in anterior surgery: A review and a new use in extracapsular surgery. *Am. Intraocular Implant Soc. J.,* 8:148–154.
45. Hruby, K. (1961): Hyaluronsaure als Glaskorperersatz bei Netzhautablosung. *Klin. Monatsbl. Augenheilkd.,* 138:484–496.
46. Hull, D. S., Green, K., Boyd, M., and Wynn, H. R. (1977): Corneal endothelial bicarbonate transport and the effect of carabonic anhydrase inhibitors on endothelial permeability and fluxes and corneal thickness. *Invest. Ophthalmol. Vis. Sci.,* 16:883–892.
47. Hultsch, E. (1980): The scope of hyaluronic acid as an experimental intraocular implant. *Ophthalmology,* 87:706–712.
48. Hultsch, E. (1983): Low molecular weight hyaluronic acid in experimental anterior surgery: An alternative to Healon. *Ophthalmology,* 90 (Suppl.):102.
49. Jacob, T. J. C., and Duncan, G. (1982): Glucose-induced membrane permeability changes in the lens. *Exp. Eye Res.,* 37:445–453.
50. Kaufman, H. F., and Katz, J. V. (1976): Endothelial damage from intraocular lens insertion. *Invest. Ophthalmol. Vis. Sci.,* 15:996–1000.
51. Kaye, G. I., Mishima, S., Cole, J. D., and Kaye, N. W. (1968): Studies on the cornea. VII. Effects of perfusion with a Ca^{++}-free medium on the corneal endothelium. *Invest. Ophthalmol. Vis. Sci.,* 7:53–66.
52. Kinoshita, J. H., Kador, P., and Catiler, M. (1981): Aldose reductase in diabetic cataracts. *J.A.M.A.,* 246:257–261.
53. Kinsey, V. E., and Cogan, D. G. (1942): The cornea. III. Hydration properties of excised corneal pieces. *Arch. Ophthalmol.,* 28:272–278.
54. Kinsey, V. E., and Cogan, D. G. (1942): The cornea. IV. Hydration properties of the whole cornea. *Arch. Ophthalmol.,* 28:449–463.
55. Lolley, R. N. (1983): Metabolism of retinal rod outer segment. In: *Biochemistry of the Eye,* edited by R. E. Anderson, pp. 178–188. American Academy of Ophthalmology, San Francisco.

56. Mac Rae, S. M., Edelhauser, H. F., Hyndiuk, R. A., Burd, E. M., and Schultz, R. O. (1983): The effects of sodium hyaluronate, chondroitin sulfate, and methylcellulose on the corneal endothelium and intraocular pressure. *Am. J. Ophthalmol., 95:*332–341.
57. Matsuda, M., Tano, Y., Inaba, M., Sato, M., Inoue, Y., and Manabe, R. (1983): Corneal complications after pars plana vitrectomy using SMA_2 for an intraocular irrigating solution. *Folia Ophthalmol. Jpn., 34:*1424–1428.
58. McCarey, B. E., Edelhauser, H. F., and Van Horn, D. L. (1973): Functional and structural changes in the corneal endothelium during in vitro perfusion. *Invest. Ophthalmol. Vis. Sci., 12:*410–417.
59. McEnerney, J. K., and Peyman, G. A. (1977): Simplification of glutathione-bicarbonate-Ringers solution: Its effect on corneal thickness. *Invest. Ophthalmol. Vis. Sci., 16:*657–666.
60. Merrill, D. L., Fleming, T. C., and Girard, L. J. (1960): The effects of physiologic balanced salt solutions and normal saline on intraocular and extraocular tissues. *Am. J. Ophthalmol., 49:*895–898.
61. Meyer, K., and Palmer, J. W. (1934): The polysaccharide of the vitreous. *J. Biol. Chem., 107:*629–634.
62. Miller, D. M., O'Connor, P., and Williams, J. (1977): Use of Na-hyaluronate during intraocular lens implantation in rabbits. *Ophthalmic Surg., 8:*58–61.
63. Miller, D. M., and Stegman, R. (1981): Use of sodium hyaluronate in human IOL implantation. *Ann. Ophthalmol., 13:*811–815.
64. Moorhead, L. C., Redburn, D. A., Merritt, J., and Garcia, C. (1979): The effects of intravitreal irrigation during vitrectomy on the electroretinogram. *Am. J. Ophthalmol., 88:*239–245.
65. Negi, A., Honda, Y., and Kawano, S. (1980): Comparative studies on intraocular irrigating solutions. *Folia Ophthalmol. Jpn., 31:*1452–1459.
66. Negi, A., Honda, Y., and Kawano, S. (1981): Effects of intraocular irrigating solutions on the electroretinographic b-wave. *Am. J. Ophthalmol., 92:*28–37.
67. Ng, M. C., and Riley, M. V. (1980): Relation of intracellular levels and redox state of glutathione to endothelial function in the rabbit cornea. *Exp. Eye Res., 30:*511–517.
68. Otori, T., Hohki, T., Nakao, Y., Akena, K., Ikeda, M., Yamamoto, M., and Yamamoto, Y. (1981): Studies on the intraocular irrigating solution for ophthalmic surgery: Report 2: Reappraisal of the role of bicarbonate concentration. *Acta Soc. Ophthalmol. Jpn., 85:*1237–1242.
69. Otori, T., Hohki, T., Yamamoto, Y., Yamamoto, M., and Ikeda, M. (1980): Physiological studies on the intraocular irrigating solution for ophthalmic surgery: A preliminary report. *Acta Soc. Ophthalmol. Jpn., 84:*1272–1277.
70. Pape, G., and Balazs, E. A. (1980): The use of sodium hyaluronate (Healon) in human anterior segment surgery. *Ophthalmology, 87:*699–705.
71. Pape, L. G. (1980): Intracapsular and extracapsular techniques of lens implantation with Healon. *Am. Intraocular Implant Soc. J., 6:*342–343.
72. Passo, M., and Ernest, J. V. (1985): Intraocular pressure following cataract surgery using Healon. *Arch. Ophthalmol. (in press).*
73. Peyman, G. A., Sanders, D. R., and Ligara, T. (1979): Dextran 40 containing infusion fluids and corneal swelling: A specular microscopic study. *Arch. Ophthalmol., 97:*152–155.
74. Polack, F. M., De Mong, T., and Santaelli, H. (1981): Sodium hyaluronate (Healon) in keratoplasty and IOL implantation. *Ophthalmology, 88:*425–431.
75. Riley, M. V. (1982): Transport of ions and metabolites across the corneal endothelium. In: *Cell Biology of the Eye,* edited by D. S. McDevitt, pp. 53–95. Academic Press, New York.
76. Riley, M. V. (1983): The chemistry of the aqueous humor. In: *Biochemistry of the Eye,* edited by R. E. Anderson, pp. 79–95. American Academy of Ophthalmology, San Francisco.
77. Riley, M. V., Meyer, R. F., and Yates, E. M. (1980): Glutathione in the aqueous humor of human and other species. *Invest. Ophthalmol. Vis. Sci., 19:*94–96.
78. Smolin, G., and Thoft, R. (1983): Scientific foundations and clinical practice. In: *The Cornea,* edited by G. Smolin and R. Thoft, pp. 21–24. Little, Brown, Boston.
79. Soll, D., Harrison, S., Arturi, F., and Clinch, T. (1980): Evaluation and protection of corneal endothelium. *Am. Intraocular Implant Soc. J., 6:*239–242.
80. Stegman, R., and Miller, D. (1981): Protective function of sodium hyaluronate in corneal transplantation. *J. Ocular Ther. Surg., 1:*28–31.
81. Stern, M. E., Edelhauser, H. F., Pederson, H. J., and Staatz, W. D. (1981): Effects of

ionophores X537A and A23187 and calcium-free medium on corneal endothelial morphology. *Invest. Ophthalmol. Vis. Sci.,* 20:497–507.

82. Struve, C. A., Gage, T. D., Bishop, D. W., and Rock, R. L. (1961): Saline versus balanced salt solution in intraocular surgery: A double blind study. *Am. J. Ophthalmol.,* 51:159.
83. Waltman, S. R., Carroll, D., Schemmelpfenning, W., and Okun, E. (1975): Intraocular irrigating solutions for clinical vitrectomy. *Ophthalmic. Surg.,* 6:90–94.
84. Widder, W. (1960): Hyalurononsosure alsa Glaskorperemplantat bei Netzhautablosung. Experimentelle Grundlagen. *Albrecht von Graefes Arch. Klin. Ophthalmol.,* 162:416–429.
85. Wiederholt, M., and Koch, M. (1979): Effect of intraocular irrigating solutions on intracellular membrane potentials and swelling rate of isolated human and rabbit cornea. *Invest. Ophthalmol. Vis. Sci.,* 18:313–317.
86. Whikehart, D. R., and Edelhauser, H. F. (1978): Glutathione in rabbit corneal endothelia: The effects of selected perfusion fluids. *Invest. Ophthalmol. Vis. Sci.,* 17:455–464.
87. Winkler, B. S., Simson, V., and Benner, J. (1977): Importance of bicarbonate in retinal function. *Invest. Ophthalmol. Vis. Sci.,* 16:766–768.

Commentary

Viscous Solutions in Anterior Segment Surgery

The lecture given by Professor Joaquín Barraquer was so outstanding in its presentation as to dwarf any written comment. Herein Barraquer demonstrates the usefulness of Healon® in keratoplasty, cataract surgery, and in glaucoma surgery. His surgical skills employing Healon® were, in certain moments, breathtaking.

In the days when intracapsular cataract extraction was the rule, experienced observers knew that the best postoperative gauge of intraoperative trauma was the appearance of the cornea. As biomicroscopy was refined with the use of specular microscopy, demonstrations of surgical damage to the endothelium of the cornea necessarily led to application of a "viscous" surgery to the anterior segment. Air, widely used previously, seemed to produce its own form of damage. Hyaluronic acid, its derivatives, and other "gags" (glycoaminoglycosans) were initially studied as vitreous substitutes, and, later, as aqueous substitutes (2).

In the United States, and, in Spain, Healon® has been very popular in anterior segment surgery. It is expensive, not widely available, may be difficult to dilute, and, in certain instances necessary to remove, but its overall utility proved. Several ophthalmologists have used methyl cellulose in balanced salt, and, some for almost 10 years, with good results (1, 2). Other viscous materials have been tried, but, in the U.S.A., Healon® has the head start. It should be noted as well that the use of Healon®, particularly in the closed eye, may help preserve the blood-ocular barrier, by preserving transmural pressure relationships. In this way it may also be useful at times to stem intraocular bleeding.

The Editors

REFERENCES

1. Aron-Rosa, D., Cohn, H. C., Aron-J-J, Bouquety, C. (1983) Methylcellulose instead of Healon® in extracapsular surgery with intraocular lens implantation. *Ophthalmology,* 90:1235–1238.
2. Balazs, E. A., Freeman, M. I., Klöti, R., Meyer-Schwickerath, G., Regnault, F., Sweeney, D. B. (1972): Hyaluronic acid and replacement of vitreous and aqueous humor. *Mod. Probl. Ophthalmol.,* 10:3–21.
3. Fechner, P. U., and Fechner, M. U. (1983): Methylcellulose and lens implantation. *Br. J. Ophthalmol.,* 67:259–263.

Surgical Pharmacology of the Eye,
edited by M. Sears and A. Tarkkanen.
Raven Press, New York © 1985.

Viscous Solutions in Anterior Segment Surgery

Joaquín Barraquer

Instituto Barraquer, Barcelona 21, Spain

SUMMARY: Healon® makes anterior segment surgery easier and safer. We use it in the majority of our cases.

Healon® is a high molecular weight, non-inflammatory fraction of sodium hyaluronate, which forms a viscoelastic solution in water at physiological pH and ionic strength, making it a very appropriate substitute for aqueous humor and vitreous in ophthalmic surgical procedures. The viscous nature of Healon® provides mechanical protection for cell layers such as the corneal endothelium and other intraocular structures which are exposed to mechanical damage during surgery. It does not flow out of the open anterior chamber, it helps to separate the tissues like a fluid spatula, it lubricates the tissue, and facilitates hemostasis. In penetrating keratoplasty, it is particularly useful in complicated cases (trauma, burns etc.), protecting the graft endothelium, facilitating the operative maneuvers and contributing to hemostasis. In congenital cataract operations it prevents trauma to the intraocular structures and permits the performance of a very complete extracapsular extraction, using classical, simple instruments. It is also useful in intracapsular extraction to protect the corneal endothelium. In glaucoma surgery, the injection of Healon® into the anterior chamber is very convenient to avoid pre- and postoperative collapse of the anterior chamber.

Viscosurgery has rapidly become an essential part of various surgical procedures. It may still be gaining momentum. The author started using sodium hyaluronate (Healon®) in March 1981 and has used it in more than 600 cases. In this chapter ingenious ways of using Healon® in anterior segment surgery are presented.

In this chapter we present our opinion concerning "viscosurgery"[1] and our personal experience with sodium hyaluronate in anterior segment surgery. We started using this substance in March 1981, and as of November 1983 I have used it in more than 600 cases. This does not include the operations done by my associates, who have also used this substance. Sodium hyaluronate has been used in a large variety of cases ranging from the simple objective of protecting the corneal endothelium in intracapsular cataract extraction to avoid decompensation of the endothelium (for instance, in cases of cornea

---

[1] Term coined by E. A. Balazs in 1979 to indicate procedures in which viscoelastic solutions are employed.

guttata, etc.) to its use in dramatic cases of ocular injuries requiring very complex interventions: removal of the traumatic cataract, combined with foreign body extraction, vitrectomy, reconstruction of the iris diaphragm, and keratoplasty, just to state a few examples.

If sodium hyaluronate were not available, many intraocular maneuvers that are now considered relatively easy would be impossible to perform, or if they were attempted, trauma to the ocular structures and tissues would be much more important. In all our cases we used the preparation commercially available, called Healon®, and before going on to discuss our personal experience we summarize its characteristics.

SODIUM HYALURONATE (HEALON®)[2]

Healon® is a viscoelastic, high-molecular-weight, nonflammable fraction of sodium hyaluronate. Sodium hyaluronate is a polysaccharide (glycosaminoglycan) that has a repeating unit of sodium glucuronate and N-acetylglucosamine. The molecular weight of Healon® is greater than 1 million. In physiologic salt solution, the long molecular chain forms a random loose-coil configuration.

Sodium hyaluronate forms a viscoelastic solution in water, at physiologic pH and ionic strength. Its viscoelastic nature makes Healon® a suitable substitute for aqueous humor and vitreous in ophthalmic surgical procedures. Healon® can be passed through a thin cannula (27-gauge) because the molecules can easily deform.

The viscosity of Healon® (10 mg sodium hyaluronate, highly purified, dissolved in 1 ml physiologically balanced salt solution) is up to 500,000 times greater than the viscosity of the aqueous humor or balanced salt solution (BSS). Healon® is a sterile and nonpyrogenic solution containing less than 50 μg protein/ml. Sodium hyaluronate is a naturally occurring component of human aqueous humor and vitreous.

The effectiveness of Healon® as an adjunct in ophthalmic surgery is the result of its viscoelastic properties. The viscous nature of Healon® provides mechanical protection for cell layers such as the corneal endothelium and other tissues that are exposed to mechanical damage during surgery. The elastic deformations of Healon® also absorb mechanical stress and thereby may provide a protective buffer for the tissues.

Healon® does not flow out of the open anterior chamber, and therefore a deep chamber as well as other tissue spaces may be maintained during surgical manipulation. Because Healon® is viscoelastic, it is a useful tool for gently maneuvering tissues into the desired position. It helps to identify the traumatized ocular structures and permits better evaluation of the damaged tissues and possibilities of reconstruction. It works like a viscoelastic fluid spatula separating

[2] Biochemical and physical description of Healon® courtesy of Pharmacia A.B., Box 181, S-75104 Uppsala-1, Sweden.

the tissues. It also lubricates the tissues and facilitates hemostasis. It tends to escape only if accidental compression is exerted or if planned irrigation for its removal is performed. Because of these special properties it really represents a "soft" tool or instrument, which not only protects the ocular structures, preventing and avoiding excessive trauma, but also makes the operations easier and safer.

In the anterior chamber, Healon® dissolves in the newly formed aqueous humor and is slowly eliminated through Schlemm's canal. Used in the manner we are going to explain, we have not found that it causes elevation of ocular pressure as has been described by some authors.

It is supplied sterile in disposable glass syringes, delivering 0.75 ml or 0.4 ml of sodium hyaluronate (10 mg/ml) dissolved in physiologic sodium-chloride–phosphate buffer (pH 7.0 to 7.5). Each milliliter of Healon® contains 10 mg sodium hyaluronate, 8.5 mg sodium chloride, 0.28 mg disodium hydrogen dihydrate, 0.04 mg sodium dihydrogen phosphate hydrate, and water for injection. Healon® syringes are terminally sterilized and aseptically packaged, but the solution can be transferred just before use to another syringe with more reliable action, such as glass tuberculin or insulin syringes. Refrigerated Healon® should be allowed to attain room temperature (approximately 30 min) prior to use.

SODIUM HYALURONATE (HEALON®) IN ANTERIOR SEGMENT SURGERY

Although Healon® plays an important part in surgical repair of ocular trauma, unfortunately its discussion would largely surpass the limits of this chapter. In the following we discuss Healon® in keratoplasty, in cataract surgery, and in glaucoma surgery.

Sodium Hyaluronate in Keratoplasty

Standard Technique

Donor eye

The graft is obtained with the usual technique. We use a motor-driven trephine (Barraquer-Mateus, made by Grieshaber, Switzerland), which allows complete cutting of the graft, provided the pressure exerted is uniform and a very sharp trephine blade is employed.

After careful irrigation with artificial aqueous humor, the graft is placed on a drop of Healon® in a Petri dish. Sodium hyaluronate affords good protection of the endothelium of the graft until it is placed in the recipient. It also protects the graft during the suturing because a thin film of Healon® remains, coating the endothelium.

Recipient eye

After the trephination has been completed and the peripheral iridotomies or iridectomies are performed, a drop of Healon® is injected in the four quadrants to maintain the corneal endothelium separated from the iris during the suturing of the graft. The Healon® acts as a cushion between the graft and the iris and protects the endothelium during the insertion of the sutures.

In vascularized corneas, the presence of Healon® in the anterior chamber, near the bleeding point, "plugging" the bleeding vessels, is useful because it will not only aid hemostasis but also prevent adherence of the iris to the cornea.

If the ocular hypotony is very marked, the donor button may tend to fall into the anterior chamber, which makes it difficult to ascertain which is the best position for perfect coaptation. When Healon® has been injected into the anterior chamber, the graft can be maintained at the desired level, the level of the recipient. A drop of Healon® may also be applied on the anterior surface of the graft to protect it during the placement of the sutures.

For proper re-formation of the anterior chamber at the end of the procedure, air is injected slowly until the anterior chamber depth is normal. This maneuver facilitates checking the absence of anterior synechiae; any existing adhesions are easily liberated.

The Healon® persisting in the anterior chamber forms a thin layer coating the corneal endothelium and the iris. Finally, some of the air is removed and replaced by BSS.

Restoration of a normal anterior chamber depth is achieved, leaving a bubble of air in the center, surrounded by BSS in the periphery. The Healon® protecting the corneal endothelium and iris is thus "dissolved," which should prevent its causing postoperative ocular hypertension. Also, the remnants of Healon® improve coaptation of the corneal wound.

Complicated Cases

Penetrating keratoplasty in an eye with perforated ulcer

The main difficulty is the fact that the anterior chamber is collapsed, and this makes trephination more complicated. Currently in these cases we use the Strampelli pneumatizer to re-form the anterior chamber during the operation, in order to be able to perform the trephination (1). The new automated fluid-gas system of McCuen et al. (2) is of the same value for this purpose. If neither the pneumatizer nor the automated fluid-gas system is available, the area to be excised is marked with the trephine and then cut with scissors. The section starts at the perforation site, extends to the groove marked with the trephine, and then follows the groove. As fibrin formation will have caused iris to adhere to the cornea, before introducing the scissors, Healon® is injected through the perforation site all around the periphery of the anterior chamber. Healon® acts like a "soft spatula," and the iris is kept separate, avoiding interference with the resection of the corneal button. Then, to avoid trauma to the iris, the cornea is gently lifted up with forceps and scissors while the section is being made. As stated previously, the injection of Healon® into the anterior chamber makes this maneuver much easier, because the iris is kept separate from the corneal endothelium thanks to the aforementioned viscoelastic properties.

Keratoplasty in an eye with secondary glaucoma

If secondary glaucoma because of prolonged flat anterior chamber or inflammation seems likely, one must consider surgery to prevent it. Nevertheless, it may be preferable not to do it at the same time as keratoplasty, because of the danger of flattening of the anterior chamber in the postoperative period.

If Healon® is available, however, it may be possible to do a combined keratoplasty and glaucoma operation (trabeculectomy) in these cases. Healon® should be injected into the periphery of the anterior chamber before the corneal sutures are placed and in the center of the anterior chamber when the graft has been sutured. Then the trabeculectomy is performed, and more Healon® is injected through the posterior lip of the scleral flap. The Healon® together with the aqueous humor maintains the anterior chamber depth and escapes slowly through the area of the trabeculectomy, producing a filtering bleb covered by the conjunctival flap, which may be limbus-based or fornix-based.

Penetrating keratoplasty in an eye with adherent leukoma

This procedure is sometimes performed in two steps, but thanks to the use of corticosteroids and Healon®, at present it can usually be accomplished in one step. As has been stated previously, Healon®, due to its viscoelastic properties, tends to stay in the spaces into which it has been injected, which is useful in performing certain surgical maneuvers, such as cutting synechiae and resection of membranes, with minimal trauma. For the same reason, it is also helpful in facilitating adequate hemostasia. The steps in this procedure are as follows:

1. Healon® is injected to deepen the anterior chamber. Trephination is then performed. Usually, when Healon® has been employed, the entire circumference can be cut without injury to the iris, since the Healon® does not escape from the anterior chamber.
2. The anterior synechiae are freed or cut. If the anterior surface of the iris is ragged, the irregularities are cut with scissors. If the stroma is markedly altered or atrophic, it is preferable to perform a sector iridectomy. Sometimes the iris diaphragm may be "reconstructed" using Prolene sutures.
3. Peripheral iridotomies or iridectomies are performed in the usual manner.

4. If a cataract is present, it is removed or a capsulectomy is performed.

5. If necessary, a transpupillary vitrectomy is performed and a few drops of Healon® are instilled in the posterior chamber. Also, a few drops of Healon® are applied in the periphery of the anterior chamber.

6. The graft is sutured and the anterior chamber is re-formed with Healon® and artificial aqueous humor.

Iatrogenic traumatic cataract in keratoplasty

If the iatrogenic traumatic cataract is not detected until after the operation and the lens is markedly intumescent, it may lead to iridocyclitis, pupillary block, secondary glaucoma, and opacification of the graft. Extracapsular extraction must be performed immediately using the following technique:

1. A fornix-based flap is prepared and a scleral incision approximately 4 mm in length is made.

2. Healon® is injected into the anterior chamber to protect the corneal endothelium and a sector iridectomy is performed.

3. Extracapsular extraction is done by irrigation and aspiration. In the case of a hard nucleus, the incision should be enlarged to remove it with minimal trauma to the corneal endothelium. The Healon® serves as a cushion between the corneal endothelium, the cataract, and the instruments.

4. The anterior chamber is re-formed with air, Healon® mixed with BSS, or BSS alone.

5. The incision and the conjunctival flap are sutured.

Sodium Hyaluronate in Cataract Surgery

Congenital Cataract

In the course of the last few years a number of new techniques have been described for congenital cataract surgery, in order to improve the results as compared to the classic discission-aspiration procedures. Many of these techniques require complex instrumentation and equipment, difficult to handle and often delicate and costly in their maintenance. Moreover, frequently it is difficult to prevent intermittent flattening of the anterior chamber, and the turbulence produced by the irrigation-aspiration maneuvers may cause trauma to the corneal endothelium and the iris, apart from the evident risk of accidental rupture of the posterior capsule. With the use of Healon® in cataract surgery we have developed a new technique, because this substance allows performance of a number of intraocular manipulations in the anterior and posterior chambers using conventional, simple instruments. Healon® facilitates the aspiration and extraction of the lens matter, reducing considerably the trauma to the ocular structures.

The most important advantage of the use of Healon® in congenital cataract surgery is prevention of flattening of the anterior chamber during the operation. After the lens matter has been removed, the posterior capsule is carefully cleaned and a large resection of the anterior capsule is performed. Finally, a posterior capsulotomy is done, if indicated. The technique is as follows:

1. A 2-mm slanted, valve-like corneal incision is performed at the limbus. The most appropriate instrument to perform this incision is a narrow keratome or the "ultrasharp disposable knife" made by Grieshaber (No. 68109).

2. Healon® is slowly injected into the anterior chamber until the chamber is seen to be somewhat deeper than in normal conditions. This will also increase mechanically the dilation of the pupil, which is of advantage for performing the aspiration and capsulotomy (Fig. 1).

3. The anterior lens capsule is punctured in the periphery with a Haab needle or the "ultrasharp disposable knife." The opening should be small, just sufficient to admit an 18-gauge blunt-tip cannula. Care has to be taken that the location of this opening be peripheral and the penetration not excessively deep.

4. The 18-gauge cannula, connected to a vacuum unit or a syringe, is introduced into the lens capsule and "intracapsular aspiration" of the cataract is carried out (Fig. 2). If the lens matter is soft, aspiration is rapid and easy. Care has to be taken not to aspirate the anterior or the posterior capsule, which would obstruct the opening of the cannula and make aspiration of the

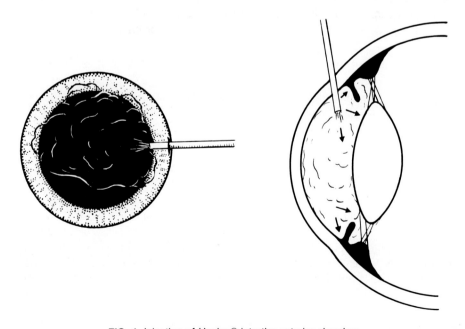

FIG. 1. Injection of Healon® into the anterior chamber.

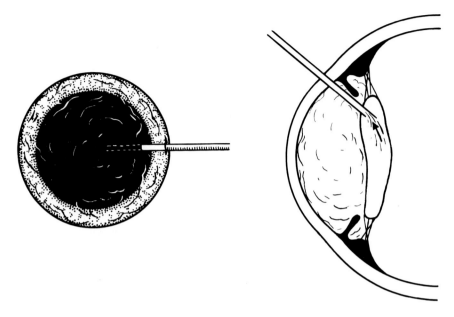

FIG. 2. "Intracapsular" aspiration of the cataract.

lens matter impossible. In cases of immature cataract, considered soft enough for aspiration, the nucleus is aspirated first and then the lens substance is aspirated until the capsule collapses, while the anterior chamber maintains its original depth thanks to the presence of Healon®.

5. A 21-gauge blunt cannula is used to irrigate the lens capsule with artificial aqueous humor,[3] completing the expulsion of the lens material that was not removed during aspiration. The "intracapsular irrigation" avoids turbulence in the anterior chamber (Fig. 3). The artificial aqueous humor and the lens remnants are eliminated without mixing with the Healon®, which remains in position, protecting the corneal endothelium and the iris.

6. The lens capsule is "refilled" with Healon® (Fig. 4). This "re-formation" of the lens permits subsequent resection of the anterior capsule without damage to the posterior capsule.

7. A large anterior capsulectomy is performed (triangular in shape, as

---

[3] The syringes used for irrigation should be glass precision syringes to ensure smooth action of the plunger. "Disposable" plastic syringes are not advisable, because considerable force has to be exerted to displace the plunger, and the action is less precise. Glass syringes must be carefully rinsed before sterilization, to prevent contamination by soap and detergents which, if they happen to get into the anterior chamber, may produce serious toxic reactions with consequent damage to the intraocular structures, principally the corneal endothelium and the iris. For increased safety, we rinse the syringe and the cannula again with BSS immediately before injecting any fluid into the eye.

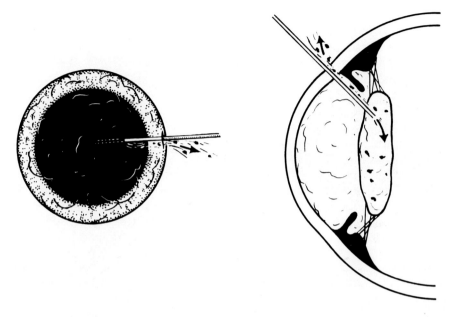

FIG. 3. "Intracapsular" irrigation to remove lens remnants.

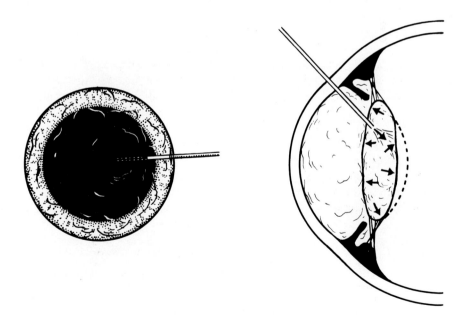

FIG. 4. "Reshaping" of the crystalline lens with Healon®.

indicated in Fig. 5). To facilitate the capsulectomy, a second limbal incision
has been performed previously, in the inferior quadrant. The capsulotomy
scissors are introduced through the limbal incisions and into the lens capsule,
to cut the anterior capsule as close as possible to the pupillary margin and
even behind it (Fig. 5). Neither the anterior nor the posterior chambers are
likely to collapse; the scissors can be easily moved without traumatizing the
endothelium, the iris, or the posterior capsule.

   8. At the end of this capsulotomy, the large triangular fragment of the
anterior capsule is removed with von Mandach forceps (Fig. 6). The anterior
chamber does not collapse (due to the presence of Healon®).

   9. The anterior chamber is irrigated with acetylcholine solution (0.5% or
1%) to constrict the pupil. The jet of acetylcholine solution may be directed
on the anterior iris surface or toward the anterior chamber angle to facilitate
miosis. This irrigation produces some dilution of the Healon® but this does
not interfere with its efficiency in protecting the corneal endothelium and
the iris.

   10. A peripheral iridectomy is essential if a posterior capsulotomy is to be
performed subsequently, either during the same intervention or as a two-stage
procedure. An additional limbal corneal incision, perpendicular to the iris
plane, is performed at the 12 o'clock meridian with the keratome or the
ultrasharp disposable knife.

   11. To perform the iridectomy, the iris is grasped near its base with Bonn

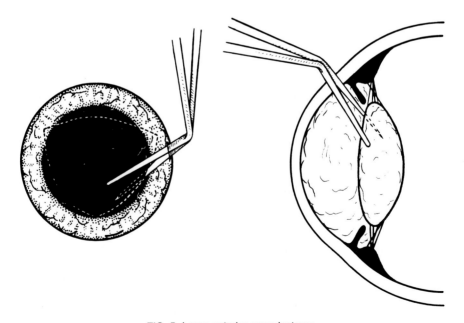

FIG. 5. Large anterior capsulectomy.

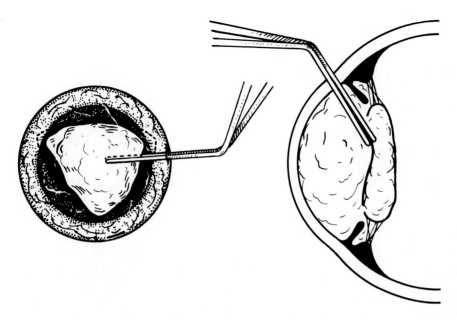

FIG. 6. Removal of the anterior capsule fragment.

forceps and is sectioned close to the incision with Barraquer scissors. The iridectomy prevents the possibility of glaucoma due to pupillary block.

12. If the posterior capsule is opaque, a posterior capsulotomy is performed in the same session. The pointed blade of the scissors penetrates through the capsule, close to the pupillary margin and is then carried to the opposite point at the pupillary margin. Subsequently, the scissors are rapidly closed and the capsule is cut (Fig. 7). Due to the presence of Healon® in the anterior chamber, the vitreous will not prolapse, provided that pressure on the globe is avoided when removing the scissors from the anterior chamber. Figure 7 also illustrates good peripheral communication between the posterior and the anterior chamber; the posterior capsule is tense and in position, without contacting the iris, owing to the presence of Healon® in the anterior and posterior chambers. Posterior capsulotomy may also be indicated in cases where the capsule is transparent but shows folds or wrinkles or to prevent formation of secondary cataract.

Figure 8 shows the situation at the end of the operation. The three incisions have been sutured applying one virgin silk (9–0) or nylon (10–0) suture to each incision. The anterior chamber is of normal depth (Healon® plus artificial aqueous humor that remained in the eye after irrigation with acetylcholine solution); there is a sufficiently large central opening in the posterior capsule. The vitreous humor near the capsulotomy forms a very small vitreous

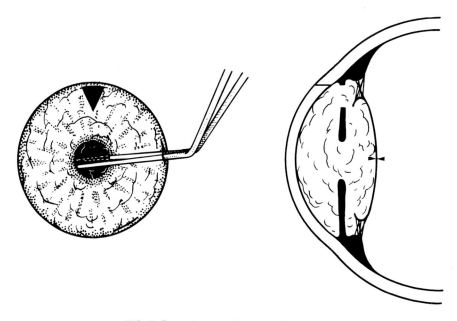

FIG. 7. Posterior capsulotomy with scissors.

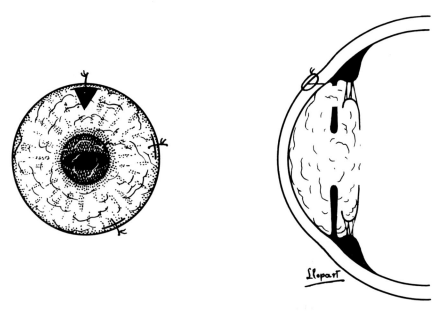

FIG. 8. Result: Peripheral iridectomy, central capsulotomy, anterior chamber of normal depth (Healon® plus BSS).

mushroom in the opening. There is a patent peripheral iridectomy to prevent a possible glaucoma due to pupillary block.

As we emphasized in the beginning, fundamentally this technique avoids trauma to the corneal endothelium, the iris, and the posterior capsule during intraocular maneuvers and allows the operation to be performed using simple, classical instruments.

Healon® is also very useful in surgery of traumatic cataract and for protection of the corneal endothelium in cases of cornea guttata when intracapsular extraction is to be performed, as well as in a number of other procedures.

Sodium Hyaluronate in Glaucoma Surgery

Healon®, due to its viscoelastic nature, is a very adequate and useful "surgical tool" to prevent collapse of the anterior chamber during glaucoma surgery and in the postoperative course.

If open-angle glaucoma does not respond to medical therapy and cannot be controlled by laser trabeculoplasty, it must be managed surgically, and at present trabeculectomy is considered the operation of choice. Also, in cases of angle-closure glaucoma in which peripheral iridectomy (which must be performed very early, before the outflow is definitely impaired) would not be sufficient, a trabeculectomy should be done as soon as possible, before the structures of the anterior chamber angle are seriously damaged by repeated episodes of subacute angle-closure mechanism.

The danger of filtering operations (including trabeculectomy) is loss of the anterior chamber, which may lead to many complications, including, of course, the most dramatic one, ciliary block glaucoma (malignant glaucoma). This complication occurs more frequently in cases of narrow anterior chamber and a certain disproportion of the crystalline lens, which is too large—a condition that is relatively frequent in angle-closure glaucoma but may also occur in open-angle glaucoma in the presence of a narrow angle.

Technique

1. A large conjunctival flap is dissected, either limbus-based or fornix-based. Since 1980 we have used a fornix-based flap which, in our opinion, is easy to perform and has certain advantages.

2. A scleral trapdoor is prepared, passing through the central third of the scleral thickness, and the dissection is continued up to 0.5 mm inside the limbus, following carefully the same plane in the tissues until the cornea is reached. The disposable, angled (60°) ultrasharp pyriform knife, made by Grieshaber (No. 681.21), is very useful in preparing the scleral flap.

3. Before the anterior chamber is entered, it may be useful to insert several preplaced scleral nylon sutures (10–0) in the scleral flap. These sutures are left without tying.

4. In the corneal portion of the trapdoor an incision is performed penetrating into the anterior chamber (Fig. 9). The diamond knife is very appropriate, because it permits making the incision with minimal pressure, thus avoiding flattening of the anterior chamber due to loss of aqueous humor while the incision is being completed.

5. Immediately after the incision has been made, Healon® is injected (Fig. 10) so that the anterior chamber not only does not collapse, but its depth may even be increased if desired.

6. The trabeculectomy is performed as usual; we prefer a Walser scleral punch for this.

7. Subsequently a peripheral iridectomy is performed. If accidental pressure on the globe is carefully avoided, the anterior chamber will not collapse during these maneuvers. The aqueous humor flows out from the posterior chamber through the iridectomy and the trabeculectomy, whereas the Healon® remains in the anterior chamber.

8. The preplaced sutures are tied, and the knots are buried under the scleral flap.

9. If it is considered appropriate, 0.1 cc Healon® may be injected through the scleral opening after the sutures have been tied, in order to increase the depth of the anterior chamber (Fig. 11) and to have a thin coating of Healon®

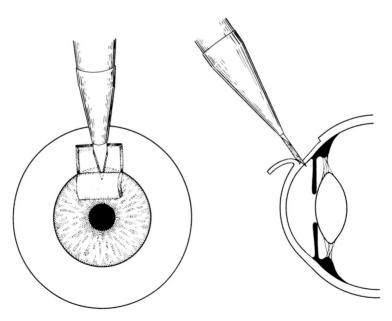

FIG. 9. Opening the anterior chamber with the diamond knife. The preplaced sutures are not shown in the drawing.

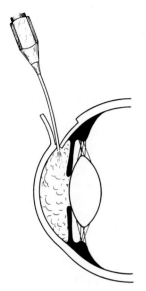

FIG. 10. Injection of Healon® to avoid collapse of the anterior chamber.

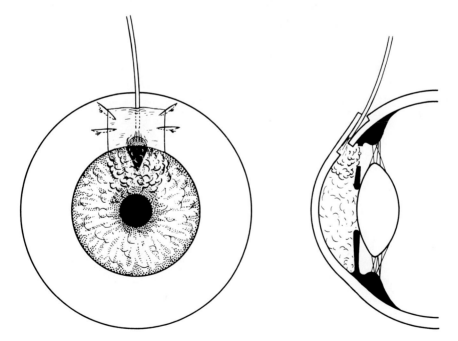

FIG. 11. Additional injection of Healon® after tying the sutures.

on the surfaces and edges of the scleral trapdoor to facilitate the draining of the aqueous humor.

10. The Healon® maintains the anterior chamber depth, and the aqueous humor is draining through the new outflow facility, i.e., the trabeculectomy (Fig. 12).

11. The conjunctival flap is sutured, taking care that the area of the scleral opening is adequately covered. A few drops of Healon® are placed between the conjunctiva and the sclera to keep them separate and facilitate the formation of a filtering bleb, which is usually diffuse and not very prominent (Fig. 13).

In the postoperative course the Healon® dissolves in the aqueous humor and disappears slowly from the anterior chamber. Since the outflow through the trabeculectomy opening is easy, the sodium hyaluronate, used in this way, does not produce serious ocular hypertension, and there is no doubt that it contributes considerably to reduced incidence of flat anterior chamber in the postoperative course. For the same reason, Healon® is very useful in the prevention and management of ciliary block or malignant glaucoma.

The best way to prevent this complication is to suture the scleral opening carefully, restore the anterior chamber with Healon®, apply 1% atropine to produce adequate relaxation of the ciliary body, and use local and general corticosteroids to inhibit the inflammatory reaction. If in spite of these precautions ciliary block glaucoma develops, osmotherapy must be started immediately (intravenous mannitol, or preferably, lyophilized urea), the pupil must be dilated using 4% atropine and 10% phenylephrine, and the doses of corticosteroids should be increased (60 mg prednisolone in intramuscular injection and frequent instillation of dexamethasone eye drops). If the problem does not resolve within a few hours, immediate *reintervention* is imperative, as follows:

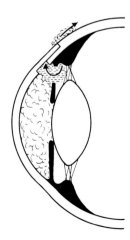

FIG. 12. Aqueous humor draining through the trabeculectomy.

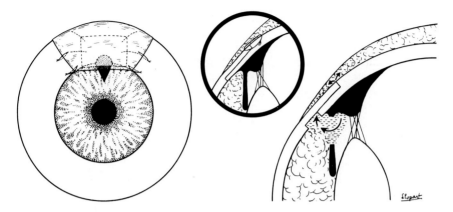

FIG. 13. Diffuse filtration under the conjunctival flap. In the circle, the nylon suture with the knot buried into the sclera and the conjunctiva covering the area of filtration are illustrated at high magnification.

1. Posterior sclerotomy at the level of the pars plana ciliaris.
2. Vitrectomy and aspiration of the aqueous humor that is retained behind and/or in the vitreous humor.
3. Re-formation of the anterior chamber with Healon®.
4. Keeping the pupil dilated with 4% atropine for a prolonged period of time.

REFERENCES

1. Barraquer, J., and Rutllán, J. (1984): *Microsurgery of the Cornea. An Atlas and Textbook.* Ediciones Scriba, Barcelona.
2. McCuen, B. W., Jr., Bessler, M., Hickingbotham, D., and Isbey, E., III (1983): Automated fluid-gas exchange. (Letter to the editor.) *Am. J. Ophthalmol.,* 95:717.

This chapter refers essentially to my personal experience, and no additional references are made to other publications. An extensive bibliography has been published in the book *Healon® (Sodium Hyaluronate). A Guide to Its Use in Ophthalmic Surgery* (1983), edited by Miller and Stegman; John Wiley & Sons, New York, and we refer the reader to this excellent publication.

Commentary

The Use of Hyaluronic Acid in Complicated Retinal Detachments

In retinal detachment surgery, intravitreal sodium hyaluronate, Healon®, can be used to maintain the volume of the globe when a large amount of subretinal fluid must be drained. Its slow turnover, about 0.5 μg/24 hr, in the rabbit vitreous body (3), makes it suitable for this purpose. Proliferative vitreoretinopathy (PVR) presents a more difficult challenge. Retinal pigment epithelial cells undergo metaplasia behaving like fibroblasts. Retinal astrocytes also participate in the proliferative process growing along the inner and outer retinal surfaces to form membranes. The authors have studied the outcome of PVR patients classified according to the prescription of the Retina Society Terminology Committee and treated by intravitreal Healon® injection and scleral buckling. The intraoperative high success rate of 78% declined to 60% at two weeks and to 34% at three months postoperatively. At this stage in grade C-1 50% were attached, in grades C-2 through D-1 30% whereas in grade D-2 none were attached. These results agree well with the final success reported by other procedures. The fibrous metaplasia of the retinal pigment epithelium and astrocytic proliferation continued in spite of the ingenious and time-consuming efforts of the surgeons. The authors restrict the use of Healon® in combination with scleral buckling as the possible first step in the treatment of PVR for grades C-1 to D-1. For arresting the disease process other means must be found. Of the cystostatic agents, intravitreal and/or subconjunctival injections of fluorouracil or newer agents (1) may offer some faint glimmer of hope (2).

The Editors

REFERENCES

1. Blumenkranz, M. S., Hajek, A., Hernandez, E., and Hartzer, M. (1985): Flourouridine: A second generation ocular antimetabolite. *Invest Ophthalmol. Vis. Sci. ARVO Suppl.,* 26(11): 285.
2. Blumenkranz, M. S., et al. (1982): *Am. J. Ophthalmol.,* 94:458–467.
3. Laurent, U. B. G., and Fraser, J. R. E. (1983): *Exp. Eye Res.,* 36:493–504.

Surgical Pharmacology of the Eye,
edited by M. Sears and A. Tarkkanen.
Raven Press, New York © 1985.

The Use of Hyaluronic Acid in Complicated Retinal Detachments

Edmund Gerke, Gerhard Meyer-Schwickerath,
and Achim Wessing

University Eye Hospital, D-4300 Essen 1, Federal Republic of Germany

In retinal detachment surgery, fixed retinal folds and dense vitreous strands existing preoperatively or developing postoperatively represent the main cause for failure in permanent reattachment.

Various surgical techniques have been used to overcome this complication, which has been referred to as massive vitreous retraction (MVR), massive preretinal retraction (MPR), massive periretinal proliferation (MPP), and most recently proliferative vitreoretinopathy (PVR). In addition to scleral buckling procedures, most surgeons use internal retinal tamponades by injecting air or gas; however, silicone oil (1,2) and hyaluronic acid (3) have been recommended. These substances have been injected with and without vitrectomy and with vitrectomy and epiretinal membrane removal. Recently an encircling procedure without internal tamponade and vitrectomy but with high indentation of the scleral buckle was recommended (4).

A comparison of the success rates of different surgical techniques remains difficult, since few authors have defined precisely the retinovitreal situation. Using the new PVR classification (5), which standardizes the grading of PVR according to different stages, we hope to elucidate the success rates and the complications of one particular therapeutic approach, i.e., intravitreal injection of Healon® in combination with scleral buckling.

The rationale for the use of Healon® is based on its capability to push into position the immobile retinas in PVR and at the same time not seep into the subretinal space, even in cases of large retinal holes. Also, Healon® slowly disappears out of the vitreous cavity, thus maintaining the retina in the reattached position for the time needed for the development of chorioretinal scars.

PATIENTS

More than 200 eyes with various retinal problems were operated on with a combination of intravitreal Healon® injection and scleral buckling. We retrospectively selected those eyes that had preoperative PVR of grades C-1, C-2,

C-3, D-1, and D-2. A total of 73 eyes qualified for this study. Eighteen eyes had grade C-1, 17 had grade C-2, 16 had grade C-3, 20 had grade D-1, and 2 had grade D-2. Forty-four eyes (60%) had undergone previous unsuccessful surgery—37, once; 7, twice; and 4, three times. In 10 eyes (14%) perforating or contusion injury was the underlying cause of the detachment. Twenty eyes (27%) were aphakic. Two eyes had giant tears. The patients were examined 2 weeks and 3 months after the operation. Seven patients were not seen in our clinic at the 3-month follow-up, but their examination reports were provided by the referring physicians. Four patients were lost to the 3-month follow-up but were known to have detachments at the 2-week examination. These eyes were also regarded as detached for the 3-month control.

SURGICAL PROCEDURE

In all 73 eyes an encircling element was applied, with a final constriction of about 20 mm or more. Posteriorly located retinal tears were closed by additional scleral plombs (silicone, silastic sponge, or dura mater) or intrascleral and episcleral pockets. Supplementary scleral infolding was carried out in 4 eyes. Ten eyes had already undergone scleral infolding in a previous procedure. Coagulation of the tears and holes was achieved by cryopexy, by diathermy in few cases, or by xenon photocoagulation at the end of the operation, when the retina was attached. Prior to the injection of Healon® through the pars plana, subretinal fluid was drained. Ringer's solution was injected in 16 eyes in an attempt to push back the retina. The situation, however, remained unchanged in all 16 cases, so in a second step, Healon® was used. The injection technique was changed over the 4-year period of this study, from an injection into the center of the vitreous cavity to an injection into the posterior third of the vitreous cavity close to the retina, the latter technique being applied in the majority of cases. The rationale for this was to push back the retina and simultaneously push forward the vitreous strands and membranes. In the majority of cases, after the injection of 1 to 2 ml Healon®, the retina at the posterior pole was reattached, with vitreous strands and membranes well in front of the retina. The injection needle was withdrawn from the vitreous cavity and the final length of the encircling element was fixed. Further injection of Healon® in most cases was necessary to achieve complete attachment. In general, vitreous membranes continued to come forward and toward the periphery during this procedure, with the retina often being remarkably smooth. The amount of the injected Healon® varied from 1.0 to 5.5 cc, depending on the volume of the eye, the combined buckling procedures, and the amount of subretinal fluid. The aim of the injection was considered to be achieved when the retina was completely attached. The average injected quantity in the 73 eyes was 2.4 ± 0.4 cc.

RESULTS

Intraoperatively, in 57 of the 73 eyes (78%) complete reattachment of the retina was achieved. At the examination 2 weeks later, 13 retinas had detached, so that at that time the rate of complete reattached retinas was 60%. At the 3-month postoperative examination, the retina was found to be completely attached in 25 eyes (34%). The success rate at this time was different according to the grade of PVR. In grade C-1, 50% were completely attached, in grade C-2 through D-1 the rate was 30%, whereas in grade D-2 none were attached (Table 1). Although the retinas were attached, the visual acuities in the 25 eyes were poor: 2 eyes, 20/200; the majority (15 eyes), between 10/200 and 6/200; 4 eyes, finger counting; and 4 eyes, hand movements (Table 2).

Intraoperative complications during the maneuver of intraocular injection of Healon® occurred in 3 eyes. In one case a retinal tear was created due to a firm adhesion between two adjacent retinal folds. In 2 eyes Healon® penetrated through a retinal tear into the subretinal space. Tiny epiretinal hemorrhages were seen in some eyes at the end of the injection. They were, however, absorbed at the 2-week examination. Intraocular pressure was found to be higher than 30 mmHg in 7 eyes during the postoperative period. Two of these eyes were phakic and 3 were aphakic. In one aphakic eye with pressure elevation to 60 mmHg, anterior vitrectomy was performed, which led to a normal intraocular pressure. The remaining eyes returned to normal pressure under local medication and intermittent administration of Diamox®. Two eyes developed cataracts but also showed clinical signs of string syndrome. Another eye with string syndrome had corneal opacification. In 3 of the 25 eyes with attached retina 3 months after the operation, minimal flare in the anterior chamber was seen. Flare within the vitreous, however, was absent in all 25 eyes at the 3-month control. Within the second through the tenth postoperative day, the vitreous in approximately 10% of the 73 eyes became hazy to a moderate degree, but it did not prevent visibility of the major fundus details.

TABLE 1. *Completely attached retinas in relation to grade of PVR and follow-up time (73 eyes)*

Grade PVR	Intraoperative (%)	Postoperative (%)	
		2 Weeks	3 Months
C-1	16/18 (39)	13/18 (72)	9/18 (50)
C-2	13/17 (76)	8/17 (47)	5/17 (29)
C-3	12/16 (75)	12/16 (75)	5/16 (31)
D-1	15/20 (75)	11/20 (55)	6/20 (30)
D-2	1/2 (50)	0/2 (0)	0/2 (0)
Totals	51/73 (78)	44/73 (60)	25/73 (34)

TABLE 2. *Visual acuity of successfully treated eyes*

Visual acuity	Gonvers (silicone) (%)	Grey & Leaver (silicone) (%)	Grizzard & Hilton (encircling) (%)	Machemer (vitrectomy) (%)	Present study (Healon®) (%)
>20/200	2/12 (17)	8/51 (15) ⎫	3/16 (19)	6/17 (35)	0
20/200	3/12 (25)	7/51 (14) ⎭		3/17 (18)	2/25 (8)
10/200–6/200	7/12 (58)	0	5/16 (31)	0	15/25 (60)
CF	0	22/51 (43)	7/16 (44)	6/17 (35)	4/25 (16)
HM	0	10/51 (20)	1/16 (6)	0	4/25 (16)
LP	0	4/51 (8)	0	2/17 (12)	0

CF, counting fingers; HM, hand motions; LP, light perception.

DISCUSSION

Comparison of success rates in surgery of retinal detachment complicated by PVR is difficult, because often the grade of this complication is not precisely defined; therefore, the study by Pruett et al. (3) on two different techniques both with the use of hyaluronic acid (Hyvisc®), does not precisely describe the preoperative findings. The authors could achieve a 16% final success rate in "retinal detachments judged inoperable by standard surgical techniques" by a combined technique of scleral buckling and injection of hyaluronic acid close to the optic disc. A slightly higher final success rate of 18% resulted in a combined technique of open-sky vitrectomy and replacement of the vitreous by hyaluronic acid. In a multiple-center study (6) on the intraocular injection of Healon®-H in eyes that had "extremely severe vitreoretinal pathology," the degree of which was not specified, the long-lasting success rate was 50%. In his article, Machemer (7) reports on 47 eyes that were operated on by vitrectomy, membrane peeling, and, in most cases, with gas injection, using a very precise classification of MPP. The 6-month success rate in eyes with four different stages of MPP (corresponding to PVR of grade C-1 to D-3) was 36%. Similar results were recorded by Grizzard and Hilton (4). These authors, however, performed scleral-buckling procedure alone, with marked constriction of the encircling element. The percentage of reattachment after 6 months in 46 eyes with PVR of grade C-1 through D-2, excluding grade D-3, was 34.7%. This success rate is mainly due to very good results in the C-1 and C-2 grades, whereas the percentage of reattached retinas in the C-3 and D-1 grades is low (23.5%), compared with the results of Machemer (37%) (7) and those of our study (30.5%). Using silicone oil injection, Scott (8) could achieve a success rate of 79% (126 eyes) in a series of 160 eyes. Since he included eyes with "prefibrotic stage," the results are very difficult to compare. This also holds true for the study by Grey and Leaver (1), who applied a similar technique with a success rate of 55%. Recently, Gonvers (2) reported on 21 eyes operated on by vitrectomy, removal of epiretinal membranes, disseminated photocoagulation, and temporary use of intraocular silicone. The success rate was 57%.

Whatever the surgical technique, it is a common observation that the intraoperative rate of completely reattached retinas is by far higher than the corresponding rate a few months later. In the present study, the overall rate declines from a 78% success intraoperatively to a 34% rate at three months. Machemer (7) found 68% and 36%, respectively, at 6 months. The disease process causing the proliferative vitreoretinopathy is not stopped by any of the surgical techniques; this may be the reason that the use of intraocular Healon® in combination with scleral buckling has a final success rate similar to other procedures. Although injection of silicone oil has a reported higher success rate when the parameter of visual acuity is used as a standard, it should be remembered that often the inferior retina redetaches. Therefore, on an anatomical basis, these success rates cannot be compared.

According to our results, injection of Healon®, on the other hand, does not seem an adequate method, neither for eyes with PVR of grade D-2, none of which had a reattached retina 3 months later in the present study, nor for eyes with PVR of grade D-3, which were not treated in this study. In these cases injection of silicon oil after vitrectomy seems to be indicated.

Healon®, however, has a very low complication rate in both the intraoperative manipulation and the postoperative course. We therefore recommend the use of Healon® in combination with scleral-buckling procedures as a possible first step in the treatment of PVR of grades C-1 to D-1 (especially C-3 and D-1), before silicone oil injection is considered. The use of Healon® in these cases might also be considered after performing a vitrectomy and removing epiretinal membranes.

ACKNOWLEDGMENT

The authors thank Dr. R. Machemer, Durham, North Carolina, and Dr. G. Blankenship, Miami, Florida, for helpful discussions, Reba Hurtes for her editorial work, and Charlaine Rowlette for typing the manuscript.

REFERENCES

1. Grey, R. H. B., and Leaver, P. K. (1979): Silicone oil in the treatment of massive preretinal retraction. I. Results in 105 eyes. *Br. J. Ophthalmol.,* 63:355–360.
2. Gonvers, M. (1982): Temporary use of intraocular silicone oil in the treatment of detachment with massive periretinal proliferation; preliminary report. *Ophthalmologica,* 184:210–218.
3. Pruett, R. C., Schepens, C. L., and Swann, D. A. (1979): Hyaluronic acid vitreous substitute. A six-year clinical evaluation. *Arch. Ophthalmol.,* 97:2325–2330.
4. Grizzard, W. S., and Hilton, G. F. (1982): Scleral buckling for retinal detachments complicated by periretinal proliferation. *Arch. Ophthalmol.,* 100:419–422.
5. The Retina Society Terminology Committee. (1983): The classification of retinal detachment with proliferative vitreoretinopathy. *Ophthalmology,* 90:121–125.
6. Balazs, E. A., Freeman, M. I., Kloti, R., Meyer-Schwickerath, G., Regnault, F., and Sweeney, D. B. (1972): Hyaluronic acid and replacement of vitreous and aqueous humor. *Mod. Probl. Ophthalmol.,* 10:3–21.
7. Machemer, R. (1977): Massive periretinal proliferation: A logical approach to therapy. *Trans. Am. Ophthalmol. Soc.,* 75:556–586.
8. Scott, J. D. (1975): The treatment of massive vitreous retraction by the separation of pre-retinal membranes using liquid silicone. *Mod. Probl. Ophthalmol.,* 15:285–290.

Commentary

Strabismus

In this chapter, both erudite as well as practical, Art Jampolsky has very appropriately emphasized the close cooperation between the surgeon and anesthesiologist so that active, as well as passive, components contributing to muscle tonus can be evaluated and managed properly. The author desires increased knowledge of muscle tonus during surgery to enhance the surgical result.

Surgical leashes have become a valuable addition to strabismus surgery. Surgery has been made easier, especially when reoperation is required. Not only can fine tuning be done but also an undesirable alignment can be changed. Patients with thyroid orbital disorders and candidates for vertical muscle surgery are especially well suited. The indications for the use of botulinus toxin have also become better defined. What may not be appreciated is that the work was based on early observations of the action of the toxin by Thesleff (2) and, later, first applied to the eye, intramuscularly by Dr. Carl Kupfer (1) of our National Eye Institute, NIH.

The Editors

REFERENCES

1. Kupfer, C. (1958): Selective block of synaptic transmission in ciliary ganglion by Type A Botulinus toxin in rabbits. *Proc. Soc. Exp. Biol. Med.,* 99:474–476.
2. Thesleff, S. (1973): Functional properties of receptors in striated muscle. In: *Drug Receptors,* edited by H. P. Rang, pp. 121–133. University Park Press, Baltimore.

Surgical Pharmacology of the Eye,
edited by M. Sears and A. Tarkkanen.
Raven Press, New York © 1985.

Strabismus

Arthur Jampolsky

Smith-Kettlewell Institute of Visual Sciences, San Francisco, California 94115

SUMMARY: Current surgical management of strabismus requires the special application of pharmacological knowledge and agents presurgically, at surgery and immediately postsurgically. This demands much greater teamwork between the anesthesiologist and the strabismus surgeon.

Strabismus alignment surgery now depends on identification and better understanding, as well as quantification and control of complete oculorotary muscle relaxation to complete rotary elimination of the active innervational components. This will allow the separation and control of the mechanical (passive) factors vs. the innervational (active) factors of strabismus alignment.

There are two unique anesthetic requirements: (a) that succinylcholine be avoided as an induction agent, since there is a sustained oculorotary muscle contracture response for more than 20 min, and (b) that pancuronium be used to assure complete muscle relaxation. The purpose of these requirements is to allow the surgeon to assess reliably the mechanical elements with forceps forced-traction maneuvers, forceps spring-back maneuvers, muscle length-force change measurements during surgery, and at the completion of surgery.

The anesthetic agent should be chosen to allow adequate surgical anesthesia with complete muscle relaxation during surgery, with the goal of complete postoperative recovery of the oculorotary muscle tonus, and full alertness in those instances where postoperative suture adjustments are to be made.

The pharmacological management of strabismus by injecting oculinum (botulism) neurotoxin directly into an eye muscle, in order to produce a temporary paralysis, ushers in a new treatment modality.

The strabismus surgeon now extends his important diagnostic tests, and important treatment assessment methods, into the surgical anesthetic process. There must be the utmost cooperation with the anesthesiologist, and careful consideration of the agents used before, during, and extending into the immediate postoperative period.

Current surgical management of strabismus requires the special application of pharmacologic knowledge and agents presurgically, at surgery, and immediately postsurgically. This demands much greater teamwork between the anesthesiologist and the strabismus surgeon. To understand the full nature of this statement, it is good to review briefly the problems and the reasons why such teamwork is necessary.

The strabismus management problem, simply stated, is to diagnose accurately the ocular misalignment in *alert* humans and to alter surgically the alignment, so that in the final result the *fully alert* human will have the eyes satisfactorily aligned. In other words, there is a balance of all the orbital and muscle forces that affect ocular alignment.

What are these forces? These are the *passive* (mechanical) forces of the muscles and the globe-orbit, and the *active* (innervational) forces of the muscles. All of these forces must be balanced so that the eyes are aligned in the alert state. Why the emphasis on the fully alert human? As will be seen, the innervational tonus of the oculorotary muscles is sensitively affected by any alterations in the state of alertness, and sensitively affected by drugs, often in a paradoxical fashion (compared to other skeletal muscles). We shall return to this point.

Permit me to state the conclusions at the outset. Manipulation and alteration of the mechanical balancing forces now take place *at* surgery, under anesthesia, wherein there must be an elimination (and separation) of all innervational tonus factors. And further, in many cases surgery is extended into the postoperative recovery period, when the patient has recovered full alertness and return of all normal innervational tonus forces, to be added to the altered mechanical balancing forces for the net alignment result. Since the oculorotary muscles are exquisitely sensitive to a wide variety of pharmacologic agents, very careful attention must be paid to what preoperative medications are used, what induction medications are—and are not—to be used, what anesthetic and auxiliary medications are to be used during surgery, and what postoperative medications are—and are not—to be used, with an eye toward full alertness for the postoperative period of assessment of alignment and alteration of muscle positions. Thus, it is absolutely essential that one be able to understand and manipulate both the passive (mechanical), and active (innervational) forces, as well as understand the pharmacologic effects on these forces.

Let us first illustrate the goals and problems with two practical examples of strabismus management: first, an essentially mechanical strabismus with purely passive (mechanical) forces to be adjusted for alignment of the two eyes, and second, strabismus management of essentially innervational (active) forces. This comparison will point out management differences for passive versus active force balancing during surgery and immediately after surgical anesthesia.

Example 1

An adult patient with constant unilateral exotropia is characteristic of what may be considered to be an essentially mechanical strabismus. The exact amount of misalignment may be measured very accurately by simple objective methods in the office or clinic, preoperatively. At surgery, under full anesthesia, when all of the active (innervational) forces have been eliminated, the degree of ocular misalignment is unchanged from that measured preoperatively during the alert state. The presence or absence of active muscle innervational forces plays little role. Thus, the surgeon may align the eyes at surgery, reliably assessing the mechanical ocular deviation (by the spring-back test to be described), with good confidence that the alignment surgically attained under anesthesia will be the alignment that the patient will have when he is again fully alert postoperatively.

This is because the alignment is unaffected by the anesthesia (before, during, or after), since the active innervational factors are unimportant in this essentially mechanical strabismus.

Example 2

An essentially active innervational strabismus exists in an infant with cerebral palsy and esotropia. The esodeviation measured preoperatively may completely disappear under deep surgical anesthesia, and in fact, the eyes may become exotropic with anesthetic elimination of the innervational factors. The surgeon traditionally attempted to solve this problem by mechanically altering the alignment under surgical anesthesia, hoping to correct by just the right amount the to-be-returned innervational forces when the patient was fully alert again, postoperatively. Hardly a scientific task, often requiring multiple surgical procedures for incremental approximations.

Traditionally, the strabismus surgeon was admonished to make a preoperative clinical diagnosis and to devise a surgical plan often based on a formula that equates millimeters of surgical muscle repositioning to prism diopters of alignment effect—as if there were always a uniform and predictable relationship, which of course there is not. By no means are all strabismus cases purely mechanical, and thus a single treatment method (or formula) will fail in a significant number of cases.

ANESTHESIA FOR STRABISMUS SURGERY

One of the major current problems is that the strabismus surgeon can in no way depend on the anesthetic depth as completely eliminating all of the active (innervational) factors. Everyone is aware that under the early stages of anesthesia, the eyes drift inward and upward, and finally, after long saturation with the anesthetic agents, settle down and become more stable.

It has been shown that even under general anesthesia, the oculocardiac reflex may be activated by conjunctival manipulation. Thus, it is important to add topical anesthesia (conjunctival drops) even though the patient is under general anesthesia. Additionally, it has been shown that the oculocardiac reflex (slowing of the heart rate by pulling on an ocular muscle, especially the medial rectus) is mediated not via the eye muscle per se, nor the globe per se, but indirectly through tension on the Gasserian ganglion. But all of the muscles and the globe may be completely extirpated, and tension on the remaining retro-orbital tissues may produce a slowing of the heart rate. The medial rectus muscle simply has a straighter shot in effective pull. The oculocardiac reaction may be ameliorated and prevented by good oxygenation and atropinization during anesthesia.

If succinylcholine has been used as an induction agent, there will result a sustained contraction of all of the oculorotary muscles that will last approximately 20 min (Fig. 1). This action of the oculorotary muscles in response to

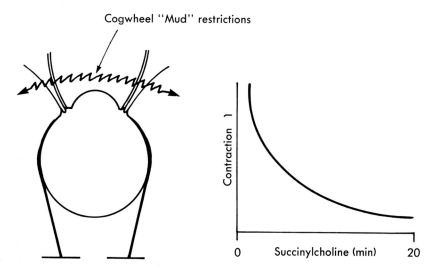

Cogwheel "Mud" restrictions

FIG. 1. Succinylcholine, as usually administered during anesthesia, has an effect on the oculorotory muscles that lasts 20 min. This is in distinct contrast to the effect on other skeletal muscles.

succinylcholine differs markedly from the reaction of other skeletal muscles. It is well known that the respiratory muscles resume their adequate functioning within a few minutes after succinylcholine administration. Not so for the oculorotary muscles, whose sustained contraction is marked for 8 to 10 min, and a residual measurable effect lasts for 20 min. Since modern strabismus surgical procedures demand that the surgeon assess the purely mechanical forces at the very beginning of surgery, and alter the treatment plan according to the mechanical findings during surgery, it is absolutely imperative that all of the oculorotary muscles are relaxed, i.e., there is *no* active innervational tonus force.

Since many anesthesiologists routinely use succinylcholine during induction for strabismus surgery, we simply avoid using those uncooperative anesthesiologists who insist on continuing this procedure. It is as important, and simple, as that.

So at the outset it may be stated that there are two unique anesthetic requirements: (a) succinylcholine be avoided as an induction agent, and (b) pancuronium be used to assure muscle relaxation (Fig. 2). The purpose of these two requirements is to allow the surgeon to assess reliably the passive mechanical elements with forceps forced-traction maneuvers, forceps spring-back maneuvers, and the change of muscle length-force measurements during surgery and at the completion of surgery.

The anesthetic agent should be chosen to allow adequate surgical anesthesia with complete muscle relaxation during surgery, with the goal of postoperative

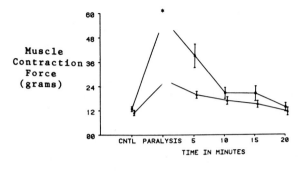

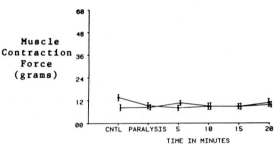

FIG. 2. Change in the force required to forceps-rotate the globe following succinylcholine 1 mg/kg i.v. Note that the effect lasts for 20 min in the oculorotary muscles. Also note that temporal rotation, which tests the medial rectus contracture (*upper curve*), is more marked than nasal rotation, which tests the lateral rectus contraction. (From ref. 1, with permission.)

complete recovery of the oculorotary muscle tonus, and full alertness in those instances where postoperative muscle adjustments are to be made.

The mode and rate of induction of the general anesthesia is of great importance. It is my strong clinical impression, that a quick jolting induction of anesthetic agents produces a vasodilatation of the conjunctival and scleral vessels, leading to unnecessary bleeding during the entire strabismus surgical procedure. Instillation of topical vasoconstrictors only partially ameliorates this unnecessary status.

It is *absolutely essential* that the strabismus surgeon is able to assess the purely passive mechanical elements by absolutely controlling *all* of the active innervational forces, which can only be done with the close cooperation of the anesthesiologist, together with the agents used as described above. The reasons for this are discussed in the following section.

THE FORCEPS FORCED-TRACTION RESTRICTION TEST (FORCED-DUCTION)

The forceps forced-traction restriction test assesses mechanical restrictions to rotations at the beginning of surgery (under muscle-relaxation anesthesia), during surgery, and at the end of surgery. It measures not only the muscle-restrictive forces but also the conjunctiva, surrounding tissue, and global restricting forces.

Under anesthesia, the globe is grasped at the limbus with forceps, and rotations are manually made in the arc of rotation of the globe, feeling relative or complete restrictions to rotation. The surgeon seeks to feel any restrictive force between the forceps at the limbus, in the area away from which the forced rotation is made. One rotates the globe away from the line of force to be tested, as in stretching a rubber band (Fig. 3). In other words, to test a restrictive force in the medial aspect of the globe, one abducts the eye with forceps placed at the nasal limbus. The forceps should engage as little conjunctiva as possible at the limbus, and the arc of rotation of the globe should be maintained during the test. The surgeon must avoid the error of pushing the globe back into the orbit during the forceps rotation, which artifactually relaxes tension force measured.

The causes and locations of restrictions are several. Although the majority of restrictions are caused by stiff muscles, a great many restrictions are caused by nonmuscle tissue (e.g., conjunctiva, subconjunctival tissue, Tenon's fascia, and orbital tissue). Subtleties of forceps manipulation will help the surgeon immensely in diagnosing relative as well as absolute restrictions if the method of performing the test is refined and the arc of rotation is well maintained.

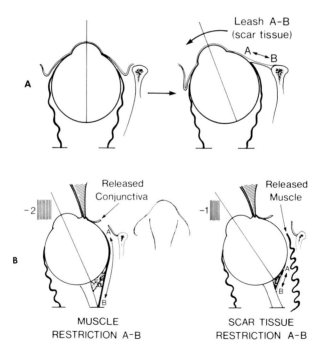

FIG. 3. A: Leash (*A-B*) due to the conjunctiva. **B:** Release of the conjunctiva allows better forceps rotation though there is still incomplete release of restriction. The remaining restriction is further released when the muscle is severed. Residual orbital scar may continue to restrict motion. (From ref. 2, with permission.)

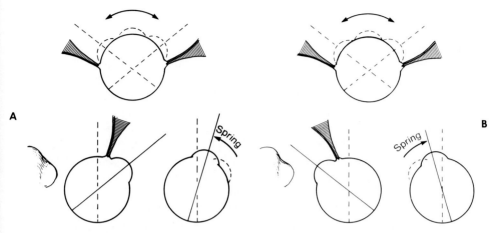

FIG. 4. Dynamic spring forces. **A:** Spring-back balance test. The globe is rotated to and fro six to eight times and then quickly released from a mid-abducted position (approximately 30°). The examiner notes the spring-back end point. **B:** After several more rotations, the spring-back is released from the opposite direction (midadducted position). The examiner notes the midpoint bisecting the spring-back zone and also the breadth of the spring-back zone. (From ref. 3, with permission.)

It is especially important to learn whether the restriction is operative in the primary zone, since in most surgical instances this restriction will effect a habitual head turn position when alert, and the primary zone restriction must be released.[1]

THE FORCEPS SPRING-BACK FORCE BALANCE TEST

The spring-back balance test is a method of aiding the strabismus surgeon in judging the balanced mechanical aligning forces at the time of strabismus surgery under anesthesia (i.e., the alignment result). It is especially useful in mechanical strabismus (see example 1, cited earlier), or in those cases in which the active muscle tonus return is reasonably balanced to the agonist-antagonist muscles, that the spring-back balance test at the time of surgery provides a useful alignment guide (Fig. 4).

The force-balance test assesses the effect of releasing a restricting muscle from the globe and at the same time assesses the ability of the antagonist muscle to unbalance the forces, a lot or a little, toward the opposite direction. Thus, both agonist and antagonist spring forces may be assessed at the beginning of surgery, during surgery, and especially at the end of surgery to assess the final results.

---

[1] In some instances, the surgeon deliberately creates a restriction in the primary zone for "fixation-duress" purposes, and the surgeon must be able to assess these directly at the time of surgery.

The globe is grasped at the nasal limbus, in the same fashion as one does for the forceps forced-traction test. It is rotated to and fro in the desired plane (let us say horizontally) about six or eight rotations, and then quickly released from a temporalward rotation position (approximately 30° to 45°). The globe springs back to rest in a slightly abducted position. In theory, ideally the globe would spring back to the straight-ahead position (assessed for each eye). The globe is then grasped at the opposite temporal limbus and rotated six or eight times back and forth. It is now released from a nasalward rotation position and its spring-back position is noted. Theoretically idealized, the globe should spring back to the ortho position. In actuality, one simply determines the midpoint of the zone of the two spring-backs. The straight-ahead position may be marked on the upper lid or may be estimated.

This test mechanically stretches out and loads all of the mechanical spring coils just prior to globe release, and one can measure the globe's final spring back, rest position after a few seconds, and the breadth or narrowness of the zone of the spring-back from either direction. Additionally, the velocity of the globe's spring-back may be assessed. The spring-back zone breadth can be easily demonstrated to be large if both medial and lateral rectus muscles are detached from the globe, thus effectively eliminating the major spring coil opposing forces. During this circumstance, there is a much slower spring-back, of relatively modest degree, from each direction. The globe "sits" where it is put, since opposing muscle forces have been detached. However, if, without the muscles attached to the globe, the spring-back balance rest position is biased to one side, then one may or may not wish to make appropriate adjustments at the time, depending on the final goal and objectives. Similarly, a slightly wider than normal zone of spring-back in the actual initial assessment of a patient (under anesthesia) would suggest opposing weaker than normal forces. Furthermore, a smaller than normal zone with fast spring-backs would suggest opposing stiff muscles. It indicates that when the globe is rotated in either direction, the tight springs are further tightly coiled, and the opposing tighter-than-normal springs keep the spring-back zone small.

In our example of adult constant unilateral exotropia (a mechanical strabismus), if the spring-back balance test does not show alignment at the conclusion of surgery (whether unilateral or bilateral surgery has been performed), one had best consider doing more surgery in order to complete the alignment at the time of general anesthesia spring-back balance test assessment, since the example is one of an essentially mechanical nature.

In summarizing these two tests, it is important to emphasize the difference between the forced-traction test for mechanical *restriction* analysis and the spring-back *balance of forces* test for alignment assessment. Neither test can be reliably performed unless all active innervational muscle tonus has been dissipated and controlled under general anesthesia (with pancuronium).

MUSCLE LENGTH CHANGE–FORCE CHANGE MEASUREMENTS

Muscle stiffness characteristics may now be directly assessed at the time of surgery. The modern strabismus surgeon may reposition such abnormal muscles so as to optimize balanced alignment for the primary position and for eye rotations. Again, the surgeon must be absolutely certain that such measurements of the important muscle-force-balancing components are performed under conditions that assuredly eliminate all active innervational tonus. During prolonged reoperation procedures, this assurance must be maintained throughout by the anesthesiologist's choices of pharmacologic agents.

Eye muscles are mechanically analogous to rubber bands. Some are stiff, relatively inelastic, and some are slack. For every millimeter of length change by repositioning the muscle (whether strengthening or weakening it) there is a wide variety of *force* change, depending on how much or how little the muscle is stretched and, most important, the stiffness of the muscle. All muscles are certainly not the same (Fig. 5).

The intrasurgical measurement of the length-change–force-change relationship of individual muscles may be directly assessed by a device designed by my colleague Dr. Carter Collins (Fig. 6). The muscle tension force is measured by a strain gauge incorporated into a forceps, which moves the eye (A. B. Scott, M.D., C. C. Collins, Ph.D.). The length change of the muscle during this force assessment is measured as the distance between the forceps (with a minimicrophone in the forceps) and the temporally placed ultrasonic detection apparatus (a miniature sonar device). The linear muscle stretch and relaxation distance is monitored in this fashion to give a simultaneous muscle-length–muscle-tension force curve displayed on an oscilloscope in a dynamic fashion. Accurate quantitative measurements of muscle characteristics and the effective forces around the all-important primary position can be assessed, altered, reassessed, and accurately balanced. This is especially important with abnormal muscles, which occur in both normal and reoperated patients.

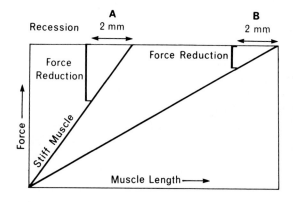

FIG. 5. Difference in force reduction by the same 2-mm recession of a stiff short muscle (*A*) and a normal muscle (*B*). There is considerably more force reduction (effectiveness) for the same 2-mm recession of a short stiff muscle. Equal amounts of recession may produce vastly different effects, depending on the muscle characteristics as well as the status of the opposing muscle. Diagram by Carter C. Collins, Ph.D. (From ref. 2, with permission.)

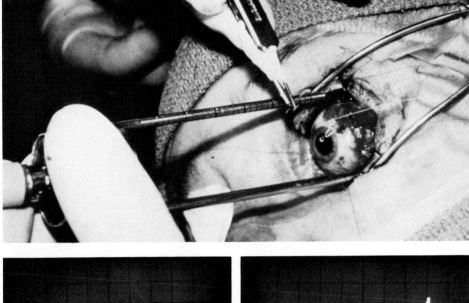

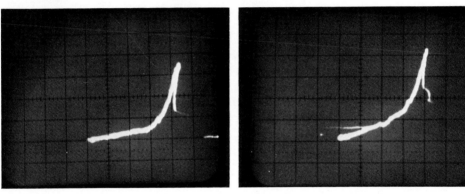

FIG. 6. Top: The forceps with tension strain gauge and microphone (an ultrasonic muscle length-detection device, designed by Carter C. Collins, Ph.D., at the Smith-Kettlewell Institute of Visual Sciences). This device is in current use during surgery, in order to quantify the length-force curves. **Bottom:** Length-force curves may be displayed on an oscilloscope (*left*, stiff muscle; *right*, normal muscle).

Clinically, for some time, the experienced surgeon has been able to "feel" the relative muscle stiffness by pulling directly on the sutures in the detached muscle. The surgeon can accurately determine the maximum allowable advancement of an abnormally stiff muscle before unacceptable restriction is produced. The assistant rotates the globe in an acceptable opposite rotation posture and holds it in this position while the surgeon pulls up on the short stiff muscle until all of the slack is taken up. Additionally, the surgeon may note the indentation sign of the sutures running over the sclera, revealing a limiting tight muscle position, which the surgeon may easily feel. The muscle is then released slightly to the point where the surgeon feels the beginning of

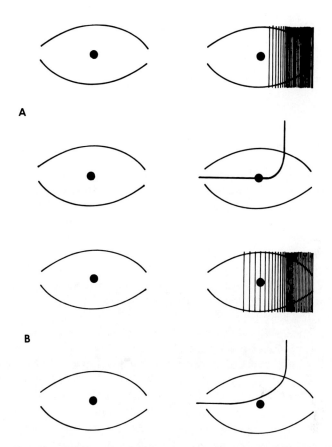

FIG. 6. Cont. The clinical diagramatic representation of graded restrictions (not quantified): **(A)** an abrupt tether; **(B)** less abrupt tether, some of the restrictive forces being active in the primary position. The *upper parts* are the usual representations recorded at the time of examination, a shaded area becoming more dense in the extreme field of abduction of the left eye. The *lower parts* depict another method, simulating the muscle length-force tension curve of the antagonist muscle (MR) in this case. Both methods show the relative abruptness of the leash effect. This clinically unquantified but useful method may now be quantified by the above methods shown in the photographs. (From ref. 2, with permission.)

the muscle tightness, as it is drawn forward and/or observes the indentation sign of the muscle sutures on the sclera. Any further muscle advancement (or resection) would create an unacceptable leash, limiting rotations. Thus, the surgeon fixes the limiting rotation at this juncture and/or assures that the muscle position will not restrict rotation.

Thus, the surgeon first fixes the allowable restriction by taking out all the slack of the muscle, in doing a so-called dynamic forced-traction test at the time of surgery. And under these conditions (no active innervational tonus) the surgeon can predict that this same acceptable rotational restriction will continue into the postoperative alert status.

The next step then is to balance the primary position force of this now repositioned muscle with its antagonist. This is done by the spring-back balance test assessment. For mechanical strabismus cases, such adjustment of acceptable rotational restrictions (taking up the slack of the muscles), and spring-back balancing of the alignment of *each* eye separately, is the current optimal strabismus surgical management technique.

ACTIVE (INNERVATIONAL) COMPONENT ASSESSMENT

Let us now consider the problem of surgical management of the strabismus patient, where it is not essentially a mechanical strabismus but has a large active innervational component, with special reference to anesthetic agents. Let us examine a "worst-case" example of unilateral sixth nerve (lateral rectus) complete paralysis. In this instance, any balancing of the passive mechanical forces at the time of surgery, even perfect alignment, will result in a very gross misalignment when the patient is again alert, postoperatively. The innervation will have returned to the still active medial rectus muscle of the involved eye, but no innervation whatsoever will return to the dead lateral rectus muscle, thus re-creating a marked esotropia during the alert awake status, regardless of the mechanical surgical balanced alignment that was done under anesthesia. One solution to this problem is to completely eliminate the activity of the medial rectus muscle by recession far back of the equator, thus balancing zero opposing forces of the medial and lateral rectus muscles, so that when innervation does return during the alert stage, the mechanical balance at the time of surgery will be the same as the mechanical balance during the alert stage; balancing opposing dead forces converts the case into a purely mechanical strabismus. However, the medial rectus must be recessed so far back, and sewed in position, that it will have no effective pull on the globe whatsoever. Stable alignment in the primary position is the goal, with compromised rotations.

There is another, better alternative. One may rebalance the muscles post-operatively by putting the active medial rectus muscle on an "adjustable suture," which the surgeon may manipulate and reposition after the patient is completely awake and fully recovered from all of the anesthetic agents. This is balanced by a newly fashioned antagonist force by transposition of one-half of the superior and inferior rectus muscles, preferably on an adjustable suture.

Such adjustable sutures are now common practice (Fig. 7). Modification of older adjustable surgical techniques with modern techniques has made it entirely possible to place adjustable muscle sutures in one or more muscles in adults (and in many children) under general anesthesia (stage I). When the patient is fully alert, in the immediate postsurgical period (a few hours after surgery or the next morning—stage II), under office-clinical conditions with the patient sitting up in bed, the surgeon adjusts the balance of forces so as to gain a perfectly desired alignment result before the patient leaves the hospital.

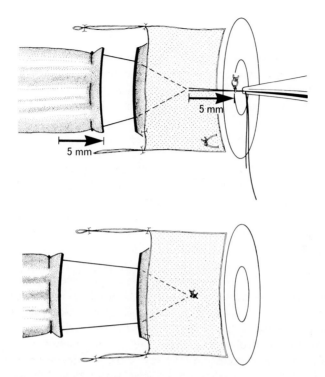

FIG. 7. Adjustable sutures allow the muscle to "hang loose" from the insertional stump, with alterations in the muscle position made postoperatively by means of a sliding constricting knot **(top)** shown next to the forceps that hold the muscle sutures. These adjustable muscle sutures are placed at the time of general anesthesia (stage I). Postoperatively **(bottom)**, under topical conjunctival drop anesthesia, the fully alert patient has the alignment of the eyes and rotations assessed by usual clinical methods. The muscle sutures are then tied in place, *after* the desired result has been obtained. (The dotted area indicates a recessed conjunctiva, bare-sclera technique, stage II.)

It is important to note that stage II is performed under topical (conjunctival drops) anesthesia and now demands a fully alert patient. As we will see, normal alertness may differ markedly from the apparent full alertness induced postoperatively by chemical reversal of anesthetic agents. Thus, the adjustable strabismus surgical technique encompasses the mechanical balancing of forces at the time of surgery (stage I), with sutures so placed and constructed that one or more abnormal muscles may be *again* repositioned postoperatively with the patient fully alert and attending to real-life targets (stage II).

We have discussed how important it is under general anesthesia for the surgeon to be certain that there is continued elimination of all of the active innervational components, and complete muscle relaxation, it order to surgically deal with the mechanics. Now, during stage II of postoperative adjustment and repositioning of muscles, it is equally imperative that *all* of the normal active innervational tonus is present. There must be no compromise with full normal alertness and natural fixation of targets in the primary position and in different fields of gaze.

It is therefore optimal for the anesthesiologist to use no preoperative sedatives and to use agents at the time of surgery that will be dissipated as completely as possible, for full postoperative alertness. Similarly, it is a problem for the strabismus surgeon to prevent nurses, interns, and residents from giving obtunding drugs to the patient during the postoperative period. *Any* agents of the morphine family, the barbiturate family, etc., do indeed significantly affect the natural active innervational tonus of the very sensitive oculorotary muscles. One allows only such things as aspirin, codeine, etc., to be given for pain in order to assure complete alertness. "Just a touch" of evening barbiturate may last into the next morning, and full natural alertness will *not* be present, thus potentially compromising the entire goal of adjusting muscle placement.

ALERTNESS AND ACTIVE INNERVATIONAL MUSCLE TONUS

The oculorotary muscles are exquisitely sensitive to a variety of diseases and to a very wide variety of pharmacologic agents. Often the sensitivity to pharmacologic agents is paradoxical and opposite to the reaction of other skeletal muscles.

Clinicians are well aware of the very early involvement of oculorotary muscles in thyroid, diabetic, and myesthenic myopathies. There is very early involvement of the oculorotary muscles compared to other skeletal muscles.

Similarly, a wide variety of pharmacologic agents act in a wide variety of ways and at different locations, affecting oculorotary muscle tonus, usually in the direction of an esodeviation shift. Thus, relative hypoxia, alcohol, barbiturates, etc., all document that the cartoons are correct: one does get cross-eyed under these conditions. The medial rectus muscle forces are increased relative to the lateral rectus muscle forces, presumably due to a relative lowering of inhibitory control of the higher centers over the lower centers. The induced misalignments are in the direction of esotropia, because the medial and lateral rectus muscles are not equal and opposite forces, like leather or purely mechanical rubber bands. Equal amounts of innervational tonus arriving at the globe (however induced) produce *more* contraction force of the medial rectus than of the lateral rectus muscles. Similarly, elimination of all of the active innervation in a normal person allows the medial rectus muscles to give up more tonus force than the lateral rectus muscles do, resulting in a diminishing esodeviation, or a resulting exodeviation. After death, the eyes are normally slightly exotropic, because the normal medial rectus muscles give up more force than the normal lateral rectus muscles do, resulting in a slight exotropic misalignment. Similarly, inattention and less than optimal alertness result in a significant alteration of muscle tonus and alignment.

The pontine reticular formation (PRF), of course, is involved in the state of alertness. Relative to eye movements, it has been shown by my colleague,

Dr. E. L. Keller at the Smith-Kettlewell Institute, that single-neuron recordings in the monkey reveal several categories of neural activity that are closely and differentially correlated with various types of eye movements (4). Dr. Keller has shown by such techniques that a fully motivated monkey (well trained), fixating a target light, has a maximum saccadic velocity under these conditions. Without such a target display, the interested but not fully motivated monkey makes spontaneous saccadic movements to objects of interest, with lower maximum saccadic velocities of abnormally long duration. As the monkey became less alert, the saccadic velocity became diminished. Thus there is "a continuous scale of central nervous system alertness from fully alert and motivated, to drowsy" (4).

The laboratory monkey investigation by Dr. Keller is entirely compatible with the work done by clinical ophthalmologists on alert humans, by the Smith-Kettlewell research group. The alert clinician can easily observe a slowed saccade, and may especially note the "floating saccade" observed in attempted saccades by a paretic muscle. Thus, the observed saccadic velocity of an attempted eye movement is an important and valid clinical index of the state of alertness.

A strabismus surgeon can easily detect the presence of a slower saccade during the postoperative strabismus muscle adjustment (stage II), during which full alertness and full return of active tonus *must* be present. A slower than normal saccadic eye movement reveals that the anesthetic agents have not been fully dissipated and/or that some well-intentioned recovery room or ward nurse or medical assistant has administered some "mild" sedative agent. This postpones the adjustment procedure. Pharmacologic reversal of anesthetic agents by Narcan®, etc., gives apparent alertness, but our experience has taught us that this is not always equivalent to full natural alertness. Parenthetically, it should be remarked that physostigmine uniquely reverses anesthetic agents to a degree not observed with other agents.[2]

It is curious that in abnormally high levels of alertness (as in hyperkinetic children) there is a higher than normal incidence of esotropia (the medial rectus tonus wins over the lateral rectus tonus). And further, it is well known that hyperkinetic children may react oppositely to sedatives. Indeed, much of importance needs to be learned about the alerting mechanism, eye muscle tonus, general skeletal muscle tonus, and their pharmacologic control.

FUTURE CONSIDERATIONS

Ideally, it would be advantageous for the strabismus surgeon to be able to turn on fully and turn off completely the active tonus components *during*

---

[2] We have seen two postoperative strabismus patients who have had complete absence of the saccadic system, lasting into the next postoperative day, after uneventful and usual general anesthesia. Only physostigmine, after other agents had been tried, immediately reestablished the saccadic system. We have reason to believe that profound psychologic factors were present in both instances, "as if" there were disability of the attention and saccadic mechanism.

surgery. If the surgical procedure could be made painless, while the patient was completely anesthetized, and the active innervational components could be manipulated in such a fashion that full alertness could be turned on or off, then all strabismus patients should be cured with one surgical procedure. Nitrous oxide anesthesia has the advantage of being water soluble (rather than fat soluble) and thus allows rapid alterations of the anesthetic state, with minimal lingering anesthetic-alertness effects. It is thus optimal for stage II muscle adjustment procedures. Nitrous oxide combined with fentanyl is considered by some to be an ideal stage I anesthetic agent combination.

I would like to entice neuropharmacologists with a problem/solution of reflexively stimulating eye movements during deep surgical anesthesia. Caloric stimulation of the vestibulo-ocular reflex, while under anesthesia, would produce yoked innervational patterns of eye rotations and would allow instant assessment of balanced or imbalanced eye movements. One "should" be able to cause the eyes to reflexively move to the right or to the left with caloric stimulation of each ear, independently, under present-day general anesthetics. Unfortunately, such caloric stimulation is ineffectual under halothane (of course, without muscle relaxants), even under light general anesthesia, and I so wish to report this unexpected repeatable finding. This basic reflex eye movement would be helpful, if a general anesthetic agent could be used that would allow this assessment of actively and briefly stimulating eye movements by ear calorics, to assess muscle repositioning and balanced alignment results.

Succinylcholine produces a *sustained* contracture of *all* eye muscles— curiously, with electrical silence (no recordable EMG). It is far from the idealized normal return of active innervational components that might be used beneficially during surgery. Thus, this method of attempting to elicit eye movements during surgery, has a differential effect on eye muscles (1) (Fig. 2), probably because of muscle differences in cross-sectional area and the reaction to unusual induced innervation by pharmacologic agents.

We need to know more about the precise mechanism of action of physostigmine on the alerting mechanism and its more dependable action in neutralizing agents used during anesthesia. This will lead to other useful pharmacologic agents.

There is a yet unresolved important secret in the paradoxical reaction of hyperkinetic (hyper-alert) children to usual sedatives, relative to the alerting mechanism. Such children have a much higher incidence of esotropia.

A significant advance has been made in the pharmacologic management of strabismus by the introduction of oculinum (botulism) neurotoxin directly into an eye muscle in order to produce a temporary paralysis. This technique has been devised by my colleague at the Smith-Kettlewell Institute, Dr. Alan B. Scott. It is now widely accepted and used in strabismus management and in management of other nonoculorotary muscles, such as the facial muscles involved in intractable blepharospasm.

In strabismus, one can alter the spring-back position of rest by temporarily inducing a paralysis in one muscle. The dose-related effect of the paralysis is guided into the muscle site under topical conjunctival drop anesthesia by means of a double-barreled electromyographically guided needle. The auditorily monitored needle site can be determined as being within the muscle into which the botulism is injected.

The temporary paralysis allows the antagonist muscle to obtain some degree of contracture. The neurotoxin paralysis is completely reversible with time alone. This alters the basic deviation because of residual mechanical contracture of the antagonist muscle of the agonist-antagonist muscle pair. The injection and contracture-producing process may be repeated at intervals.

This is being used in adults as well as children with strabismus. In blepharospasm, an injection into the muscles apparently interrupts the spasm site, often with permanent cure of this debilitating condition. Such imaginative uses of pharmacologic agents will become more and more common in the management of strabismus, as well as other muscle diseases.

Progress in strabismus realignment surgery will depend on identification and better understanding, as well as quantification and control of (a) complete oculorotary muscle relaxation, and (b) complete restoration and/or elimination of the active innervational components. This will allow separation and control of the mechanical (passive) versus the innervational (active) factors of strabismus alignment.

Pharmacologic quantification and control of these factors will put us closer to the goal of satisfactory balanced alignment, with balanced rotations, in one strabismus surgical procedure.

I hope I have made it apparent that the strabismus surgeon now extends his important diagnostic tests and important treatment assessment methods into the surgical anesthetic process. There must be the utmost cooperation with the anesthesiologist and careful consideration of the agents used before and during surgery and extending into the immediate postoperative period.

ACKNOWLEDGMENT

This research was supported in part by USPHS R01 EY03915 and The Smith-Kettlewell Eye Research Foundation.

REFERENCES

1. France, N. K., France, T. D., Woodburn, J. B., and Burbank, D. P. (1980): Succinylcholine alteration of the forced duction test. *Ophthalmology,* 87:1282-1287.
2. Jampolsky, A. (1978): Surgical leashes, reverse leashes in strabismus surgical management. In: *Strabismus Symposium, Transactions of the New Orleans Academy of Ophthalmology,* pp. 244-268. C. V. Mosby, St. Louis.
3. Jampolsky, A. Spring-back balance test in strabismus surgery. In: *Strabismus Symposium, Transactions of the New Orleans Academy of Ophthalmology,* pp. 104-111. C. V. Mosby, St. Louis.
4. Keller, E. L. (1974): Participation of medical pontine reticular formation in eye movement generation in monkey. *J. Neurophysiol.,* 37:316-319.

Commentary

Pharmacology of Corneal Surgery

One of the most talented corneal surgeons on earth has given us the benefit of his expertise in this chapter to show us how pharmacology may serve as an important adjunct to corneal surgery.

Meticulous attention to surgical detail is possible with microsurgical techniques and tools, but improvements in drug design and utilization have paralleled the surgical advance. The appropriate use of corticosteroids, hyaluronate, nonsteroidal agents, irrigating solutions, and immunosuppressive agents all deserve emphasis. The use of hyaluronate, a polysaccharide with a molecular weight of more than a million not only protects the corneal endothelium in difficult cases but makes the operative maneuvers easier and safer in a great many instances. Of course, in all cases, preoperative attention to the level of intraocular pressure is essential for the success of penetrating keratoplasty.

Advances in eye bank procedures have also contributed greatly to the success of corneal transplantation. Rapid enucleation, attention to biomicroscopy and specular microscopy of the donor material, together with early use, are important features. Short term storage in tissue culture media, TC 199, dextran, and appropriate antibiotics, (the McCarey-Kaufman technique) is perhaps the most useful but improvements are on the horizon. [For example see, Cipolla, L., Whitehouse, A., Eiferman, R., and Schultz, G. (1985): Stimulation of human corneal endothelial cell mitosis *in vitro* by human cord serum. *Invest. Ophthalmol. Vis. Sci. ARVO Suppl.,* 26(1):16.]

This is a most complete chapter and should be carefully studied and evaluated.

The Editors

Surgical Pharmacology of the Eye,
edited by M. Sears and A. Tarkkanen.
Raven Press, New York © 1985.

Pharmacology of Corneal Surgery

Ali A. Khodadoust

Yale University School of Medicine, New Haven, Connecticut 06510

Advancement in pharmacology has contributed to the evolution of corneal surgery in recent years. Tranquilizers, sedatives, and analgesic agents have provided comfort and relaxation for the patient and indirectly for the surgeon. The discovery of long-acting anesthetic agents has enabled surgeons to perform microsurgery under well-controlled and optimal conditions. Antiseptic agents have provided a more dependable sterility, and antibiotics as prophylactic or therapeutic agents have helped in the prevention or control of postoperative infection. More recently, the introduction of irrigating and protective solutions for corneal endothelial cells has enabled corneal surgeons to be more aggressive in undertaking the most complicated surgical tasks in the reconstruction of the anterior segment of the eye (Figs. 1–3).

The cornea, because of its position and its avascular nature, differs from other tissues in its wound-healing and in its response to various pharmaceutical agents. Despite being a privileged site in hosting foreign tissue as a graft, allograft rejection is the leading cause of corneal graft failure. The introduction of anti-inflammatory and immunosuppressive agents has played an important role in the control of corneal graft rejection. The pharmacology of corneal surgery, particularly that of corneal transplantation, is not limited to the pre-, intra-, or immediate postoperative period. This subject, in some instances, must be applied for the life of the patient. It is therefore the responsibility of any ophthalmologist who provides postoperative care for such patients to be familiar with the best pharmacologic agents available for the management of late postoperative complications. In this chapter we discuss pharmacology as applied to corneal surgery in terms of the agents used in our practice (including more than 2,000 corneal grafts) and their side effects.

ANATOMIC CONSIDERATIONS

There are three anatomic features that make the cornea different from other vascularized tissue in its response to pharmaceutical agents as applied to surgery. These features are corneal avascularity, anatomic position, and transparency.

Absence of blood vessels in the cornea has caused some reduction of the natural defense of this tissue. The wound-healing is slow, and the tissue,

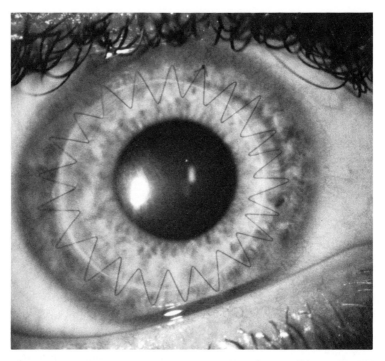

FIG. 1. Phakic penetrating corneal graft (10 days postoperative) in a 25-year-old patient with keratoconus. The patient received 60 mg oral prednisone from the second postoperative day, topical corticosteroid every 4 hr from the fifth postoperative day, and topical chloramphenicol 4 times a day. The anterior chamber was free of ray and cells; there is minimum congestion of bulbar conjunctiva.

specifically its central portion, is less accessible to medications administered systemically.

After any surgical procedure there is a disruption of the continuity of the corneal epithelium. This, plus the reduction of corneal sensation, further reduces the defense of this tissue at the immediate postoperative period. These factors make the role of prophylactic and therapeutic antibiotic therapy, as well as the role of antiseptic agents, highly critical in any corneal surgery. Slow avascular wound-healing makes the cornea more susceptible to the inhibitory effects of some of the topically applied medication in its wound-healing. These features can readily explain the chronic nature of bacterial, viral, and fungal infections of the cornea as compared to similar infections in other vascularized tissues of the body.

Anatomic position, on the other hand, has made the cornea readily accessible to topically applied drugs and agents targeted at the cornea itself or to the tissues within the eye. In this connection, the toxic effect of topically applied medications for either purpose on the corneal wound has to be considered.

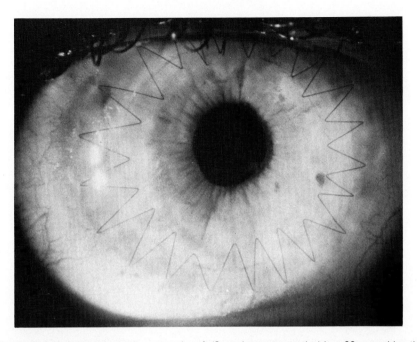

FIG. 2. Pseudophakic penetrating corneal graft (2 weeks postoperative) in a 66-year-old patient with Fuchs' endothelial dystrophy and cataract. The patient received prophylactic oral antibiotic therapy for 5 days, oral prednisone and topical chloramphenicol from the second postoperative day, and topical corticosteroid from the sixth postoperative day. Air was used as a cushion between the graft and the posterior chamber intraocular lens during surgery. Vision uncorrected, 20/40; corneal thickness, 0.55 mm.

The maintenance of corneal transparency, especially its central portion, is one of the goals of any surgical procedure on the cornea. In this connection, the reduction of the inflammatory process by anti-inflammatory agents has been considered. Anti-inflammatory agents, on the other hand, do retard corneal wound-healing. Titration of these agents for each particular disease condition is an art that can be gained only through experience.

Any surgical procedure or laceration of the cornea results in a transection of the corneal nerve. Anesthetic cornea, like any exposed and denervated tissue of the body, is more prone to injury and infection. A more rigid follow-up and sometimes prophylactic use of antibiotics before epithelial regeneration and recovery of corneal sensation should be considered.

PHYSIOLOGIC CONSIDERATIONS

The drugs applied topically on the corneal surface in the form of solutions or ointments must cross the cornea to affect its deeper portion or the anterior chamber of the eye. Knowledge of corneal permeability to a variety of

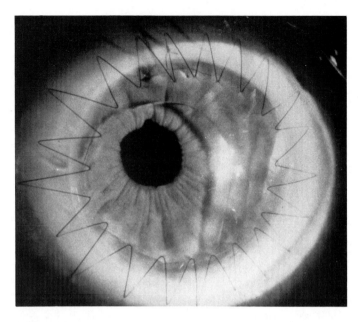

FIG. 3. Pseudophakic penetrating corneal graft (6 weeks postoperative) in a 75-year-old patient with advanced aphakic bullous keratopathy and vitreous in the anterior chamber. The patient had an anterior vitrectomy, anterior chamber intraocular lens, and an 8-mm penetrating graft. Air was used as a cushion between the graft and the anterior chamber lens. Vision uncorrected, 20/20; corneal thickness, 0.57 mm.

therapeutic agents helps in their proper selection, concentration, and the frequency of use. For a drug to pass through the intact cornea, it should be bipolar, i.e., both water and lipid soluble. This is because the lipid-soluble compound (nonpolar) can pass through the epithelium and endothelium, and the water-soluble (polar) compound can pass through the corneal stroma (75,128). A marked enhancement of permeability of the cornea to various drugs follows any surgical or traumatic insult to the cornea, especially those involving disruption of corneal epithelium or endothelium (15). Topical anesthetic and surface-tension-reducing agents enhance corneal permeability (98). When rapid action of miotic or mydriatic drugs is needed prior to corneal surgery or in the immediate postoperative period, application of these agents will enhance penetration of these drugs (46).

DRUGS AND CORNEAL WOUND-HEALING

Avascular healing of the corneal wound is slower than vascularized healing (51); thus, the inhibitory effect of a variety of conditions on its wound-healing is more noticeable. A number of systemic conditions such as debilitating diseases, malnutrition, hypoproteinemia, vitamin A and vitamin C deficiency, antineoplastic and immunosuppressive therapy are associated with retardation of wound-healing (112). We have seen 360-degree wound dehiscence of corneal graft 9 to 12 months postoperatively after suture removal in malnourished and hypoproteinemic individuals. Systemic corticosteroid therapy for a short period of time has a negligible effect, but its use topically has a profound inhibitory effect on corneal wound-healing (5,89,110). This effect of topical corticosteroid therapy is dose-related (54). Topical use of corticosteroids was found not to influence wound-healing if treatment was delayed until the seventh postoperative day (69). In corneal transplantation, we initiate systemic corticosteroids from the second postoperative day, and we delay topical treatment 5 to 6 days. At this time the graft is usually covered by epithelium and there is minimal interruption of wound-healing. As soon as all inflammation clears up, we rapidly taper and stop the therapy within 2 to 3 weeks. We do not recommend a maintenance dose of topical steroid therapy.

All antiviral agents with the exception of idoxuridine (IDU) retard corneal wound-healing, and their effect, similar to the corticosteroid, is dose-related (53). There are instances of corneal transplantation for herpetic keratitis in which antiviral agents must be added as long as the patient is on topical or systemic corticosteroid therapy. IDU has been shown to protect the cornea against steroid activation of the disease and seems to be a preferred agent (72). These patients need special postoperative care. Steroid therapy should be reduced or stopped as soon as possible, and suture removal must be delayed.

β-Irradiation, used for the prevention or obliteration of corneal vascularization, does retard corneal wound-healing (88,96). Its excessive use should be avoided if one plans corneal transplantation.

Epithelial denudation has a profound inhibitory effect on the stromal wound-healing; conversely, stromal healing can be assisted by rapid epithelialization of the corneal surface (34,51). A number of agents used topically at the immediate postoperative period interfere with epithelial healing and indirectly retard stromal repair. Most of the topical anesthetic solutions including proparacaine, benoxinate, cocaine, butacaine, and tetracaine would retard epithelial wound-healing (48,58,84). Their excessive use, postoperatively, should be avoided. A variety of antiseptics commonly used as preservatives or therapeutic agents, such as zinc sulfate, thimerosal (Merthiolate®), merbromin (Mercurochrome®), or benzalkonium chloride (Zephiran®), similarly delay epithelial healing (13,85).

Antibiotics used topically as prophylactic or therapeutic measures in the immediate postoperative period do not significantly interfere with mitosis or epithelial migration (83). However, in high concentrations, they do delay epithelial wound-healing. Bacitracin at a concentration of 1,000 U/ml has been shown to inhibit epithelial healing (85), and at a concentration of 10,000 U/ml, it was found to be toxic to the epithelium (103,132). Neomycin at a therapeutic concentration (3.5 mg/ml) does not influence wound-healing (83), but allergic reaction with punctate keratopathy has frequently been observed

(42,44). Higher concentrations of neomycin (8 mg/ml) do slightly retard epithelial wound-healing (103). Gentamicin at a concentration of 3 mg/ml does not alter wound-healing, but 10 mg/ml slightly retards epithelial repair (103). Subconjunctival (20 mg) gentamicin or its topical use at a concentration of 14 mg/ml may be toxic to the cornea (67). Ophthalmologists have been warned of the toxic effect of bacitracin, 10,000 U/ml, gentamicin sulfate, 8 to 15 mg/ml, and neomycin, 5 to 8 mg/ml (132). Chloramphenicol at therapeutic concentrations has been shown to be nontoxic to the rabbit corneal epithelium (103). Penicillin, polymyxin B, erythromycin, vancomycin, and sulfonamide in high concentrations delay epithelial wound-healing, but none of these agents has a significant effect in therapeutic concentrations.

There is no specific drug available for the acceleration of corneal wound-healing in humans. However, in experimental corneal wounds, a marked enhancement of repair has been observed by topical application of mesodermal growth factor (115,121) and vitamin A acid (123).

PREOPERATIVE EVALUATION AND MEDICATION

Whether the operation will be performed under general or local anesthesia with or without a standby, a thorough knowledge of the patient's past medical history and present medical condition should be obtained by the surgeon. For elective corneal surgery, this knowledge is best obtained prior to admission, and for emergency cases, at the time of admission. A telephone call to the patient's family physician or internist will facilitate proper preoperative care of the patient, especially those with multiple systemic disorders. Any elective corneal surgery should be postponed in the presence of uncontrolled systemic diseases such as diabetes mellitus, angina, hypertension, cardiac failure, pulmonary disease, genitourinary or gastrointestinal disorders, or thyroid abnormalities. The selection of a proper preoperative medication and its optimum dose should be tailored to each patient. Full knowledge of all the medications the patient is receiving will prevent some side effects of drug interaction, particularly in older patients. Topical epinephrine or phenylephrine can precipitate a hypertensive crisis in patients on monoamine oxidase inhibitors; the average dose of premedication can cause a profound vasodepressive effect in patients taking tranquilizers. The physical and emotional stress of the operation can lead to acute adrenal cortical insufficiency and shock in patients on chronic corticosteroid therapy.

In general or local anesthesia with a standby, the surgeon and the anesthesiologist should be in constant consultation with each other in each case, although the anesthesiologist is responsible for writing the preoperative medications. If local anesthesia is used, the surgeon is responsible for writing preoperative orders and medications. In either case, the objective of premedication is to have a relaxed, alert, and cooperative patient upon arrival in the operating room. A few minutes of discussion with the patient regarding the nature of the operation, including the sequence of events in the operating room, prior to or immediately after admission is helpful. Such patients are extremely relaxed and cooperative and readily responsive to the average premedication. Older patients generally do not need as much premedication as do younger patients, and overpremedication in elderly individuals causes more delirium and agitation.

Preoperative medication basically consists of three classes of drugs: sedative-hypnotic agents, analgesics, tranquilizers, and antiemetics. They can be used as sole agents or in combination with other classes. There are several drugs in each class, and every physician has his or her own preference. However, the following agents are the most popular.

Sedative-Hypnotic Agents

Intermediate-acting barbiturates (3 to 6-hr duration) are the most commonly used agents. In this class, secobarbital (Seconal®) or pentobarbital (Nembutal®) have been used for preoperative sedation. The dosage, depending on the patient's age, weight and general condition, varies from 50 to 300 mg. It is usually given 1 to 3 hr before surgery. Barbiturates are not recommended in older patients because they can cause disorientation, delirium, and restlessness. Chloralhydrate is the best substitute for barbiturates in elderly patients. It can be used orally from 750 to 2,000 mg, 1 to 2 hr prior to surgery. Phenothiazines potentiate the effect of barbiturates, and when used in combination, the dosage should be reduced by one-half.

Analgesics

The best and the most commonly used drug in this class is meperidine hydrochloride (Demerol®), a synthetic opiate. It can be used in doses of 50 to 100 mg orally or intramuscularly 1 hr before surgery. It is used with barbiturates and/or phenothiazines because it does not have any sedative or hypnotic effect. Because of the depressing effects of Demerol® on the cardiovascular and respiratory system, its dosage should be accurately assessed in elderly patients.

Tranquilizers and Antiemetics

Phenothiazine groups have been used extensively to alleviate apprehension and to control nausea and vomiting, both pre- and postoperatively in ophthalmology. They all potentiate the action of barbiturates and opiates, and the dosage should be reduced to half when used in combination with either one. The most common drugs of the phenothiazine group used as premedications are promethazine (Phenergan®) 25 to 100 mg, triflupromazine (Vesprin®) 5 to

10 mg, perphenazine (Trilafon®) 10 to 15 mg, and diazepam (Valium®) 5 to 10 mg. All of these medications can be used intramuscularly.

Typical premedication for elective corneal surgery in our practice is as follows: Nembutal® or Seconal® 35 to 100 mg by mouth 2 hr before surgery (for older patients, chloral hydrate, 750 to 1,000 mg p.o.); Demerol®, 50 to 100 mg, and Phenergan®, 25 to 50 mg, intramuscularly 1 hr before surgery.

CARBONIC ANHYDRASE INHIBITORS AND HYPEROSMOTIC AGENTS

The reduction of intraocular pressure by carbonic anhydrase inhibitors and osmotic agents for corneal surgery is sometimes necessary. In routine phakic penetrating or lamellar grafts or in small corneal lacerations without excessive elevation of intraocular pressure, we have not used any of these agents. However, in corneal grafts combined with cataract extraction, in aphakic or pseudophakic eyes with or without intraocular lens insertion, in large corneal lacerations, in repair of wound dehiscence, in patients with borderline intraocular pressure, and in children (below the age of 14), preoperative use of these agents is indicated.

Carbonic Anhydrase Inhibitors

There are a number of agents available in this group. They include acetazolamide (Diamox®) 250 mg, dichlorphenamide (Daranide®) 50 mg, ethoxyzolamide (Cardaze®) 125 mg, and methazolamide (Neptazane®) 50 mg. These agents should not be used in patients with severe electrolyte imbalance, cirrhosis of the liver, or adrenal failure. Before using these agents, the serum potassium should be checked in all patients who have been using thiazide derivatives and in those patients on digitalis. If the serum potassium is low, potassium chloride should be used to correct the condition.

For premedication, whenever indicated, we ordinarily use 500 mg Diamox® (2 tablets of 250 mg) orally 2 hr prior to surgery or intravenously 10 to 30 min before surgery.

Osmotic Agents

There are several hyperosomotic agents available and, depending on the preference of the surgeon, any one of these may be used.

Glycerol (1 to 1.5 ml/kg) is a good agent used orally with fruit juice (150 to 200 ml of 50% solution for the average patient) (50). It is nontoxic and does not promote diuresis; therefore, catheterization is not necessary. However, it is not as effective as other agents that can be used intravenously. It may produce nausea, vomiting, hyperglycemia, and glycosuria.

Mannitol (1 to 2 g/kg) is the most common agent used in intraocular surgery (1,99). In the average patient, 250 ml of 20% solution can be used over a period of 20 to 30 min. Maximum effect is attained between 20 and 90 min. It is a sugar alcohol that does not penetrate the cell wall and is therefore confined to extracellular space. It is as effective as urea in lowering intraocular pressure. Timing is important; if given too soon prior to surgery, rebound rise in intraocular pressure occurs; if given too late, there is no effect on intraocular pressure during surgery. It should be started about 1 hr prior to surgery. If crystals are present, the solution should be warmed before injection.

Urea (1 to 1.5 g/kg) is used as a 30% solution in 10% fructose intravenously over 30 to 45 min. The maximum effect is attained about 60 min after start of the infusion. Subcutaneous extravasation causes necrosis and sloughing of underlying tissue, and its use is contraindicated in severe renal or hepatic failure.

Hyperosmotic agents should not be used in individuals who are dehydrated. The side effect of these agents consists of headache, nausea, and dizziness, distressing frequency of micturition, and marked diuresis; catheterization is desirable. These agents also induce thirst and can cause an overload of the cardiovascular system and acute failure in patients with borderline cardiovascular insufficiency. Although rare, intracranial hemorrhage has been reported with these agents (86). Hyperosmotic agents can be used in combination with carbonic anhydrase inhibitors.

ANESTHESIA IN CORNEAL SURGERY

Corneal surgeons have their own preference as to the type of anesthesia used for each case of corneal surgery. Some prefer general anesthesia for most cases, including removal of corneal graft sutures; others use general anesthesia for major surgeries and local anesthesia for minor surgeries. In our experience, most elective corneal surgeries and some of the traumatic cases can satisfactorily be performed with local anesthesia. Local anesthesia causes less disturbance of body function, lower incidence of both ocular and systemic complications, less postoperative observation, and, above all, less nausea and vomiting. In addition, it is less expensive. However, there are instances of a definite need for general anesthesia. These include apprehensive and uncooperative patients, patients with large corneal lacerations, patients with large descemetocele or perforated ulcers, and children. We also prefer general anesthesia in patients addicted to narcotics and in patients with inflamed and congested eyes or orbital tissue, because in either of these cases, local infiltration of anesthetic agents does not provide adequate anesthesia. Judgment of the patient's cooperation preoperatively is sometimes difficult. One practical way is to observe the patient's response to the first topically applied anesthetic solution in his conjunctival cul-de-sac. Overreactive patients are generally not the best candidates for a major surgical procedure under local anesthesia.

Topical and Local Anesthesia

We use topical anesthesia for superficial corneal procedures when prolonged anesthesia and ocular immobility are not essential, i.e., corneal irrigation, removal of superficial foreign body, suture removal, tattooing of small leukomas, small superficial keratectomies, scraping or debridement of corneal ulcers, etc. We use local infiltrative anesthesia (lid and retrobulbal block) for the following conditions: penetrating corneal grafts or any corneal surgery involving the opening of the anterior chamber and nonpenetrating corneal surgeries in which ocular immobility is essential, such as lamellar cornea grafts; large keratectomies; tattooing of large leukomas; deeply embedded intracorneal foreign bodies, etc. Local anesthesia can safely be used for small corneal lacerations, at the discretion of the surgeon.

The most commonly used topical anesthetic agents are as follows:

1. *Proparacaine hydrochloride,* 0.5% (Ophthaine®, Ophthetic®, and Alcaine®) is the least irritating and the most commonly used agent that possesses the least drug sensitivity (16). It provides good anesthesia within 6 to 20 sec and lasts for 10 to 20 min.

2. *Pontocaine* (tetracaine), 0.5 to 2% provides more effective anesthesia for the same length of time as proparacaine hydrochloride but irritates, causes a transient superficial epithelial lesion, and delays corneal wound-healing (58).

3. *Cocaine,* 1 to 4% is an excellent agent that provides prolonged and potent topical anesthesia (12). It penetrates the cornea readily and may give a good anesthesia for the iris. The corneal toxicity of this agent manifesting as superficial grayish pits and irregularities is, however, significant (four times as much as proparacaine) (10).

To avoid irritation and the burning sensation of tetracaine or cocaine, a drop of proparacaine hydrochloride can be used prior to the administration of either of these agents.

Injectable Anesthetics

There are several injectable anesthetic agents available for corneal surgery (124). The most common agents we have used with or without epinephrine and hyaluronidase are the following:

1. *Lidocaine* (Xylocaine®), 0.5 to 4%. This is the most common and the most popular anesthetic agent used in ophthalmology, including corneal surgeries. Its safe dose is 3 to 4 mg/kg body weight without epinephrine and up to 7 mg/kg body weight with epinephrine. Onset of anesthesia is about 5 to 10 min and lasts for 2 hr without epinephrine and 2 to 3 hr with epinephrine. We have been using 2% solution for both lid block and retrobulbar injection. Some surgeons prefer to use 1% for lid block and 2% or 4% for retrobulbar

injection. The duration of anesthesia and akinesia of lidocaine is, however, short for longer surgical procedures.

2. *Bupivacaine* (Marcaine®, Sensorcaine®) is a long-acting anesthetic agent recently introduced in ophthalmology (27,63). It has enabled surgeons to perform the most sophisticated corneal surgeries, which would require longer operating time under local anesthesia. It comes in 0.25%, 0.5% and 0.75%, and its maximum safe dose in adults is 250 mg with epinephrine, 200 mg without epinephrine. It is four times more toxic than lidocaine. The onset of anesthesia and akinesia is slower than lidocaine but it lasts for 3 to 6 hr (74). It does not diffuse into the tissue readily and produces some pain when injected.

3. *Hyaluronidase* (Wydase®). Hyaluronidase hydrolyzes the hyaluronic acid, thus permitting faster spread of the solution into the tissue. It also potentiates the hypotony (94). We use 6 to 10 turbidity reducing units (TRU). Since this agent contains a minute quantity of bovine plasma protein, it can potentially cause a hypersensitivity reaction, although we have not seen this.

4. *Epinephrine.* Most of the local anesthetic agents (except cocaine) dilate the vessels. This leads to rapid absorption of the anesthetic agent and thus reduces the duration of its anesthetic effect. Adding epinephrine to the anesthetic solution will cause a constriction of blood vessels, thus reducing its absorption and prolonging anesthesia (43). The recommended dose of epinephrine is less than 1 mg (1 ml of 1/1000). Use of epinephrine in an individual with hypertension, coronary artery disease, thyrotoxicosis or, in general, anesthesia with cyclopropane and halothane is prohibited. Also, the addition of epinephrine is not recommended by some surgeons in combination with bupivacaine since bupivacaine provides long-lasting anesthesia (28).

In a double-blind clinical study, Chin and Almquist (28) compared bupivacaine 0.75% with epinephrine and/or hyaluronidase and lidocaine 2% with epinephrine and hyaluronidase as to the onset and duration of surgical anesthesia and akinesia. No significant difference was noted in the onset time of anesthesia between bupivacaine and lidocaine with epinephrine and hyaluronidase, but bupivacaine with ephinephrine was slow in attaining akinesia and anesthesia. Mean duration of akinesia was 11 hr with bupivacaine and 4 hr with lidocaine. Anesthesia with bupivacaine lasts about 8 hr, compared to 2 hr with lidocaine.

For surgical procedures of short duration (up to 1 hr), we have used 2% lidocaine with epinephrine and hyaluronidase, and for longer procedures, a mixture of 2% lidocaine and 0.75% bupivacaine in equal volume with epinephrine and hyaluronidase is used. This mixture used for both retrobulbar and van Lindt akinesia provides a rapid, painless, and long-lasting anesthesia for most corneal grafts and reconstructive surgery of the anterior segment of the eye. In outpatient surgery we use lidocaine 2% for lid block and the mixture of lidocaine and bupivacaine for retrobulbar injection.

DIAGNOSTIC AGENTS IN CORNEAL SURGERY

A number of diagnostic agents have been used preoperatively for evaluation of patients undergoing corneal surgery, intraoperatively to evaluate the integrity of the wound, or postoperatively to follow the course of corneal wound-healing.

Sodium fluorescein (solution of 0.5% to 2%, or fluorescein strip) is used preoperatively to evaluate the lacrimal system both for dry eye and for the obstruction of the lacrimal damage system. Intraoperatively, fluorescein has been used to stain the knife or the suture for demarcation of the tracts by some surgeons. At the completion of the surgery, if the wound is leaking and the site cannot be identified, fluorescein dissolved in a balanced salt solution may be injected into the anterior chamber through a separate Ziegler incision. The wound can be visualized with the operating microscope to detect the site of leakage. Postoperatively, fluorescein can be used to follow the course of epithelial wound-healing or to assure proper fit of contact lens as well as in the evaluation of corneal epithelium after removal of the contact lens. Fluorescein cannot be used for hydrophilic contact lenses because the dye will stain the lens. In these instances, fluorescein derivatives with larger molecular weight such as fluorexon can be used (114). Fluorescein can be used for a Seidel test postoperatively if the anterior chamber is shallow and there is some suspicion of wound leakage. A drop of sodium fluorescein is placed in the conjunctival cul-de-sac, and the patient is examined with cobalt blue light. A slight pressure on the globe may be necessary to see the leakage if the eye is excessively soft.

Rose bengal, a derivative of fluorescein, used in 1% solution, stains the devitalized epithelium and is a more sensitive agent to evaluate the dry eye preoperatively (102). Similar to fluorescein, this can also be used to stain the herpetic keratitis. It is more irritating than fluorescein but no preliminary use of topical anesthesia is required.

Methylene blue, 0.5%, is another agent that can be used intraoperatively for staining the knife or suture tracts as demarcation lines, or it can be used postoperatively to evaluate the course of epithelial wound-healing. The staining of methylene blue in the tissue lasts longer than fluorescein or rose bengal. It is more irritating than rose bengal and should be preceded by topical anesthesia.

TISSUE ADHESIVES IN CORNEAL SURGERY

Eastman 910 (methyl 2-cyanoacrylate monomer) was first used on an experimental animal eye as an alternative to suturing the conjunctival flap (41). It provided a suitable strength but was too toxic to the tissue. Subsequently, the alkiderivative of the cyanoacrylate became available and was better tolerated by living tissues (52). Although these agents are still under Food and

Drug Administration investigation, they have been used as an immediate therapy to seal off perforated corneal ulcers or descemetoceles (17,56,66). They are generally known as surgical glues, and the commercial grade adhesive is called Krazy Glue®; the so-called medical grade adhesive is manufactured by Braun in West Germany and also by Tri-hawk Company in Canada (histacryl glue).

A tissue adhesive for closure of the corneal wound was first used in 1968 (130), and since that time numerous studies have shown its efficacy in corneal perforations or impending perforations (61,62,66,126,131). These agents, although not ideal, can be used as an alternative to conjunctival flap or corneal graft in cases of perforated corneal ulcers. The application of a tissue adhesive is technically simple. It can be applied under topical anesthesia, under slit lamp, or at bedside. It is best done with the patient in supine position under the operative microscope. The epithelium is denuded from the base of the ulcer, the surface is dried with a weck-cell sponge, and a small drop of tissue adhesive is placed immediately over the perforated site. Within 5 to 10 min, the tissue adhesive is dry, the chamber will start to form, and at this time the cornea may be covered by a soft bandage lens. The tissue adhesive can stay in place for 1 day to more than 1 year. It can easily be removed by a pair of fine forceps prior to the definitive surgical procedure, such as conjunctival flap or corneal graft when the ulcer has healed with the growth of vessels.

Aside from corneal ulcers, the tissue adhesive has rarely been used for the closure of leaking wounds postoperatively (127). Its use as an alternative to the sutures (sutureless corneal graft) is contraindicated because the living tissue cannot be fused with a nonbiodegradable synthetic material. The glue is toxic and leads to necrosis of the tissue at interface. Toxicity of the surgical glues have been extensively reviewed by Refojo and his co-workers in 1971 (113). There is a high incidence of failure and leakage after application of the glue, but it can be repeated. The glue leads to corneal vascularization, and if it enters into the anterior chamber, it will cause cataract formation. Healon® has been recently used to form the chamber prior to the application of surgical glue (60,82).

PROTECTIVE SOLUTIONS IN CORNEAL SURGERY

The transparency of the cornea depends to a great extent on the integrity of corneal endothelial cells (93). Mechanical or chemical injuries to this single layer of cells during the course of surgical procedure have a detrimental effect. A simple mechanical contact of endothelial cells to the intraocular lens (71) or rubbing these cells against the lens or iris during the course of corneal transplantation has been shown to cause a loss of cells or a reduction of the number of cells postoperatively (19). To avoid this complication, a variety of viscose solutions have been used as physical buffers between the corneal endothelium and its underlying tissue or devices. Some of these agents have recently become popular for clinical use and some have been used on experimental animals only. These agents include mucopolysaccharides (sodium hyaluronate and chondroitin sulfate), air, methylcellulose, serum albumin, and gamma globulin.

Sodium Hyaluronate

Sodium hyaluronate (Healon®) has a high molecular weight (10^6) and is a viscoelastic polymer naturally found in the vitreous, umbilical cord, joint fluid, and rooster comb. As a 1% solution, it is a clear viscose fluid, nontoxic and nonantigenic. It can be irrigated through a 30-gauge cannula. This solution was initially introduced to protect the corneal endothelium against the mechanical and electrostatic trauma of intraocular lens during its insertion (70,91,92). Subsequently, it has been used in a variety of surgical procedures on the anterior as well as posterior segments of the eye (6,70,100,101,109,125). Corneal surgeons have different opinions as to the limits of its use in corneal surgery. It has been used on the anterior chamber of both donor and recipient eyes prior to trephinization or scissor incision of corneal button in penetrating keratoplasties in order to keep the endothelium away from the iris and the lens. It has also been used on the anterior chamber of recipient eyes before transferring the donor button in aphakic and pseudophakic eyes. Its prime indication in corneal surgery is in aphakic keratoplasties to keep the vitreous away and in triple procedures to keep the intraocular lens away from the corneal endothelium during the course of surgery (Fig. 3). Healon® has been used in large perforated corneal ulcers both in experimental animals and in humans prior to the application of a tissue adhesive as a spacing agent to keep the intraocular content away from the perforated site and the tissue adhesive (60,82). Commercially, Healon® is obtained from the comb of the rooster and is made by Pharmacia in Sweden. After the completion of surgery, Healon® can be removed from the anterior chamber by aspiration combined with its simultaneous replacement by balanced salt solution. It also can be left in the eye, but there is a dose-related elevation of intraocular pressure lasting for 2 to 4 days (7). Technically, there is also some problem with handling the suture material once it gets involved with the solution.

Chondroitin Sulfate

Chondroitin sulfate is another mucopolysulfate found in human tissues, including the corneal stroma. It has a molecular weight of 5×10^4, and in 1% solution similar to Healon®, it is a clear viscose solution, nontoxic and nonantigenic. This solution has recently been introduced as a protective solution for corneal endothelial cells. Its use in human eye bank eyes and in experimental animals has been claimed to be superior to sodium hyaluronate in protecting the corneal endothelial cells during the traumatic insertion of intraocular lens (59). This agent has therapeutic qualities in corneal wound-healing and does not cause elevation of intraocular pressure once it is left in the anterior chamber.

Air has been used as a cushion between the cornea and its underlying tissue (18). It is preferred by some surgeons because it is readily available and visible during the course of surgery. A large air bubble and prolonged exposure of endothelial cells to air can damage the cells (40). A large or medium-size air bubble should be replaced by a balanced salt solution after completion of the surgery to prevent pupillary block, but a small air bubble can be left in the anterior chamber.

Methylcellulose (1% in 0.04 9% Salt Solution)

This agent has recently been advocated by Aron-Rosa and her co-workers (3) for the insertion of intraocular lens. They claim methylcellulose to be superior to air for protection of the corneal endothelial cells. There is no elevation of intraocular pressure when this solution is left in the anterior chamber, but a 1.5 or 2% solution is associated with an elevation of intraocular tension.

Bovine serum albumin and gamma globulin have been used in experimental animals and found to be less effective than chondroitin sulfate (59). None of these agents has been recommended for human use.

IRRIGATING SOLUTIONS IN CORNEAL SURGERY

Irrigation of the cornea during the course of surgery can damage the endothelial cells and lead to postoperative stromal edema. We have avoided using any irrigation during the course of uncomplicated corneal surgery such as phakic or aphakic penetrating keratoplasties or in combined corneal graft and intracapsular cataract extraction. There are, however, instances in which the cornea or the anterior chamber must be irrigated. These instances include irrigation of the lens cortex in extracapsular cataract extraction, irrigation of blood, irrigation of the donor button, or irrigation during the course of anterior vitrectomy in aphakic corneal grafts. In these instances, the selection of the proper solution for irrigation is important, to minimize endothelial damage and subsequent corneal edema.

The ideal irrigating solution should match the normal aqueous humor in its chemical composition, osmolarity, pH and, for prolonged irrigation, nutrient material. Endothelial damage and postoperative corneal edema had been among the major complications of prolonged intraocular irrigation during the course of extracapsular cataract extraction or vitrectomy (20,90). In recent years, however, significant progress has been made in the chemical composition of these solutions. This has led to the introduction of new solutions that can be used more safely in a variety of intraocular procedures including corneal surgery.

There are three irrigating solutions commonly used for corneal surgery: physiologic saline, lactated Ringer's solution, and balanced salt solution (BSS). More recently, glutathione-bicarbonate Ringer's solution (BSS Plus) has been added to the list.

Physiologic saline (0.9% sodium chloride) has been the first irrigating solution used for the cornea and anterior segment during the course of corneal surgery and is still being used in some areas where there is no access to the newer agents. This solution causes the destruction of endothelial cells of the cornea, a separation of the apical junction, and rapid swelling of the corneal stroma (37,39). Physiologic saline can be used for irrigation of the cornea and conjunctival cul-de-sac prior to surgery but it should not be used for irrigation of the anterior chamber or the corneal button.

Lactated Ringer's solution contains potassium, calcium, and lactated ions. It maintains the corneal endothelial cells for a longer time when used in perfusion chamber experiments as compared to physiologic saline, but it too causes ultrastructure changes and damage to the endothelium within 1 hr, resulting in corneal edema (39). This solution can be used if there is no access to the more physiologic preparations.

BSS is the most widely accepted solution for irrigation in corneal surgery. This solution contains sodium, potassium, and calcium chloride in addition to magnesium and acetate-citrate buffer system. It was formulated on the basis that it maintained normal rabbit corneal endothelial cells in tissue culture (73). This solution, however, does not contain any energy source and is slightly hypotonic to the aqueous humor. It is superior to both physiologic saline and lactated Ringer's solution in supporting endothelial cells. An investigation on perfusion experiments has shown the endothelial change to occur only after 2 hr of continuous exposure to this solution (39). It is commercially available, but once the container is opened, it cannot be reused, because no preservative is added to the solution.

Dextrose-glutathione-bicarbonate Ringer's solution (BSS Plus) has recently been introduced and is used mainly for prolonged intraocular irrigation (35,37). This solution was initiated by an accidental finding of Dikstein and Maurice (31,32), who noted that the addition of glutathione to bicarbonated Ringer's solution improved the endothelial pump in the cornea undergoing temperature reversal. Its calcium is essential for the maintenance of endothelial cell function, and its bicarbonate buffer system is the same as normal aqueous humor. Glucose is a substrate for aerobic cellular metabolism, and glutathione protects the cellular enzyme that is essential for maintaining intercellular tight junction. In early experiments, reduced glutathione and adenosine was used (37,87). However, it was shown that oxidized glutathione alone was as effective as a combination of both agents (38). Protective properties of BSS Plus for corneal endothelial cells have been shown to be superior to BSS during the course of vitrectomy or extracapsular cataract extraction both in laboratory animals and in humans (35,37,39,129). However, this solution is unstable and is commercially provided in two parts that must be mixed in the operating room prior to use.

SUTURE MATERIAL IN CORNEAL SURGERY

Two types of suture material are commonly used in corneal surgery, silk and nylon. We have been using 8/0 or 9/0 virgin or black silk as a cardinal suture for corneal grafts, and have removed them at the completion of wound closure by monofilament nylon sutures. The use of silk sutures as a definitive suture for corneal surgery is not recommended because it can bind to gamma globulin and cause toxicity. It also attracts vascularization and tends to cause an inflammatory reaction by activating polymorphonuclear leukocytes and monocytes and causing a fibroblastic response (95). Although the inflammatory response enhances wound-healing in corneal grafts, it increases the incidence of allograft rejection. For corneal lacerations, especially those extending to the center of the cornea, this suture can lead to the formation of a dense scar and reduction of vision.

Monofilament nylon sutures are the best and most often recommended for any type of corneal surgery (79). They are available in sizes 8–0 to 14–0. We have been using 10–0 suture because it provides enough tensile strength, is easy to work with, and within a short period of time postoperatively will be covered by the epithelium (Fig. 1). Monofilament nylon sutures cause minimal tissue reaction and do not attract blood vessels unless the suture loops get loose or the knots are exposed (4,9). Because of minimum inflammatory response, the corneal wound-healing is relatively slow, but the sutures can be left in place for a long time. We usually remove them within 6 months to 1 year postoperatively. Should the suture loop become loose and attract the blood vessels, it can be removed within 2 to 3 months postoperatively. But leaving this suture material in the cornea for an extended period of time (more than 2 years) will lead to progressive disintegration and loss of its tensile strength.

MIOTICS, MYDRIATICS, AND CYCLOPLEGICS IN CORNEAL SURGERY

Proper use of miotics, mydriatics, and cycloplegic agents at different stages of corneal surgery helps to prevent complication and alleviate pain.

Pilocarpine 2% to 4% is the most commonly used miotic agent preoperatively in all cases of elective lamellar and penetrating corneal grafts in phakic and aphakic eyes. The constricted pupil will guide the surgeon in positioning the trephine in the center of the cornea, and in penetrating grafts, it protects the lens during the course of surgical procedure. For planned intracapsular cataract extraction and corneal grafts with or without anterior chamber intraocular lens, we do not use any miotics or mydriatics preoperatively. Retrobulbar injection of anesthetic agents usually provides adequate pupillary dilation for lens extraction, and the pupil can readily be constricted by miotics intraoperatively.

Intraoperatively, a miotic agent (carbachol 0.01% in BSS) is used to constrict the pupil immediately after intracapsular cataract extraction, before insertion of the anterior chamber intraocular lens, or before insertion of the donor tissue. For planned extracapsular cataract extraction and posterior chamber intraocular lens, miotics are used after insertion of the lens and before transfer of donor tissue.

Preoperative use of mydriatics and cycloplegics is not indicated in elective penetrating or lamellar corneal grafts. However, in the presence of active keratitis, corneal ulcer or iritis, these agents should be used. In combined corneal grafts and extracapsular cataract extraction, maximum pupillary dilation is essential for adequate anterior capsulotomies and irrigation of the lens cortex after delivery of the lens nucleus. In these instances, short-acting mydriatic agents such as Neo-Synephrine® combined with Mydriacyl® are used as a premedication. Long-acting mydriatic agents such as atropine are not recommended because the pupil will be more resistant to the miotic action of carbachol intraoperatively. Should the pupil constrict, we have been using epinephrine in the anterior chamber (1:10,000 dilution) intraoperatively.

At the immediate postsurgical period, for any type of penetrating or lamellar grafts, corneal lacerations, or nonpenetrating large corneal surgeries, we usually dress the eye with 1% atropine solution. We then continue the treatment daily thereafter, until all inflammation has cleared in the anterior chamber. Topical application of phenylephrine postoperatively, especially in the presence of epithelial defect, is not recommended because, in the presence of epithelial defect, there is a marked enhancement of drug penetration into the cornea leading to a toxic effect on keratocytes and endothelial cells (2,36,47,55).

ANTIBIOTICS IN CORNEAL SURGERY

1. *Preoperative.* Use of antibiotics as prophylactic agents in elective corneal surgery preoperatively is controversial. Topical antibiotics are routine; some surgeons use systemic and some use subconjunctival antibiotics prior to surgery (45). Certainly all patients with perforating corneal injuries or perforating corneal ulcers need a full dose of intravenous antibiotics soon after admission, and any source of infection around the eye, including the ocular adnexa, should be treated prior to any elective corneal surgery.

2. *Intraoperative.* There is no indication for intraoperative use of antibiotics in elective corneal surgery. However, irrigation of the anterior chamber with an antibiotic solution in certain cases of endophthalmitis with perforated corneal ulcers has been suggested (80). In our experience, the intravenous administration of antibiotics during the course of surgery provides adequate concentration of the drug in the aqueous humor in such instances. At the

completion of surgery, most surgeons routinely inject antibiotics such as gentamicin, subconjunctivally. We have been using gentamicin in all instances of penetrating corneal grafts in aphakic eyes, as well as in all combined procedures of corneal graft and cataract extraction with or without intraocular lens. In uncomplicated phakic penetrating grafts, we have not used subconjunctival antibiotics.

3. *Postoperative.* The use of postoperative topical and/or systemic prophylactic antibiotic therapy in elective corneal surgery is as controversial as its use preoperatively. We have not used systemic antibiotics routinely in uncomplicated elective penetrating or lamellar corneal grafts in phakic eyes. However, in aphakic corneal grafts or in combined corneal grafts and cataract extraction or specifically those with anterior vitrectomy, we have used systemic antibiotic therapy for the first five days postoperatively. As long as the corneal graft is denuded of epithelium or the sutures are exposed, we have been using topical prophylactic antibiotic therapy postoperatively. As soon as the area is covered by epithelium, we usually stop the antibiotics. This regimen seems to reduce the incidence of a stitch abscess, which is a common complication at the immediate postoperative period.

ANTI-INFLAMMATORIES AND CORTICOSTEROIDS IN CORNEAL SURGERY

Some degree of iritis is frequently seen after any penetrating corneal surgery, but corneal surgeons are usually familiar with the extent of postoperative inflammation in any given surgical procedure. Mild to moderate iritis in most cases can be managed by cycloplegics and topical use of corticosteroids. In corneal grafts, however, even mild iritis will influence the incidence of graft rejection reaction, and every attempt should be made to suppress the postoperative inflammation. Nonsteroidal anti-inflammatory agents such as antihistamines, aspirin, indomethacin, and acetaminophen as agents for reduction of postoperative inflammation in corneal surgery have not become widespread. Corticosteroids are the most commonly used agents for suppression of postoperative inflammation. We have routinely used subconjunctival injection of dexamethasone (Decadron®) at the completion of surgery in all cases of penetrating and lamellar corneal grafts that receive subconjunctival gentamicin. From the second postoperative day, providing there are no signs or symptoms of intraocular infection, systemic corticosteroid therapy is initiated at a dose of 60 to 80 mg prednisone daily. As soon as the graft is covered by the corneal epithelium (average 4 to 6 days), topical corticosteroids are initiated every 2 to 3 hr during the waking hours. Once all the inflammation in the anterior segment has cleared up, both systemic and topical corticosteroids are reduced and stopped within 7 to 10 days (Fig. 1).

Severe to moderate postoperative aseptic iritis can sometimes mimic a clinical picture of septic endophthalmitis. These cases need reexamination within 6 to 12 hr to reevaluate the postoperative inflammation. Suspected cases of endophthalmitis should be treated immediately with intravenous antibiotics after obtaining a smear and culture from the lid margin and conjunctival cul-de-sac. Within 12 hr the reaction in the anterior chamber and vitreous is reevaluated, and if the condition is static or improving, systemic corticosteroid therapy will then be initiated. If the reaction is worse, we usually tap the anterior chamber and vitreous for identification of the offending organism and then change the antibiotic therapy accordingly.

NONSTEROIDAL IMMUNOSUPPRESSIVE THERAPY

Although corticosteroids are still the most effective and most commonly used agents for the prevention and control of allograft rejection in corneal transplantation, there are instances of fulminating allograft rejection that are nonresponsive to corticosteroid therapy. These include corneal grafts in heavily vascularized corneas, previous history of graft rejection, and some primary graft rejections with fulminating courses. There are also instances in which prolonged use of corticosteroid therapy is not indicated because of the presence of glaucoma or the formation of cataracts. In these instances, the use of nonsteroidal immunosuppressive agents seems to be the next alternative. There are a number of agents available and commonly used for control of graft rejection in kidney, heart, and liver transplants. Some of these have been used on an experimental trial, but none have adequately been tried for human corneal graft rejection.

Cyclosporin A is a peptide metabolite of the fungi *Trichoderma polysporum rifai* and *Cylindrocarpon lucidom booth.* The immunosuppressive property of this agent has been recognized both in man and in a variety of experimental animals (11,29). Its systemic use in man has been associated with the development of lymphomas and nephrotoxicity. It specifically affects the T-cells and delays skin graft rejection, but because of its toxic effect, its systemic use in man for nonessential organ transplants has been discouraged. This agent, used intramuscularly, retrobulbarly, and topically in experimental animals, has been shown to be effective in prolonging corneal graft survival (65,68,117,118). No information is available on its use in human corneal transplantation, but the results of its topical use in experimental animals are encouraging. In the near future, this agent may prove to be useful in the control of allograft rejection reaction in humans.

Azathioprine (Imuran®) is a major purine analog and has a potent immunosuppressive property in experimental corneal xenografts (77,78). But because of its toxicity, it has not been used in human corneal grafts.

Methotrexate is a folic acid analog and has been used in cancer chemotherapy because of its inhibitory effect on DNA synthesis. Although it does have a specific suppressive effect on humoral immune response and has been used for treatment of uveitis unresponsive to corticosteroids (76), clinical improvement of corneal graft rejection has been reported (133).

Antilymphocyte sera or its IgG fraction as an antilymphocyte antibody has been found to have immunosuppressive properties. Although some beneficial effect in experimental corneal grafts has been reported (111,116,122), its effect in human corneal grafts is questionable.

CHEMICAL INJURIES OF THE CORNEA

The cornea, because of its anatomic position, is vulnerable to chemical injuries. The outcome of these injuries is dependent on two factors: the severity of injury and the rapidity of proper medical or surgical therapy. The severity of chemical injury depends on concentration of the chemical and the duration of exposure. Rapid and proper management of chemical injuries is the prime responsibility of any ophthalmologist.

Chemical agents are basically classified into acid and alkali. The extent of corneal damage inflicted by acids is usually less than that inflicted by alkali of the same concentration and duration of exposure. This is because the protein of corneal epithelium precipitates on contact with acid and prevents further penetration of chemical agents to the corneal stroma and into the anterior chamber. Although the cornea may have a ground-glass appearance after exposure to the acid, the lesion is mainly superficial. Alkali and very strong acids rapidly penetrate the cornea and enter into the anterior chamber. This leads to the destruction of the corneal stroma and the intraocular tissues. Exposure of the conjunctiva to alkali leads to thrombosis of conjunctival and episcleral vessels leading to ischemia and subsequent necrosis of these tissues. A variety of drugs and agents for management of this condition have recently been introduced; some are currently under investigation and some have proved to be useful additions to the preexisting mode of therapy (104). The general approach to the management of chemical injury of the eye is summarized below with special emphasis on the role of new pharmaceutical agents.

Initial Care

The goal is immediate dilution of the chemical agent in the anterior segment of the eye by the following:

1. Irrigation of cornea and conjunctival cul-de-sac by any rapidly available clean and inert solution. In the emergency room or in the clinic, any of the intravenous solutions such as saline or lactated Ringer's solutions can be used.

2. Removal of any sticky solid chemical agents (lime or paste) by forceps or cotton-tipped applicator.

3. Paracentesis of the anterior chamber (in severe alkali burns) and its reformation by BSS or its irrigation by phosphate buffer (14,26,57). Paracentesis can be performed in the emergency room under topical anesthesia; one need not wait to have the patient taken to the operating room.

4. Continuous irrigation of conjunctival cul-de-sac and the cornea by

connecting the intravenous tubing to the inflow channel of a scleral shell placed in the conjunctival cul-de-sac for 2 to 3 hr.

Following these initial steps, atropine 1% twice a day, topical antibiotics (chloramphenicol or gentamicin) four to six times a day plus analgesics for the pain should be used.

Intermediate Treatment

For prevention of symblepharon, corneal ulceration, and perforation, all patients with moderate to severe chemical injuries must be admitted on an emergency basis.

The cornea and bulbar conjunctiva, once denuded from the epithelium, plus leakage of plasma protein, rich in fibrinogen, set the stage for adhesion. In severe cases, it results in symblepharon and total obliteration of conjunctival cul-de-sac. The fibrin strands should be removed and lysed with a cotton-tipped applicator daily, and in severe cases, the bulbar conjunctiva may be separated from tarsal conjunctiva mechanically by the insertion of a plastic or methylmethacrylate ring. Persistent epithelial defects of the cornea should be managed by the insertion of therapeutic semirigid contact lens to encourage reepithelialization.

When the cornea and perilimbal area are involved in chemical injuries, corneal perforation and ulceration is a common problem. Collagenase has been isolated from the alkali-burned cornea, and it seems to play an important role in the pathogenesis of these ulcers (25). Based on this observation, an attempt has been made to inhibit this enzyme by chelating the calcium that is required for the enzyme activity (104). A variety of agents have been tried (21–24,64). The most promising ones are as follows:

1. *L-cysteine* (0.2 M solution in 0.9% sodium chloride) is used as a drop four to five times daily, initiated 7 days after injury and continued until the cornea is covered by epithelium. Cysteine is an irreversible inhibitor of collagenase and attaches to the enzyme in addition to chelating the calcium. It has been used both in experimental animals subjected to alkali burn as well as in humans and has been claimed to prevent ulceration and enhance epithelialization of the ulcer (119).

2. *Acetylcysteine* (Mucomyst® 10% to 20%) is more stable and more available than cysteine. It appears to inhibit collagenase, and its topical application, similar to cysteine, has been shown to reduce the incidence of corneal ulcer after alkali burn in animals (119). The effect of acetylcysteine in severe alkali burns in humans has been discouraging (106).

3. *EDTA* (0.2 M calcium EDTA in polyvinyl alcohol), one drop every 2 hr during waking hours for 2 weeks, has been shown to enhance healing of the corneal ulcers of nonspecific etiology and to have some beneficial effect in inhibiting the progress of corneal ulcerations from alkali burns (120).

Topical corticosteroids for the first week are recommended for reducing inflammation, but because of their inhibitory effect on fibroblast proliferation in healing progress, their prolonged use can retard wound-healing (33).

4. *Ascorbic acid.* The transport process in the ciliary epithelium provides an excessive amount of ascorbic acid in the aqueous humor (20 times the plasma level). Ascorbic acid is important for the production of collagen in the healing of the wound (8). It acts as a co-factor in hydroxylation of proline. Fibroblasts of scorbutic cornea cannot extrude mature collagen. Recently it was shown that there is a marked reduction in aqueous humor ascorbate of alkali-burned rabbit eyes (81). This observation led to a series of investigations showing that topical or subcutaneous ascorbate will reduce the incidence of corneal ulceration and perforation in moderate to severely burned corneas (81,107,108). Ascorbate can be used as a 10% solution topically or by subcutaneous injection. This will reverse the process of scorbutic cornea of alkali burn and enhances the wound-healing. In extreme alkali burns, ascorbic acid does not have any effect on the outcome in experimental animals.

5. *Citric acid.* In experimental rabbits with severe and extreme alkali-burned eyes, topical application of 10% citric acid, initially used as a placebo for ascorbic acid, was noted to cause a marked reduction of corneal ulcerations and perforation as compared to a control group (105,106). Citric acid causes reduction of polymorpholeukocytes and, apparently, chelates calcium in the extracellular space, and it interferes with the production of activated calcium-binding protein and inhibition of many intracellular processes (104).

The effect of ascorbic and citric acid on moderately severe to severe alkali burns of the human eye is currently being investigated (104). Investigators used either agent as a 10% solution hourly for 14 hr a day, with 2 g of the agents orally every 6 hr as a random clinical trial.

A number of anabolic steroids such as androgen, as well as progesterone hormones, have been tried in experimental alkali burns, and the results are encouraging (30,97). Apparently, these hormones enhance wound-healing by stimulation of general protein synthesis, especially from the corneal fibroblasts.

Mild to moderate chemical injuries usually result in some stromal haze and some reduction of visual acuity, but the majority of moderate to severe cases result in symblepharon formation, densely vascularized corneal scars. These complications necessitate extensive reconstruction surgery 1 to 2 years after the chemical burn. The prognosis for corneal graft in these cases is poor because of extensive vascularization, dry eye, and secondary glaucoma.

ALLOGRAFT REJECTION REACTION

All patients receiving a corneal graft should be alerted to the signs and symptoms of allograft rejection reaction. Should congestion or redness of the eye occur, with reduction of vision, the patient should report immediately to his or her ophthalmologist. The presence of ciliary congestion, keratic precipitates, or endothelial rejection line on the graft, with graft edema, represents the early sign of allograft rejection reaction. Initial therapy in these instances consists of topical corticosteroid therapy every hour; the patient will then be reevaluated within 24 hr. The reduction of keratic precipitates and graft edema or disintegration of endothelial rejection line are indications that topical corticosteroids have effectively controlled the rejection process. Should the reaction worsen, the patient should be treated with systemic as well as daily subconjunctival injections of corticosteroids in addition to topical steroids, and the course of the rejection has to be monitored daily. More than 70% of the cases with allograft rejection reaction can be controlled successfully by topical corticosteroid therapy (Fig. 4A,B,C). In 20% to 25% of the cases, systemic as well as subconjunctival corticosteroids are needed. In the remaining 5% to 10% of the cases, the process of rejection reaction is so fulminating that neither topical nor systemic or subconjunctival corticosteroids can control the rejection process.

Short-term systemic corticosteroid therapy is usually safe, provided the patient does not have an active peptic ulcer or a history of it. In this instance, it is best to use an antacid while the patient is on steroid therapy. Hyperosmolar, hyperglycemic, nonketotic coma (a serious and often lethal condition) has been reported in three previously healthy patients after a short course of oral corticosteroids (49). In over 20 years of its use in more than 2,000 corneal grafts, I have not observed such a complication as the result of oral steroids at the immediate postoperative period.

SPECIFIC CONSIDERATIONS

Corneal Grafts and Glaucoma

Elective corneal transplantation is contraindicated in the presence of elevated intraocular pressure. Combined corneal graft and any type of glaucoma operation in phakic or aphakic eyes is not a sound practice. If the intraocular pressure cannot be controlled with minimum medical therapy (i.e., with either miotics, timolol, or epinephrine), some sort of glaucoma operation should be performed prior to corneal transplantation. Even borderline glaucoma tends to worsen after corneal transplantation. There are, however, instances of glaucoma developing after corneal grafts. Topical use of corticosteroids postoperatively also leads to an elevation of intraocular pressure in steroid responders.

Intraocular pressure can safely be measured by applanation or pneumotonometer at any time postoperatively. We routinely check the intraocular pressure on all the grafts on the third or fourth day postoperatively prior to initiation of topical corticosteroid therapy. If the intraocular pressure is normal, the tension will be checked once a week as long as the patient is on topical

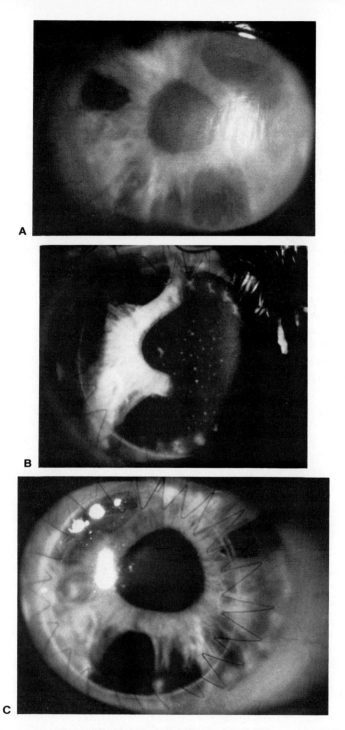

FIG. 4A: Preoperative picture of patient with advanced endothelial decompensation and a history of multiple filtering operation. Intraocular tension was 18 mm Hg without medication. **B:** Three months after an 8-mm penetrating corneal graft, vision dropped from 20/30 to 20/70. There were scattered mutton fat keratic precipitates on the graft endothelium associated with moderate graft edema. The patient was treated with topical corticosteroids every hour. **C:** The same graft as **B,** 4 days later, showing a marked reduction of keratic precipitates and improved vision of 20/30. Intraocular pressure was 32 mm Hg. Corticosteroid therapy was tapered within 10 days and maintained to 1 drop twice a day for 2 weeks, then once a day for 4 weeks. Tension was controlled with Timoptic® twice a day.

corticosteroid therapy. Transient elevation of intraocular pressure up to 30 mm Hg seen in some of the aphakic eyes with large grafts will usually return to normal as soon as postoperative iritis subsides. In corticosteroid responders, as soon as the topical steroid is reduced, the intraocular pressure also will return to normal. Should the tension remain high for more than 1 week to 10 days, we use topical timolol 0.5% every 12 hr. Diamox® or epinephrine can be added if the intraocular pressure cannot be controlled. Use of miotics at the immediate postoperative period in the presence of iritis is not recommended.

In our experience, there is a high incidence of secondary glaucoma after the corneal graft or conjunctival flap for perforated corneal ulcers. In these cases, if the elevated intraocular pressure cannot be controlled with maximum medical therapy, we are forced into trabeculectomy in the phakic eyes and cyclocryotherapy in aphakic eyes.

Corneal Grafts and Herpetic Keratitis

One main indication for lamellar or penetrating corneal transplantation is the corneal scar or nonhealing corneal ulcer of herpetic origin. Use of systemic and topical corticosteroid therapy postoperatively predisposes these individuals to recurrence of herpetic keratitis. As a prophylactic measure, we routinely use topical antiviral agents as long as these patients are on topical corticosteroid therapy. We have been using IDU 1 drop four to five times a day and continue this treatment for 3 days after cessation of corticosteroid therapy. IDU apparently has the least inhibitory effect on corneal wound healing (53).

Should active herpetic keratitis appear on the graft postoperatively, the patient should be treated in the same way as for herpetic keratitis in ungrafted eyes. These eyes should be watched very closely for the signs and symptoms of graft rejection reaction. The presence of combined graft rejection and active herpetic keratitis is a therapeutic challenge for the ophthalmologist. In such cases, the patient should be treated initially with a heavy dose of systemic corticosteroids (60 to 80 mg prednisone) combined with topical antiviral agents. As soon as the herpetic lesion is under control, topical or subconjunctival steroids may be initiated while continuing the antiviral agents. As soon as the allograft rejection is under control, the corticosteroid therapy should be tapered rapidly to the minimum possible dose. Antiviral agents should be continued as long as the patient is on the corticosteroid therapy.

Both corticosteroids and antiviral agents have an inhibitory effect on the corneal wound-healing. Patients should be watched carefully for the wound dehiscence, and suture removal must be delayed.

Corneal Grafts and Active Corneal Ulcers

Patients with active corneal ulcers (bacterial or fungal) are not the best candidates for corneal transplantation. These cases are best managed with medical therapy. Conjunctival flap is a preferred initial treatment for nonhealing ulcers, and the use of surgical glue for perforated ulcers should be considered. Once the infection and inflammation are under control, corneal transplantation can be performed within 6 months to 1 year as elective surgery. Because of inflammation of anterior segment and soft eye, corneal grafts in eyes with active or perforated ulcers are technically difficult and are subject to a higher incidence of secondary glaucoma and graft rejection. The use of anti-inflammatory agents in these cases may mask the signs and symptoms of recurrence of corneal ulcer at postoperative period.

REFERENCES

1. Adams, R. E., Kirschner, R. J., and Leopold, I. H. (1963): Ocular hypotensive effect of intravenously administered mannitol. A preliminary report. *Arch. Ophthalmol.,* 69:55–58.
2. Antoine, M. W., Edelhauser, H. F., and O'Brien, W. J. (1984): Pharmacokinetics of topical ocular phenylephrine Hcl. *Invest. Ophthalmol. Vis. Sci.,* 25:48–54.
3. Aron-Rosa, D., Cohn, H. C., Aron, J. J., and Bouquety, C. (1983): Methylcellulose instead of Healon in extracapsular surgery with intraocular lens implantation. *Ophthalmology,* 90:1235–1238.
4. Aronson, S. B., and Moore, T. E., Jr. (1969): Suture reaction in the rabbit cornea. *Arch. Ophthalmol.,* 82:531–536.
5. Ashton, N., and Cook, C. (1951): Effect of cortisone on healing of corneal wounds. *Br. J. Ophthalmol.,* 35:708–717.
6. Balazs, E. A., and Freeman, M. I. (1972): Hyaluronic acid and replacement of vitreous and aqueous humor. *Mod. Probl. Ophthalmol.,* 10:3–21.
7. Balazs, E. A., and Gibbs, D. A. (1970): The rheological properties and biological function of hyaluronic acid. In: *Chemistry and Molecular Biology of the Intracellular Matrix,* edited by E. A. Balazs, pp. 1241–1253. Academic Press, New York.
8. Barnes, M. J. (1975): Function of ascorbic acid in collagen metabolism. *Ann. N.Y. Acad. Sci.,* 285:264–277.
9. Basu, P. R., and Hasany, S. M. (1971): A histochemical study on corneal suture reactions. *Can. J. Ophthalmol.,* 6:328–431.
10. Behrendt, T. (1956): Experimental study of corneal lesions produced by topical anesthesia. *Am. J. Ophthalmol.,* 41:99–105.
11. Bell, G., Easty, D. L., and McCullough, K. G. (1981): Controlled trial of cyclosporin A (cy A) in homograft reactions in laboratory animals. *Invest. Ophthalmol. Vis. Sci., 20(ARVO Suppl.)*:2.
12. Bellows, J. G. (1934): Surface anesthesia in ophthalmology. Comparison of some drugs used. *Arch. Ophthalmol.,* 12:824–832.
13. Bellows, J. G. (1946): Influence of local antiseptics on regeneration of corneal epithelium of rabbits. *Arch. Ophthalmol.,* 36:70–81.
14. Bennett, T. O., Peyman, G. A., and Rutgard, J. (1978): Intracameral phosphate buffer in alkali-burns. *Can. J. Ophthalmol.,* 13:93–95.
15. Berkowitz, R. A., Klyce, S. D., Salisbury, J. D., and Kaufman, H. E. (1981): Fluorophotometric determination of the corneal epithelial barrier after penetrating keratoplasty. *Am. J. Ophthalmol.,* 88:332–335.
16. Boozan, C. W., and Cohen, I. J. (1953): Ophthaine. A new topical anesthetic for the eye. *Am. J. Ophthalmol.,* 36:1619–1621.
17. Boruchoff, S. A., Refojo, M., Slansky, H. H., Webster, R. G., Freeman, M. I., and Dohlman, C. H. (1969): Clinical application of adhesives in corneal surgery. *Trans. Am. Acad. Ophthalmol. Otolaryngol.,* 73:499–505.
18. Bourne, W. M., Brubaker, R. F., and O'Fallon, W. M. (1979): Use of air to decrease endothelial cell loss during intraocular lens implantation. *Arch. Ophthalmol.,* 97:1473–1475.
19. Bourne, W. M., and O'Fallon, W. M. (1978): Endothelial cell loss during penetrating keratoplasty. *Am. J. Ophthalmol.,* 85:760–766.

20. Brightbill, F. S., Myers, F. L., and Bresnick, G. H. (1978): Post vitrectomy keratopathy. *Am. J. Ophthalmol.,* 85:651–655.

21. Brown, S. I., Akiya, S., and Weller, C. A. (1969): Prevention of the ulcers of the alkali-burned cornea. Preliminary studies with collagenase inhibitors. *Arch. Ophthalmol.,* 82:95–97.

22. Brown, S. I., and Hook, C. W. (1971): Treatment of corneal destruction with collagenase inhibitors. *Trans. Am. Acad. Ophthalmol. Otolaryngol.,* 75:1199–1207.

23. Brown, S. I., Tragakis, M. P., and Pearce, D. B. (1972): Treatment of the alkali-burned cornea. *Am. J. Ophthalmol.,* 74:316–320.

24. Brown, S. I., and Weller, C. A. (1970): Collagenase inhibitors in prevention of ulcers of alkali-burned cornea. *Arch. Ophthalmol.,* 83:352–353.

25. Brown, S. I., Weller, C. A., and Wassermann, H. E. (1969): Collagenolytic activity of alkali burned corneas. *Arch. Ophthalmol.,* 81:370–373.

26. Burns, R. P., and Hikes, C. E. (1979): Irrigation of the anterior chamber for the treatment of alkali-burns. *Am. J. Ophthalmol.,* 88:119–120.

27. Carolan, J. A., Cerasoli, J. R., and Houle, T. V. (1974): Bupivacaine in retrobulbar anesthesia. *Ann. Ophthalmol.,* 6:843–847.

28. Chin, G., and Almquist, H. T. (1983): Bupivacaine and lidocaine retrobular anesthesia. *Ophthalmology,* 90:369–372.

29. Coster, D. J., Shepherd, W. F. I., Chin Fook, T., Rice, N. S. C., and Jones, B. R. (1979): Prolonged survival of corneal allografts in rabbits treated with cyclosporin A. *Lancet,* 2:688.

30. Crabb, C. V. (1977): Endocrine influence on ulceration and regeneration in the alkali-burned cornea. *Arch. Ophthalmol.,* 95:1866–1870.

31. Dikstein, S. (1973): Efficiency and survival of the corneal endothelial pump. *Exp. Eye Res.,* 15:639–644.

32. Dikstein, S., and Maurice, D. M. (1972): The metabolic basis to the fluid pump in the cornea. *J. Physiol. (Lond.),* 221:29–44.

33. Donshik, P. C., Berman, M. B., Dohlman, C. H., Gage, J., and Rose, J. (1978): Effect of topical corticosteroids on ulceration in alkali-burned corneas. *Arch. Ophthalmol.,* 96:2117–2120.

34. Dunnington, J. H., and Weimar, V. L. (1959): Influence of the epithelium on the healing of corneal incision. *Am. J. Ophthalmol.,* 45:89–95.

35. Edelhauser, H. F., Gonnering, R., and van Horn, D. L. (1978): Intraocular irrigating solutions: a comparative study of BSS plus and lactated Ringer's solutions. *Arch. Ophthalmol.,* 96:516–520.

36. Edelhauser, H. F., Hine, J. E., Pederson, H., van Horn, D. L., and Schultz, R. O. (1979): The effect of phenylephrine on the cornea. *Arch. Ophthalmol.,* 97:937–947.

37. Edelhauser, H. F., van Horn, D. L., Hyndiuk, R. A., and Schultz, R. O. (1975): Intraocular irrigating solutions: their effect on the corneal endothelium. *Arch. Ophthalmol.,* 93:648–657.

38. Edelhauser, H. F., van Horn, D. L., Miller, P., and Pederson, H. J. (1976): Effect of thiol-oxidation of glutathione with diamide on corneal endothelial function, junctional complexes and microfilaments. *J. Cell Biol.,* 68:567–578.

39. Edelhauser, H. F., van Horn, D. L., Schultz, R. O., and Hyndiuk, R. A. (1976): Comparative toxicity of intraocular irrigating solutions on the corneal endothelium. *Am. J. Ophthalmol.,* 81:473–481.

40. Eiferman, R. A., and Wilkins, E. L. (1981): The effect of air on human corneal endothelium. *Am. J. Ophthalmol.,* 92:328–331.

41. Ellis, R. A., and Levine A. (1963): Experimental sutureless ocular surgery. *Am. J. Ophthalmol.,* 55:733–741.

42. Epstein, S. (1958): Dermal contact dermatitis from neomycin. *Ann. Allergy,* 16:268–280.

43. Everett, W. G., Vey, E. K., and Finlay, J. W. (1961): Duration of oculomotor akinesia of injectable anesthetics. *Trans. Am. Acad. Ophthalmol. Otolaryngol.,* 65:308–314.

44. Fedukowicz, H., Wise, G. N., and Zaret, M. M. (1955): Toxic conjunctivitis due to antibiotics. *Am. J. Ophthalmol.,* 40:849–856.

45. Fine, M. (1979): Postoperative management of corneal grafts. In: *Symposium on Medical and Surgical Diseases of the Cornea. Transactions of the New Orleans Academy of Ophthalmology,* pp. 179–197. C. V. Mosby, St. Louis.

46. Forman, A. R. (1980): A new low-concentration preparation for mydriasis and cycloplegia. *Ophthalmology,* 87:213–215.

47. Fraunfelder, F. T., and Scafidi, A. F. (1978): Possible adverse effects from topical ocular 10% phenylephrine. *Am. J. Ophthalmol.,* 85:447–453.
48. Friedenwald, J. S., and Buschke, W. (1944): Influence of some experimental variables on the epithelial movements in the healing of corneal wounds. *J. Cell Comp. Physiol.,* 23:95–107.
49. Fujikawa, L. S., Meisler, D. M., and Nozik, R. A. (1983): Hyperosmolar hyperglycemic nonketotic coma. A complication of short-term systemic corticosteroid use. *Ophthalmology,* 90:1239–1241.
50. Galin, M. A., Binkhorst, R. D., and Kwilko, M. L. (1968): Ocular dehydration. *Am. J. Ophthalmol.,* 66:233–235.
51. Gasset, A. R., and Dohlman, C. H. (1968): The tensile strength of corneal wounds. *Arch. Ophthalmol.,* 79:595–602.
52. Gasset, A. R., Hood, C. L., Ellison, E. D., and Kaufman, H. E. (1970): Ocular tolerance to cyanoacrylate monomer tissue adhesive analogues. *Invest. Ophthalmol. Vis. Sci.,* 9:3–11.
53. Gasset, A. R., and Katzin, D. (1975): Antiviral drugs and corneal wound healing. *Invest. Ophthalmol. Vis. Sci.,* 14:628–630.
54. Gasset, A. R., Lorenzetti, D. W. C., Ellison, E. M., and Kaufman, H. E. (1969): Quantitative corticosteroid effect on corneal wound-healing. *Arch. Ophthalmol.,* 81:589–591.
55. Geroski, D. H., and Edelhauser, H. F. (1978): Corneal metabolism: Endothelial response to epithelial scraping, topical anesthesia, and phenylephrine. *Invest. Ophthalmol. Vis. Sci.,* 17(ARVO Suppl.):211.
56. Ginsberg, S. P., and Polack, F. M. (1972): Cyanoacrylate tissue adhesive in ocular disease. *Ophthalmic Surg.,* 3:126–132.
57. Grant, W. M. (1950): Experimental investigation of paracentesis in the treatment of ocular ammonia burns. *Arch. Ophthalmol.,* 44:399–404.
58. Gundersen, T., and Liebman, S. D. (1944): Effect of local anesthetics on regeneration of corneal epithelium. *Arch. Ophthalmol.,* 31:29–33.
59. Harrison, S. E., Soll, D. B., Shayegan, M., and Clinch, T. (1983): Chondroitin sulfate: A new and effective protective agent for intraocular lens insertion. *Ophthalmology,* 89:1254–1260.
60. Hirst, L. W., and Juan, E. D. (1982): Sodium hyaluronate and tissue adhesive in treating corneal perforations. *Opthalmology,* 89:1250–1253.
61. Hirst, L. W., Smiddy, W. E., and Stark, W. J. (1982): Corneal perforations: Changing methods of treatment, 1960–1980. *Ophthalmology,* 89:630–634.
62. Hirst, L. W., Stark, W. J., and Jensen, A. D. (1979): Tissue adhesives: New perspectives in corneal perforations. *Ophthalmic Surg.,* 10:58–64.
63. Holekamp, T. L. R., Arribas, N. P., and Boniuk, I. (1979): Bupivacaine anesthesia in retinal detachment surgery. *Arch. Ophthalmol.,* 97:109–111.
64. Hook, C. W., Brown, S. I., Iwanij, W., and Nakanishi, I. (1971): Characterization and inhibition of corneal collagenase. *Invest. Ophthalmol. Vis. Sci.,* 10:496–503.
65. Hunter, P. A., Wiehelmus, K. R., Rice, N. S. C., and Jones, B. R. (1981): Cyclosporin A applied topically to the recipient eye inhibits corneal graft rejection. *Clin. Exp. Immunol.,* 45:173–177.
66. Hyndiuk, R. A., Hull, D. S., and Kinyoun, J. L. (1974): Free tissue patch and cyanoacrylate in corneal perforation. *Ophthalmic Surg.,* 5(2):50–55.
67. Jones, D. B. (1980): Strategy for the initial management of suspected microbial keratitis. In: *Symposium on Medical and Surgical Diseases of the Cornea,* pp. 111–112. C. V. Mosby, St. Louis.
68. Kana, J. S., Hoffmann, F., Buchen, R., Krolik, A., and Wiederholt, M. (1982): Rabbit corneal allograft survival following topical administration of cyclosporin A. *Invest. Ophthalmol. Vis. Sci.,* 22:686–690.
69. Kara-Jose, N., Lorenzetti, D. W. C., McAuliffe, R., and Conti, T. (1972): Time response effect of corticosteroid on corneal wound healing. *Can. J. Ophthalmol.,* 7:48.
70. Kaufman, H. E. (moderator); Bourne, W. M., and Byron, H. M. (1983): Protection of corneal endothelium during IOL surgery. A symposium. *The CLAO Journal,* 9(2):97–101.
71. Kaufman, H. E., and Katz, J. I. (1976): Endothelial damage from intraocular lens insertion. *Invest. Ophthalmol. Vis. Sci.,* 996–1000.
72. Kaufman, E. H., and Maloney, E. D. (1962): IDU and hydrocortisone in experimental herpes simplex keratitis. *Arch. Ophthalmol.* 68:396–398.
73. Kaye, G. I., Mishima, S., and Cole, J. D. (1968): Studies on the cornea. VII. Effect of

perfusion with a Ca^{++} free medium on the corneal endothelium. *Invest. Ophthalmol. Vis. Sci.,* 7:53–66.

74. Kennerdell, J. S., Rydze, D., and Robertson, M. (1976): Comparison of retrobulbar marcaine and combined marcaine-carbocaine in ophthalmic surgery. *Ann. Ophthalmol.,* 8:1236–1240.

75. Kishida, K., and Otori, T. (1980): A quantitative study on the relationship between transcorneal permeability of drugs and their hydrophobicity. *Jpn. J. Ophthalmol.,* 24:251–259.

76. Lazar, M., Weiner, M. J., and Leopold, I. H. (1969): Treatment of uveitis with methotrexate. *Am. J. Ophthalmol.,* 67:383–387.

77. Leibowitz, H. M., and Elliott, J. H. (1966): Chemotherapeutic immunosuppression of the corneal graft reaction. I. Systemic antimetabolites. *Arch. Ophthalmol.,* 75:826–835.

78. Leibowitz, H. M., and Elliott, J. H. (1966): Chemotherapeutic immunosuppression of the corneal graft reaction. II. Combined systemic antimetabolite and topical corticosteroid therapy. *Arch. Ophthalmol.,* 76:338–344.

79. Lemp, M. A. (1976): Cornea and sclera. Annual review, corneal wound healing. *Arch. Ophthalmol.,* 94:473.

80. Leopold, I. H. (1964): Antibiotics and antifungal agents. Problems and management of ocular infections. *Invest. Ophthalmol. Vis. Sci.,* 3:504–511.

81. Levinson, R. A., Paterson, C. A., and Pfister, R. R. (1976): Ascorbic acid prevents corneal ulceration and perforation following experimental alkali burns. *Invest. Ophthalmol. Vis. Sci.,* 15:986–993.

82. Maguen, E., Nesburn, A. B., and Nacy, J. I. (1984): Combined use of sodium hyaluronate and tissue adhesive in penetrating keratoplasty of corneal perforations. *Ophthalmic Surg.,* 15:55–57.

83. Marr, W. G., Wood, R., and Grieves, M. (1954): Further studies on the effect of agents on regeneration of corneal epithelium. *Am. J. Ophthalmol.,* 37:544–548.

84. Marr, W. G., Wood, R., Senterfit, L., and Singelman, S. (1957): Effect of topical anesthetics on regeneration of corneal epithelium. *Am. J. Ophthalmol.,* 43:606–610.

85. Marr, W. G., Wood, R., and Storck, M. (1951): Effect of some agents on regeneration of corneal epithelium. *Am. J. Ophthalmol.,* 34:609–612.

86. Marshall, S., and Hinman, F. (1962): Subdural hematoma following administration of urea for diagnosis of hypertension. *J.A.M.A.,* 182:813–814.

87. McCarey, B. E., Edelhauser, H. F., and van Horn, D. L. (1973): Functional and structural changes in the corneal endothelium during in vitro perfusion. *Invest. Ophthalmol. Vis. Sci.,* 12:410–417.

88. McDonald, J., and Wilder, H. (1953): The effect of beta radiation on corneal healing. *Am. J. Ophthalmol.,* 40:170–179.

89. McDonald, T. O., Borgmann, A. R., Roberts, M. D., and Fox, L. G. (1970): Corneal wound-healing. I. Inhibition of stromal healing by three dexamethasone derivatives. *Invest. Ophthalmol. Vis. Sci.,* 9:703–709.

90. Michels, R., and Ryan, S. (1975): Results and complications of 100 consecutive cases of pars plana vitrectomy. *Am. J. Ophthalmol.,* 80:24–29.

91. Miller, D., O'Connor, P., and William, J. (1977): Use of Na-hyaluronate during intraocular lens implantation in rabbit. *Ophthalmic Surg.,* 8:58.

92. Miller, D., and Steggmann, R. (1981): Use of hyaluronate in human implantation. *Ann. Ophthalmol.,* 13:811.

93. Mishima, S., and Kudo, T. (1967): In vitro incubation of rabbit cornea. *Invest. Ophthalmol. Vis. Sci.,* 6:329–339.

94. Moore, D. C. (1950): An evaluation of hyaluronidase in local and nerve block analgesia: A review of 519 cases. *Anesthesiology,* 11:470–484.

95. Moore, T. E., Jr., and Aronson, S. B. (1969): Suture reaction in the human cornea. *Arch. Ophthalmol.,* 82:575–579.

96. Morrison, D. R., Kanai, A., and Gasset, A. R. (1971): Beta radiation inhibition of corneal healing. I. Tensile strength and ultrastructure change. *Invest. Ophthalmol. Vis. Sci.,* 10:826–839.

97. Newsome, D. A., and Gross, J. (1977): Prevention by medroxyprogesterone of perforation in the alkali-burned rabbit cornea: Inhibition of collagenolytic activity. *Invest. Ophthalmol. Vis. Sci.,* 16:21–31.

98. O'Brien, C., and Swan, K. (1942): Carbaminoylcholine chloride in the treatment of glaucoma simplex. *Arch. Ophthalmol.*, 27:253–263.
99. O'Keefe, M., and Nabil, M. (1983): The use of mannitol in intraocular surgery. *Ophthalmic Surg.*, 14:55–56.
100. Pape, L. G. (1980): Intracapsular and extracapsular technique of lens implantation with Healon. *Am. Intraocular Implant Soc. J.*, 6:342–343.
101. Pape, L. G., and Balazs, E. A. (1980): The use of sodium hyaluronadate (Healon) in human anterior segment surgery. *Ophthalmology*, 87:699–705.
102. Passmore, J. W., and King, J. H., Jr. (1955): Vital staining of conjunctiva and cornea. *Arch. Ophthalmol.*, 53:568–574.
103. Petroutsos, F., Guimaraes, R., Giraud, J., and Pouliguen, Y. (1983): Antibiotics and corneal epithelial wound-healing. *Arch. Ophthalmol.*, 101:1775–1781.
104. Pfister, R. R. (1983): Chemical injuries of the eye. *Ophthalmology*, 90:1246–1253.
105. Pfister, R. R., Haddox, J. L., and Paterson, C. A. (1982): The efficacy of sodium citrate in the treatment of severe alkali burns of the eye is influenced by the route of administration. *Cornea*, 1:205–211.
106. Pfister, R. R., Nicolaro, M. L., and Paterson, C. A. (1981): Sodium citrate reduces the incidence of corneal ulceration and perforations in extreme alkali-burned eyes—acetylcysteine and ascorbate have no favorable effect. *Invest. Ophthalmol. Vis. Sci.*, 21:486–490.
107. Pfister, R. R., and Paterson, C. A. (1980): Ascorbic acid in the treatment of alkali-burns of the eye. *Ophthalmology*, 87:1050–1057.
108. Pfister, R. R., Paterson, C. A., and Hayes, S. A. (1978): Topical ascorbate decreases the incidence of corneal ulceration after experimental alkali burns. *Invest. Ophthalmol. Vis. Sci.*, 17:1019–1024.
109. Polack, F. M., DeMong, J., and Santella, H. (1981): Sodium hyaluronadate (Healon) in keratoplasty and intraocular lens implantation. *Ophthalmology*, 88:425–431.
110. Polack, F. M., and Rosen, P. N. (1967): Topical steroids and tritiated thymidine uptake. Effect on corneal healing. *Arch. Ophthalmol.*, 77:400–404.
111. Polack, F. M., Townsend, W. M., and Waltman, S. (1972): Antilymphocyte serum and corneal graft rejection. *Am. J. Ophthalmol.*, 73:52–55.
112. Pollack, S. V. (1982): Wound healing. IV. Systemic medications affecting wound healing. *J. Dermatol. Surg. Oncol.*, 8-II:667–672.
113. Refojo, M. F., Dohlman, C. H., and Koliopoulos, J. (1971): Adhesives in ophthalmology: A review. *Surv. Ophthalmol.*, 15:217–236.
114. Refojo, M. F., Miller, D., and Fiore, A. S. (1972): A new fluorescent stain for soft hydrophilic lens fitting. *Arch. Ophthalmol.*, 87:275–277.
115. Rich, L. F., Weimar, V. L., Squires, E. L., and Haraguchi, K. H. (1979): Stimulation of corneal wound-healing with mesodermal growth factor. *Arch. Ophthalmol.*, 97:1326–1330.
116. Ring, J., Dechant, W., Seifert, J., Lund, O. E., Greite, J. H., Stefani, F. H., and Brendel, W. (1978): Immunosuppression with antilymphocyte globulin (ALG) in the treatment of ophthalmic disorders. *Ophthalmic Res.*, 10:82–97.
117. Salisbury, J. D., and Gebhardt, B. M. (1981): Suppression of corneal graft rejection by cyclosporine A. *Arch. Ophthalmol.*, 99:1640–1643.
118. Shepherd, W. F. I., Coster, D. J., Chin Fook, T., Rice, N. S. C., and Jones, B. R. (1980): Effect of cyclosporin A on the survival of corneal graft in rabbits. *Br. J. Ophthalmol.*, 64:148–153.
119. Slansky, H. H., Berman, M. B., Dohlman, C. H., and Rose, J. (1970): Cysteine and acetylcysteine in the prevention of corneal ulceration. *Ann. Ophthalmol.*, 2:288–291.
120. Slansky, H. H., Dohlman, C. H., and Berman, M. B. (1971): Prevention of corneal ulcers. *Trans. Am. Acad. Ophthalmol. Otolaryngol.*, 75:1208–1211.
121. Smith, R. S., Smith, L. A., Rich, L., and Weimar, V. (1981): Effect of growth factors on corneal wound-healing. *Invest. Ophthalmol. Vis. Sci.*, 20:222–229.
122. Smolin, G. (1968): Suppression of corneal graft reaction by antilymphocyte serum. *Arch. Ophthalmol.*, 79:603–610.
123. Smolin, G., and Okumoto, M. (1981): Vitamin A acid and corneal epithelial wound-healing. *Ann. Ophthalmol.*, 13:563–566.
124. Snow, J. C. (1972): *Anesthesia in Otolaryngology and Ophthalmology.* Charles C Thomas, Springfield, IL.

125. Stegmann, R., and Miller, D. (1981): Protective function of sodium hyaluronate in corneal transplantation. *J. Ocular Therapy & Surgery,* 28:31.
126. Straatsma, B. R., Allen, R. A., Hale, P. N., and Gomez, R. (1963): Experimental studies employing adhesive compounds in ophthalmic surgery. *Trans. Am. Acad. Ophthalmol. Otolaryngol.,* 67:320–333.
127. Streit, S., Ackerman, J., and Kanarek, I. (1981): Cyanoacrylate. *Ann. Ophthalmol.,* 13:315–316.
128. Waltman, S. R. (1981): The cornea. In: *Adler's Physiology of the Eye,* 7th ed., edited by R. A. Moses, p. 51. C. V. Mosby, St. Louis.
129. Waltmann, S. R., Carrol, D., Schimmelpfennig, W., and Okun, E. (1975): Intraocular irrigating solutions for clinical vitrectomy. *Ophthalmic Surg.* 6(4):90–94.
130. Webster, R. G., Jr., Slansky, H. H., and Refojo, M. F. (1968): The use of adhesive for the closure of corneal perforations: Report of two cases. *Arch. Ophthalmol.,* 80:705–709.
131. Weiss, J. L., Cot, P. W., Lindstrom, R. L., and Doughman, D. J. (1983): The use of tissue adhesive in corneal perforation. *Ophthalmology,* 90:610–615.
132. Wilson, F. M. (1979): Adverse external ocular effects of topical ophthalmic medications. *Surv. Ophthalmol.,* 24:57–88.
133. Wong, V. G. (1969): Immunosuppressive therapy of ocular inflammatory diseases. *Arch. Ophthalmol.,* 81:628–637.

Commentary

Pharmacology of Cataract Surgery

Stark and co-authors have written a marvelous, terse document for all cataract surgeons. The authors state that "in spite of dramatic changes, cataract surgery remains a procedure whose outcome depends upon meticulous attention to detail". Actually, it is probably just because of these dramatic changes, not in spite of them, that continued meticulousness is required for perfection in cataract surgery (see Preface). The challenge of good science in ophthalmology is ever present to produce a top surgical product.

We favor Stark's emphasis on appropriate utilization of drugs. A few comments: For those surgeons preferring methods of extracapsular extraction that utilize large quantities of infusion fluid, the presence of bicarbonate and GSH (glutathione) certainly reduces corneal edema by reducing endothelial cell damage and cell loss (see chapters by Woog and Albert, and Edelhauser and Mac Rae). In addition, steroid plus non-steroidal pretreatment may be more effective in maintaining the health of corneal endothelium than nonsteroidal prophylaxis alone (1). Phenylephrine is useful and certainly less dangerous in the 2.5% topical solution compared with the 10% solution recommended by the authors. Readers should nonetheless note Stark's meticulous attention to detail of his experienced preoperative, intraoperative, and postoperative use of drugs. Please note the section on postoperative use of steroids, especially Stark's prolonged use of topical therapy.

On local anesthesia, the readers should note comments about mixtures and compare these with the opinion of our anesthesia expert N. M. Greene (*this volume*). One of us has found that simple retrobulbar bupivacaine with the usual (Honan) ocular compression thereafter obviates the need in almost all instances for a lid block. Should a lid block be necessary, 2% xylocaine can be used. The prolonged action of bupivacaine means that the operated eye may require a cover until appropriate lid and corneal reflexes are restored (a few hours later).

Stark has been negative on the UV absorbing implants because of their potential toxicity if damaged after neodymium-YAG laser capsulotomy. Release of toxic substances may occur after high energy intensity. With new work by Stark (2), low energies, 1-2 mJ, do not seem to be associated with damage to ocular cells, as determined by tissue culture. These lenses are in a developmental

471

stage (March 1985) and this development must continue. Information about the hazards of UV light to the unprotected aphakic eye becomes more precise with each passing year. More needs to be learned about the pros and cons of susceptibility of the aphakic eye to short wavelength light. Certainly in the operating theater where the eye is essentially imprisoned by the illumination of the surgical microscope, steps must be taken to eliminate both thermal and phototoxic damage. Built in filters and/or simple corneal covers must be utilized, and, operating time under damaging illumination reduced. (For example, McIntyre has described a simple opaque "eclipse" filter that can be operated by a lever attached to the surgical microscope.)

We are in the debt of Stark and his collaborators for a precise, succinct dissertation on how to achieve great results with the procedure of extracapsular cataract extraction.

The Editors

REFERENCES

1. Macdonald, J. M., and Edelhauser, H. F. (1985): The corneal endothelial barrier—the effect of anti-inflammatory agents during intraocular inflammation. *Invest. Ophthalmol. Vis. Sci. ARVO Suppl.,* 26(10):320.
2. Terry, A. C., Stark, W. J., Newsome, D. A., Maumenee, A. E., and Pina, E. (1985): Tissue toxicity of laser-damaged intraocular lens implants. *Ophthalmology,* 92:414–418.

Surgical Pharmacology of the Eye,
edited by M. Sears and A. Tarkkanen.
Raven Press, New York © 1985.

Pharmacology of Cataract Surgery

Walter J. Stark, Arlo C. Terry, David Denlinger,
Manuel Datiles, and Isabel DeLeon

The Wilmer Institute, The Johns Hopkins Hospital, Baltimore, Maryland 21205

With the increasingly frequent use of intraocular lenses, the movement toward extracapsular extraction techniques, and new instrumentation designed to facilitate these changes, the skilled intracapsular cataract surgeon may feel hopelessly outdated. Ten years ago intraocular lenses were somewhat a curiosity, the intracapsular procedure was state of the art (extracapsular techniques had been abandoned years earlier), and patients were satisfied with vision provided by aphakic spectacles. Today more than 75% of all cataract operations performed in the United States are done with an intraocular lens, and the extracapsular technique is used in more than 50% of all procedures performed (44). The ophthalmic surgeon who has somehow managed to keep abreast of most of these changes has doubtless experienced frustration in selecting the particular surgical technique, instrumentation, and intraocular lens that best suit his or her needs.

In spite of dramatic changes, cataract surgery remains a procedure whose outcome depends largely on meticulous attention to detail. For example, the medicines used before, during, and after surgery may determine the success of the procedure itself. Inadequate preparation of an eye for surgery may compromise the surgical result, and a surgeon who is frequently faced with a poorly dilated pupil or positive vitreous pressure should reexamine the preoperative routine.

The purpose of this chapter is to present our pharmacologic management of patients before, during, and after extracapsular cataract surgery. Numerous other regimens are doubtless equally as effective, but it is hoped that the following will provide ideas that will assist the surgeon in developing his or her own best method.

SEDATION FOR LOCAL ANESTHESIA

Local anesthesia for ophthalmic procedures is associated with a lower mortality rate than is general anesthesia (11,14,20,33,34). In addition, pulmonary and embolic complications, nausea, vomiting, and bleeding are all less frequent with local anesthesia (19). With proper preoperative sedation, local anesthesia is associated with minimal discomfort; we therefore prefer it for the vast majority of our patients. We reserve general anesthesia for children and uncooperative or noncommunicative patients.

Most sedative regimens for local anesthesia consist of narcotics, sedatives, tranquilizers, and anticholinergic agents separately or in combination. We have found a combination of fentanyl and diazepam gives satisfactory results.

Fentanyl

Fentanyl (Sublimaze®) is a synthetic opioid estimated to be 80 times more potent than morphine sulfate (21). The precise site and mechanism of the analgesic action of fentanyl and other opioids remain uncertain, but central nervous system effects include analgesia, sleep, respiratory depression, cough suppression, miosis, nausea, and vomiting. The analgesia produced is such that one may be aware of the pain stimulus but will not perceive it as painful (21).

Ventilatory depression is due to a decrease in the responsiveness of the respiratory center to increases in carbon dioxide tension (21), but the moderate increase in carbon dioxide is well tolerated, provided oxygenation of arterial blood is maintained. The plastic head drape represents an added threat to adequate oxygenation, and we inspect the drape at regular intervals during the procedure to be certain it is not covering the patient's nose. In addition, the patient is frequently asked if the supplemental air is sufficient.

Fentanyl exerts a direct depressant effect on the cough center in the medulla, which may result in accumulation of secretions, aspiration, airway obstruction, and atelectasis (25). At the beginning of each procedure, we instruct the patient to inform us if he needs to cough or clear his throat. This allows us to select the most expeditious moment for an increase in vitreous pressure.

Nausea and vomiting seldom occur with the small doses of fentanyl used for sedation in ophthalmic cases, and antiemetics are effective in controlling these side effects. The nausea and vomiting are caused by direct stimulation of the chemoreceptor zone for emesis located in the medulla (25,42).

Diazepam

Diazepam (Valium®) is a colorless, crystalline compound belonging to the benzodiazepine group of minor tranquilizers. It acts by hindering interneuronal transmission at the spinal cord level while depressing the limbic system at the supraspinal level (43). Besides sedation, one of the more desirable central nervous system effects of diazepam is the production of anterograde amnesia (50). The sedative effects of diazepam are enhanced by concomitant use of fentanyl, and the dosage of both should be reduced significantly and administered in small increments.

Our usual preoperative sedative regimen consists of 5 to 10 mg diazepam given orally 1 hr prior to surgery. The amount given depends on the patient's age, weight, and physical and psychological state. We avoid the use of diazepam in patients older than 80 years, as we have found responses varying from respiratory depression to paradoxical hyperexcitation in this age group.

When the patient arrives in the operating suite, intravenous fentanyl and diazepam are administered by the anesthetist to achieve the desired level of sedation. Fentanyl is injected first, the usual dosage ranging from 25 to 100 μg. Next intravenous diazepam is given in 1.0-mg increments, the total dose seldom exceeding 2.5 mg. (Patients older than 80 years are given fentanyl only.)

LOCAL ANESTHETIC AGENTS

The ideal local anesthetic agent combines a short onset of action with a long duration and minimal toxicity. The short onset of action allows early evaluation of the adequacy of akinesia and anesthesia, and the long duration allows ample time for use of the preoperative pressure-lowering device without fear that anesthesia may wear off prematurely.

Unfortunately, the ideal local anesthetic agent does not exist, but the one we prefer is a 1:1 mixture of 0.75% bupivacaine (Marcaine®) and 2% lidocaine. Bupivacaine reliably provides surgical anesthesia for up to 5 hr and prevents postoperative pain for 12 hr or longer (7,23). In our experience, the major drawback to the use of bupivacaine alone is the slow onset of anesthesia, delaying surgery if injection of additional anesthetic becomes necessary.

Lidocaine, on the other hand, has an onset of action of 4 to 6 min (7), but when lidocaine is used alone, prolonged pressure-reducing devices cannot be used, and patients may experience pain or discomfort in the early postoperative period. A mixture of bupivacaine and lidocaine results in rapid onset of anesthesia together with long duration, thereby capitalizing on the virtues of both.

We inject 4 to 6 ml of the bupivacaine-lidocaine mixture in a modified Van Lindt technique to achieve lid akinesia, following which a 3-ml retrobulbar injection is given. Additional anesthetic is occasionally necessary, but only rarely does the total dose injected exceed 12 ml. We have not encountered any difficulty with respiratory depression caused by retrobulbar bupivacaine as reported by others (37,40).

Hyaluronidase

The mucolytic enzyme hyaluronidase depolymerizes interstitial hyaluronic acid, allowing fluids to diffuse more freely through tissues. When combined with local anesthetic agents, the enzyme permits larger quantities of anesthetic to be safely injected, increases the effective area of anesthetic action (23), and significantly decreases the induction time (30). Hyaluronidase also enhances the hypotony produced by retrobulbar anesthesia (23).

In a double-blind study of 55 postoperative patients in 1978, Roper and Nisbet (36) reported an increased incidence of cystoid macular edema associated with the use of hyaluronidase as an adjunct to retrobulbar anesthesia. They postulated a potentiation of intraocular inflammation as the cause of their observation. Kraff and co-workers (27), however, found no significant difference in the rate of cystoid macular edema proved by fluorescein angiography or in postoperative visual results with or without hyaluronidase in 609 patients who underwent cataract extraction. In addition, Havener (23) points out that because there is no hyaluronic acid in capillary walls, hyaluronidase does not affect capillary permeability.

In our own experience, hyaluronidase has had no deleterious effect on the incidence of clinically significant cystoid macular edema, which remains at 0.3% in cases performed by Walter J. Stark and A. Edward Maumenee at the Wilmer Institute. We therefore believe that hyaluronidase is a safe and effective adjunct to local anesthesia and continue to use it routinely.

PRESSURE-LOWERING AGENTS

Obtaining a soft eye preoperatively is of paramount importance in any type of cataract procedure. In extracapsular cataract extraction, a soft eye allows maintenance of the anterior chamber, thereby facilitating anterior capsulotomy, aspiration of cortex, and intraocular lens implantation. In addition, expression of the nucleus is accomplished in a more controlled fashion and there is much less chance of vitreous loss.

The most effective pressure-lowering measure in our preoperative armamentarium is the gentle continuous external compression provided by the Honan balloon. We routinely apply this device for a minimum of 15 min prior to proceeding with surgery and seldom find we need to employ pharmacologic agents as an adjunct in lowering intraocular pressure. The Honan balloon not only reduces vitreous volume, but more important, it decompresses the orbit.

In the rare patient for whom mechanical means have failed to adequately lower the intraocular pressure, we administer 1½–2 g/kg mannitol intravenously over a short period of time. Caution with the use of hyperosmotic agents must be taken in patients with poorly controlled diabetes mellitus or cardiovascular compromise, and provision for emptying the bladder during the operative procedure should be anticipated. In our experience, preoperative carbonic anhydrase inhibitors are ineffective in achieving a "surgically soft" eye.

Immediately postoperatively, we administer timolol topically in an effort to blunt or prevent the normal postoperative pressure rise. Timolol is continued twice daily postoperatively until the intraocular pressure normalizes (seldom more than 48 hr).

PREOPERATIVE MYDRIASIS

One of the most important prerequisites for extracapsular cataract extraction is good pupillary dilatation. A wide pupillary opening allows creation of an anterior capsulotomy large enough to permit expression (or phacoemulsification) of the nucleus without difficulty. Adequate mydriasis facilitates irrigation and aspiration of cortical material by allowing direct visualization. Finally, insertion of the intraocular lens and discission of the posterior capsule (if desired) are more readily accomplished through a well-dilated pupil.

Atropine

Because we consider adequate mydriasis to be essential, we begin dilating the pupil with atropine the evening prior to surgery. Atropine 1% is instilled again a few hours before surgery.

Atropine sulfate is a potent long-acting parasympatholytic (also termed anticholinergic or antimuscarinic) agent, a representative of the belladonna alkaloids. It blocks postganglionic cholinergic nerve endings on smooth muscles and glands. The block is relative and can be overcome with pilocarpine or physostigmine if present in sufficient concentration (23).

In the eye, atropine causes mydriasis by blocking the parasympathetic nerve endings on the sphincter muscle of the iris. The mydriasis is maximal in 30 to 40 min and lasts for 7 to 12 days; cycloplegia is maximal in 1 to 3 hr and lasts about 2 weeks (23).

Untoward reactions include contact dermatitis, conjunctivitis, delirium or toxic psychoses, facial and truncal rash, hyperthermia, tachycardia, and palpitations (17,21). Reactions may be treated by discontinuation of the drug, but with more severe reactions, administration of subcutaneous physostigmine (1.0 mg) may be necessary (21).

Homatropine Hydrobromide

Homatropine hydrobromide is a parasympatholytic, semisynthetic belladonna alkaloid similar to atropine in its effect but weaker and safer. A 5% solution of homatropine produces maximal mydriasis in 10 to 30 min and may last for up to 4 days (21). Cycloplegia is maximal at 30 to 90 min, lasting for 10 to 48 hr. Homatropine is only one-fiftieth as toxic as atropine, and its side effects are infrequent and mild.

As part of our preoperative mydriatic regimen, we instill 1 drop of 5% homatropine to the operative eye every 15 min beginning 2 hr prior to surgery, stipulating that a total of 6 doses be given.

Phenylephrine Hydrochloride

Phenylephrine hydrochloride is a synthetic, direct-acting sympathomimetic amine that has a powerful α-receptor stimulant effect with little β-receptor effect (21). In the eye, phenylephrine acts directly on the dilator muscle of the iris, causing mydriasis without cycloplegia. The 10% solution produces maximal mydriasis at 20 to 60 min and lasts from 3 to 7 hr. Because intense light stimulation continues to cause pupillary constriction in the presence of phenylephrine, this drug is generally used in combination with a cyclo-plegic agent.

The most common side effect to the use of this medication is acute hypertension following systemic absorption from the nasal mucosa. Blood pressures higher than 210/110 have been reported following use of 10% phenylephrine drops (41,49).

In normotensive or well-controlled hypertensive patients, we routinely instill 2.5% phenylephrine preoperatively (along with homatropine) every 15 min beginning 2 hr prior to surgery. (A maximum of 6 doses is given.)

Pierce's Solution

Pierce's solution is a combination of 0.5% phenylephrine hydrochloride, 0.4% homatropine hydrobromide, and 1% procaine hydrochloride, stabilized by sodium citrate, sodium bisulfite, benzyl alcohol, and sodium chloride (Table 1).

A subconjunctival injection (0.3 to 0.5 ml) of this solution is given immediately following the retrobulbar injection in normotensive patients whose dilatation is marginal. We find this solution a very helpful adjunct in maintaining mydriasis throughout the operation.

Intraocular Epinephrine

In most cases, preoperative mydriatics together with retrobulbar anesthesia provide good intraoperative mydriasis, but when these measures prove inade-quate, we find it helpful to augment mydriasis by introducing diluted 1:1,000 intracardiac epinephrine directly into the anterior chamber. This can be accomplished in one of two ways. In order to assure maintenance of mydriasis throughout the procedure, 0.4 ml of intracardiac epinephrine can be added to the 500-ml container of balanced salt solution used for irrigation and aspiration of the cortex.

A more concentrated solution of intracardiac epinephrine can be injected directly into the anterior chamber when wider dilatation is needed. For this

TABLE 1. *Formula for Pierce's solution*

Ingredient	Amount	Ingredient	Amount
Phenylephrine hydrochloride	2.5 g	Sodium citrate	2.0 g
Homatropine hydrobromide	2.0 g	Benzyl alcohol	5.0 ml
Procaine hydrochloride	5.0 g	Sodium chloride	1.34 g
Sodium bisulfite	0.5 g	Distilled water	500.0 ml

purpose we dilute 1:1,000 intracardiac epinephrine (Parke-Davis) to 1:8,000 using balanced salt solution. The dilution reduces the toxicity of the epinephrine and the buffer to the corneal endothelial cells.

As noted by Edelhauser and associates (15) any solution intended for intraocular use should have a low buffer capacity in order to minimize endothelial toxicity. We have found the Parke-Davis 1:1,000 intracardiac epinephrine to be suitable for this purpose. A 1:10,000 intracardiac epinephrine is also available from Parke-Davis, but the sodium bisulfite buffer is similar in concentration to that of the 1:1,000 solution. Use of the undiluted 1:10,000 solution, therefore, results in greater endothelial toxicity, because the endothelial cells are exposed to greater concentrations of the toxic bisulfite buffer.

POSTOPERATIVE MYDRIASIS

Extracapsular cataract extraction generally produces a significant anterior chamber reaction, and we believe it is important to keep the pupil moving in order to prevent formation of posterior synechiae in the early postoperative period. The presence of a posterior chamber lens implant seems to protect against the formation of synechiae, but in patients who have undergone extracapsular extraction without such an implant, we routinely use 1% tropicamide and 2.5% phenylephrine twice daily to prevent formation of posterior synechiae.

Tropicamide

Tropicamide (Mydriacyl®) is a rapid-acting parasympatholytic agent that produces mydriasis and incomplete cycloplegia. A 1% solution produces maximal mydriasis in 15 to 30 min that persists for 4 to 6 hr (21). Cycloplegia (incomplete) is maximal at 20 to 25 min and lasts about 6 hr. Aside from a burning sensation experienced on instillation, side effects from the use of tropicamide are unusual.

INTRAOPERATIVE MIOTICS

In 1949, Amsler and Verrey (1) suggested the use of intraoperative acetylcholine in cataract surgery after observing its rapid miotic effect. Schimek (39), Harley and Mishler (22), and Rizzuti (35) have subsequently reported acetylcholine to be useful in intracapsular cataract extraction to protect the vitreous face, to prevent iris incarceration into corneoscleral sutures, and to aid in reposition of prolapsed iris in conventional iridectomies.

In extracapsular cataract extraction, intraoperative miosis is likewise useful in preventing iris incarceration into sutures. In addition, miosis is also helpful in determining proper centration of the pseudophakos and in demonstrating the absence of restriction of pupillary action, which may be caused by incarceration of a capsular remnant into the wound or by pupillary capture of the pseudophakos.

Acetylcholine (Miochol®) and carbachol (Miostat®) are the two miotics currently available for intraocular use. Douglas (12) has shown that there is no appreciable difference in the degree of miosis produced by either of these agents at 2 and 5 min after instillation, but he concurred with the findings of Beasley (2,3) that carbachol has a significantly longer duration of action.

We routinely instill carbachol at the end of any procedure where the pupillary diameter is greater than 4 mm. When a primary posterior capsulotomy is performed, carbachol is instilled after the capsulotomy. We prefer carbachol to acetylcholine primarily because of the longer duration of miosis it provides.

IRRIGATING SOLUTIONS

Compared with intracapsular cataract extraction, extracapsular procedures require more prolonged periods of intraocular irrigation in order to accomplish removal of cortical lens material. The effect of extended irrigation on the corneal endothelium has been a subject of great concern, and various solutions have been used in the past for intraocular irrigation. Edelhauser and colleagues (16) compared the effect of several of these solutions on the corneal endothelium and concluded that the solutions that most closely resemble normal human aqueous in terms of organic and inorganic constituents, pH, and osmolality are likely to cause the least amount of damage to the corneal endothelium.

At the Wilmer Institute we routinely use balanced salt solution (BSS) and have been unable to detect any corneal complications related to its use in more than 1,000 consecutive extracapsular procedures. Stark and Michels (*unpublished data*) found no statistically significant difference in endothelial cell loss or in the incidence of late corneal decompensation when using either of these solutions for vitrectomies in diabetics. BSS is less expensive, more stable, and requires less preparation than BSS-plus or similar more "physiologic" solutions.

SODIUM HYALURONATE

Sodium hyaluronate (Healon®) is a viscoelastic jelly that has gained rapid acceptance in anterior segment surgery primarily because of the protection it affords the corneal endothelium during intraocular manipulations. It is commonly used as an adjunct for a variety of surgical procedures, including trabeculectomy, penetrating keratoplasty, cataract extraction, and repair of traumatic wounds of the anterior segment (32). In extracapsular cataract extraction, sodium hyaluronate maintains the anterior chamber during anterior capsulotomy and intraocular lens insertion, while affording excellent visualization for these procedures.

We fill the anterior chamber with sodium hyaluronate immediately on entering the eye, which allows us to perform the anterior capsulotomy without irrigation. Just prior to insertion of the intraocular lens, we refill the anterior chamber with this agent, which maintains the chamber and "lubricates" the implant, thus reducing the possibility of endothelial damage. Sodium hyaluronate pushes the posterior capsule posteriorly while allowing the iris to come forward. The space created permits insertion of the posterior chamber lens haptic into the ciliary sulcus.

Despite claims to the contrary (29), we have found that leaving the anterior chamber filled with sodium hyaluronate at the end of the procedure often results in significant postoperative intraocular pressure elevation. For this reason we routinely aspirate the bulk of sodium hyaluronate remaining in the anterior chamber prior to closing the eye.

INTRAOCULAR LENSES

The polymethylmethacrylate used in the manufacture of intraocular lenses is of uniformly high quality and appears to be stable for extended periods of time within the human eye. Recently, however, several manufacturers have introduced intraocular lenses containing ultraviolet-absorbing materials. The manufacturers claim these lenses block transmission of ultraviolet light in the 300- to 400-nm wavelength, a range that is presumably toxic to the retina.

To our knowledge, there have been no well-controlled studies demonstrating the retinal toxicity of daily exposure to ultraviolet light in the 300- to 400-nm range. We are concerned about the incorporation of potentially toxic materials into intraocular lenses; the same protection is safely provided by the use of ultraviolet-absorptive spectacles.

Discission of the opaque posterior capsule using the neodymium-YAG laser frequently results in damage to the intraocular lens (47). Because of the potential toxicity of ultraviolet-absorbing compounds released within the eye, the Food and Drug Administration has recently issued a warning to physicians regarding the use of the neodymium-YAG laser for posterior capsulotomy in eyes implanted with ultraviolet-absorptive lenses (45).

ANTIBIOTICS AND CATARACT SURGERY

Although no definitive study convincingly demonstrates the effectiveness of prophylactic antibiotics in ophthalmic procedures, Christy and Sommers (5) have presented evidence showing that topical and subconjunctival antibiotics may decrease the incidence of postoperative bacterial endophthalmitis. Locatcher-Khorazo and associates (28) have shown that the most common source of bacteria resulting in postoperative endophthalmitis is the normal flora of the conjunctiva and eyelids, and for this reason good preoperative lid hygiene seems to be a logical starting place in prophylaxis against endophthalmitis.

In addition to lid hygiene, our current approach to antibiotic prophylaxis consists of topical broad-spectrum antibiotics beginning 1 day prior to surgery. At the end of each surgical procedure 20 mg of garamycin and 50 mg of cefazolin is given subconjunctivally and a topical antibiotic-steroid combination is instilled postoperatively for approximately 1 month.

Widespread use of prophylactic antibiotics raises the issue of selection of resistant bacterial strains, but the presumed beneficial effect in terms of decreasing the incidence of postoperative bacterial infections outweighs the possible risks in the minds of most surgeons. An excellent review of this subject has been provided by Starr (46).

POSTOPERATIVE STEROIDS

The value of topical and/or periocular steroids following cataract extraction has long been a subject of controversy. Clinical studies have yielded variable results with no convincing data supporting the efficacy or lack thereof. Burde and Waltman (4) and Mustakallio and co-workers (31) found that routine use of topical corticosteroids 3 times daily did not reduce inflammation, whereas Corboy (6) arrived at the opposite conclusion. Havener (23) does not favor the use of corticosteroids following uncomplicated intracapsular cataract extraction but feels that they may be of value in extracapsular extraction.

To compound the problem further, most studies available address the issue of corticosteroid use following intracapsular cataract extraction without pseudophakos. In 1982 approximately 60% of cataract operations in the United States were performed using an extracapsular technique, and more than 75% were done with a pseudophakos (44).

Because implantation of a pseudophakos and extracapsular extraction may both be associated with an increased amount of postoperative inflammation, we routinely use postoperative steroids. All patients are followed for steroid-induced intraocular pressure elevation with closer follow-up given to those with a history of diabetes mellitus, chronic open-angle glaucoma, or a family history of glaucoma. In patients who experience significant pressure elevation, we have found that switching to fluorometholone derivatives is helpful.

Our practice is to inject 4 mg dexamethasone subconjunctivally at the end of each procedure and to instill topical 0.1% dexamethasone in a steroid-antibiotic combination 4 times daily beginning the first postoperative day. The frequency of topical dexamethasone is usually decreased to twice daily at 2 weeks and to once daily at 1 month postoperatively. If topical steroid therapy is needed beyond 6 weeks postoperatively, fluorometholone is used.

PROSTAGLANDIN INHIBITORS

Recently we completed a prospective, randomized, controlled clinical trial of prostaglandin synthetase inhibitor, p-hydroxyephedrine (Suprofen®), to determine its effects on surgically induced miosis, postoperative inflammation, and cystoid macular edema (10).

We found that the pupils remained very slightly larger during surgery in eyes treated with a 1% solution of p-hydroxyephedrine compared with eyes receiving a placebo. No statistically significant difference in the incidence of cystoid macular edema or postoperative inflammation was detected, but our patients were also treated with corticosteroids postoperatively as discussed above.

The findings support the hypothesis that prostaglandins are involved in surgically induced miosis (13,38,48), but miosis apparently is not completely blocked by prostaglandin synthetase inhibitors. Recent studies of surgically induced miosis implicate neural mechanisms and substance P (believed to be a peptide neurotransmitter released on antidromic nerve stimulation). Studies are currently underway to clarify this clinically important phenomenon.

MEDICAL PREVENTION OF CATARACT FORMATION

Recent research that may reduce the future need for cataract surgery deserves mention in a discussion of the pharmacology of cataract surgery. Kinoshita and co-workers (26) at the National Eye Institute have shown that sorbitol accumulation within the lens of diabetic animals is responsible for cataract formation. The sorbitol is produced by the action of the enzyme aldose reductase on glucose. Excess glucose is converted into sorbitol within the lens fibers resulting in an osmotic imbalance. Water is imbibed by the lens causing swelling and rupture of lens fibers, which results in cataract formation.

Blocking the aldose reductase with potent aldose reductase inhibitors can prevent or reverse cataract formation in laboratory animals (8,24). Clinical trials are currently being planned to study the effect of aldose reductase inhibitors in human diabetics, and it is hoped that these studies will show a reduction in the incidence and rate of cataract formation in the diabetic. In addition to cataractogenesis, aldose reductase has been implicated in the pathogenesis of diabetic neuropathy (18), retinopathy (51), and epitheliopathy (9).

Although current research on the pharmacologic intervention of cataractogenesis centers on the diabetic population, in the future medical management of cataracts in the general population may become a reality. It is estimated that if cataract formation could be delayed by 10 years, the need for cataract surgery would be reduced by 40% to 50%.

ACKNOWLEDGMENTS

This work was supported in part by the Bernard Davis and the Mary Jammer White Research Funds.

REFERENCES

1. Amsler, M., and Verrey, F. (1949): Mydriase et myose directes et instances par les mediateurs chimiques. *Ann. Oculist.*, 182:936–937.
2. Beasley, H. (1971): Carbachol is an effective miotic in cataract surgery. *Tex. Med.*, 67:79–80.
3. Beasley, H. (1971): Miotics in cataract surgery. *Trans. Am. Ophthalmol. Soc.*, 69:237–244.
4. Burde, R. M., and Waltman, S. R. (1972): Topical corticosteroids after cataract surgery. *Ann. Ophthalmol.*, 4:290–293.

5. Christy, N. E., and Sommers, A. (1979): Antibiotic prophylaxis of postoperative endophthalmitis. *Ann. Ophthalmol.,* 11:1261–1265.
6. Corboy, J. M. (1976): Corticosteroid therapy for the reduction of postoperative inflammation after cataract extraction. *Am. J. Ophthalmol.,* 82:923–927.
7. Crandall, D. C. (1982): Pharmacology of ocular anesthetics. In: *Biomedical Foundations of Ophthalmology,* vol. 3, edited by T. D. Duane and E. A. Jaeger, chap. 35. Harper & Row, Philadelphia.
8. Datiles, M., Fukui, H., Kuwabara, T., and Kinoshita, J. (1982): Galactose cataract prevention with sorbinal, an aldose reductase inhibitor: A light microscopic study. *Invest. Ophthalmol. Vis. Sci.,* 22:174–179.
9. Datiles, M., Kador, P., Fukui, H., Hu, T. S., and Kinoshita, J. (1983): Corneal re-epithelialization in galactosemic rats. *Invest. Ophthalmol. Vis. Sci.,* 24:563–569.
10. Datiles, M., Stark, W. J., Fagadau, W., Maumenee, A. E., deFaller, J., and Klein, P. (1983): Pseudophakic CME: Clinical trial of a new prostaglandin synthetase inhibitor. *Ophthalmology, (submitted).*
11. Donlon, J. V. (1983): Anesthesia for eye, ear, nose, and throat surgery: In: *Anesthesia,* edited by Miller, R. D., pp. 1265–1321. Churchill Livingstone, New York.
12. Douglas, G. R. (1973): Comparison of acetylcholine and carbachol following cataract extraction. *Can. J. Ophthalmol.,* 8:75–77.
13. Duffin, M., Camras, C., Gardner, S., and Pettit, T. (1982): Inhibitors of surgically induced miosis. *Ophthalmology,* 89:966–978.
14. Duncalf, D., Garter, S., and Carol, B. (1970): Mortality in association with ophthalmic surgery. *Am. J. Ophthalmol.,* 69:610–615.
15. Edelhauser, H. F., Hyndiuk, R. A., Zeeb, A., and Schultz, R. O. (1982): Corneal edema and the intraocular use of epinephrine. *Am. J. Ophthalmol.,* 93:327–333.
16. Edelhauser, H. F., Van Horn, D. L., Hyndiuk, R. A., and Schultz, R. O. (1975): Intraocular irrigating solutions: Their effect on the corneal endothelium. *Arch. Ophthalmol.,* 93:648–657.
17. Ellis, P. P. (1977): *Ocular Therapeutics and Pharmacology.* C. V. Mosby, St. Louis.
18. Fargius, J., and Jameson, S. (1981): Effects of aldose reductase inhibitor treatment in diabetic polyneuropathy—a clinical and neurophysiological study. *J. Neurol. Neurosurg. Psychiatry,* 44:991–1002.
19. Frayer, W. C., and Jacoby, J. (1983): Local anesthesia: In: *Clinical Ophthalmology,* vol. 5, edited by Thomas D. Duane, chap. 2. Harper & Row, Philadelphia.
20. Gartner, S., and Billet, E. (1958): A study on mortality rates. *Am. J. Ophthalmol.,* 45:847–849.
21. Goodman, L. S., and Gilman, A. (1970): *The Pharmacological Basis of Therapeutics.* Macmillan, Toronto.
22. Harley, R. D., and Mishler, J. E. (1966): Acetylcholine in cataract surgery. *Br. J. Ophthalmol.,* 50:429–433.
23. Havener, W. H. (1983): *Ocular Pharmacology.* C. V. Mosby, St. Louis.
24. Hu, T.-S., Datiles, M., and Kinoshita, J. (1983): Reversal of galactose cataract with sorbinal in rats. *Invest. Ophthalmol. Vis. Sci.,* 24:640–644.
25. Hug, C. C. (1981): What are the roles of narcotic analgesics in anesthesia? *Refresh. Courses Anesthesiol.,* 9:71–81.
26. Kinoshita, J., Kador, P., and Datiles, M. (1981): Aldose reductase in diabetic cataract. *J.A.M.A.,* 246:257–261.
27. Kraff, M. C., Saunders, D. R., Jampol, L. M., and Lieberman, H. L. (1983): Effect of retrobulbar hyaluronidase on pseudophakic cystoid macular edema. *Am. Intra-Ocular Implant Soc. J.,* 9:184–185.
28. Locatcher-Khorazo, D., Sullivan, N., and Gutierrez, E. (1967): *Staphylococcus aureus* isolated from normal and infected eyes. *Arch. Ophthalmol.,* 77:370–377.
29. Miller, D., and Stegmann, R. (1974): Use of sodium-hyaluronate in anterior segment surgery. *J. Am. Intra-Ocular Implant Soc.,* 6:613–615.
30. Mindel, J. S. (1978): Value of hyaluronidase in ocular surgical akinesia. *Am. J. Ophthalmol.,* 85:643–646.
31. Mustakallio, A., Kaufman, H. E., Johnston, G., Wilson, R. S., Roberts, M. D., and Harter, J. C. (1973): Corticosteroid efficacy in postoperative uveitis. *Ann. Ophthalmol.,* 5:719–730.
32. Pape, L. G., and Balazs, E. A. (1980): The use of sodium hyaluronate (Healon) in human anterior segment surgery. *Ophthalmology,* 87:699–705.

33. Petrusak, J., Smith, R. B., and Breslin, P. P. (1973): Mortality rate related to ophthalmological surgery. *Arch. Ophthalmol.,* 89:106–109.
34. Quigley, H. A. (1974): Mortality associated with ophthalmic surgery: A twenty year experience. *Am. J. Ophthalmol.,* 77:517–524.
35. Rizzuti, A. B. (1967): Acetylcholine in surgery of the lens, iris, and cornea. *Am. J. Ophthalmol.,* 63:484–486.
36. Roper, D. L., and Nisbet, R. M. (1978): Effect of hyaluronidase on the incidence of cystoid macular edema. *Ann. Ophthalmol.,* 10:1673–1677.
37. Rosenblatt, R. M., May, D. R., and Barsoumian, K. (1980): Cardiopulmonary arrest after retrobulbar block. *Am. J. Ophthalmol.,* 90:425–427.
38. Sawa, M., and Masuda, K. (1976): Topical indomethacin in soft cataract aspiration. *Jpn. J. Ophthalmol.,* 20:514–519.
39. Schimek, R. A. (1961): The use of intraocular acetylcholine in anterior segment surgery. *An. Inst. Barraquer.,* 2:687–688.
40. Smith, J. L. (1981): Retrobulbar marcaine can cause respiratory arrest. *J. Clin. Neuro. Ophthalmol.,* 1:171–172.
41. Solosko, D., and Smith, R. B. (1972): Hypertension following 10% phenylephrine ophthalmic. *Anesthesiology,* 36:187–189.
42. Stanley, T. H. (1979): Pros and cons of using narcotics for anesthesia. *Refresh. Courses Anesthesiol.,* 7:203–212.
43. Stanley, T. H. (1981): Pharmacology of intravenous non-narcotic anesthetics. In: *Anesthesia,* edited by R. D. Miller, Chap. 16, Churchill Livingstone, New York.
44. Stark, W. J., and Streeten, B. (1983): The anterior capsulotomy of extracapsular cataract extraction. *Ophthalmology, (in press).*
45. Stark, W. J. (1983): Meeting of the Ophthalmic Device Advisory Panel, Food and Drug Administration, November, 1983.
46. Starr, M. B. (1983): Prophylactic antibiotics for ophthalmic surgery. *Surv. Ophthalmol.,* 27:353–373.
47. Terry, A. C., Stark, W. J., Maumenee, A. E., and Fagadau, W. (1983): Neodymium YAG laser for posterior capsulotomy. *Am. J. Ophthalmol.,* 96:716–720.
48. Waitzman, M. B., and King, C. D. (1967): Prostaglandin influences on intraocular pressure and pupil size. *Am. J. Physiol.,* 212:329–334.
49. Wilensky, J. T., and Woodward, H. J. (1970): Acute systemic hypertension after conjunctival instillation of phenylephrine hydrochloride. *Am. J. Ophthalmol.,* 70:729–732.
50. Wilson, J., and Ellis, F. R. (1973): Oral premedication with lorazepam: A comparison with heptabarbitone and diazepam. *Br. J. Anaesth.,* 45:738–744.
51. Yajima, Y., Akagi, Y., Kador, P., and Kuwabara, T. (1982): Immuno-histochemical demonstration of aldose reductase in the human eye. *Invest. Ophthalmol. Vis. Sci.,* 22A(ARVO Abstracts):286.

Commentary

Pharmacology of Glaucoma Surgery

The candor of these presentations by Professors Krieglstein and Leydhecker is remarkable and to them we owe our gratitude.

In filtration surgery, in experienced hands, the two causes of failure and/or complication are either the excessive scarring or excessive thinning of the conjunctiva and/or Tenon's capsule. In the latter case, avoidance of excision of Tenon's is desirable in many instances. Else within a few years a thinned infection-susceptible bleb results. In the former case the following points need to be remembered: the underside of Tenon's is a glistening, smooth surface ordinarily gliding easily over the sclera below it. Tenon's capsule therefore needs to be replaced with the least disturbance. It needs to be sutured or caught within the conjunctival suture when the edges of the latter are reapposed, whether after a limbal or a fornix-based flap. (If the latter, a corneal groove is appropriate for aid in suturing the flap to the cornea.) The edges of cut or torn Tenon's capsule and/or conjunctiva are not only what delimit the bleb but also what encourage a progressively encroaching scar on the filtration site.

Even with these mechanical precautions filtration can sometimes fail at these external sites. Not without hope, we commend the extension of the preoperative measures for extracapsular cataract extraction to glaucoma surgery. Preoperative treatment of the patient with steroids and/or indomethacin not only for hours but for several days, elimination of irritating drugs, and maintenance of intraoperative intraocular pressure so as to avoid the paracentesis effect (here, the use of viscosurgery, if necessary) are among our recommendations.

Among recent thoughts on this subject have been the idea that a disrupted blood ocular barrier may bring growth factors to the aqueous to stimulate fibroplasia at the filtration site (2) and that the use of steroid by injection, preoperatively (1), may be preventative. Probably enough serum issues from the cut edges of episcleral tissue anyway without involving aqueous factors for fibroplasia, but, the preservation of transmural pressure relations, that is the elimination of the paracentesis effect, is paramount. Regarding steroid *injections,* one always has the risk of hemorrhage after an injection, an unhappy prospect near a filtration site.

A prospective randomized clinical trial of these and the aforementioned preoperative measures in glaucoma filtration surgery would be useful.

The Editors

REFERENCES

1. Ciangiacomo, J., Dueker, D., and Adelstein, E. H. (1985): The effect of preoperative subconjunctival triamcinolone on glaucoma filtration. *Invest. Ophthalmol. Vis. Sci. ARVO Suppl.,* 26(11):126.
2. Herschler, J., Claflin, A. J., and Fiorentino, G. (1980): The effect of aqueous humor on the growth of subconjunctival fibroblasts in tissue culture and its implications for glaucoma surgery. *Am. J. Ophthalmol.,* 89:245–249.

Surgical Pharmacology of the Eye,
edited by M. Sears and A. Tarkkanen.
Raven Press, New York © 1985.

Pharmacology of Glaucoma Surgery: The Clinical Pharmacologist's Point of View

G. K. Krieglstein

*University Eye Hospital Würzburg, Kopfklinikum, D-8700 Würzburg,
Federal Republic of Germany*

Glaucoma surgery deals with a variety of ocular disorders distinguished by the mechanism whereby aqueous outflow is impeded at the chamber angle. Pharmacotherapy usually precedes the indication for operation and will overlap with it in many cases. To bring out the best possible surgical results, accompanying conservative measures have to be considered and may be subdivided into pharmacologic requisites devoted to the presurgical situation, to surgery itself, and to postsurgical care.

PHARMACOTHERAPY SUPPORTING THE PRESURGICAL SITUATION

Drug actions in the presurgical phase are primarily aimed at (a) having a soft eye for the procedure regardless of untreated intraocular pressure (IOP) level; (b) reducing the paracentesis effect; and (c) preventing early scarring of the intended site of infiltration.

Hypotensive Agents Used Prior to Surgery

Performing an antiglaucomatous operation on eyes with high pressure bears a series of risks, such as acute choroidal effusion, expulsive hemorrhage, postoperative flat chamber, or ciliary block glaucoma. To achieve a favorable starting IOP level, agents that decrease vitreous volume are to be preferred to agents reducing aqueous flow [unlike cataract surgery, mechanical compression of the globe should be avoided because of the higher risk of expulsive hemorrhage (29)]. In this respect osmotic agents are given priority over carbonic anhydrase inhibitors. One should definitely avoid long-lasting flow reduction with β-blockers because of untoward effects on the filtration mechanism.

For surgery under retrobulbar anesthesia, peroral osmotic agents may be useful if the problem of nausea is considered. Glycerol is given perorally together with fruit juice at a dosage of 1 to 1.5 g/kg (11). The time course of response meets the surgical requirement, with hypotension beginning 10 min after application and peaking 30 min thereafter, with a maximum duration of 5 hr (11). One should be careful with diabetics in a borderline metabolic situation (3). Alternatively, 1.5 g/kg isosorbide may be used in a 50% solution, which was claimed to have fewer side effects than glycerol (3). Intravenously administered hyperosmotic agents such as mannitol give a greater hypotensive effect than oral ones (22). Two grams per kilogram body weight of a 20% solution of mannitol is usually used as a preoperative dosage (34). For the best response the administration should be from 30 min and 60 min prior to the procedure (22). Serious side effects may turn up in patients with reduced renal function (9). Glycerol may be also used intravenously, however, at a very low infusion rate (28).

If untreated IOP level requires it, acetazolamide at a dose of 250 mg or 500 mg may be given intravenously, which causes a prompt reduction of pressure (6). Sustained-release preparations of carbonic anhydrase inhibitors should not be used prior to filtration surgery. In chronic angle-closure glaucoma with very high preoperative IOP, intravenous application of 40 mg furosemide will reduce vitreous volume together with an instantaneous IOP decrease.

Presurgical Treatment of Acute Angle-Closure Glaucoma

Successful surgery of acute angle-closure glaucoma strongly depends on quick relief of angle block. The longer the acute pressure rise persists, the less responsive is the eye to emergency drug treatment. The immediate application of pilocarpine 0.5% to 1% four times at 15-min intervals is most important. This will pull the basal iris out of the chamber angle. The inevitable concomitant ischemic iritis should be treated with topical steroids such as 0.1% dexamethasone or 1% prednisolone eye drops four times on the day of the attack. If the miotic property of pilocarpine fails, miosis may be supported by 0.5% thymoxamine eye drops (31). One should be careful with excessive use of pilocarpine because this again may provoke pupillary block. With initiation of topical therapy 500 mg acetazolamide, i.v., should be given as well. If there is no significant IOP drop within 1 hr, osmotic agents such as glycerol or mannitol at adequate doses (Table 1) may be added (27). Small quantities of alcohol (i.e., 20 cc brandy) also have an IOP-lowering effect (13). Because of the extreme pain to the patient, an analgesic is necessary. Repeated doses of 600 to 1,000 mg aspirin are helpful and also advantageous with respect to prostaglandin-induced disruption of the blood-aqueous barrier. After termination of angle block, a differentiation between angle closure and open-angle glaucoma with narrow angles can be made using the thymoxamine test (30). Since this α-adrenergic blocker will produce miosis without affecting aqueous dynamics, the pressure will be within normal range in a pure angle-closure glaucoma in this respect. Presurgical pharmacologic testing may help to design the adequate surgical procedure.

TABLE 1. *Presurgical conservative treatment of acute angle-closure glaucoma*

Topical treatment	Systemic treatment
0.5%–1% pilocarpine (4 doses, every 15 min) 0.1% dexamethasone 0.5% thymoxamine (optional)	500 mg acetazolamide, i.v. 1–1.5 g/kg oral glycerol (optional) 500 ml 20% mannitol, i.v. (optional) 600 mg aspirin, p.o.

Treatment Designed to Lessen the Surgical Trauma

A major contribution of pharmacology to ophthalmic surgery is the prevention of secondary postsurgical inflammation. Inflammation is mainly induced by surgery itself, and by the paracentesis effect (4), mediated by the liberation of prostaglandins from the anterior uvea. Prostaglandin-linked ocular inflammation can be prophylactically treated by nonsteroidal anti-inflammatory agents (18). These compounds inhibit a cyclooxygenase, whereas anti-inflammatory steroids decrease the availability of arachidonic acid for prostaglandin synthesis (10). One of the effective prostaglandin inhibitors to be used on the eye is indomethacin (12), which penetrates the eye well, and the levels reached in the eye by topical application considerably exceed aqueous levels after systemic administration. Favorable effects of indomethacin pretreatment on the postoperative inflammation have been proved for different operations, such as cataract extraction, cyclocryotherapy, or trabeculectomy (12). But one has to keep in mind that once the inflammation is present, prostaglandin inhibitors seem to be of little value; they inhibit the synthesis of prostaglandins but cannot antagonize the effects of prostaglandins after their release from the uvea (21). Pretreatment with 0.5% indomethacin eye drops over 24 hr before surgery (4 to 5 doses) will bring out the desired clinical effect (16). The advantages for glaucoma surgery are obvious: There will be less risk of postoperative hypotony, which may cause macular damage or choroidal effusion; there will be less pronounced secondary aqueous secretion that may obstruct filtration pathways; there will be less development of posterior synechiae; and there will be less incidence of postoperative hypertension requiring additional medication.

The ocular inflammation due to the tissue damage of the operation may be better controlled by steroids. To have effective tissue levels already present at the time of surgery, we treat the patient with 50 mg fluocortolone perorally on the day prior to surgery (in addition to prostaglandin inhibitors).

AGENTS USED DURING SURGERY

There are only a few compounds adjuvant to the procedure itself: sodium hyaluronate for viscosurgery, acetylcholine and epinephrine to control pupil motility, and vasopressin derivatives as hemostatics.

Viscosurgery Using Sodium Hyaluronate (Healon®)

Healon® is a highly purified noninflammatory fraction of sodium hyaluronate, which is used in microsurgery of the eye because of its viscoelastic properties (1). Its biophysical behavior and ocular tolerance protect cells from mechanical trauma during surgery, maintain tissue spaces (most important for glaucoma surgery), ensure separation of tissues, and permit manipulation in ocular compartments (1). In a prospective study we have realized that Healon® is useful in filtration surgery of open-angle glaucoma. Blocking the trabeculectomy opening of the anterior chamber with a Healon® plug (Fig. 1) prevents loss of aqueous during surgery. Re-formation of original chamber depth is faster after Healon® than in a matched control group; the incidence of flat chambers and hypotonic complications is less frequent. In cyclodialysis the cleft can be kept open by filling in Healon® (Fig. 2); less postoperative hypotony and fewer severe hemorrhages may occur. It can be of great help in goniotomy for visualization of the angle recess in the hyperopic eye, and it diminishes the chances for hemorrhages (33). In angle-closure glaucoma surgery, Healon® is capable of breaking angle synechiae and deepening the peripheral angle (26). Filling of the sub-Tenon's fascia at the filtration site prepares the filtering bleb and will prevent an excess of aqueous collection in the first postoperative days (26). When using Healon® in peripheral iridectomy, the logic is primarily to break goniosynechiae (24). In full thickness filtration operations without scleral flaps, Healon® is advantageous in prevention of chamber loss (25). However, one should not forget that there may be considerable Healon®-mediated

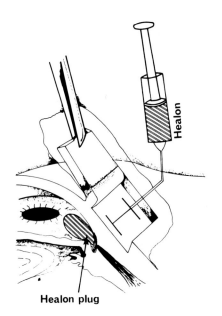

FIG. 1. Preservation of the anterior chamber volume prior to trabeculectomy by blocking the corneoscleral incision with a Healon® plug from inside.

Healon plug

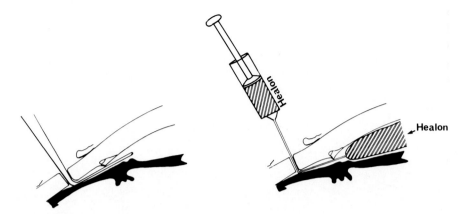

FIG. 2. Widening the cyclodialysis cleft with Healon®. After formation of the cyclodialysis cleft with a spatula **(left)** the peripheral chamber and the opening of the cleft is filled with Healon® **(right)**.

pressure rises in the first 1 or 2 postoperative days, which may detract from its advantages.

Control of Pupillary Diameter

Iris constriction is most often required during antiglaucomatous surgery; e.g., for pulling out the iris from a corneoscleral incision, holding open a cyclodialysis cleft, or pulling the iris out of the chamber recess during goniotomy. When prompt miosis of short duration is needed, acetylcholine is the cholinergic agent of choice (2). Intraocular instillation of a 1:100 concentration will give the desired effect. Pilocarpine or eserine would give intense miosis of longer duration, but they create severe postoperative pain. If intraoperative miosis of longer duration than achievable with acetylcholine is needed, carbachol 0.01% can be applied intracamerally (15). Still, because of its short half-life time within the eye, acetylcholine has the best therapeutic ratio to produce intraoperative pupillary constriction. There are very few indications for pupil dilation during glaucoma surgery, and if they occur, all agents at disposal have to be used with great caution on the open eye. If filtration surgery has to be combined with cataract extraction (especially with extracapsular procedures), maintenance of pupil dilation can be achieved by epinephrine instillation 1:16,000 to 1:96,000 into the anterior chamber (7). However, the use of epinephrine of any concentration is strictly contraindicated during anesthesia with Fluothane®.

Hemostatic Treatment During Surgery

Epinephrine or related compounds are of limited value as vasoconstrictors to stop extra- or intraocular hemorrhage (34). Systemic risks are too great in intubation anesthesia; also, reactive hyperemia after vasoconstriction can cause late relapses of hemorrhages. We found the therapeutic ratio of vasopressin-like agents superior, and therefore prefer ornithine vasopressin as vasoconstrictor applied intracamerally. Dosages required to exert hemostatic action do not cause cardiovascular effects (8).

POSTOPERATIVE MEDICAL CARE

In uncomplicated glaucoma surgery, postoperative treatment is primarily of prophylactic value. The topical medication in the first days after surgery usually consists of a steroid, an antibiotic, and a mydriatic or miotic (Table 2) (5,32). Although prophylactic antibiotic treatment is very much debated (11), we prefer gentamicin topically for 4 to 5 days postoperatively, until wound closure would hardly permit ascending infection of the anterior chamber. We chose gentamicin since it is highly effective on gram-negative organisms (especially *Pseudomonas*) ubiquitous in large hospitals. For treatment of inevitable postoperative inflammation 1% prednisolone drops or ointment should be preferred because of its good intraocular penetration (11). If there is a history of failure of glaucoma surgery, we add 40 mg fluocortolone systemically. Should the specific situation require very potent anti-inflammatory treatment, dexamethasone may be given subconjunctivally. Prostaglandin-inhibitor treatment initiated presurgically should be continued over at least 10 days after surgery. A promising approach to prevent early scarring of the filtering bleb was reported recently with 5-fluorouracil, an antimetabolite (19). Applying it subconjunctivally up to a total dose of 21 mg in patients with poor prognosis, IOP control could be achieved in the majority of patients.

In case of development of flat chamber and to prevent posterior synechiae we give atropine 1% twice daily over 5 days in all filtration procedures. In those operations in which miosis is required at the same time (such as goniotomy or cyclodialysis) we give pilocarpine 1% four times daily.

Postoperative Flat Chamber

One of the major challenges of glaucoma surgery is the management of postoperative hypotony associated with a flat anterior chamber. After careful

TABLE 2. *Postoperative drug treatment*
in uncomplicated glaucoma surgery

Filtration surgery	Cyclodyalysis/ goniotomy
1% atropine, b.i.d.	1% pilocarpine, q.i.d.
1% prednisolone, q.i.d.	1% prednisolone, q.i.d.
0.5% gentamicin, b.i.d.	0.5% gentamicin, b.i.d.

exclusion of an external fistula or an open cyclodialysis cleft with ciliary body detachment (requiring surgical measures of the first line) some conservative attempts can be made. Taking into consideration that the underlying mechanism inhibits aqueous secretion caused by the surgical trauma, water loading with quick infusion of an electrolyte infusion or intake of 1 liter of tea within a short time often stimulates aqueous production and restores the anterior chamber (17). This would also be indicated in primary overfiltration together with mechanical compression of an excessive filtering bleb. Some authors (5) combine the water-loading of the eye with preceding carboanhydrase inhibitors. When aqueous production catches up again or overfiltration is stopped, one should avoid misdirection of flow by maximum mydriasis and ciliary body relaxation. We found the combination of 1% cyclopentolate with 10% phenylephrine very effective, and in some cases (after careful exclusion of systemic risk factors) we apply a cotton sponge soaked with the drugs to the cul-de-sac of the affected eye. Parallel to that, systemic steroids are indicated to stop choroidal effusion (32). Finally, visual acuity is a good guide when conservative treatment is to be replaced by an adequate surgical intervention (14). Refilling the anterior chamber with Healon® is more successful than refilling with air or salt solution (Fig. 3).

Ciliary-Block Glaucoma

The development of a shallow anterior chamber together with high IOP after glaucoma surgery characterizes ciliary-block glaucoma. The forward displacement of the lens to get in touch with the ciliary processes is accompanied by a misdirection of aqueous flow with consequent pooling of aqueous behind the lens. Resolute mydriasis with cycloplegia is the first measure to be taken in this condition; 1% atropine or 1% cyclopentolate with 10% phenylephrine four times daily may be the most effective regimen for obtaining the best

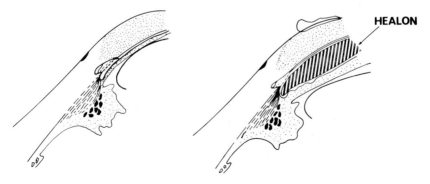

FIG. 3. Re-formation of a postoperative flat chamber by the use of Healon®. In the postoperative flat chamber (**left**) a peripheral incision of the chamber is made and filled with Healon® to restore original chamber depth (**right**).

TABLE 3. *Conservative management of ciliary-block glaucoma*

Topical treatment	Systemic treatment
1% cyclopentolate, q.i.d.	50 mg fluocortolone
10% phenylephrine, q.i.d.	2 ml/kg oral glycerol
1% prednisolone, q.i.d.	250 mg acetazolamide, q.i.d.
	600 mg aspirin, q.i.d.

mydriasis possible. In order to act on ciliary body edema, steroids should be given both topically and systemically. Systemic hypotensive drugs are aimed at the reduction of the vitreous volume (hyperosmotic agents) and at the reduction of high IOP by transiently decreasing aqueous flow (carboanhydrase inhibitors) (20). A guideline for the conservative treatment of ciliary-block glaucoma is given in Table 3.

Postoperative Hemorrhage

Postoperative hyphema is one of the more frequent complications of glaucoma surgery. Many disputes can be found in literature about conservative efforts to accelerate clearance of hyphemas (11). Subconjunctival injection of streptokinase, streptodornase, or fibrinolysin can increase the rate of absorption (23). Fresh blood clots will be most effectively treated by irrigation of the anterior chamber with fibrinolysin, whereas 5-day-old clots can no longer be treated this way. In the early phase of postoperative hemorrhage, miotics encourage the escape of red blood cells through the trabecular meshwork. Obviously, the efficacy of all agents supposed to facilitate hyphema clearance depends on how early in the course of the problem they are instituted.

REFERENCES

1. Balazs, E. A. (1983): Sodium hyaluronate and viscosurgery. In: *Healon. A Guide to Its Use in Ophthalmic Surgery,* edited by D. Miller and R. Stegmann, pp. 5–28. John Wiley, New York.
2. Barraquer, J. I. (1964): Acetylcholine as a miotic agent for use in surgery. *Am. J. Ophthalmol.,* 57:406.
3. Becker, B., Kolker, A. E., and Krupin, T. (1967): Isosorbide. An oral hyperosmotic agent. *Arch. Ophthalmol.,* 78:147.
4. Bill, A. (1980): The physiology of the paracentesis effect and its recovery. In: *Wound Healing of the Eye and Its Complications,* edited by G. O. H. Naumann and B. Gloor, pp. 65–70. J. F. Bergmann, Munich.
5. Draeger, J., and Wirt, H. (1983): Behandlung nach Glaukom-Operationen. *Z. Prakt. Augenheilk.,* 4:321–329.
6. Drance, S. M. (1979): Use of systemic ocular hypotensive agents. In: *Symposium on Ocular Pharmacology and Therapeutics. Trans. New Orleans Acad. Ophthalmol.,* pp. 132–142. C. V. Mosby, St. Louis.
7. Duffin, R. M., Pettit, T. H., and Straatsma, B. R. (1983): Maintenance of mydriasis with epinephrine during cataract surgery. *Ophthalmic Surg.,* 14:41.
8. Goodman, L. S., and Gilman, A. (1975): *The Pharmacological Basis of Therapeutics,* 5th ed., p. 856. Macmillan, New York.

9. Grabie, M. T., Gipstein, R. M., Adams, D. A., and Hepner, G. W. (1981): Contraindications for mannitol in aphakic glaucoma. *Am. J. Ophthalmol.,* 91:265.
10. Hall, D. W. R., and Bonta, I. L. (1977): Prostaglandins and ocular inflammation. *Doc. Ophthalmol.,* 44:421–434.
11. Havener, W. H. (1978): *Ocular Pharmacology,* 4th ed., pp. 116–118. C. V. Mosby, St. Louis.
12. Katz, I. M. (1981): Indomethacin. *Ophthalmology,* 88:455–458.
13. Leydhecker, W., and Ricklefs, G. (1968): May glaucoma patients drink alcohol and coffee? *Atti. 50. Congr. Soc. Oftal. Ital. Firenze 1967,* p. 24.
14. Maumenee, A. E. (1980): Hypotony. In: *Current Ocular Therapy,* edited by F. T. Fraunfelder and F. H. Roy, pp. 448–449. W. B. Saunders, Philadelphia.
15. McDonald, T. O., Roberts, M. D., and Borgmann, A. R. (1970): Intraocular safety of carbamylcholine chloride (carbachol) in rabbit eyes. *Ann. Ophthalmol.,* 2:878.
16. Mishima, S., and Masuda, K. (1977): Clinical implications of prostaglandins and synthesis inhibitors. In: *Symposium on Ocular Therapy,* vol. 10, edited by I. H. Leopold and R. P. Burns, pp. 1–19. John Wiley, New York.
17. Neubauer, H. (1982): Die postoperative aufgehobene Vorderkammer. In: *Bücherei des Augenarztes,* vol. 94, pp. 110–119. Enke, Stuttgart.
18. Nickander, R., McMahon, F. G., and Ridolfo, A. S. (1979): Nonsteroidal anti-inflammatory agents. *Annu. Rev. Pharmacol. Toxicol.,* 19:469–490.
19. Parrish, R. K., Heuer, D. K., Gressel, M. G., Anderson, D. R., Palmberg, P. F., and Hodapp, E. A. (1983): 5-Fluorouracil and glaucoma filtering surgery. In: *Aktuelle Traumatologie in der Augenheilkunde,* 81. Tagung der Dtsch. Ophthal. Ges., Heidelberg.
20. Podos, S. M., and Ritch, R. (1980): Malignant glaucoma. In: *Current Ocular Therapy,* edited by F. T. Fraunfelder and F. H. Roy, pp. 458–459. W. B. Saunders, Philadelphia.
21. Sawa, M., and Masuda, K. (1976): Topical indomethacin in soft cataract aspiration. *Jpn. J. Ophthalmol.,* 20:514–519.
22. Shields, M. B. (1982): *A Study Guide for Glaucoma,* p. 439. Williams & Wilkins, Baltimore, London.
23. Sinskey, R. M., and Krichesky, A. R. (1962): Experimental hyphema in rabbits. *Am. J. Ophthalmol.,* 54:445.
24. Stegmann, R., and Miller, D. (1983): Peripheral iridectomy using Healon. In: *Healon. A Guide to Its Use in Ophthalmic Surgery,* edited by D. Miller and R. Stegmann, pp. 141–148. John Wiley, New York.
25. Stegmann, R., and Miller, D. (1983): Thermal sclerotomy using Healon. In: *Healon. A Guide to Its Use in Ophthalmic Surgery,* edited by D. Miller and R. Stegmann, pp. 149–160. John Wiley, New York.
26. Stegmann, R., and Miller, D. (1983): Trabeculectomy using Healon. In: *Healon. A Guide to Its Use in Ophthalmic Surgery,* edited by D. Miller and R. Stegmann, pp. 161–170. John Wiley, New York.
27. Sugar, H. S. (1974): Management of angle closure glaucoma. *Ann. Ophthalmol.,* 6:517.
28. Tarter, R. C., and Linn, J. G. (1961): A clinical study of the use of intravenous urea in glaucoma. *Am. J. Ophthalmol.,* 52:323.
29. Völcker, H. E. (1983): Expulsive Blutung—extreme Folge der akuten Bulbus-Hypotonie. *Fortschr. Ophthalmol.,* 79:417–419.
30. Wand, M., and Grant, W. M. (1978): Thymoxamine test: Differentiating angle closure glaucoma from open angle glaucoma with narrow angles. *Arch. Ophthalmol.,* 96:1009.
31. Wand, M., and Grant, W. M. (1980): Thymoxamine hydrochloride: An alpha-adrenergic blocker. *Surv. Ophthalmol.,* 25:75.
32. Wetzel, W. (1982): Postoperative Behandlung nach Glaukomoperationen. Spätkomplikationen und ihre Beseitigung. *Bücherei des Augenarztes,* 94:95–109.
33. Wirt, H., Draeger, J., and Winter, R. (1983): Erfahrungen mit Hyaluronsäure in der operativen Glaukombehandlung. In: *Aktuelle Traumatologie in der Augenheilkunde,* 81. Tagung der Dtsch. Ophthal. Ges., Heidelberg.
34. Worthen, D. M., and Quon, D. (1980): Dose response of intravenous mannitol on the human eye. Presented at Annual Meeting of Association for Research in Vision and Ophthalmology, *A.R.V.O. Abstracts,* p. 140.

Surgical Pharmacology of the Eye,
edited by M. Sears and A. Tarkkanen.
Raven Press, New York © 1985.

Pharmacology of Glaucoma Surgery: Skeptical Remarks of the Devil's Advocate

W. Leydhecker

University Eye Hospital Würzburg, Kopfklinikum, D-8700 Würzburg, Federal Republic of Germany

SUMMARY: After learning that Dr. Krieglstein had a more optimistic viewpoint on the usefulness of some of the newer drugs than I had, I decided to deliver somewhat more skeptical remarks in the role of the devil's advocate. Only a few drugs have an important place in glaucoma surgery. We need corticosteroids and prostaglandin inhibitors in order to suppress inflammation, and we need antibiotics for the treatment of infections. Besides, we need acetylcholine for an immediate miosis in the open eye, and mydriatics before, or, more often, after surgery, in order to prevent synechiae. Unfortunately, we have no drugs that will keep a cyclodialysis cleft open. We have no drug that will prevent an expulsive hemorrhage, or postsurgical hemorrhages into the anterior chamber or into the vitreous.

Professor Krieglstein and I have agreed that he should give the review and I should add some skeptical remarks in the role of the devil's advocate, after we had discussed his chapter together.

Healon® is much in fashion nowadays, and I like to use it in cataract surgery. I have some doubts if it is useful to the same extent in glaucoma surgery. In trabeculectomy procedures, the anterior chamber is re-formed anyway by the end of the operation. With my technique of iridencleisis, only one drop of aqueous is lost but never the whole of the anterior chamber. In cyclodialysis, the technique for avoiding hemorrhages is to use a perforated spatula and to perform the operation with a constant infusion of BSS into the anterior chamber under some pressure. I would not like to have Healon® in the cyclodialysis cleft where we want aqueous outflow and its absorption by the uvea. In goniotomy, the same technique of increasing the pressure in the anterior chamber by a perforated knife is employed. Even then, minor hemorrhages are often unavoidable. With Healon® and blood mixed in the anterior chamber, the visualization of the trabeculae would be more difficult than with a mixture of blood with BSS, which can be washed out more easily.

In patients with angle-closure glaucoma, the choice of the surgical technique should not mainly depend on the presence or absence of peripheral synechiae, which might be breakable by Healon®. After long contact or repeated contacts of the peripheral iris with the trabeculae these will not function normally any longer, even if there are no synechiae. Iridectomy *without* a filtering procedure, therefore, will be insufficient in approximately 30% of all such cases. The choice of the surgical technique cannot depend on breaking synechiae, and it is a decision independent of pharmacologic actions.

The value of the thymoxamine test seems doubtful. After an attack of angle-closure glaucoma, the eye is usually soft anyway, in consequence of hyposecretion of aqueous, and it is no problem to keep the intraocular pressure low until surgery, which should follow soon.

We have no means to prevent cicatrization of Tenon's fascia over a filtering wound, no pharmaceutics, and no reliable surgical means. Some patients will always develop cicatrization, even if we give them high doses of cortisone before and after surgery, or even if we excise Tenon's fascia.

The re-formation of a flat anterior chamber can be more frustrating than it sounded in Dr. Krieglstein's report. Most surgical glaucoma patients are old and unable to tolerate water loading. Its value for re-forming a flat anterior chamber is not proved in young patients either. If the eye is soft and the anterior chamber shallow but not flat, one can wait for any time. If it is flat on the periphery only, and the lens not in contact with the cornea, one can wait up to 2 weeks for any invasive therapy, and apply steroids and mydriatics. If the eye is hard and the chamber flat, we speak of malignant glaucoma, and this calls for immediate action, for atropine and phenylephrine. However, in approximately half of these patients medical therapy fails, the lens has to be removed and the vitreous dissected.

It can be very difficult to remove or to stop repeated hemorrhages into the anterior chamber. If absorption has not started within 6 days, a paracentesis should be performed in order to avoid blood staining of the cornea.

A choroidal detachment in a hypotonic eye can be a hard problem to treat. Time works better than drugs, and if the anterior chamber is not lost and the eye has no functional damage, there is no need to hurry. I would send the patient home and give him his next appointment no earlier than 2 months.

To summarize, I think that only a few drugs have an important place in glaucoma surgery, except in the treatment of acute angle-block glaucoma. These are cortisone and prostaglandin inhibitors for suppression of inflammation, antibiotics for prevention of infections, and acetylcholine for an immediate miosis during surgery. We have no specific medical treatment for postsurgical hemorrhages, choroidal effusion, or cicatrization of the filtering bleb.

Some mistakes should be mentioned. Treatment with cholinesterase inhibitors during the last three days before surgery produces a rigid iris that will not prolapse—as we wish it would—after opening of the anterior chamber, especially in iridencleisis. Any drugs suppressing aqueous production, such as carbonic anhydrase inhibitors or β-blockers, should not be given during or after surgery, because this would have an unfavorable effect on the formation of filtering bleb. Miotics after surgery are indicated only in cyclodialysis or in goniotomy in order to keep the cleft open. In all other cases, atropine is indicated immediately after surgery and during the first postsurgical week to avoid posterior synechiae, lento-ciliary block, or pupillary block.

Commentary

Pharmacology of Surgery of the Vitreous and Retina

These authors have produced an impressive document that very specifically addresses the pharmacologic challenges offered by surgery of the vitreous and retina. Arachidonic acid mediated inflammation induced by surgery is prophylactically treated by the authors with the "synergistic" effect of combined steroidal and nonsteroidal agents. They support their therapeutic approach to protection of ocular tissue with experimental documentation. The clinical implications of this section should be read and digested. On the subject of intraocular gases, the authors point out the utility of these, and, also their potential hazards, including the avoidance of the supine position to prevent cataract formation caused by apposition of the bubble to the lens. Irrigating solutions are discussed with emphasis on the requirements of pH, the presence of at least 400 mg/dl glucose, calcium, magnesium, glutathione and bicarbonate (in BSS plus) in appropriate concentrations to avoid toxic damage to tissue, especially lens and cornea. The section on fibroplasia indicates the physiological basis for current thinking about antifibroproliferative compounds. Importantly, the contribution of one of the authors (T.M.A.), namely, the role of the retinal pigment epithelium in fibroplasia, is discussed. Dosage and route of delivery for active antimetabolites remain a challenge as the search for a suitable antifibroproliferative drug and delivery continues. The next generation, beyond 5-fluorouracil, may include 5-fluorouridine [see: Blumenkranz, M. S., Hajek, A., Hernandez, E., and Hartzer, M. (1985): Fluorouridine: A second generation ocular antimetabolite. *Invest. Ophthalmol. Vis. Sci. ARVO Suppl.* 26(11):285.] Certainly the future is brighter than ever for patients with proliferative vitreoretinopathy.

The Editors

Surgical Pharmacology of the Eye,
edited by M. Sears and A. Tarkkanen.
Raven Press, New York © 1985.

Pharmacology of Surgery of the Vitreous and Retina

Thomas M. Aaberg and George A. Williams

Medical College of Wisconsin, Milwaukee, Wisconsin 53226

SUMMARY: The response of the eye to vitreous surgery depends on the basic disease state and the age of the patient. The extensive tissue manipulations required in vitreoretinal surgery precipitate an inflammatory response that manifests both intra- and postoperative complications. These responses may be mediated by the prostaglandin cycle so that prostaglandins, thromboxanes and leukotrienes have been increasingly implicated in the pathophysiology of the ocular reaction to trauma. Pharmacologic blockade of arachidonic acid therefore may ameliorate or prevent these complications. Examples of such problems include intraoperative miosis, requiring undesired lens extraction, and increased pre- and postoperative microvascular permeability giving rise to troublesome and catastrophic fibrinoid response. Topical nonsteroidal drugs, when combined with subconjunctival and retroseptal steroid drugs may additively or synergistically prevent or reduce these complications. Indomethacin inhibits the cyclooxygenase pathway while steroids inhibit the hydrolysis of arachidonic acid by phospholipase possibly preventing the diversion of arachidonic acid through the lipoxygenase pathway into the formation of leukotrienes, substances known to increase the cellular response to trauma. The combination therapy has theoretical advantages. Thus, while technical advances enable the vitreous surgeon to deal with unapproachable problems, the ultimate answer will be through an understanding of the pharmacologic basis of the disease process.

With the advent of vitrectomy, previously inoperable eyes have become salvageable and the adverse natural course of diseases such as diabetes and proliferative vitreoretinopathy has been interrupted. However, the technical advances of vitreous surgery are not without risk. Vitreous surgery exposes the eye to exogenous fluids and gases, intraocular medications, and instrumentation, and it disrupts intraocular anatomic integrity. These events have created both intraoperative and postoperative complications. Unfortunately, in some cases the recognition, understanding, and eventual elimination of these complications has lagged behind acceptance of the precipitating surgical procedures. For example, the clinical complications with intraocular solutions and gases lead to investigations disclosing the pathophysiology of their toxic side effects.

FACTORS MEDIATING THE OCULAR RESPONSE
TO VITREORETINAL PROCEDURES

Vitreoretinal procedures do not induce the same response in all eyes. The two most significant factors mediating the ocular response to vitreoretinal procedures are (a) the underlying disease state for which the surgery is performed and (b) the age of the patient. These factors may result in greatly different ocular responses among eyes undergoing the identical vitreoretinal procedure.

The importance of the precipitating disease state is most evident in diabetes. Diabetic eyes manifest different responses to vitreoretinal procedures and their complications than do nondiabetic eyes. In particular, diabetic eyes have an increased tendency to develop iris neovascularization and subsequent neovascular glaucoma following vitrectomy, especially if the lens is removed or absent (1,2). Iris neovascularization also occurs following vitrectomy if a rhegmatogenous retinal detachment develops. Nondiabetic eyes subjected to identical events do not manifest postoperative neovascularization as often. Thus, diabetic vitrectomy, which is an effective and beneficial procedure for the complications of proliferative retinopathy, results in complications that are mediated by the underlying disease process.

The increased incidence of postoperative iris neovascularization in diabetes probably reflects the preoperative neovascular state. How and why vitreous removal and/or lens removal alters the neovascular state is uncertain. In response to chronic retinal ischemia, still ill-defined events stimulate vascular endothelial cells to proliferate and organize into neovascularization that penetrates the internal limiting lamina and apposes the posterior cortical vitreous. This stimulates premature separation of the posterior cortical vitreous resulting in traction on the neovascularization that further enhances vessel growth. This cycle of traction-enhanced neovascular growth can be interrupted by removal of the posterior vitreous. With rare exceptions, retinal neovascularization does not progress following complete vitrectomy for as long as 68 months (2,3).

Interestingly, iris neovascularization, which also reflects retinal ischemia in diabetes, is enhanced by vitrectomy, particularly if the lens is also removed (1,2). Retinal detachment in vitrectomized diabetic eyes also stimulates iris neovascularization. Why vitreous removal inhibits retinal neovascularization but stimulates iris neovascularization is not known.

The sickle hemoglobinopathies are a second example of a disease state modifying the ocular response to vitreoretinal procedures. Retinal detachment surgery in patients with sickle hemoglobinopathies presents risks not usually seen in patients with normal hemoglobin profiles. In particular, anterior segment ischemia following scleral buckling has been described (4). This is due to intravascular sickling probably secondary to venous congestion induced by encircling scleral elements. These eyes also poorly tolerate even mild increases in intraocular pressure (IOP), which would be of no pathologic significance in patients with normal hemoglobin. Thus, it is apparent that disease states such as diabetes and the sickle hemoglobinopathies are important in determining the ocular response to vitreoretinal procedures.

The age of the patient is a second factor that mediates the ocular response to vitreoretinal procedures. For example, choroidal edema following scleral buckling for retinal detachment repair is related to the extent of vortex vein obstruction, but the degree to which the edema becomes manifest is directly related to the age of the patient (5–7). Older patients develop greater choroidal edema in response to vortex vein obstruction (7) than do younger patients with similar buckles. Animal studies have also shown an age-dependent response. In young rabbits, air and sulfur hexafluoride induce reduplication of corneal endothelial cells that is not seen in older rabbits (8).

THE OCULAR RESPONSE TO EXOGENOUS COMPOUNDS IN VITREORETINAL SURGERY

Replacement of the vitreous during and following vitrectomy surgery has introduced factors that influence the ocular response to vitreoretinal surgery and the eventual therapeutic result. These replacement substances can be divided into those of (a) short-term operative and postoperative duration (i.e., infusion solutions); (b) intermediate postoperative duration (i.e., expansile gases); and (c) indefinite postoperative duration (i.e., liquid silicone). Silicone will not be discussed in this chapter since its use in the United States is limited to early experience before advanced vitrectomy techniques. Discussion will be therefore limited to short- and intermediate-duration substances.

OPERATIVE INFUSION SOLUTIONS

Edelhauser and co-workers (9), through a series of elegant studies on animal and human corneal buttons, determined that intraocular infusion solution must have several characteristics: (a) the pH must be approximately 7.4; (b) glucose must be available to allow continued metabolism of the endothelium; (c) calcium and magnesium must be present to maintain the endothelial intercellular connections; and (d) glutathione should be present in an accessible form. Deficiency in any of these characteristics reduces the corneal tolerance to the infusion solution with subsequent corneal edema and opacification.

During phakic diabetic vitrectomy, infusion solutions may also have adverse effects on the lens resulting in cataract formation. Faulborn et al. (10) reported that 36% of initially clear diabetic lenses became opacified during vitrectomy. Such cataract change typically presents as a feathery separation of lens cortical fibers. It became intuitively apparent that although current improved intraocular solutions (9) contained glucose equivalent to the nondiabetic aqueous humor, the diabetic eye was accustomed to a hyperglycemic aqueous. This concept was tested and subsequently established by Haimann and co-workers (11). They found that a balanced salt solution (BSS Plus) with glucose concentration of 400 mg/dl prevented the formation of operative cataract in both diabetic rabbits and humans (11,12). Lensectomy becomes necessary when operative cataract formation significantly compromises visualization. The adverse clinical consequences of lensectomy in diabetic vitrectomy are well known. Lensectomy increases the postoperative incidence of iris neovascularization and neovascular glaucoma (1,2). By diminishing the intraoperative incidence of cataract formation, glucose-fortified infusion solutions have diminished another disease-mediated complication of vitreoretinal surgery.

INTERMEDIATE-DURATION VITREOUS REPLACEMENT

Although various substances have been tried as vitreous substitutes without widespread clinical acceptance (i.e., sodium hyaluronate, methylcellulose), gases have been utilized most frequently, the most common being sulfur hexafluoride (SF_6) (13). The physiologic expansile properties of SF_6 arise from the movement of nitrogen, oxygen, and carbon dioxide (the first being the only significant factor) from the blood into the SF_6 bubble (14). At the same time there is gradual diffusion of SF_6 from the bubble into the blood until there is an equilibration of all component partial pressures between the bubble and blood (Fig. 1) (14). A 100% SF_6 bubble expands within the eye 2.3 times the injected volume, reaching its final volume at a time dependent on the initial volume injected (14). In the rabbit, 0.85 cc of 100% SF_6 reached its maximum volume in 48 hr (14). The bubble slowly disappears over a period of 1-1/2 to 2-1/2 weeks. Other compounds, particularly the perfluorinated hydrocarbons and xenon gases, are less soluble than SF_6 and expand more slowly and persist within the eye for longer periods of time (15,16).

The adverse side effects of vitreous gas substitutes are determined by two factors: (a) the rate of expansion (and consequently the IOP rise) and (b) the toxicity of constant gas/tissue contact. The rise in IOP following gas injection is dependent on the amount and rate of expansion of the gas and the outflow facility of the eye. Concentrations of SF_6 greater than 18% are expansile and therefore may increase IOP. Killey et al. (17) demonstrated that despite continued expansion of a 100% SF_6 bubble, IOP stabilized 8 to 12 hr after injection of 100% SF_6 because of the linear relationship between outflow facility and IOP. However, in eyes with diminished facility of outflow, even minimal expansion may result in large increases in IOP. The wide variation in outflow facility and the difficulty in accurately determining the intraocular concentration of gas makes prediction of postoperative IOP very difficult. Excessive elevation of IOP can result in central retinal artery closure or optic nerve infarction. Abrams (18) has documented an 11% incidence of these complications using SF_6. He therefore recommends that the IOP be checked at 2, 6, and 12 hr postinjection (19).

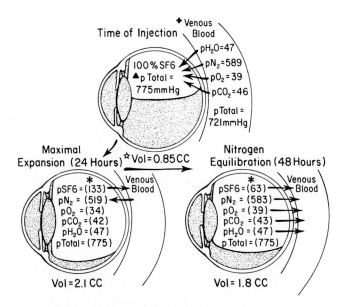

FIG. 1. Gas dynamics of an intravitreal SF_6 gas pocket. (Modified from ref. 14.)

The toxicity of direct gas-tissue contact appears to be negligible for the retina (20). However, there are toxic effects of SF_6 on the cornea and lens. Constant contact of SF_6 with the cornea damages the endothelium (8) and also may cause cataract formation, which makes positioning important in patients with intraocular gas. Aphakic patients may develop keratopathy or angle closure when in a supine position because of the anterior movement of the gas. Similarly, a supine position in a phakic patient may cause a cataract. Patients with intraocular gas must be instructed to avoid the supine position.

PHARMACOLOGIC AND MECHANICAL MODIFICATION OF PATHOPHYSIOLOGICAL RESPONSE TO VITREORETINAL TISSUE

Mechanical Modifications

Vitrectomy surgery for reattachment of the retina involved in the advanced states of proliferative vitreoretinopathy (PVR), previously referred to as massive periretinal proliferation (MPP), requires the mechanical removal of epiretinal and subretinal membranes and the hydraulic reattachment of the retina by pressurized air/fluid exchange. This creates an air-filled vitreous cavity milieu that alters ocular response to concurrent treatment modalities, such as photo-coagulation, cryotherapy, and antiproliferative compounds.

Vitreous membrane formation in the human is primarily a proliferation of cells. The cells initially proceed as a monolayer but then form a multilayered structure. As a monolayer, the cells are transparent except for variable pigment content. As the cell layer becomes increasingly stratified and as the myofibro-blastic elements contract, the membrane becomes ophthalmoscopically visible. Collagen is synthesized and added to the membrane structure. The neural retina of the embryonic chick synthesizes vitreous collagen similar to type II collagen (native human vitreous collagen) (21,22). In addition to this fibrillar collagen, which can be produced by proliferative neural derived cells, basement membrane (type IV) is a product of glial cells (Müller cells in intact retina) (23). Since these two morphologic types of collagen are present in the vitreous, it is not surprising that neural cells can secrete two types of collagen during embryogenesis and during ectopic proliferation along membranous structures.

DIFFUSE EPIRETINAL MEMBRANE AS A COMPONENT OF PVR

Contractile membranes covering the entire epiretinal surface are rare without actual retinal hole formation. Once a retinal break is present, pigment epithelial proliferation may ensue. Typically, pigment epithelium does not proliferate through intact retina but requires a full-thickness retinal break. In such an event, proliferation of pigment epithelial and glial cells proceeds on the inner and outer surfaces of the detached retina; hence, the term periretinal prolifer-ation or, more recently, PVR.

Pigment Epithelial Proliferation

In the cat, investigators have demonstrated that the loss or disruption of the normal metabolic exchange between pigment epithelium and photoreceptors appears to be the stimulus for the dedifferentiation of pigment epithelial cells and the resulting proliferative response (24). If the experimentally detached cat retina accurately reflects the time course of the response in other mammalian retinas, then this proliferative response occurs much sooner than had been previously reported. Labeled nuclei were noted at 24 hr after sensory retinal detachment. This is significant because the adult mammalian retinal pigment epithelium is mitotically inactive (24). The response is confined only to the zone of detachment and may continue even after retinal reattachment.

Aaberg and Machemer (25) first proposed and identified participation of the pigment epithelium in PVR. They showed that pigment epithelial cells extended around the edges of retinal tears from the subretinal space to form a monolayer of proliferation on the internal retinal surface. Near the retinal hole the epiretinal monolayer closely resembled *in situ* pigment epithelial cells, i.e., were cuboidal, with internally directed villi and spherical pigment granules. As the cells proliferated further from the hole, extending as an epiretinal monolayer, they underwent metaplasia, taking on a flattened appearance and losing both their internal villi and pigment granules. Although the cells undergo many cellular divisions, pigment is not renewed during the division, so the pigment content is very low (26). Eventually the pigment epithelial cells could not be distinguished from fibrocytes. Machemer and Laqua (26) further postulated that cells derived from pigment epithelium were responsible, at least in part, for retroretinal as well as pre- or epiretinal membrane formation.

Retinal pigment epithelial cells transplanted into the vitreous cavity in diffusion chambers undergo several forms of transformation: first into macrophages and then into spindle-shaped cells with collagen production and having epithelial cell characteristics (27). DNA replication as shown by autoradiography and loss of pigment granules indicated proliferation of the cells. These results further support the hypothesis that retinal pigment epithelial cell proliferation and transformation play a major role in the formation of collagen-containing membranes as found in proliferative vitreoretinopathy. In the vitreous cavity the cells are ophthalmoscopically visible in clusters like "tobacco dust." Those cells undergoing metaplasia multiply as fibroblast-like cells forming clusters and tissue membranes on surfaces such as the inner retinal surface, posterior vitreous surface, outer retinal surface, and even on the posterior lens surface. These cell clusters and tissue membranes are clinically visible as an opaque appearance to the retinal surface and occasional areas of pigmentation.

Astrocyte Proliferation

Retinal astrocytes show an increasing participation in the proliferative process as the epiretinal and vitreous membranes become established in the eye with a chronically detached sensory retina. These cells migrate through the internal and external limiting membranes of the retina and form localized membranes that sometimes cover large areas. The fibroblastic cells form fibrocytes and migrate toward cell-free spaces along available surfaces, which serve as templates for cellular adherence. As the cells move forward they become stretched, forming tensile or contractile forces (28).

Cytoplasmic filaments are found in both the metaplastic pigment epithelial cells and the proliferating astrocytic cells (29). Although the exact function of the cytoplasmic filaments is not known, it has been postulated that they are contractile (30).

Membrane Contraction

The temporal sequence of cellular proliferation, membrane formation, and membrane contraction is quite constant. Variation appears to depend on the size and number of retinal holes and thus the extent of the pigment epithelial cell "inoculum." Characteristically, contraction occurs 6 to 8 weeks after repair of a retinal detachment, which is performed 1 to 2 weeks after onset of the retinal detachment.

The fibroblast is a pluripotent cell adapting to different situations by changing morphologic, biochemical, and functional features. Thus, during wound healing there is a transformation of local fibroblasts and fewer differentiated cells into myofibroblasts (31), the same occurrence as in periretinal membranes. These transformed fibroblasts acquire contractile apparatus responsible for the mechanism of membrane contraction. A fibrillar system develops in the transformed fibroblasts—not the few fibrils seen in normal fibroblasts but bundles of parallel fibrils resembling those of smooth-muscle cells (32). The fibrils measure 40 to 80 Å in diameter (rarely, 100 to 120 Å) and are usually arranged parallel to the long axis of the cell. There are numerous intercellular connections between membrane tissue fibroblasts (32). These connections, together with a well-defined layer of material having the structural characteristics of a basal lamina, allow the membrane tissue to contract as a sheet-like structure.

Pharmacologically the transformed fibroblasts (myofibroblasts) contract and relax like smooth muscle (33). Cellular strips contract in response to 5-hydroxytryptamine, angiotensin, vasopressin, norepinephrine, bradykinin, epinephrine, and prostaglandin $F_{1\alpha}$. The cells fix antiactin and antimyosin antibodies, supporting the possibility that a mechanism involving an interaction between actin and myosin is responsible for the contraction.

It therefore now appears that the forces producing membrane contraction lie in the proliferative tissue. A relationship between intracytoplasmic filaments and cellular motion, development of tension and intracytoplasmic movements, has been proposed for a wide spectrum of cells. In proliferative membrane tissue, the contraction of a single myofibroblast is then transmitted as synchronized responses to the other cells and the secondary collagen stroma produced by the fibroblasts. The end result is massive membrane contraction.

Although contractile forces are exerted early in the development of the membranes, initially the changes are clinically not detectable. Contraction along vitreous scaffolds usually goes undetected. On the surface of the retina a slight tortuosity of blood vessels may herald the presence of future contraction. As the contractile forces become stronger than the structural force of the retina, retinal folds develop and an immobile detached retina occurs.

The role of collagen in the process of contraction has been debated. It is known, however, that collagen does not contract, as such, and only undergoes shortening when denatured (34). Therefore, the proliferative cells are implicated in producing the contractile forces, whereas the collagen, which is responsible for the whitish appearance of the intravitreal tissue, contributes to the stabilization of the contracted membrane. Membranes are not condensations of preexisting vitreous collagen. The collagen present in the membrane, other than the scaffold on which it grows, is new or secondary collagen.

Classification of PVR or MPP

The recent reclassification by the American Retina Society has subdivided PVR into four grades (minimal, moderate, marked, and massive) (35).

Grade A

Grade A findings are encountered in practically all rhegmatogenous retinal detachments, although these same clinical manifestations, when progressive, may be the harbinger of relentless cellular proliferation. Vitreous haze and pigment clumps mark this category.

Grade B

In grade B the proliferating cells are forming clumps or masses, and focal wrinkling of the retina occurs.

Grade C

In grade C, contraction is already beginning, giving rise to fixed retinal folds, i.e., star folds. Although the full extent of grade C may not be clinically appreciated, the critical point is that once contraction of the membranes begins, cellular proliferation has now developed over most, if not all, available surfaces. Grade C is subdivided as follows: C-1, no more than one quadrant of fixed folds; C-2, between one and two quadrants of fixed folds; C-3, between two and three quadrants of fixed folds.

Opacification of the vitreous gel progressively increases at this grade as diffuse cellular proliferation and membrane formation on the posterior vitreous hyaloid surface increases. The posterior membrane may have round or oval dehiscences, with anteroposteriorly oriented strands that are under considerable tension decreasing the mobility of the vitreous gel.

The preretinal component may be more clinically suggestive than apparent at this grade. Irregular reflexes on the retinal surface, ("cellophane appearance") secondary to wrinkling of the internal limiting membrane, characterize the development of large, thin epiretinal membranes. Vessels become less visible and more tortuous as the retina becomes less mobile with a fixed configuration of folds. An important clinical consequence of this manifestation of early PVR is that the anatomic geography of the subretinal fluid may no longer be determined by location of the retinal hole, since the epiretinal and anterior-posterior vitreal forces may now be the main causative forces in the production of the retinal detachment.

Grade D

Grade D refers to fixed folds in all four quadrants. Grade D represents a progression of architecture, mainly in the dynamics of contracture and increasing collagen deposition, fixing the contracted retinal folds. The ophthalmoscopic appearance of vitreous, epiretinal, and subretinal membranes becomes more pronounced. The posterior vitreous membranes become very rigid and prominent. The anterior vitreous is heavily opacified, with strands and pigmented cell clusters. The volume of the anterior vitreous space is reduced as liquefied vitreous is forced posteriorly through gaps in the posterior vitreous membrane, with the retina, in turn, pulled increasingly toward the center of the vitreous cavity. This explains the anterior-posterior orientation of the vitreous strands.

Very typical of grade D is the development of a circumferential equatorial rigid retinal fold caused by rigid organization of the vitreous base by proliferating cells. The equatorial retina is pulled toward the optic axis by contraction of these proliferating cells causing: (a) the retina to detach beyond the ora serrata, and (b) drape-like retinal folds pointing toward the disc from the contracted equatorial retina. Because the proliferating membrane extends forward along the vitreous base over the pars plana, contracting axially as it proceeds forward, it is necessary at the time of vitrectomy surgery to make relaxing cuts through this membrane anteriorly over the ora serrata. If this is not accomplished, the retina is held taut in clothesline fashion by the contracted vitreous base, and subretinal fluid leaks anteriorly after subsequent scleral buckling with failure of the operation.

When all of the posterior retinal surface is folded, with the posterior vitreous plane contracted, a typical funnel-shape configuration of PVR D-3 results. In grade D-1 there is a wide funnel. Grade D-2 refers to a narrow funnel. In grade D-3 the funnel is closed so that the optic disc is no longer visible. The anterior retina is fixed centrally by the contracted vitreous membrane to such an intense degree that the resulting funnel precludes any view of the optic disc, i.e., "closed funnel." Because of the decreased transparency of the irregular retinal surface, subretinal membranes (strands) may not be visualized, although they are present in most cases and are the same as the vitreous membrane (strands), hence the term proliferative vitreoretinopathy (PVR) or massive periretinal proliferation (MPP). The subretinal membranes also contract. Anteriorly, when retinal detachment progresses beyond the ora serrata, this membrane is termed "ringschwiele." Posteriorly the subretinal membranes become fenestrated as they contract, forming long taut strands. In general, subretinal membranes do not adhere as strongly to the retina as epiretinal membranes, but they may be very taut, preventing retinal reattachment unless they are surgically severed.

The vital question, as yet unanswered, is why certain eyes with rhegmatogenous retinal detachment develop PVR. Certainly the basis for PVR, dispersion of pigment epithelial cells throughout the vitreous body, is present in essentially all eyes with rhegmatogenous retinal detachment. Only a small percentage (probably 5% to 8%) of such eyes develop a membranous proliferation that encompasses the entire available retinal surface and contracts to form PVR

D-3. Why proliferation aborts at a subclinical stage is the unknown. When such an answer is available, it may well serve as a key to future therapy of the problem.

Surgical Therapy

Removal of the epiretinal membranes, as well as the anterior-posterior transvitreal bands, is the goal in the treatment of retinal detachment complicated by PVR (36). This can be accomplished by using liquid silicone to dissect bluntly the membranes from the retina by the hydraulic injection force. Silicone then fills the vitreous cavity, completely forcing the retina back to the pigment epithelium (37). This technique, while successful in some cases, has the potential disadvantages of leaving the proliferative tissue within the vitreous cavity, leaving the vitreous opacities, and risking the toxicity of the liquid silicone.

The advanced techniques of vitrectomy have made actual removal of proliferative tissue from the eye a promising reality. The initial step in the operative procedure posterior vitrectomy is releasing all anterior/posterior traction including as much circumferential vitreous base traction as possible. Tangential epiretinal traction is then released by either stripping or segmenting epiretinal membranes releasing all fixed folds (38). A test for adequate release of traction is performed by exchanging the vitreal infusion solution with air by a constant air infusion pump (39). This pressurized air insufflation of the vitreous cavity hydraulically reattaches the retina by allowing drainage of subretinal fluid (SRF) through a preexisting posterior retinal hole or a deliberately created retinotomy.

If the retina does not totally flatten, residual traction, either epiretinal or subretinal, is present. If the residual traction is due to subretinal proliferative material, additional retinotomies are performed and the subretinal bands removed. At this point, the retina is anatomically in the correct position, although it is maintained by a most unnatural condition, i.e., pressurized air infusion. Once the retina is reattached, an adhesive modality is necessary to initiate cellular adhesion between sensory retina and pigment epithelium. Cryotherapy can be performed transsclerally or internally but is less desirable from a technical and functional aspect than endophotocoagulation. Since xenon endophotocoagulation cannot be utilized in an air-filled cavity, argon endophotocoagulation is the preferred modality (40). Argon burns are placed confluently around all premarked retinal holes, and a triple row of burns is placed confluently on the buckle and posteriorly, creating a demarcation line that will delimit any recurrent anterior detachment secondary to unrelieved vitreous base traction. Photocoagulation of retina in contact with air, rather than fluid, creates potential hazards. Without a fluid heat-sink to dissipate tissue heat during the photocoagulation process, excessive treatment is possible, resulting in immediate retinal dissolution or late necrosis. This hole formation can result in repeat retinal detachment. Use of long-duration (0.5 sec) burns of low energy, preferably with the blue wavelength filtered out to minimize inner layer damage, may diminish hole formation. Positioning of the patient postoperatively is necessary to continue the tamponade of the retinal holes by air until the reaction is of adequate strength (3 to 4 days).

The success of the above procedure is dependent on the ability to prevent reproliferation of epiretinal or subretinal membranes. Prevention of reproliferation depends on pharmacologic inhibition of cellular proliferation. Many compounds have been considered and experimentally evaluated. Tano et al. (41) have examined the use of triamcinolone acetonide, blocking mitotic activity and creating an inhibitory effect on the growth of fibroblasts. Although possibly useful as an adjunctive agent, steroids do not prevent reproliferation to the degree necessary for long-term success. Recent data by Blumenkranz et al. (42), utilizing 5-fluorouracil, appears to be the scientific breakthrough that was necessary (7). Fluorouracil inhibits thymidylate synthetase and interferes with DNA synthesis, thereby halting cellular proliferation. A 1-mg intravitreal injection of fluorouracil is effective in an experimental model of PVR. Fluorouracil decreased the rate of tractional retinal detachment from 36.8% to 5.2% at 1 week and from 73.6% to 31.5% at 4 weeks. Thus, the inhibition was less as time increased in the postoperative period, corresponding to clinical observations that fluorouracil-treated eyes develop proliferation at a later time and to a lesser degree (38). An additional point of interest was that intraocular neovascularization was reduced from 36.8% in controls to 5.2% in treated eyes, a possible consideration for diabetic cases developing iris neovascularizations after vitrectomy (42). When supplemented by 10 mg subconjunctival injections of fluorouracil, the inhibitory effect was enhanced. This report has led to an ongoing clinical study that appears to confirm the experimental studies (*unpublished data*).

The optimal dosage and route of administration for fluorouracil remains to be determined. Both subconjunctival and intravitreal administration has been suggested. In rabbits, subconjunctival injection of 6.25 mg fluorouracil results in peak aqueous levels of 69.5 μg/ml and peak vitreous levels of 10.5 μg/ml (43). Intravitreal injections, of course, result in higher levels and have a greater risk of toxicity. In rabbits, after vitrectomy and lensectomy, intravitreal injection of 0.5 mg fluorouracil every 24 hr for 7 days resulted in no clinical histologic or electrophysiologic evidence of toxicity (44). Higher dosages and more frequent administration resulted in significant toxicity (45). Electrophysiologic and histologic studies in vitrectomized rabbits suggest that levels as high as 250 μg/ml are well tolerated (45). However, the toxicity of fluorouracil in air-filled eyes is not known. The study of the pharmacokinetics and toxicity of fluorouracil in humans will require well-designed protocols to ascertain the optimal use of this agent. Nonetheless, preliminary clinical experience suggests that a single 1-mg intravitreal injection at the end of surgery, supplemented by daily 10-mg subconjunctival injections for 5 days, will produce a marked reduction in intraocular proliferation (*unpublished data*). Additional therapy with other agents, such as corticosteroids, may provide adjunctive therapy to retard proliferation in PVR surgery.

ARACHIDONIC-ACID-MEDIATED COMPLICATIONS OF VITREORETINAL SURGERY

Prostaglandins, thromboxanes, and more recently, leukotrienes have become increasingly implicated in the pathophysiology of ocular disease. It is apparent that these arachidonic acid (AA) derivatives are important in vitreoretinal diseases and surgery. Aberration of normal prostaglandin metabolism in diseases such as diabetes may contribute to their vitreoretinal manifestations. Also, prostaglandin release during surgical trauma may mediate various intraoperative or postoperative complications. The following paragraphs review prostaglandin-mediated phenomena in vitreoretinal surgery, discussing possible beneficial pharmacologic manipulation of AA metabolism.

Prostaglandins are labile compounds of relatively short biologic half-life, produced in response to a variety of stimuli. They are most active locally at the site of their production and are then degraded. Thus, sustained prostaglandin activity requires continued local prostaglandin production. The primary prostaglandin precursor is AA, a polyunsaturated fatty acid that is bound (esterified) to membrane phospholipids. Initiation of prostaglandin synthesis requires hydrolysis of AA from esterification sites in membrane phospholipids by phospholipases. The major phospholipase is phospholipase A_2 which cleaves AA from phosphatidylcholine, phosphatidylinositol, phosphatidylserine, and phosphatidylethanolamine. A second enzyme, phospholipase C, is active in platelets, removing inositol from phosphatidylinositol and leaving a diacylglyceride that requires a diglyceride lipase for AA release. Phospholipases are activated by a variety of chemical and mechanical stimuli, including surgical trauma, thereby resulting in AA release. Corticosteroids affect prostaglandin (PG) production through inhibition of phospholipase activity by an unknown mechanism that requires protein synthesis.

Following release from phospholipids, the majority of AA is reacylated back to phospholipids. The remainder is metabolized via two pathways (46). The lipoxygenase pathway results in the formation of hydroperoxyeicosatetraeinoic acid (HPETE) and the leukotrienes (47). The leukotrienes are important inflammatory mediators that affect microvascular permeability, chemotaxis, and PMN lysozyme release. Slow-reacting substance of anaphylaxis, SRS-A, consists of leukotrienes. Recently, leukotriene production and slow-reacting substance-like activity have been demonstrated in rabbit uvea (48). These compounds may be important mediators of intraocular leukocyte responses and inflammation.

The lipoxygenase pathway may act independently or, as in some tissue systems, in conjunction with the second pathway of AA metabolism, the PG synthetase complex. This microsomal complex mediates two enzymatic functions. The first is mediated by cyclooxygenase (CO), which adds molecular oxygen to AA and cyclizes it to the cyclic endoperoxide PGG_2. Nonsteroid anti-inflammatory agents affect PG synthesis by blocking CO activity (49). PGG_2, in turn, is acted on by the second enzyme of the complex, peroxidase, converting PGG_2 to PGH_2 with subsequent release of oxygen radicals. PGH_2 represents the primary precursor for subsequent prostaglandin and thromboxane (TX) production. Which specific PG or TX is produced is dependent on tissue-specific localization of several enzymes. Isomerases and reductases convert PGH_2 to one or more of the classic or primary prostaglandins (PGE_2, $PGF_{2\alpha}$, PGD_2). In endothelial cells prostacyclin synthetase produces prostacyclin. In platelets, TXA_2 is produced by TX synthetase; in mast cells and basophils an isomerase produces PGD_2. Thus, formation of PGH_2 derivatives is a tissue-specific event. Ocular tissue can convert AA into all of the above prostaglandins, thromboxanes, and leukotrienes (48,50).

The exact physiologic role of arachidonic derivatives in ocular disease remains to be elucidated. It is known that some prostaglandins such as PGF, $PGF_{2\alpha}$ can cause increased intraocular pressure, miosis, and increased vascular permeability (51). The precise role of other arachidonic derivatives, such as prostacyclin, TXA_2, and the leukotrienes in ocular disease is not yet known. However, they appear to be crucial factors in the ocular inflammatory response. An understanding of the ocular activities of these individual compounds and their composite ocular effects should provide significant insight into ocular pathophysiology.

We will now discuss possible applications of AA metabolism to vitreoretinal surgery and suggest possible therapeutic pharmacologic intervention.

The tissue insult of vitreoretinal surgery induces an inflammatory response that is at least in part mediated by AA derivatives. Ambache (52) described formation of a lipid soluble compound in the aqueous following mechanical iris stimulation that produced miosis, increased intraocular pressure, and increased vascular permeability. Subsequent studies identified this compound as a mixture of prostaglandins (53).

Surgically induced increases in PG generation occur in human aqueous following anterior segment surgery (54), ciliary body cryopexy, and iris photocoagulation (55). Presumably, the mechanical trauma of surgery activates phospholipases with subsequent PG release. The physiologic sequelae of intraoperative PG release can pose significant problems for the vitreoretinal surgeon. The extensive tissue manipulations required in vitreoretinal surgery may precipitate an inflammatory response that manifests both intraoperative and postoperative complications. Pharmacologic blockade of AA metabolism may ameliorate or prevent these complications.

Intraoperative miosis resulting from PG release is a significant complication to the vitreoretinal surgeon. In phakic vitrectomies, miosis may enhance lenticular or media opacities preventing adequate visualization and necessitating lensectomy. We have noted intraoperative miosis to be a particular problem in diabetic vitrectomies. In patients with preoperatively marginally clear lenses, miosis may require lensectomy resulting in an increased incidence of neovascular glaucoma. Thus, a PG-mediated intraoperative complication may resut in significant postoperative complications. Miosis is also a problem in diabetic patients undergoing lensectomy prior to posterior vitrectomy. The anterior segment trauma of lensectomy may result in significant miosis, denying the surgeon optimal visualization for posterior techniques.

Topical indomethacin diminishes intraoperative miosis during extracapsular cataract extraction (56). Indomethacin blocks cyclooxygenase, thereby preventing subsequent PG production (54). We believe that topical indomethacin diminishes miosis during vitrectomy and use it routinely.

Following vitrectomy, diabetic patients and older patients have a tendency to develop a marked fibrinoid response with the formation of fibrin membranes in the anterior chamber, across the pupillary space, and posteriorly. This is particularly common following fluid-air exchanges. Although usually a transient event, these membranes may complicate postoperative management by decreasing visualization or increasing IOP. Fibrin deposition into the eye reflects increased microvascular permeability. In diabetics, the exaggerated fibrin response results from an already compromised blood-aqueous barrier and hyperfibrinogenemia. Surgically induced PG generation further enhances microvascular permeability in diabetes. Sanders et al. (57) have shown that topical 1% indomethacin diminishes microvascular leakage following cataract surgery. We feel topical indomethacin has a similar beneficial effect following vitreoretinal surgery.

Another complication of vitrectomy surgery that may be PG-mediated is bleeding from small vessels. This bleeding may be due to increased intraocular levels of prostacyclin. Prostacyclin is a potent endogenous antiplatelet agent and vasodilator. There are very high levels of prostacyclin derivatives in secondary aqueous (58). It is reasonable to speculate that high levels of prostacyclin produced locally in the eye could compromise platelet function and maintain vasodilation in ocular vascular beds, resulting in the recurrent bleeding problems encountered clinically. Inhibition of prostacyclin by topical indomethacin could prove beneficial in this problem.

It is apparent that topical indomethacin may be of value in prevention or amelioration of AA-mediated surgical complications. However, despite high aqueous levels of indomethacin, following topical administration (59), ocular prostaglandin generation is not completely inhibited (60). For this reason we also use topical, subconjunctival, and retroseptal steroids in conjunction with topical indomethacin. This provides inhibition of PG production at two sites: (a) inhibition of phospholipase by corticosteroids and, (b) inhibition of cyclooxygenase by indomethacin. These effects are probably synergistic (61). In addition, selective inhibition of cyclooxygenase activity by topical indomethacin with continued production of AA may present new problems. If cyclooxygenase is blocked, AA may be shunted into the lipoxygenase pathway with subsequent production of leukotrienes. This has been shown in animal models (48,61). The result is that the chemotactic leukotrienes increase the leukocytic cellular response. Thus, topical indomethacin increases the cellular response to inflammation. Considering the mitogenic potential of leukocytes, this response may be detrimental in entities such as PVR.

The vitreoretinal surgeon thus is confronted with ocular pathology that is modified by a variety of pharmacologically mediated processes interrelating the underlying disease state and the basic tissue-aging state. Although technical advances in instrumentation enable the surgeon to deal with previously unapproachable problems, as well as handling a variety of difficult complications, the ultimate answer will be through the understanding of the physiologic and pharmacologic basis of disease processes.

REFERENCES

1. Aaberg, T. M. (1981): Pars plana vitrectomy for diabetic traction retinal detachment. *Ophthalmology,* 88:639.
2. Rice, T. A., Michels, R. G., Maguire, M. G., and Rice, E. F. (1983): The effect of lensectomy on the incidence of iris neovascularization and neovascular glaucoma after vitrectomy for diabetic retinopathy. *Am. J. Ophthalmol.,* 95:1.
3. Rice, T. A., Michels, R. G. (1980): Long-term anatomic and functional results of vitrectomy for diabetic retinopathy. *Am. J. Ophthalmol.,* 90:297.
4. Ryan, S. J., and Goldberg, M. F. (1969): Anterior segment ischemia following scleral buckling in sickle cell hemoglobinopathy. *Am. J. Ophthalmol.,* 81:512–517.
5. Aaberg, T. M. (1975): Experimental serous and hemorrhagic uveal edema associated with retinal detachment surgery. *Invest. Ophthalmol. Vis. Sci.,* 14:243.
6. Aaberg, T. M., and Maggiano, J. M. (1979): Choroidal edema associated with retinal detachment repair: Experimental and clinical correlation. *Mod. Probl. Ophthalmol.,* 20:6.
7. Packer, A. J., Maggiano, J. M., Aaberg, T. M., et al. (1983): Serous choroidal detachment after retinal detachment surgery. *Arch. Ophthalmol.,* 101:1221–1224.
8. Van Horn, D. L., Edelhauser, H. F., and Aaberg, T. M. (1972): In vivo effects of air and sulfur hexafluoride gas on rabbit corneal endothelium. *Invest. Ophthalmol. Vis. Sci.,* 11:1028.
9. Edelhauser, H. F., Van Horn, D. L., Schultz, R. O., and Hyndiuk, R. A. (1976): Comparative toxicity of intraocular irrigating solutions. *Am. J. Ophthalmol.,* 81:474.
10. Faulborn, J., Conway, B. T., and Machemer, R. (1978): Surgical complications of pars plana vitreous surgery. *Ophthalmology,* 851:116–125.
11. Haimann, M. H., Abrams, G. W., Edelhauser, H. F., and Hatchell, D. L. (1982): The effect of intraocular irrigating solution on lens clarity in normal and diabetic rabbits. *Am. J. Ophthalmol.,* 94:594.
12. Haimann, M. H., and Abrams, G. W. (1984): Prevention of lens opacity in diabetic vitrectomy. *Ophthalmology,* 91:116–121.
13. Aaberg, T. M., Abrams, G. W., and Edelhauser, H. F. (1977): Intraocular sulfur hexafluoride: An experimental and clinical correlation. *New and Controversial Aspects of Vitreoretinal Surgery,* edited by A. McPherson, p. 393. C. V. Mosby, St. Louis.
14. Abrams, G. W., Edelhauser, H. F., Aaberg, T. M., and Hamilton, L. H. (1974): Dynamics of intravitreal sulfur hexafluoride gas. *Invest. Ophthalmol. Vis. Sci.,* 13:863.
15. Lincoff, A., Lincoff, H., Solorgano, C., and Iwanoto, T. (1982): Selection of xenon gas for rapidly disappearing retinal tamponade. *Arch. Ophthalmol.,* 100:996.
16. Lincoff, H., Mardirossian, J., and Lincoff, A. (1980): Intravitreal longevity of three perfluorocarbon gases. *Arch. Ophthalmol.,* 98:1610.
17. Killey, F. P., Edelhauser, H. F., and Aaberg, T. M. (1980): Intraocular fluid dynamics.

Measurements following vitrectomy and intraocular sulfur hexafluoride administration. *Arch. Ophthalmol.*, 98:1448.

18. Abrams, G. W., Swanson, D. E., Iabates, W. E., and Goldman, A. I. (1982): Results of sulfur hexafluoride gas in vitreous surgery. *Am. J. Ophthalmol.*, 94:165.
19. Abrams, G. W. (1983): Results of sulfur hexafluoride gas in vitreous surgery. Reply to letter to editor. *Am. J. Ophthalmol.*, 96:406.
20. Fineberg, E., Machemer, R., Sullivan, P., Norton, E. W. D., Hamasaki, D., and Anderson, D. (1975): Sulfur hexafluoride in owl-monkey vitreous cavity. *Am. J. Ophthalmol.*, 79:67.
21. Newsome, D., Linsenmayer, T., and Trelstad, R. (1976): Vitreous body collagen. Evidence for a dual origin from the neural retina and hyalocytes. *J. Cell. Biol.*, 71:59.
22. Von der Mark, K., von der Mark, H., Timpl, R., and Trelstad, R. (1977): Immunofluorescent localization of collagen types I, II and III in the embryonic chick eye. *Dev. Biol.*, 59:75–85.
23. Uga, S., and Smelser, G. (1973): Electron microscopic study of the development of retinal mullerian cells. *Invest. Ophthalmol. Vis. Sci.*, 12:295.
24. Anderson, D. H., Stern, W. H., Fisher, S. K., Erickson, P. A., and Borgula, G. A. (1981): The onset of pigment epithelial proliferation after retinal detachment. *Invest. Ophthalmol. Vis. Sci.*, 21:10.
25. Aaberg, T. M., and Machemer, R. (1970): Correlation of naturally occurring retinal detachments with long-term retinal detachment in the owl-monkey. *Am. J. Ophthalmol.*, 69:640.
26. Machemer, R., and Laqua, H. (1975): Pigmented epithelial proliferation in retinal detachment (massive periretinal proliferation). *Am. J. Ophthalmol.*, 80:1.
27. Mueller-Jensen, K., Machemer, R., and Azarnia, J. (1975): Autotransplantation of retinal pigment epithelium in intravitreal diffusion chamber. *Am. J. Ophthalmol.*, 80:530.
28. Machemer, R., Van Horn, D., and Aaberg, T. M. (1978): Pigment epithelial proliferation in human retinal detachment with massive periretinal proliferation. *Am. J. Ophthalmol.*, 85:181.
29. Van Horn, D. L., Aaberg, T. M., Machemer, R., and Fenzl, R. (1977): Glial cells proliferation in human retinal detachment with massive periretinal proliferation. *Am. J. Ophthalmol.*, 84:383.
30. Newsome, D. A., and Kenyon, R. (1973): Collagen production in vitro by the retinal pigmented epithelium of the chick embryo. *Dev. Biol.*, 32:387–400.
31. Gabbiani, G., Hirschel, B. J., Ryan, G. B., Statkov, P. R., and Majno, G. (1972): Granulation tissue as a contractile organ. A study of structure and function. *J. Exp. Med.*, 135:719.
32. Gabbiani, G., Ryan, G. B., and Majno, G. (1971): Presence of modified fibroblasts in granulation tissue and their possible role in wound contraction. *Experientia*, 27:549.
33. Majno, G., Gabbiani, G., Hirschel, B. J., Ryan, G. B., and Statkov, P. R. (1971): Contraction of granulation tissue in vitro: Similarity to smooth muscle. *Science*, 173:548.
34. Peacock, E. E., and Van Winkle, W. (1970): *Surgery and Biology of Wound Repair*, p. 49. W. B. Saunders, Philadelphia.
35. The Retina Society Terminology Committee. (1983): The classification of retinal detachment with proliferative vitreoretinopathy. *Ophthalmology*, 90:121–125.
36. Machemer, R., and Aaberg, T. M. (1979): *Vitrectomy*, 2nd ed., pp. 86–89. Grune & Stratton, New York.
37. Scott, J. D. (1975): The treatment of massive vitreous retraction by the separation of preretinal membranes using liquid silicone. *Mod. Probl. Ophthalmol.*, 15:285.
38. Meredith, T. A., Kaplan, H. J., and Aaberg, T. M. (1980): Pars plana vitrectomy techniques for relief of epiretinal traction by membrane segmentation. *Am. J. Ophthalmol.*, 89:408–413.
39. Hueneke, R. L., and Aaberg, T. M. (1983): Instrumentation for continuous fluid-air exchange during vitreous surgery. *Am. J. Ophthalmol.*, 96:547–548.
40. Fleischman, J. A., Swartz, M., and Dixon, J. A. (1981): Argon laser endophotocoagulation. *Arch. Ophthalmol.*, 99:1610–1613.
41. Tano, Y., Chandler, D., and Machemer, R. (1980): Treatment of intraocular proliferation with intravitreal injection of triamcinolone acetonide. *Am. J. Ophthalmol.*, 90:810.
42. Blumenkranz, M. S., Ophir, A., Claflin, A. J., and Hajek, A. (1982): Fluorouracil for the treatment of massive periretinal proliferation. *Am. J. Ophthalmol.*, 94:458.
43. Rootman, J., Tisdall, J., Gudauskas, G., and Ostry, A. (1979): Intraocular penetration of subconjunctivally administered 14C-fluorouracil in rabbits. *Arch. Ophthalmol.*, 97:2375.
44. Stern, W. H., Guerin, C. J., Erickson, P. A., et al. (1983): Ocular toxicity of fluorouracil after vitrectomy. *Am. J. Ophthalmol.*, 96:43–51.

45. Barrada, A., Peyman, G. A., and Greenburg, D. (1983): Toxicity of antineoplastic drugs in vitrectomy infusion fluids. *Ophthalmic Surg.,* 14:845–847.
46. Kuehl, F. A., and Egan, R. W. (1980): Prostaglandins, arachidonic acid and inflammation. *Science,* 210:978.
47. Samuelson, B. (1980): Leukotrienes, a new group of biologically active compounds including SRS-A. *Trends Pharmacol. Sci.,* 9:227.
48. Kulkarni, P. S., and Srinivasan, B. D. (1983): Synthesis of slow reacting substance-like activity in rabbit conjunctiva and anterior uvea. *Invest. Ophthalmol. Vis. Sci.,* 24:1079–1085.
49. Vane, J. R. (1971): Inhibition of prostaglandin synthesis as a mechanism of action for aspirin-like drugs. *Nature,* 231:232.
50. Bhattacherjee, P., Kulkarni, P. S., and Eakins, K. E. (1979): Metabolism of arachidonic acid in rabbit ocular tissue. *Invest. Ophthalmol. Vis. Sci.,* 18:172.
51. Waitzman, M. B., and King, C. D. (1967): Prostaglandin influences on intraocular pressure and pupil size. *Am. J. Physiol.,* 212:329.
52. Ambache, N. (1957): Properties of irin, a physiological constituent of the rabbit's iris. *J. Physiol.(Lond.),* 135:114.
53. Ambache, N., and Brummer, H. C. (1968): A simple chemical procedure for distinguishing E from F prostaglandins with application to tissue extracts. *Br. J. Pharm. Chemother.,* 33:162.
54. Miyake, K., Sugiyama, S., Norimatsu, I., and Ozawa, T. (1978): Prevention of cystoid macular edema after lens extraction by topical indomethacin. Radioimmunoassay measurement of prostaglandins in the aqueous during and after lens extraction procedures. *Albrecht v. Graefes Arch. Klin. Exp. Ophthalmol.,* 209:83.
55. Chavis, R. M., Vygantas, C. M., and Vygantas, A. (1976): Experimental inhibition of prostaglandin-like inflammatory response after cryotherapy. *Am. J. Ophthalmol.,* 82:310.
56. Sawa, M., and Masuda, K. (1976): Topical indomethacin in soft cataract aspiration. *Jpn. J. Ophthalmol.,* 20:514.
57. Sanders, D. R., Kraff, M. C., Lieberman, H. L., et al. (1982): Breakdown and reestablishment of blood-aqueous barrier with implant surgery. *Arch. Ophthalmol.,* 100:588.
58. Ledbetter, S. R., Hatchell, D. L., and O'Brien, W. J. (1981): Differential effect of secondary aqueous humor from rabbit and cat on DNA synthesis of cultured bovine corneal endothelial cells. *Curr. Eye Res.,* 1:723.
59. Sanders, D. R., Goldstick, B., Kraff, M. C., et al. (1983): Aqueous penetration of oral and topical indomethacin in humans. *Arch. Ophthalmol.,* 101:1614.
60. Kulkarni, P. S., and Srinivasan, B. D. (1981): Effect of topical and intraperitoneal indomethacin on the generation of PGE$_2$-like activity in rabbit conjunctiva and iris ciliary body. *Exp. Eye Res.,* 33:121.
61. Kulkarni, P. S., Bhattacherjee, P., Eakin, K. E., and Srinivasan, B. D. (1981): Antiinflammatory effects of betamethasone phosphate, dexamethasone phosphate and indomethacin on rabbit ocular inflammation induced by bovine serum albumin. *Curr. Eye Res.,* 1:43.

Commentary

Radiation Therapy in the Management of Ocular
and Adnexal Tumors

Current choices of radiation therapy in the management of ocular and adnexal malignancies are brilliantly summarized by Dr. Char. There is controversy about the management of choroidal melanomas. The trend now appears to be "conservative". The author points out that for small and medium sized melanomas (less than 15 mm in diameter, less than 5 mm thick) several treatment modalities are available, brachytherapy and charged particles. Thick tumors and those situated 4–8 mm from the optic nerve and fovea are, perhaps, best treated with charged particles without delivering significant amounts of radiation to either of these structures while other tumors in this group may be successfully treated with simple and cheap radioactive plaque therapy.

Other non-radiation treatment modalities to these tumors include surgical excision, xenon-beam or laser photocoagulation and/or cryotherapy. For large melanomas (over 15 mm in diameter, and 5 mm in thickness) only charged particle irradiation can be employed. The visual acuity in these eyes is usually poor so that the other treatment of choice with a functioning second eye is certainly enucleation. Of the 500 patients so far treated with charged particles 10% of the eyes have developed neovascular glaucoma, especially when very large tumors were treated. Scleral melt, lack of tumor control, lid telangiectasia, increased subretinal fluid, lash loss, closure of the lacrimal drainage system and other complications have also been observed. At the moment this treatment modality is available in San Francisco (helium ions) and in Boston (proton beam) as well as in Lausanne, Switzerland. The cost of the equipment (up to 2 million U.S. dollars) plus the required personnel will limit this treatment to a few centers in the world. Perhaps, one-eyed patients with malignant melanoma of the choroid would make a priority group for this treatment.

A prospective randomized treatment trial is now beginning in the United States to determine whether preenucleation irradiation will alter the incidence of metastatic disease. A total dose of 20 Gy was selected. Of the 30 patients with large uveal melanomas treated so far 14% developed metastases within a mean follow-up of 25 months. This low figure may certainly justify a larger prospective randomized trial.

Two additional points: First, the immune status of any patient will need to be uncovered to evaluate truly the short as well as long term events after any treatment; i.e. metastases. Second, ocular melanoma is a life-threatening disease. Responsible safe management of the *patient* as well as his or her eye is indicated.

The Editors

Surgical Pharmacology of the Eye,
edited by M. Sears and A. Tarkkanen.
Raven Press, New York © 1985.

Radiation Therapy in the Management of Ocular and Adnexal Tumors

Devron H. Char

*Ocular Oncology Unit, Department of Ophthalmology, University of California,
San Francisco, California 94143*

SUMMARY: Diagnosis and treatment of most ocular and adnexal tumors are straightforward. All extraocular lesions should be biopsied prior to treatment with any form of radiation. Lacrimal gland masses should have an en bloc excision or fine needle biopsy. Incisional biopsy does not adversely effect prognosis for other adnexal malignancies.

Most intraocular tumors can be correctly diagnosed with noninvasive techniques; rarely is fine needle biopsy necessary in an atypical case.

The choice of a radiation modality depends on the expertise of the clinician, the location of the tumor, whether the lesion is focal or diffuse, and, with certain intraocular tumors, the requirement for precise localization of the radiation to avoid visually destructive radiation vasculopathy.

Radiation techniques are useful in the management of many lid, conjunctival, intraocular, and orbital tumors. Some adnexal tumors such as sebaceous carcinoma are better treated surgically. Circumscribed lid or conjunctival tumors can often be managed with surgery and/or cryotherapy avoiding potential radiation complications. Newer radiation techniques with charged particle beams appear to have improved the treatment for uveal malanoma; however, data including long term follow up are limited.

Certain issues about radiation treatment of eye and adnexal are unresolved. In some systemic malignancies preoperative radiation has been effective in the prevention of matastasis. For poor risk uveal melanoma a cooperative, multicenter trial of preenucleation irradiation has been organized. Similarly, the relative efficacy and morbidity of radioactive plaques versus charged particles (protons or helium ions) in the therapy for uveal melanoma remains to be determined.

Experimental approaches combining radiation therapy with other modalities for management of ocular malignancies include radiation sensitizing agents, hyperthermia, monoclonal antibodies, and photochemotherapy. Further research must be performed before a clinical role for these therapies can be defined.

A number of radiation therapy advances have improved our ability to treat lid, orbital, conjunctival, and intraocular tumors. There are a myriad of excellent reviews on radiobiology and ocular effects of ionizing and particle radiation (1–3). Newer aspects of clinically relevant, ocular radiation oncology include trials of preenucleation radiation for poor-risk melanoma, brachytherapy (radioactive plaques), charged-particle irradiation (helium ions or protons) to treat uveal melanomas; photon external-beam irradiation for thyroid ophthalmopathy and orbital pseudotumor; and experimental approaches using hypoxic cell sensitizers as well as radionuclides linked to antitumor monoclonal antibodies.

Radiation can be delivered in the form of waves, photons, or particles. Radiation results in intracellular ionization with DNA and cytoplasmic alterations manifest as immediate and delayed cell damage (4–5). The two most accepted terms for the clinical description of irradiation dose are rads and grays (Gy). A rad is the absorption of 100 ergs of energy by 1 g of absorbing material. The revised term for dose is the gray; a gray (Gy) equals 100 rads. Low voltage (85 to 140 kV) or orthovoltage (180 to 400 kV) can be used to deliver superficial ionizing radiation to the skin. Megavoltage machines (greater than 1 million electron volts) have skin-sparing effects and deliver maximum dose at a finite depth relative to the dermis.

A number of factors can biologically modify the effect of radiation. The use of fractionated radiation doses increases tumor effect while sparing normal tissue (6,7). Normal tissues usually have more effective reparative properties and a greater ability to repopulate than tumor tissue. In addition, relatively hypoxic tumor cells can be more effectively treated by increasing dose fractionation to allow reoxygenation of these cells between fractions. Alternatively, chemicals that are radiation sensitizers can be given to increase tumor cells' susceptibility to radiation; on a molecular level, these agents simulate the effect of cell oxygenation and may have the greatest application to hypoxic tumor cells such as vitreous seeding in retinoblastoma (8,9). Some malignancies such as melanomas appear to be relatively hypoxic and have an unusual propensity to repair sublethal damage; such tumors may be more susceptible to high dose fractions of radiation (10). Treatment simulation is performed prior to patient irradiation with any form of external beam. The major therapeutic effect of radiation is to alter the reproductive integrity of a tumor cell. Clinical, ultrasound, or radiologic evidence of tumor response is usually delayed; radiation-induced DNA damage is manifest as tumor destruction when malignant cells enter mitosis. The intermitotic phases of different malignancies are variable, and objective signs of tumor shrinkage can often be delayed for between 1 and 24 months after treatment (4).

LID TUMORS

Basal cell carcinomas account for more than 90% of lid malignancies (11). The proper role for radiation in the management of lid carcinoma is dependent on the surgical expertise of the ophthalmologist and the interest and experience of the radiation therapist. Approximately 60% of basal cell carcinomas are focal localized (nodular) lesions; surgery with frozen-section control, Mohs' chemosurgery, cryotherapy, or radiation therapy should eradicate over 95% of such tumors (11). In our ocular oncology unit, we have tended to advocate radiation therapy in debilitated patients with diffuse tumors, or in patients with very large diffuse tumors in whom presurgical radiation may produce sufficient shrinkage to allow a definitive resection. Ionizing radiation can be delivered to lid carcinomas using a number of techniques (12–15). Orthovoltage, electron, or photon irradiation with shielding of the cornea and lens have all been used with excellent therapeutic response. Basal cell carcinoma are usually treated with 15 fractions of 3 Gy orthovoltage radiation (total dose 45 Gy) over a 3-week period.

The incidence of treatment complications after radiation therapy for lid carcinomas is approximately 10% to 12%. Eyelash loss and telangiectatic skin changes are routinely seen. Significant radiation to the globe can result in keratitis, corneal perforation, scleral melting, or loss of the eye (13–16). Keratinization of the lid can occur with secondary ocular irritation and corneal scarring; this is more likely to occur if the central upper lid is treated. Treatment of the medial canthal area often results in canalicular or punctal occlusion; it is often advisable to intubate the lacrimal system of such patients with small silicone tubes prior to treatment (16). In addition to basal cell carcinomas, a number of other malignant lid tumors can be treated using radiation; these include malignant melanoma, sebaceous carcinoma, squamous cell carcinoma, and metastatic lid tumors. Treatment techniques are similar; however, a higher dose and different fractionation schedules are used for some of these tumors.

CONJUNCTIVAL TUMORS: MELANOMA AND SQUAMOUS CELL CARCINOMA

Most focal conjunctival melanomas or squamous cell carcinomas can be treated with either surgery with frozen-section control of margins or a combination of surgery and cryotherapy (11). All suspicious conjunctival lesions should be biopsied. Often a scraping with cytologic analysis can be diagnostic; if a focal lesion is present, an excisional biopsy with frozen-section control should be performed. At the time of surgery, if there is microscopic disease at the edge of the resection, adjunctive double freeze-thaw cryotherapy can be used.

Focal conjunctival melanomas have been successfully treated with radiation (17). However, we and others have found the results with surgery alone or surgery with cryotherapy are comparable to radiation, without the ionizing radiation complications. Indications for radiation therapy in conjunctival melanomas include diffuse malignant degeneration of acquired conjunctival melanosis, or treatment for an incompletely excised melanoma or squamous cell carcinoma. Radiation can be delivered either with external beam (ortho-voltage or electrons) or using brachytherapy such as strontium 90 or other types of β-radiation radioactive plaques such as iridium 192 or ruthenium 106

(11,17). Contraindications for radiation include benign lesions, bulky tumors of the fornix, intraocular invasion, or orbital involvement. Squamous cell conjunctival carcinomas have almost no metastatic potential. Focal lesions should be surgically resected; if there is tumor noted at the edges of resection, adjunct cryotherapy should be given.

Unfortunately, some patients first present to their ophthalmologist with a diffuse conjunctival carcinoma simulating a chronic unilateral conjunctivitis. In patients with conjunctival carcinoma involving the palpebral and bulbar conjunctiva, 60 Gy of photon irradiation can control tumor; however, the majority of such cases eventually require surgical removal of the eye and conjunctiva (anterior orbital exenteration) secondary to wide-field ocular radiation complications such as dry eye or scleral or corneal perforation. Conjunctival lymphoid lesions respond well to irradiation; benign lymphoid lesions generally require less than 20 Gy, lymphomas are treated with 30 to 40 Gy (18).

UVEAL TUMORS: MELANOMA AND METASTATIC LESIONS

There have been a number of improvements in the radiation therapy of uveal melanomas since the initial treatment attempts in 1929 (19). Unfortunately, a number of issues remain unresolved including at what stage in the natural history of uveal melanomas treatment should occur and what is the best means of doing so. A number of clinical trials are ongoing, including preenucleation irradiation of poor-risk uveal melanomas, and attempts to destroy tumors with preservation of vision using either brachytherapy or charged-particle (helium ion or proton) irradiation.

PREENUCLEATION IRRADIATION

In a number of body sites, preoperative irradiation appears to decrease tumor-related mortality (20). There are no prospective randomized studies available that have compared the efficacy of adjunctive radiotherapy versus enucleation alone in the prevention of uveal melanoma metastasis. Patients have been treated with preoperative, intraoperative, and postoperative irradiation in uncontrolled trials (21-27).

We have performed a phase I-II study in poor-risk, large uveal melanomas (>15 mm in diameter or >5 mm in thickness) to determine the morbidity associated with five 4 Gy fractions of photon irradiation prior to enucleation (28). The choice of this radiation protocol is empiric. *In vitro* and *in vivo* studies demonstrate that some melanomas are relatively hypoxic and have a large capacity to repair sublethal damage (29). Larger than conventional radiation fractions (4 Gy versus 2 Gy) may be more effective in destroying such cells, and this is one reason why we chose large fraction (4-Gy) irradiation. The choice of a total dose of 20 Gy of photon irradiation was selected because it has been successful in the management of other tumors, it is relatively safe, it can be delivered in 5 consecutive days for out-of-town referral patients, and it appears to be a reasonable starting point. A prospective randomized treatment trial is beginning in the United States to determine whether preoperative irradiation significantly alters the incidence of metastasis versus treatment with enucleation alone. Although it can be standardized for a national trial in a more reproducible manner than an investigation of different types of surgical techniques, there are a number of potential pitfalls to this therapeutic approach (28). First, it is unclear what dose and fractionation schedule is necessary to sterilize uveal melanomas; it is possible that the treatment protocol chosen will be inadequate. Second, preoperative irradiation has been most effective in tumors in which there is a high incidence of local recurrence and nodal disease; this is not the case for uveal melanoma. Third, if uveal melanomas have subclinical metastasis prior to discovery and treatment of the intraocular lesion, this form of treatment will not be efficacious.

We have treated 30 large uveal melanomas with preenucleation irradiation with a mean follow-up of approximately 25 months (range 3 to 70 months). We have had essentially no significant morbidity. Fourteen percent of patients have developed metastases. This relatively low figure suggests to us that a prospective randomized treatment trial should be performed.

BRACHYTHERAPY

As mentioned above, after the initial treatment of a uveal melanoma with local radiotherapy in 1929, Stallard and co-workers treated a large number of patients using cobalt plaques (30,31). A number of investigators have observed a high incidence of radiation complications associated with cobalt plaques, especially with tumors treated at or posterior to the equator of the eye (32–34). Other brachytherapy protocols have been developed to attempt to decrease the radiation morbidity associated with cobalt plaques. Radon seeds, gold 198, ruthenium 106, and iodine 125 have all been used as radioactive plaques (35–38). Lommatzsch and co-workers (37) have used ruthenium 106 plaques to treat small and medium-size melanomas with relatively good results. They observed a 91% 5-year survival and retention of the eye in 62% of cases. The strong beta and relatively absent gamma component of this type of plaque generally limits its use to tumors generally less than 5 mm in thickness.

A number of investigators following the pioneering work of Sealy have attempted to use ^{125}I plaques in the treatment of uveal melanoma (38,39). ^{125}I has a much softer gamma emission spectrum (27 to 35 keV) than cobalt, which results in less spread of radiation to non-tumor-containing portions of the eye. It is safer for operating room personnel since it can be stopped with 0.2 mm of gold foil, unlike cobalt 60, which requires 11 mm of lead to decrease its dose to 50%. While ^{125}I has a half-life of only 60 days, it is widely available commercially in the United States, unlike ruthenium, which is currently not routinely available. The results of different forms of uveal melanoma brachytherapy demonstrate that approximately 90% of patients are alive without tumor dissemination, although follow-up is short (37,40).

There are significant complications with all forms of ocular radiation. We predicted that almost all medium or large choroidal melanomas behind the equator treated with cobalt plaques would develop visually destructive radiation retinopathy (34). In short-term follow-up, nearly 40% of patients treated with cobalt plaques have developed visually significant radiation retinopathy or optic neuropathy (34,40). All forms of radiation (radioactive plaques or charged-particle irradiation) have produced some radiation complications, including vasculopathy, neovascular glaucoma, and loss of eyes. The relative complication rates of these techniques are unclear. We have begun a morbidity study to determine the complication rate of ^{125}I versus helium ion irradiation in our institution.

CHARGED PARTICLE IRRADIATION

There are a number of potential physical and biologic properties of charged-particle irradiation that may be advantageous in the management of uveal melanomas (41). Charged particles, including helium ions and protons, have an inherent Bragg peak effect. The lateral and distal edges of the helium ion beam are sufficiently sharp that radiation dose decreases from 100% to 0% in less than 3.0 mm; no form of brachytherapy can be as sharply focused. In addition, heavy ions have high linear energy transfer (LET); this property may prove to be more efficacious in the treatment of relatively hypoxic tumors such as melanoma (42).

Approximately 500 patients have been treated with charged-particle irradiation either in San Francisco (helium ions) or in Boston (proton beam) for ciliary body, choroidal, or iris-ciliary-body melanomas (41,43,44). Similar results have been reported with both therapies. More than 90% of treated patients have had either medium (3 to 5 mm in thickness and 10 to 15 mm in diameter), or large (>15 mm in diameter or >5 mm in thickness) melanomas. More than 95% of treated eyes have been retained, and tumor shrinkage usually occurs within 2 to 18 months of therapy. Final visual acuity is dependent on tumor location and to a lesser degree on tumor size. Treatment of uveal melanoma eyes with either radioactive plaques or external-beam irradiation require that both the tumor and a 2-mm surround of normal uvea and retina be included in the radiation field to avoid a "marginal miss." If a tumor is within 3 to 4 mm from the nerve or fovea, regardless of the radiation technique used, a full tumor dose is delivered to these structures, and radiation-induced vision decrease usually results. Eyes containing tumors farther than 5 mm from the fovea or nerve usually will retain good vision when treated with charged-particle irradiation.

Unfortunately, a number of complications have been observed after proton- or helium-ion therapy (45). Approximately 10% of eyes have developed neovascular glaucoma, especially when very large tumors are treated. Scleral melt, lack of tumor control, lid telangiectasia, increased subretinal fluid, lash loss, closure of the lacrimal drainage system, and other complications have also been observed.

The relative efficacy of charged-particle irradiation versus radioactive-plaque therapy is undetermined. In tumors less than 3 to 4 mm from the nerve or the fovea either treatment modality probably results in a similar incidence of visually destructive radiation retinopathy, although the onset of radiation retinopathy may be delayed for as long as 20 years after treatment. In two groups of uveal melanoma patients, charged-particle irradiation has theoretic and practical advantages over radioactive plaques. Patients with relatively thick tumors between 4 and 8 mm from the optic nerve or the macula are probably better treated with charged-particle irradiation. As radioactive plaques are used to treat progressively thicker tumors, there is increasing lateral radiation scatter, which will produce foveal radiation retinopathy or optic neuropathy. In contrast, tumors 4 to 8 mm from the nerve or the fovea can be treated with charged-particle irradiation without delivering significant amounts of radiation to either of these structures. A second group of patients in whom charged particles may prove to have greater efficacy are those with uveal melanomas that are greater than 9 to 10 mm in thickness. In order to treat such tumors with radioactive plaques, sufficient radiation has to be delivered to the sclera and the entire eye, with a very high incidence of radiation complications; it is likely that the incidence of complications in such patients treated with charged-particle irradiation will be significantly less.

These excellent short-term results with alternative radiation therapies may or may not reflect better tumor control than with enucleation (46). Our definitions of tumor size and our ability to detect early tumors have changed dramatically over the last 10 years. There is an absence of prospective randomized treatment data, and it is unclear in those reports from single institutions in which some patients were radiated and others enucleated, why patients were placed in one or another treatment group. There are some theoretic reasons why ocular irradiation could result in decreased melanoma-related mortality. In some animal models significantly less mortality is observed when eyes are not removed; traumatic enucleation and T-cell immunosuppression are required to produce metastasis in a B16 murine melanoma model (47). It is unlikely that a lesser degree of ocular manipulation, as was proposed by Zimmerman, is an isolated, paramount factor in determining mortality from enucleation (48). Placement of either radioactive plaques or marker rings for charged-particle irradiation entails at least as much surgical manipulation as occurs with a standard enucleation. Since the short-term mortality associated with these alternative therapies may be less than that after enucleation, other explanations must be sought.

A number of technical issues are unresolved regarding the use of radiation therapy techniques in uveal melanoma management. The fraction size, fraction number, and total dose with preoperative irradiation, radioactive plaques, or charged-particle therapy, remain unclear. Similarly, the long-term complication rates with the latter two types of modalities need better delineation; ocular radiation vasculopathy with visual loss can occur as late as 20 years after therapy. Prospective randomized treatment trials are starting to delineate these issues.

UVEAL METASTASIS

Radiation therapy plays a major role in the management of many metastatic choroidal tumors. Unfortunately, as many as 40% of patients with metastatic choroidal tumors present to their ophthalmologist prior to the discovery of the primary neoplasm (49). If possible, it is useful to determine the primary source of a choroidal metastasis since histologic considerations will affect the choice of therapy. Photocoagulation, radiation therapy, and chemotherapy have all been used to treat uveal metastases; their relative advantages and disadvantages depend upon the location, histology, and the disease status of the patient (50–54). In patients who are diagnosed with an ocular lesion prior to the detection of the primary malignancy, determination of the systemic neoplasm's histologic type is useful. If the tumor is responsive to chemotherapy, observation without direct ocular intervention is reasonable (51). Similarly, in a patient who develops an active small, isolated, focal metastasis of the posterior pole that affects vision, treatment with photocoagulation can be performed. We generally refrain from treating diffuse lesions or those inside the temporal arcade with photocoagulation since there is more visual loss with this modality than with radiation therapy. Radiation therapy is used on tumors inside the temporal arcade, lesions with a marked degree of subretinal fluid, and those patients who have failed or are not candidates for chemotherapy. Photon irradiation, generally using a lateral port to spare the lens, is given over 4 to 6 weeks with a total dose of approximately 30 to 50 Gy. Patients with widespread systemic disease can be treated more rapidly; their demise precedes the onset of radiation complications, which are more likely to occur with larger-fraction, shorter-duration therapy. Overall, approximately 85% of uveal metastasis can be successfully treated with conventional radiation therapy.

RETINOBLASTOMA

Radiotherapy plays an important role in the management of both localized and extraocular retinoblastoma (55). Unfortunately, more than 95% of unilateral retinoblastomas are sufficiently large at the time of diagnosis to preclude alternative therapy; these eyes usually have no visual potential and are best treated by enucleation. Radiation therapy of intraocular retinoblastoma can be performed for small or medium tumors using radioactive plaques or, in larger tumors, with external-beam photon irradiation.

The use of radioactive plaques (^{125}I, cobalt, or ruthenium) is indicated in a patient with a solitary retinoblastoma too large for either photocoagulation or cryotherapy, or a patient who has developed a large recurrence after alternative therapy (55). We routinely consider external-beam irradiation in retinoblastoma patients who have multiple tumors posterior to the equator, large symmetrical bilateral retinoblastomas, or smaller tumors inside the temporal arcades.

The choices of radiation fields, fractionation, and dose for treatment of retinoblastoma are unresolved (56–58). American oncology centers have tended to use lateral radiation ports, fraction sizes of approximately 1.8 to 2 Gy, and a total dose of between 35 and 45 Gy over a 4- to 6-week period. The rationale for this approach is that most large tumors occur behind the equator of the eye, and treatment can be given without a substantial risk of cataract formation. As would be expected, tumors at or anterior to the equator will not respond to this radiation technique; small tumors in this location are treated with triple freeze-thaw cryotherapy. In many European centers, anterior irradiation ports are used to treat retina. The disadvantage of this approach is that lens opacities uniformly develop, although these can be surgically removed at a later date.

In our experience, the lateral port approach is excellent as long as supplemental cryotherapy is given to lesions anterior to the equator. This approach is contraindicated if there is diffuse vitreous seeding or if one of the anterior tumors has overlying vitreous involvement. Such patients do not respond well to cryotherapy. Vitreous involvement is a poor prognostic sign; these retinoblastoma cells are hypoxic, and experimental data demonstrate a potential role for hypoxic cell sensitizers in these cases (8,9). Similarly, in other desperate cases of advanced bilateral disease, it is our anecdotal clinical impression that an additive effect can occur with radiation and systemic chemotherapy.

Overall radiation results with stage I to III retinoblastomas posterior to the equator are excellent both for vision and survival. A second course of external-beam irradiation has almost a 90% complication rate associated with its use (55). Even with conventional lateral field irradiation at 45 Gy we have observed rare cases of radiation retinopathy and hypopituitarism (55,59). Usually patients are treated with less than 2 Gy per fraction to decrease the likelihood of radiation vasculopathy (60).

Local radiation can be used for recurrent orbital or CNS disease; for osseous metastasis, radiation can be used to control pain.

INTRAOCULAR LYMPHOMA ("OCULAR RETICULUM CELL SARCOMA")

In middle-aged or older patients who present with either diffuse uveitis or vitreitis the diagnosis of intraocular lymphoma (ocular reticulum cell sarcoma) should strongly be considered. Approximately 90% of patients develop eye and orbital nervous system involvement; lymphoma in these locations can occur simultaneously, first in the eye, or initially in the CNS. The ocular and CNS lesions should receive radiation; early lesions respond rapidly; however, most patients succumb to recurrent CNS disease (61). We have produced a number of long-term remissions with intrathecal chemotherapy and irradiation, and all patients currently are treated with both modalities (62).

ORBITAL TUMORS

Photon irradiation has been used to treat a number of orbital tumors including orbital rhabdomyosarcoma, orbital metastases, lymphoma, sinus carcinomas with contiguous orbital involvement, "pseudotumor," thyroid ophthalmopathy, and advanced adenoid cystic carcinoma of the lacrimal gland (63–69).

A number of investigators in the United States have used low-dose (20-Gy) photon irradiation to treat either orbital pseudotumor or thyroid ophthalmopathy (70–73). Although some complications have been reported secondary to improper technique, using anterior lateral wedge pair ports, we have observed no significant morbidity in approximately 100 patients treated at our institution. Treatment with both orbital pseudotumor or thyroid ophthalmopathy has been most effective in patients with acute inflammatory disease. Patients with thyroid optic neuropathy often have a transient response but later have a recurrence and require surgical decompression of the optic nerve.

In orbital rhabdomyosarcoma the relative importance of chemotherapy versus irradiation is unclear. Some institutions have treated children with radiation alone, chemotherapy alone, or a combination of both. If a combination of chemotherapy and irradiation is used, the additive effects of daunomycin and radiation should be anticipated and careful coordination established to avoid ocular toxicity (66,67).

EXPERIMENTAL APPROACHES

A number of interesting investigational approaches to treat intraocular and orbital malignancies are being studied. A Swedish group has developed a "gamma knife," that allows the treatment of tumors with much greater focusing ability than conventional external beam irradiation (74). This approach is less expensive to develop than a charged-particle facility and may mitigate the deficiencies associated with radioactive-plaque treatment.

In a number of laboratories, investigators have developed monoclonal antibodies against tumor-associated antigens (75). We have produced antiretinoblastoma monoclonal antibodies and have demonstrated that conjugation of these antibodies with the cell poison ricin can result in specific retinoblastoma toxicity *in vitro* (76). It is conceivable that conjugation with either antiretinoblastoma or antimelanoma antibodies with radioactive isotopes could also be used to treat a number of tumors.

Although not ionizing radiation therapy, another approach in the management of intraocular and orbital tumors is the use of photochemotherapy. Hematoporphyrin derivative is selectively taken up by tumor tissue; activation of the compound results in a marked increase in tumor cell death at a lower dose of laser energy than required for conventional photocoagulation of tumors (77). Early results in both animal models and human tumors using hemato-porphyrin derivative and laser therapy have been promising; however, significant ocular toxicity has been observed. Similarly, early results demonstrate the possible efficacy of hyperthermia and its therapeutic application to eye and orbital tumors; however, there is a paucity of ocular data (78). Probably both hyperthermia and photodynamic therapy, if they have a role, will be used as adjuncts to radiation to decrease radiation dose and morbidity.

CONCLUSIONS

Radiation therapy can be used to treat a number of ocular and adnexal tumors. In most ocular oncology centers the majority of focal lid and conjunctival tumors are treated with nonradiation techniques. Diffuse lid or conjunctival tumors are amenable to various types of radiation therapy.

External-beam radiation and brachytherapy play a major role in the management of both uveal melanomas and retinoblastomas. While the relative efficacy of various types of radiation in the management of these intraocular malignancies is unclear, many eyes can be successfully treated with tumor destruction and retention of vision using radiation oncologic techniques.

In the management of orbital tumors, radiation therapy has a major impact in the treatment of rhabdomyosarcoma; difficult cases of thyroid ophthalmopathy and benign orbital lymphoid tumors (pseudotumor) are also well treated with radiation.

ACKNOWLEDGMENTS

This research was supported in part by an unrestricted grant from That Man May See and NIH research grants EY01441 and EY03675. Dr. Char is a recipient of the Robert C. McCormick Scholar Award from Research to Prevent Blindness, Inc for 1984.

REFERENCES

1. Merriam, G. R., Jr., Szechter, A., and Focht, E. F. (1972): The effects of ionizing radiations on the eye. *Front. Radiat. Ther. Oncol.,* 6:346.
2. Chan, R., and Shuhoosky, L. (1976): Effects of irradiation on the eye. *Radiology,* 120:673.
3. Parsons, J., Fitzgerald, C., and Hood, I. (1983): The effects of irradiation on the eye and optic nerve. *Int. J. Radiat. Oncol. Biol. Phys.,* 9:609.
4. Hellman, S. (1982): Principles and practice of oncology. In: *Cancer,* edited by V. T. DeVita, pp. 103–131. J. B. Lippincott, Philadelphia.
5. Thompson, L. H., and Suit, H. D. (1969): Proliferation kinetics of X-irradiated mouse L cells studied with time lapse photography—II. *Int. J. Radiol. Med.,* 15:347–362.
6. Withers, H. R., Peters, L. J., Thames, H. D., and Fletcher, G. H. (1982): Hyper-fractionation. *Int. J. Radiat. Oncol. Biol. Phys.,* 8:1807–1809.
7. Aristizabal, S., Caldwell, W. L., and Avila, J. (1971): The relationship of time-dose fractionation factors to complications in the treatment of pituitary tumors by irradiation. *Int. J. Radiat. Oncol. Biol. Phys.,* 2:667.

8. Wardman, P., Clarke, E. D., Flockhart, I. R., and Wallace, R. G. (1978): Rationale for the development of improved hypoxic cell radiosensitizers. *Br. J. Cancer,* 37(Suppl 3):1–5.

9. Rootman, J., Josephy, D., Adomat, H., and Palcic, B. (1982): Ocular absorption and toxicity of a radiosensitizer and its effect on hypoxic cells. *Arch. Ophthalmol.,* 100:468.

10. Doss, L. L., Memula, N. (1982): The radio responsiveness of melanoma. *Int. J. Radiat. Oncol. Biol. Phys.,* 8:1131.

11. Char, D. H. (1980): The management of lid and conjunctival malignancies. *Surv. Ophthalmol.,* 24:679.

12. Treatment of eyelid tumours. Editorial. (1976): *Br. J. Ophthalmol.,* 60:793.

13. Lederman, M. (1976): Radiation treatment of cancer of the eyelids. *Br. J. Ophthalmol.,* 60:794.

14. Gladstein, A. H. (1978): Radiotherapy of eyelid tumors. In: *Ocular and Adnexal Tumors,* edited by F. A. Jakobiec, pp. 508. Aesculapius, Birmingham, AL.

15. Grosch, E., and Lambert, H. E. (1979): The treatment of difficult cutaneous basal and squamous cell carcinomata with electrons. *Br. J. Radiol.,* 52:472.

16. Call, M. B., and Welham, R. A. N. (1981): Epiphora after irradiation of medial eyelid tumors. *Am. J. Ophthalmol.,* 92:842.

17. Lonnatzsch, T. K. (1978): Beta-ray treatment of malignant epibulbar melanoma. *Albrecht v. Graefes. Arch. Klin. Ophthalmol.,* 209:111.

18. Kim, Y., and Fayos, J. (1976): Primary orbital lymphoma: A radiotherapeutic experience. *Int. J. Radiat. Oncol. Biol. Phys.,* 1:1099–1105.

19. Char, D. H. (1978): Management of small choroidal melanomas. *Surv. Ophthalmol.,* 22:377–386.

20. Roswit, B., Higgins, G. A., Humphrey, E. W., and Robinette, C. D. (1973): Preoperative irradiation of operable adenocarcinoma of the rectum and rectosigmoid colon. *Radiology,* 108:359.

21. Burch, R. E., and Camp, W. E. (1943): Results of irradiation of malignant melanomas of the uveal tract. *Trans. Am. Acad. Ophthalmol. Otolaryngol.,* 47:335.

22. Lommatzsch, P., and Dietrich, B. (1976): The effect of orbital irradiation on the survival rate of patients with choroidal melanoma. *Ophthalmologica,* 173:49.

23. Van Peperzeel, H. (1980): Radiation therapy: Before or after enucleation. *Doc. Ophthalmol.,* 50:71.

24. Vannas, S. (1959): Zur Prognose der Malignen Geschwulste der Aderhaut. *Klin. Mbl. Augenheilk.,* 135:678.

25. Kleberger, E. (1965): Bemerkungen zu der Arbeit von J. Sobanski, L. Zeydler und J. Goetz: Uber die Thereapie des Intraokularen Melanoma Malignum. *Klin. Mbl. Augenheilk,* 147:880.

26. Sobanski, J., Pruszczynski, A., Wozniak, L., Zeydler-Grzedzielewska, L., Szusterowska-Martin, E., Szaniawski, W., and Czyzewski, J. (1972): Beurteilung der Behandlungsergebnisse der Schiedener Morphologischer Typen des Malignen Aderhautmelanoms. *Klin. Mbl. Augenheilk.,* 161:387.

27. Sobanski, J., Zeydler, L., Goetz, J. (1965): Uber Ber die Therapie des Intraokularen Melanoma Malignun. *Klin. Mbl. Augenheilk.,* 146:70.

28. Char, D. H., and Phillips, T. L. (1984): Pre-enucleation irradiation of uveal melanoma. *Br. J. Ophthalmol., (submitted for publication).*

29. Hornsey, S. (1978): The relationship between total dose, number of fractions, fraction size in the response of malignant melanoma in patients. *Br. J. Radiol.,* 51:905.

30. Moore, R. F. (1930): Choroidal sarcoma treated by the intra-ocular insertion of radon seeds. *Br. J. Ophthalmol.,* 14:145.

31. Stallard, H. B. (1966): Radiotherapy for malignant melanoma of the choroid. *Br. J. Ophthalmol.,* 50:147.

32. Bedford, M. A., Bedotto, C., and MacFaul, P. A. (1970): Radiation retinopathy after the application of a cobalt plaque. *Br. J. Ophthalmol.,* 54:505.

33. MacFaul, P. A., and Bedford, M. A. (1970): Ocular complications after therapeutic irradiation. *Br. J. Ophthalmol.,* 54:237.

34. Char, D. H., Lonn, L., and Margolis, L. (1977): Complications of cobalt plaque therapy for small choroidal melanomas. *Am. J. Ophthalmol.,* 84:536.

35. Newman, G. H., Davidorf, F. H., Havener, W. H., and Makley, T. A. (1970): Conservative management of malignant melanoma. *Arch. Ophthalmol.,* 83:21.

36. Davidorf, F. H., Makley, T. A., and Lang, J. R. (1976): Radiotherapy of malignant melanoma of the choroid. *Trans. Am. Acad. Ophthalmol. Otolaryngol.*, 81:Op849–861.
37. Lommatzsch, D. K. (1979): Radiotherapie der intraokularen tumoren, insbesondere bei aderhautmelanom. *Klin. Mbl. Augenheilk.*, 174:948.
38. Sealy, R., Buret, E., Cleminshaw, H., Stannard, C., Hering, E., Shackleton, D., Korrubel, J., Le Roux, L. M., Sevel, D., Van Oldenborgh, M., and Van Selm, J. (1980): Progress in the use of iodine therapy for tumours of the eye. *Br. J. Radiol.*, 53:1052.
39. Packer, S., and Rothman, M. (1980): Radiotherapy of choroidal melanoma with iodine-125. *Ophthalmology*, 87:582.
40. Shields, J. A., Ausburger, J. J., Brady, L. W., and Day, J. L. (1982): Cobalt plaque therapy of posterior uveal melanomas. *Ophthalmology*, 89:1201.
41. Char, D. H., Saunders, W., Castro, J. R., Irvine, A. R., Stone, R. D., Crawford, B. J., Barricks, M., Lonn, L. I., Hilton, G. F., Schwartz, A., Chen, G. T. Y., Lyman, J. R., Collier, M., Sulit, H., Straatsma, B. R., and Kaminsky, A. (1983): Charged particle therapy for choroidal melanoma. *Ophthalmology*, 90:1219.
42. Phillips, T. L., Ross, G. Y., Goldstein, L. S., Anisworth, J., and Alpen, E. (1982): In vivo radiobiology of heavy ions. *Int. J. Radiat. Oncol. Biol. Phys.*, 8:2121.
43. Char, D. H., Saunders, W. M., and Gragoudas, E. S. (1983): Charged particle (helium ion and proton) therapy for choroidal melanoma. *Ophthalmic Forum*, 1:42–44.
44. Gragoudas, E. S., Goitein, M., Verhey, L., Munzenreider, J., Suit, H. D., and Koehler, A. (1980): Proton beam irradiation. *Ophthalmology*, 87:571.
45. Char, D. H., Crawford, J. B., Castro, J. R., and Woodruff, K. H. (1983): Failure of choroidal melanoma to respond to helium ion therapy. *Arch. Ophthalmol.*, 101:236–241.
46. Seddon, J. M., Gragoudas, E. S., Albert, D. M., Hsieh, C. C., and Friedenberg, G. R. Survival after treatment of uveal melanoma: A comparison between proton irradiation and enucleation. *Am. J. Ophthalmol.*, (*in press*).
47. Niederkorn, J. Y. (1984): Enucleation in consort with immunologic impairment promotes metastasis of intraocular melanomas in mice. *Invest. Ophthalmol. Vis. Sci.*, 25:1080–1086.
48. McLean, I. W., Foster, W. D., and Zimmerman, L. E. (1982): Uveal melanoma: Location, size, cell type, and enucleation as risk factors in metastases. *Hum. Pathol.*, 13:123.
49. Ferry, A. P., and Font, R. L. (1974): Carcinoma metastatic to the eye and orbit. *Arch. Ophthalmol.*, 92:276.
50. Stephens, R. F., and Shields, J. A. (1979): Diagnosis and management of cancer metastatic to the uvea: A study of 70 cases. *Ophthalmology*, 86:1336.
51. Latson, A. D., Davidorf, F. H., and Bruce, R. A., Jr. (1982): Chemotherapy for treatment of choroidal metastases from breast carcinoma. *Am. J. Ophthalmol.*, 93:102.
52. Reddy, S., Saxena, B. S., Hendrickson, F., and Deusch, W. (1981): Malignant metastatic disease of the eye: Management of an uncommon complication. *Cancer*, 47:810.
53. Chu, F. C. N., Huh, S. H., Nisce, L. Z., and Simpson, L. D. (1977): Radiation therapy of choroid metastasis from breast cancer. *Int. J. Radiat. Oncol. Biol. Phys.*, 2:273.
54. Maor, M., Chan, R. C., and Young, S. E. (1977): Radiotherapy of choroidal metastases. Breast cancer as primary site. *Cancer*, 40:2081.
55. Char, D. H. (1983): Management of choroidal melanoma and retinoblastoma. In: *Disorders of the Vitreous, Retina and Choroid*, edited by J. J. Kanski and P. H. Morse, pp. 122–146. Butterworths, London.
56. Cassady, J. R., Sagerman, R. H., Tretter, P., and Ellsworth, R. M. (1969): Radiation therapy in retinoblastoma. *Radiology*, 93:405.
57. Freeman, C. R., Esseltine, D.-L., Whitehead, V. M., Chevalier, L., and Little, J. M. (1980): Retinoblastoma: The case for radiotherapy and for adjunct chemotherapy. *Cancer*, 46:1913.
58. Gagnon, J. D., Ware, C. M., Moss, W. T., and Stevens, K. R. (1980): Radiation management of bilateral retinoblastoma: The need to preserve vision. *Int. J. Radiat. Oncol. Biol. Phys.*, 6: 669.
59. Wara, W. M., Richards, G., Grumbach, M. M., Kaplan, S. L., Sheline, G. E., and Conte, F. A. (1977): Hypopituitarism after irradiation in children. *Int. J. Radiat. Oncol. Biol. Phys.*, 2:549.
60. Harris, J. R., and Levene, M. B. (1976): Visual complications following irradiation for pituitary adenomas and cranio-pharyngiomas. *Radiology*, 120:167.

61. Margolis, L., Fraser, R., Lichter, A., and Char, D. H. (1980): The role of radiation therapy in management of ocular reticulum cell sarcoma. *Cancer,* 45:688–692.
62. Char, D. H., Margolis, L., Newman, A. B. (1981): Ocular reticulum cell sarcoma. *Am. J. Ophthalmol.,* 91:480–483.
63. Danoff, B. F., Kramer, S., and Thompson, N. (1980): Radiotherapeutic management of optic nerve gliomas in children. *Int. J. Radiat. Oncol. Biol. Phys.,* 6:45.
64. Kim, Y. H., and Fayos, J. V. (1976): Primary orbital lymphoma: Radiotherapeutic experience. *Int. J. Radiat. Oncol. Biol. Phys.,* 1:1099.
65. Sidrys, L. A., Fritz, K. J., and Variakojis, D. (1982): Fast neutron therapy for orbital adneoid cystic carcinoma. *Ann. Ophthalmol.,* 14:104.
66. Lederman, M., and Wybar, K. (1976): Embryonal sarcoma. *Proc. R. Soc. Med.* 69:895.
67. Abramson, D. H., Ellsworth, R. M., Tretter, B., Wolff, J. A., and Kitchin, F. D. (1979): The treatment of orbital rhabdomyosarcoma with irradiation and chemotherapy. *Ophthalmology,* 86:1330.
68. Savar, D. E. (1982): High-dose radiation of the orbit. A cause of skin graft failure after exenteration. *Arch. Ophthalmol.,* 100:1750.
69. Nakissa, N., Rubin, P., Strohl, R., and Keys, H. (1983): Ocular and orbital complications following radiation therapy of perinasal sinus malignancies and review of literature. *Cancer,* 51:980.
70. Bartalena, L., Marcocci, C., Chiovato, L., Laddaga, M., Lepri, G., Andreani, D., Cavallacci, G., Baschieri, L., and Pinchera, A. (1983): Orbital cobalt irradiation combined with systemic corticosteroids for Graves' ophthalmopathy: Comparison with systemic corticosteroids alone. *J. Clin. Endocrinol. Metab.,* 56:1139.
71. Donaldson, S. S., McDougall, R., Egbert, P. R., Enzman, B. R., and Kriss, J. P. (1980): Treatment of orbital pseudotumor (opathic orbital inflammation) by radiation therapy. *Int. J. Radiat. Oncol. Biol. Phys.,* 6:79.
72. Donaldson, S. S., Bagshaw, M. A., and Kriss, J. P. (1973): Super voltage orbital radiotherapy for Grave's ophthalmopathy. *J. Clin. Endocrinol. Metab.,* 37:276–285.
73. Sergott, R. C., Glaser, J. S., and Charyulu, K. (1981): Radiotherapy for idiopathic inflammatory orbital pseudotumor. *Arch. Ophthalmol.,* 99:853–856.
74. Leksell, L. (1971): Stereotaxis and radiosurgery—an operative system. Charles C Thomas, Springfield, IL.
75. Char, D. H. (1984): Monoclonal antibodies: Current status in eye research. In: *Immunologic Ocular Disease. International Ophthalmology Clinics,* edited by M. H. Friedlaender, Little Brown, Boston, 44:3178–3183.
76. Merriam, J. C., Lyon, H. S., and Char, D. H. (1984): Toxicity of a monoclonal F(ab')^2 ricin A conjugate for retinoblastoma *in vitro. Cancer Res. (in press).*
77. Gomer, C. J., Doiron, D. R., Jester, J. B., Scirth, B. C., and Murphree, A. L. (1983): Hermatoporphyrin derivative of photoradiation therapy for the treatment of intraocular tumors: Examination of acute normal ocular tissue toxicity. *Cancer Res.,* 43:721–727.
78. Lagendijk, J. J. W. (1982): Microwave applicator for hyperthermic treatment of retinoblastoma. *Natl. Cancer Inst. Monogr.,* 61:469.

Commentary

Pharmacology of Neodymium-YAG Laser Surgery

Although the neodymium YAG laser is now used extensively for posterior capsulotomy in the human eye, there still are large gaps in our knowledge of how the ocular tissues react to this form of "noninvasive trauma". In particular, the elevation of intraocular pressure that occurs after laser capsulotomy is very largely unexplained.

While speculation is rife concerning possible mechanisms of the post treatment elevation, it still remains important to treat the eye and/or patient prophylactically. (The presence or absence of glaucoma should be determined.) Such treatment can be done with a carbonic anhydrase inhibitor or with topical timolol and carried on for as long as needed. A good many capsulotomies are done in eyes in which a good deal of cortex is present on the capsule and/or behind the iris. Such eyes are not good subjects for laser treatment. Lens-induced uveitis can be stirred by laser treatment. The prophylaxis here has to do with a clean extracapsular procedure. It is important to remove large amounts of residual lenticular cortex surgically, prior to laser capsulotomy. If the posterior capsule is intact, it should and can be cleansed by meticulous intraocular surgery. Later, if necessary, a capsulotomy can be done. Perforation of the posterior capsule by laser in the presence of cortex may subject the eye to prolonged lens induced uveitis, with the vitreous serving as a wonderful depot from which the lens antigen may never disappear unless it is removed by vitrectomy. Again, in the performance of laser capsulotomy, anticipation of laser-induced inflammation should dictate the use of preoperative steroidal and/or nonsteroidal agents.

The effect of capsulotomy on the possible subsequent development of cystoid macular edema and on the rate of reparation of cystoid macular edema is not known. Eyes with these susceptibilities demand caution. Finally, the lowest energy intensity sufficient to do the job should be utilized and care taken to avoid damage to the corneal endothelium. [See: Khodadoust, A., et al., (1984): *Am. J. Ophthalmol.* 98:144–152.]

The Editors

Surgical Pharmacology of the Eye,
edited by M. Sears and A. Tarkkanen.
Raven Press, New York © 1985.

Pharmacology of Neodymium-YAG Laser Surgery

Joseph Caprioli

*Department of Ophthalmology and Visual Science, Yale University
School of Medicine, New Haven, Connecticut 06510*

SUMMARY: The pulsed neodymium-YAG laser is an important tool for the modern ophthalmic surgeon. Much is still unknown regarding its potential toxicologic effect on the eye; therefore, caution and good judgment should be exercised in its use. Common and often unavoidable accompaniments of YAG laser treatment include inflammation, elevation of IOP, and miosis. Appropriate pharmacologic management can optimize the treatment parameters and reduce the complications.

Laser techniques using very short pulses at high energy levels were introduced to ophthalmology by Krasnov in the early 1970s. Advantages of the technique included its "cool" mode of action and a unique self-shielding effect that tended to protect structures posterior to the laser focus (33). The current surge of interest in cold ophthalmic lasers is due to the simultaneous development of the neodymium-YAG laser for ophthalmologic use by two European research groups. Fankhauser and van der Zypen of Switzerland developed and began clinical investigation of the Q-switched YAG laser (19). At approximately the same time, Aron-Rosa and colleagues introduced the mode-locked YAG laser to the ophthalmic community (1,3). Both varieties are capable of cutting nonpigmented tissue, unlike continuous-wave devices such as the argon laser. The YAG laser has been used to perform ophthalmic procedures such as anterior capsulotomy prior to cataract surgery, posterior capsulotomy after extracapsular cataract extraction, lysis of vitreous bands, synechiotomy, iridectomy, coreoplasty, cyclodialysis, trabeculoplasty, trabeculotomy, and the reopening of closed trabeculectomy sites (1–4,16,18,19,28,30,46).

The possible biochemical and mechanical consequences of intraocular YAG laser treatment are just beginning to be explored. Aside from direct damage to the tissue being treated, remote damage due to light, acoustic, or intense electric field effects (particularly regarding the corneal endothelium and retina) are of real concern (7,23,25,44). Discussion of these kinds of effects are beyond the scope of this chapter. However, even with the use of excellent technique, there are a number of common, often unavoidable accompaniments of YAG laser surgery. These include inflammation, intraocular pressure (IOP) elevation, miosis, and bleeding. We turn our attention to these side effects of laser treatment that may be pharmacologically manipulated. Assuming good technique, the best surgical results with the YAG laser will be achieved when the patient receives optimal pharmacologic management.

THE NEODYMIUM-YAG LASER

The YAG laser utilizes a solid laser medium consisting of a crystal of yttrium, aluminum, and garnet "doped" with neodymium atoms. This laser differs from that of continuous-wave lasers in that its energy is delivered in ultrashort, high-powered bursts. These extraordinary bursts of energy are currently achieved by either of two processes: Q-switching or mode locking. Both are nonmechanical techniques of releasing energy from the laser cavity. One method of Q-switching utilizes a material with special electro-optic properties that is interposed in the beam path of the laser. This material is opaque when exposed to low light intensities but bleaches and becomes transparent at high light intensities. When energy within the lasering medium builds to sufficient levels, this electro-optic assembly becomes transparent and releases the energy stored in the laser cavity; the duration of this pulse is approximately 12 nsec. The mode-locked technique also utilizes a bleachable substance placed in the laser beam path but has the unique property of returning to its opaque form only picoseconds after being bleached. The output of a typical mode-locked instrument consists of a train of pulses with a total duration of approximately 40 nsec, consisting of seven individual energy bursts each 25 psec long.

The advantages of the YAG laser include its ability to cut nonpigmented tissue and the creation of a zone of optical breakdown that limits the propagation of laser energy posterior to the point of focus. Both of these advantages are the result of a process termed *plasma formation.* The ultrashort burst of laser energy strips electrons from their atoms, creating a cloud of free electrons and a locally intense electric field, a plasma. The plasma is opaque to light, thereby limiting further penetration by the laser. In ophthalmic applications, a tiny plasma is created in the eye by the highly focusable laser. Tissue disruption is caused by a focal microexplosion and vaporization. This is in contrast to the thermal effects of a continuous-wave laser such as the argon, which requires pigmented tissue to absorb the laser energy.

The ability to cut nonpigmented tissues in a finely controlled manner without opening the globe has made the YAG laser a useful tool for ophthalmic surgeons. Its most popular application to date has been the incision of opaque posterior lens capsules after extracapsular cataract surgery. Mode-locked or Q-switched instruments can be used in the presence or absence of intraocular lens implants. The most frequent complications include increased IOP, damage to the intraocular lens, and anterior uveitis; retinal detachment following posterior capsulotomy has also been reported (36).

Iridectomy is most easily performed with the Q-switched instrument, since it is currently capable of delivering more power than the mode-locked models. The immediate postoperative course is not infrequently marked by a sudden rise of IOP to 40 mm Hg or more, usually within the first 2 hr after treatment (41,45). Other complications include pigment dispersion, hemorrhage, and focal lens opacities.

Vitreous bands to surgical wounds in aphakic or pseudophakic eyes have been severed with the YAG laser in an effort to promote resolution of cystoid macular edema (CME) and to improve visual acuity. Katzen et al. (28,29) have reported a total of 62 eyes with CME that have undergone YAG laser lysis of vitreous bands to the surgical wound. Vision in 80% of eyes improved 2 Snellen lines or more with a follow-up of 1 to 14 months. Other investigators have reported similar results in which the vitreous bands were cut with scissors or anterior vitrectomy performed (20,21,24,39). One must bear in mind, however, that the majority of patients with aphakic CME undergo spontaneous resolution with improvement in visual acuity (22). Conclusions regarding the efficacy of YAG laser treatment of aphakic CME associated with vitreous incarceration must await further study.

The use of the YAG laser in the treatment of patients with open-angle glaucoma has not been encouraging. Fankhauser (18) attempted to create cyclodialysis clefts in 31 eyes but was successful in only 1. Spaeth was successful in reopening a cyclodialysis cleft after sudden closure and marked IOP rise in 1 patient (*personal communication*). Trabeculoplasty was performed in a series of 42 eyes with poor results (18,19). Cohn and Aron-Rosa (16) have reported a single case in which a trabeculectomy site occluded by a nonpigmented membrane was reopened with reestablishment of a filtering bleb.

INFLAMMATION

Inflammation of the anterior segment is a final common response to ocular injury. The eye responds rapidly to an irritative stimulus with hyperemia, breakdown of the blood-aqueous barrier, increased IOP, and miosis. This may be followed by frank anterior uveitis, with the appearance of inflammatory cells in the anterior chamber.

Inflammation is generally associated with the release of a number of mediators including acetylcholine, bradykinin, histamine, serotonin, substance P, and prostaglandins. In the last decade the role of prostaglandins in ocular inflammation has received much attention (38,42). Irritation of the anterior uvea by a variety of noxious stimuli causes the synthesis and release of prostaglandins (11,26,37,47,48). Aspirin has been shown to prevent the blood-aqueous barrier disruption after paracentesis or laser irradiation of the iris (37). The application of prostaglandins to animal eyes produces hyperemia, disruption of the blood-aqueous barrier, increased IOP, and miosis (27). Eakins et al. (17) demonstrated that therapy of uveitis resulted in decreased levels of prostaglandins in the aqueous. Masuda et al. (34) reported elevated aqueous prostaglandin levels in patients with glaucomatocyclitic crisis or with Behçet's disease, compared to normal controls.

The pathways of arachidonic acid metabolism are schematically depicted in Fig. 1. The anti-inflammatory effects of compounds such as aspirin and indomethacin are related to the inhibition of the enzyme cyclooxygenase. Recently, another class of compounds that are products of the lipoxygenase pathway of arachidonic acid metabolism, the leukotrienes, have been implicated as mediators of the ocular inflammatory response (6,8). The nonsteroidal anti-inflammatory agents may not inhibit the lipoxygenase pathway and will therefore not diminish leukotriene production (Fig. 1). Corticosteroids, however, can inhibit both the cyclooxygenase and lipoxygenase pathways, inhibiting both prostaglandin and leukotriene synthesis.

Treatment of human ocular tissue with the YAG laser results in an acute inflammatory response of variable intensity consisting of hyperemia, increased IOP, miosis, and the appearance of aqueous flare and cell (9,18,41,46; Caprioli and Sears, *unpublished data*). The inflammatory response may be particularly severe when sectioning of the posterior capsule is performed in the presence of cortical material. A severe inflammatory reaction may also be encountered when a large number of laser applications are delivered to the eye, such as in the sectioning of an anterior vitreous band. The inflammatory reaction may result in the formation of posterior synechiae, particularly after YAG laser iridectomy (G. L. Spaeth, *personal communication*). The incision of "clean" posterior capsules are generally associated with a milder form of inflammation.

Topical corticosteroids are effective in blunting the inflammatory response after YAG surgery, particularly when treatment is begun preoperatively (Caprioli and Sears, *unpublished data*). A potent topical steroid such as dexamethasone phosphate 0.1% or prednisolone acetate 1.0% should be administered to the eye 4 and 2 hr preoperatively and continued three to four times a day for approximately 1 week postoperatively. Pilocarpine or other miotics should be avoided in the immediate postoperative period, if possible. These drugs may increase the leakiness of the blood-aqueous barrier, increase

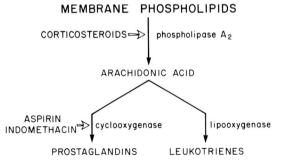

FIG. 1. Simplified scheme of the synthesis of prostaglandins and leukotrienes.

the apposition of the lens and the iris, and increase the likelihood of posterior synechiae formation.

INTRAOCULAR PRESSURE

IOP elevation after YAG laser treatment can be dramatic, with elevations to 50 mm Hg or more occurring within the first several hours postoperatively. Such elevations have been recorded after capsulotomy (anterior or posterior), iridectomy, and lysis of vitreous bands (9,10,15,41,45; Caprioli and Sears, *unpublished data;* G. L. Spaeth, *personal communication*).

A marked IOP rise in rabbits occurs within the first several hours after YAG laser irradiation of the lens or iris; this is followed by hypotony and a marked inflammatory reaction occurring 12 to 18 hr postoperatively (32). Schwartz (41) reported a mean IOP rise of 7.8 mm Hg after YAG iridectomy in a small series of patients, and Brown (9) recorded a mean peak IOP elevation of 5.7 mm Hg 15 to 60 min following posterior capsulotomy in 74 eyes. In the latter group, several patients experienced IOP elevation to 50 mm Hg. Patients with a history of glaucoma and those receiving the largest number of laser applications were most prone to this complication. Terry et al. (45) reported a postoperative increase in IOP in 28 out of 49 eyes undergoing posterior capsulotomy; in 7 of these eyes, the IOP exceeded 41 mm Hg. The peak pressure most frequently occurred 1 to 2 hr after treatment. Channell and Beckman (15) recently reported a mean IOP increase of 12 mm Hg during the first 24 hr after treatment in 33 eyes undergoing posterior capsulotomy. IOP remained elevated for several weeks in some eyes. Higher pressures were associated with larger capsulotomies and increased energy. Ruderman et al. (40) reported a case of pupillary block following posterior capsulotomy, and Shrader et al. (43) reported failure of a filtering bleb after posterior capsulotomy by occlusion of the fistula by herniated vitreous. In the vast majority of cases, however, pupillary block does not occur, and the chamber angle remains open and normal to gonioscopic examination (Caprioli and Sears, *unpublished data*).

The mechanism of the IOP rise after YAG laser treatment is unknown. It has been attributed to functional occlusion of the trabecular meshwork by particulate matter released during treatment (9). However, the pressure rise does not correlate well with the amount of material visible in the anterior chamber by slit-lamp examination. Furthermore, patients undergoing incision of a "clean" posterior capsule with only two or three laser applications can also experience a significant pressure rise. Since the postoperative IOP spike typically comes at a time when the acute irritative response is first manifested, it could be related to the synthesis and release of prostaglandins. Intracameral injection and topical application of prostaglandins have been shown to acutely raise IOP in rabbits and monkeys (5,14,27,31). Although prostaglandins increase IOP within the first hour or two after administration, they also tend to increase gross outflow facility and cause a subsequent decrease in IOP over a prolonged period, up to 20 hr (12,14,35). The acute elevation of IOP is likely caused by a rapid influx of plasmoid aqueous through the disrupted blood-aqueous barrier. The subsequent relative hypotony could in part be related to an increase in outflow facility but is certainly compatible with the fall in IOP routinely encountered in cases of acute anterior uveitis. Another possible factor in the postoperative pressure response is remote trabecular damage due to shock wave or acoustic effects. Well-designed animal research is needed to try to separate these possible factors and uncover the true cause.

The rise in IOP after YAG laser treatment can be blunted by the judicious use of topical steroids and antihypertensive agents. Brown (9) has reduced the incidence of significant pressure rise after posterior capsulotomy to less than 2% by instilling timolol 0.5% and prednisolone acetate 1.0% immediately after treatment. Prophylactic treatment of IOP elevation is indicated in patients with open-angle glaucoma and advanced optic nerve damage. Acetazolamide 500 mg orally and an oral osmotic agent such as isosorbide or glycerol should be administered preoperatively to patients in whom even a small pressure rise (5 mm Hg) may endanger a tender optic nerve. All patients should have IOP measured at 1, 2, and 3 hr after treatment, and excessive IOP elevations should be treated with timolol or one of the carbonic anhydrase inhibitors. Patients with advanced optic nerve damage from glaucoma should be admitted to the hospital so that IOP can be carefully monitored for the 24-hr period after treatment and significant pressure rises treated.

THE PUPIL

The pupillary responses to ocular trauma are discussed elsewhere in this text. However, some specific comments will be made regarding the state of the pupil and YAG laser surgery.

The performance of an adequate anterior capsulotomy with the YAG laser prior to extracapsular cataract extraction is dependent on the maintenance of good pupillary dilation throughout the procedure (Fig. 2). If special precautions are not taken to achieve this goal, the pupil can rapidly become miotic and force the surgeon to abandon the capsulotomy before its completion. Maintenance of adequate dilation can be achieved using the regimen outlined in Table 1. The same regimen has also been found to be useful preparatory to extracapsular cataract extraction (13).

Posterior capsulotomy following extracapsular extraction may be performed in the presence of a dilated pupil (Fig. 3). This allows the surgeon to inspect the topography of the entire posterior capsule and to plan the incision perpendicular to stress lines, when appropriate. Adequate dilation can be achieved routinely with tropicamide 1.0% and phenylephrine 2.5%. It is important to note the position of the pupil with respect to any eccentricity, since it is necessary to incise the posterior capsule in the visual axis.

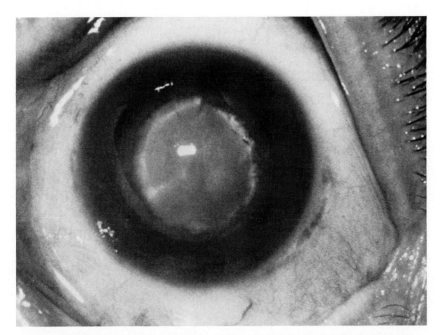

FIG. 2. YAG laser anterior capsulotomy with maintenance of a widely dilated pupil.

Some authors recommend a vigorous course of pilocarpine prior to performing YAG laser iridectomy (Fig. 4). Although such preparation is important prior to the performance of an argon laser iridectomy, it is often unnecessary with the YAG laser. If the iris is flaccid or the pupil large, a single application of a 1.0% pilocarpine solution 30 min prior to iridectomy is usually sufficient. Pilocarpine should be avoided postoperatively if possible. Its use will encourage the formation of posterior synechiae by increasing the disruption of the blood-aqueous barrier, making the pupil miotic, and by promoting the forward displacement of the lens, thereby increasing lens-iris apposition. The pupil should be widely dilated, the IOP monitored, and gonioscopy performed at the first postoperative visit 1 to several days later.

Sectioning of anterior vitreous bands to the surgical wound in aphakic eyes should be performed without dilation of the pupil. The rounding up of a peaked pupil during the procedure is a good indicator that the vitreous strand

TABLE 1. *Maintenance of adequate pupil dilation*

Time Preoperatively	Medication
4 hr	Topical prednisolone acetate 1.0%
2 hr	Topical prednisolone acetate 1.0%
1 hr	Cyclogyl 1.0% every 5 min for 4 applications
30 min	Phenylephrine 2.5% every 5 min for 4 applications

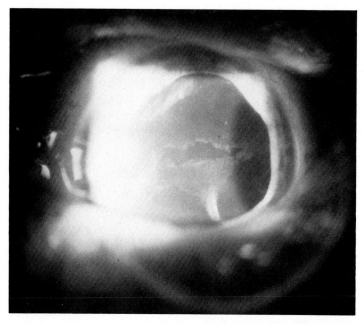

FIG. 3. Postoperative photograph of YAG laser posterior capsulotomy.

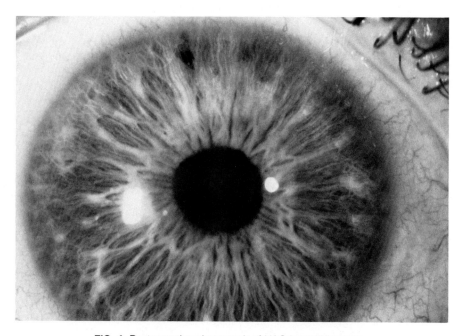

FIG. 4. Postoperative photograph of YAG laser iridectomy.

has been completely severed. In addition, the action of the sphincter of the undilated pupil serves to increase the tautness of the strand in some cases and may facilitate its lysis.

REFERENCES

1. Aron-Rosa, D. (1981): Use of a pulsed neodymium-YAG laser for anterior capsulotomy before extracapsular cataract extraction. *Am. Intra-Ocular Implant Soc. J.,* 7:332–333.
2. Aron-Rosa, D. (1983): The picosecond YAG laser in cataract surgery. In: *Pulsed YAG laser Surgery,* edited by D. Aron-Rosa, pp. 25–32. Slack Inc., Thoroughfare, NJ.
3. Aron-Rosa, D., Aron, J., Griesemann, M., and Thyzer, R. (1980): Use of the neodymium:YAG laser to open the posterior capsule after lens implant surgery. A preliminary report. *Am. Intra-Ocular Implant Soc. J.,* 6:352–354.
4. Aron-Rosa, D., Griesemann, J., and Aron, J. (1981): Use of a pulsed neodymium YAG laser (picosecond) to open the posterior lens capsule in traumatic cataract: A preliminary report. *Ophthalmic Surg.,* 12:496–499.
5. Beitch, B. R., and Eakins, K. E. (1969): The effects of prostaglandins on the intraocular pressure of the rabbit. *Br. J. Clin. Pharmacol.,* 37:158–167.
6. Bhattacherjee, P., Eakins, K. E., and Hammond, B. (1981): Chemotactic activity of arachidonic acid lipooxygenase products in the rabbit eye. *Br. J. Clin. Pharmacol.,* 73:254P–255P.
7. Bonner, R. F., Meyers, S. M., and Gaasterland, D. E. (1983): Threshold for retinal damage associated with the use of high power neodymium-YAG lasers in the vitreous. *Am. J. Ophthalmol.,* 96:153–159.
8. Borgeat, P. and Sirois, P. (1981): Leukotrienes: A major step in the understanding of immediate hypersensitivity reactions. *J. Med. Chem.,* 24:121–126.
9. Brown, G. (1983): Laser capsulotomy. In: *Laser Therapy of the Anterior Segment. A Practical Approach,* by L. Schwartz, G. L. Spaeth, and G. Brown, pp. 113–136. Slack, Inc., Thoroughfare, NJ.
10. Brown, G. (1983): Pulsed Nd:YAG laser treatment and the anterior vitreous. In: *Laser Therapy of the Anterior Segment. A Practical Approach,* by L. Schwartz, G. L. Spaeth, and G. Brown, pp. 137–147. Slack, Inc., Thoroughfare, NJ.
11. Camras, C. B., and Bito, L. Z. (1980): The pathophysiological effects of nitrogen mustard on the rabbit eye. I. The biphasic intraocular pressure response and the role of prostaglandins. *Exp. Eye Res.,* 30:41–52.
12. Camras, C. B., Bito, L. Z., and Eakins, K. E. (1977): Reduction of intraocular pressure by prostaglandins applied topically to the eyes of conscious rabbits. *Invest. Ophthalmol. Vis. Sci.,* 16:1125–1134.
13. Caprioli, J., and Spaeth, G. L. (1985): The effect of indomethacin on the maintenance of pupillary dilatation during extracapsular cataract surgery. *Ophthalmic Surg., (in press).*
14. Casey, W. J. (1974): Prostaglandin E₂ and aqueous humor dynamics in the rhesus monkey eye. *Prostaglandins,* 8:327–337.
15. Channell, M. M. and Beckman, H. (1984): Intraocular pressure changes after neodymium-YAG laser posterior capsulotomy. *Arch. Ophthalmol.,* 102:1024–1026.
16. Cohn, H. C., and Aron-Rosa, D. (1983): Reopening blocked trabeculectomy sites with the YAG laser. *Am. J. Ophthalmol.,* 95:293–294.
17. Eakins, K. E., Whitelocke, R. A. F., Bennett, A., and Martenet, A. C. (1972): Prostaglandin-like activity in ocular inflammation. *Br. Med. J.,* 3:452–453.
18. Fankhauser, F. (1983): The Q-switched laser: Principles and clinical results. In: *YAG Laser Ophthalmic Microsurgery,* edited by S. Trokel, pp. 101–146. Appleton Century Crofts, Norwalk, CT.
19. Fankhauser, F., Rousell, P., Steffen, J., Van der Zypen, E., and Chrenkova, A. (1981): Clinical studies on the efficiency of high power laser radiation upon some structures of the anterior segment of the eye. *Int. Ophthalmol.,* 3:129–139.
20. Federman, J. L., Annesley, W. H., Sarin, L. K., and Kemer, P. (1980): Vitrectomy and cystoid macular edema. *Ophthalmology,* 87:622–628.
21. Fung, W. (1980): Anterior vitrectomy for chronic aphakic cystoid macular edema. *Ophthalmology,* 87:189–193.

22. Gass, J. D. M., and Norton, E. D. W. (1969): Follow-up study of cystoid macular edema following cataract extraction. *Trans. Am. Acad. Ophthalmol. Otolaryngol.,* 73:665–682.
23. Goldman, A. I., Ham, W. T., and Mueller, H. A. (1977): Ocular damage thresholds and mechanisms for ultrashort pulses of both visible and infrared laser radiation in the rhesus monkey. *Exp. Eye Res.,* 24:45–56.
24. Iliff, C. E. (1966): Treatment of the vitreous-tug syndrome. *Am. J. Ophthalmol.,* 62:856–859.
25. Jampol, L. M., Goldberg, M. F., and Jenock, N. (1983): Retinal damage from a Q-switched YAG laser. *Am. J. Ophthalmol.,* 96:326–329.
26. Jampol, L. M., Neufeld, A. H., and Sears, M. L. (1975): Pathways for the response of the eye to injury. *Invest. Ophthalmol. Vis. Sci.,* 14:184–189.
27. Kass, M. A., Podos, S. M., Moses, R. A., and Becker, B. (1972): Prostaglandin E_1 and aqueous humor dynamics. *Invest. Ophthalmol. Vis. Sci.,* 11:1022–1027.
28. Katzen, L. E., Fleischman, J. A., and Trokel, S. L. (1983): YAG laser treatment of cystoid macular edema. *Am. J. Ophthalmol.,* 95:589–592.
29. Katzen, L. E., Lapinsky, P. T., Fleischman, J. A., and Trokel, S. (1984): YAG laser treatment of cystoid macular edema—clinical update. *Cataract,* 1:27–29.
30. Keates, R. (1983): Q-switched nanosecond pulsed Nd:YAG lasers. In: *Pulsed YAG Laser Surgery,* edited by D. Aron-Rosa, pp. 49–56. Slack, Inc., Thoroughfare, NJ.
31. Kelly, R. G. M., and Starr, M. S. (1971): Effects of prostaglandins and a prostaglandin antagonist on intraocular pressure and protein in the monkey eye. *Can. J. Ophthalmol.,* 6:205–211.
32. Khodadoust, A., Arkfeld, D., Caprioli, J., and Sears, M. L. (1984): Ocular effects of neodymium-YAG laser. *Am. J. Ophthalmol.,* 98:144–152.
33. Krasnov, M. M. (1976): Q-switched lasers (cool) in ophthalmology. *Int. Ophth. Clin.,* 16:29–44.
34. Masuda, K., Izawa, Y., and Mishima, S. (1973): Prostaglandins and uveitis: A preliminary report. *Jpn. J. Ophthalmol.,* 17:166–170.
35. Masuda, K., and Mishima, S. (1973): Effects of prostaglandins on inflow and outflow of the aqueous humor in rabbits. *Jpn. J. Ophthalmol.,* 17:300–309.
36. McPherson, A. R., O'Malley, R. E., and Bravo, J. (1983): Retinal detachment following late posterior capsulotomy. *Am. J. Ophthalmol.,* 95:593–597.
37. Neufeld, A. H., Jampol, L. M., and Sears, M. L. (1972): Aspirin prevents the disruption of the blood-aqueous barrier in the rabbit eye. *Nature,* 238:158–159.
38. Perkins, E. S. (1975): Prostaglandins and the eye. *Adv. Ophthal.,* 29:2–21.
39. Robinson, D., Landers, M. B., and Hahn, D. K. (1983): An anterior surgical approach to aphakic cystoid macular edema. *Am. J. Ophthalmol.,* 95:811–817.
40. Ruderman, J. M., Mitchell, P. G., and Kraff, M. (1983): Pupillary block following Nd:YAG laser capsulotomy. *Ophthalmic Surg.,* 14:418–419.
41. Schwartz, L. (1983): Laser iridectomy. In: *Laser Therapy of the Anterior Segment. A Practical Approach,* edited by L. Schwartz, G. L. Spaeth, and G. Brown, pp. 29–58. Slack, Inc., Thoroughfare, NJ.
42. Sears, M. L., Neufeld, A. H., and Jampol, L. M. (1973): Prostaglandins. *Invest. Ophthalmol. Vis. Sci.,* 12:161–164.
43. Shrader, C. E., Belcher, C. D., Thomas, J. V., and Simmons, R. I. (1983): Acute glaucoma following Nd:YAG laser membranotomy. *Ophthalmic Surg.,* 14:1015–1016.
44. Taboada, J. (1983): Interaction of short laser pulses with ocular tissues. In: *YAG Laser Ophthalmic Microsurgery,* edited by S. Trokel, pp. 15–38. Appleton Century Crofts, Norwalk, CT.
45. Terry, A. C., Stark, W. I., Maumanee, A. E., and Fagadau, W. (1983): Neodymium-YAG laser for posterior capsulotomy. *Am. J. Ophthalmol.,* 96:716–720.
46. Trokel, S. L., and Katzen, L. E. (1983): The mode locked laser: Principles and clinical results. In: *YAG Laser Ophthalmic Microsurgery,* edited by S. Trokel, pp. 147–179. Appleton Century Crofts, Norwalk, CT.
47. Unger, W. G., Cole, D. F., and Bass, M. S. (1977): Prostaglandin and neurogenically mediated ocular response to laser irradiation of the rabbit iris. *Exp. Eye Res.,* 25:209–220.
48. Unger, W. G., Perkins, E. S., and Bass, M. S. (1974): The response of the rabbit eye to laser irradiation of the iris. *Exp. Eye Res.,* 9:367–377.
49. Van der Zypen, E., and Fankhauser, F. (1982): Lasers in the treatment of chronic simple glaucoma. *Trans. Ophthalmol. Soc. U. K.,* 102:147–153.

Commentary

Cystoid Macular Edema: Clinical Course and Characteristics

In this scholarly review of the pathogenesis of cystoid macular edema, the basis for surgical and/or pharmacological approaches to therapy is established. The increased capillary permeability occurring in the perifoveal area and elsewhere in the retina may be the result of microconcussions to the retina produced by movement of the vitreous, by vitreous detachment and secondary macula-vitreal adherences, by irritation of the iris and ciliary body by vitreous in the absence of a posterior capsule, by inflammation secondary to the breakdown of the blood ocular barrier with the release of vasoactive factors, or from deposition in the vitreous of antigenic substances (editors). Ever since the early demonstrations (3,5,6) and hypotheses (1,4) that prostaglandins may be involved in the production of leaky ocular vessels, considerable attention has been focused on these substances as mediators of the reaction. Of course, there may be several roads that lead to Rome; i.e., cofactors and other contributing causative substances (3). Furthermore, the eye like any other tissue has limited numbers of ways of expressing pathology or showing the morphologic manifestations of a lesion. Thus, "aphakic" cystoid macular edema may be the final expression of several additive or even synergistic factors resulting from a number of "toxic" causes, such as excessive operating theater illumination, producing either ultraviolet (photochemical) and/or "thermal" injury, and, the surgical trauma itself. These must be considered as multiple contributors to the pathogenesis of the lesion, factors that can certainly be ameliorated or eliminated. See also Commentary to Dr. Tso's chapter.

The Editors

REFERENCES

1. Editorial (1973): Prostaglandins. *Invest. Ophthalmol.* 12:161–164.
2. Sears, M. L., and Albert, D. (1976): Histologic studies of the blood-aqueous barrier: Preservation with indomethacin. In: *Glaukom-Symposium,* Wurzburg, edited by W. Leydhecker, pp. 94–105. Verlag, Stuttgart.
3. Symposium on aphakic cystoid macular edema (1984): The pharmacology of ocular trauma. *Surv. Ophthalmol.* Suppl. 28:525–534.
4. Tennant, J. L. (1983): Cystoid macular edema. *Ophthalmology,* Audio-Digest Foundation. 21 (15).
5. The use of aspirin and aspirin-like drugs in ophthalmology (1974): In: *Symposium on Ocular Therapy* Vol. 7, edited by I. H. Leopold pp. 104–115. C.V. Mosby, New York.
6. Whitelocke, R. A. F., and Eakins, K. E. (1973): Vascular changes in the anterior uvea of the rabbit produced by prostaglandins. *Arch. Ophthalmol.* 89:495–499.

Surgical Pharmacology of the Eye,
edited by M. Sears and A. Tarkkanen.
Raven Press, New York © 1985.

Cystoid Macular Edema: Clinical Course and Characteristics

Leila Laatikainen

*Department of Ophthalmology, Helsinki University
Central Hospital, Helsinki, 00290 Finland*

SUMMARY: CME is the accumulation of extracellular fluid in the center of the macula. It has been described in a variety of ocular diseases, particularly in retinal vascular diseases, as a complication of intraocular inflammation and following cataract or retinal detachment surgery.

   CME is caused by disruption of the blood-retinal barrier, usually due to damage of the retinal capillary endothelium, more rarely due to failure of the retinal pigment epithelium. Several pathomechanisms may play a part in various ocular conditions. In addition to primary retinal vascular disorders, intraocular inflammation seems to be an important causative factor. The predisposition of aphakic eyes to CME may depend on the loss of the barrier between the anterior part of the eye and the vitreous body. This allows both increased mechanical irritation in the eye as well as free access of chemical mediators such as PGs or PG-like substances into the vitreous and the retina. The susceptibility of the macula to cystoid changes may depend on both its anatomical features and its high metabolic activity.

Cystoid macular edema (CME) or accumulation of extracellular fluid in the center of the macula occurs as a secondary event in several entirely different disease processes (Table 1). Most frequently, CME is seen in retinal vascular diseases and following intraocular surgery.

PATHOLOGY

   In histopathologic studies of eyes with CME cystoid spaces containing eosinophilic exudate have been found mainly in the outer plexiform layer and the inner nuclear layer (12,39,47). Due to the peculiar architecture of the retina in the macular area, the largest cysts develop around the fovea in the outer plexiform layer of Henle, where the long receptor cell axons radiate outward from the foveal area (12). In some cases, cystoid spaces have also been found in the ganglion cell and nerve fiber layer (47). With increasing size of the cysts, some disruption of the nerve fibers and degeneration of the underlying receptor cells occur, and rupture of the cyst wall may finally result in lamellar macular hole formation (11,47) or more rarely in a full-thickness

TABLE 1. *The most common ocular conditions complicated*
by cystoid macular edema

Primary retinal vascular diseases	Toxic conditions
Diabetic retinopathy	Epinephrine maculopathy
Retinal venous occlusion	Photic retinopathy
Severe hypertensive retinopathy	Macular dystrophies
Radiation retinopathy	Dominant cystoid macular edema
Retinal telangiectasis (Coats' disease)	Retinitis pigmentosa
Inflammatory diseases	Vitelliform dystrophy
Chronic cyclitis	Degenerative conditions
Posterior uveitis	Senile maculopathy with or without
Nongranulomatous iridocyclitis	subretinal neovascular membrane
Nematode endophthalmitis	Long-standing serous detachment of
Behçet's syndrome	retinal neuroepithelium
Postsurgical edema	Retinal detachment
Cataract surgery	Central serous retinopathy
Retinal detachment surgery	Choroidal tumors (hemangioma,
Aphakic penetrating keratoplasty	malignant melanoma)
Vitrectomy	

defect of the retina (47). According to Tso (47), remarkable loss of photoreceptor cells and alterations in the retinal pigment epithelium are consistently seen in CME.

DIAGNOSIS OF CME

The symptoms and clinical findings of CME vary with the severity of edema. Reduction of the central visual acuity may be mild and temporary, but persistent edema or lamellar macular hole formation may result in irreversible loss of vision.

The diagnosis of macular edema is inferred from direct and indirect ophthalmoscopy and confirmed by contact lens examination or fluorescein angioscopy or angiography. The mildest cases are diagnosed by angiography only. The characteristic pattern of cystoid spaces results in the typical petaloid late hyperfluorescence of the macula (Figs. 1–5). A nonfluorescent stellate area in the center of the macula is due to accumulation of nerve fibers and luteal pigment between the cysts. In advanced cases, the nonfluorescent spot in the center may be caused by a lamellar macular hole (Fig. 3B).

In the early phases of the fluorescein angiogram, the picture varies slightly from one disease entity to another. In the primary vascular diseases, such as diabetes or retinal venous occlusion, a variable combination of dilated capillaries and areas of capillary closure are seen (Figs. 1, 2). In eyes with secondary capillary damage, retinal capillary dilatation and leakage are usually restricted to the perifoveal capillaries (Fig. 5), although in some cases the disc capillaries may leak as well. In persistent cases and in eyes in which the main cause of retinal edema is a retinal pigment epithelial failure, no dilatation or leakage may be seen in the retinal capillaries. In these eyes, defects in the underlying pigment epithelium result in a more diffuse staining of the macula (Fig. 6).

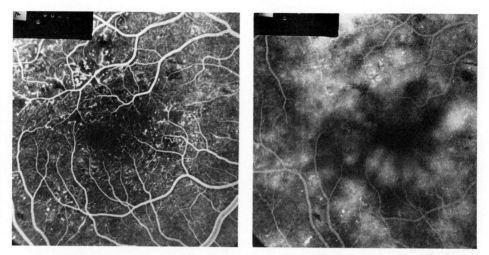

FIG. 1. Left: Fluorescein angiogram of diabetic cystoid macular edema showing areas of capillary closure, dilated capillaries and microaneurysms. **Right:** Late picture shows petaloid hyperfluorescence in the macula as well as areas of leakage around the macula.

PATHOPHYSIOLOGY OF CME IN VARIOUS CONDITIONS

In the pathophysiology of CME several factors may play a role. The two anatomic structures that are responsible for the blood-retinal barrier and control the movements of fluid into and out of the retina are the endothelium of the retinal vessels and the retinal pigment epithelium. Any significant failure of either barrier will result in intraretinal collection of fluid.

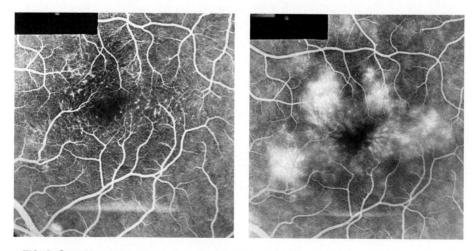

FIG. 2. Cystoid macular edema after central retinal vein occlusion. Dilated capillaries (**left**) with late intraretinal accumulation of fluorescein (**right**).

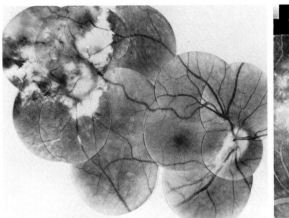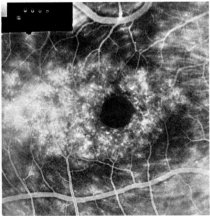

FIG. 3. Cystoid macular edema in Coats' disease. **Left:** Exudative lesion in the upper temporal periphery. **Right:** Fluorescein angiogram shows a large lamellar macular hole surrounded by dilated capillaries and accumulation of fluorescein in smaller cystoid spaces. (From ref. 43, with permission of the authors and *British Journal of Ophthalmology*.)

CME in Primary Retinal Vascular Diseases

Endothelium of the retinal vessels may be damaged by a number of mechanisms, many of which are not clearly understood. In *diabetic retinopathy* (Fig. 1), several metabolic abnormalities, most of them possibly secondary to hyperglycemia, may be blamed for endothelial cell damage and leakage of the capillaries. In the nonischemic type of *retinal venous occlusion* (Fig. 2) both veins and venules as well as macular capillaries leak fluorescein (29). In venous occlusion, endothelium of the terminal venules and capillaries may be damaged partly by increased intraluminal pressure, partly by hypoxia due to slow circulation. In *retinal telangiectasis or Coats' disease* (Fig. 3), dilated capillaries in the macula may have the same structural abnormality as the affected capillaries in the periphery, or macular edema is secondary to the peripheral exudative process (43).

CME in Inflammatory Diseases

In the primarily nonvascular diseases, damage of the vascular endothelium may be secondary to various chemical mediators. CME is a common complication in chronic cyclitis, posterior uveitis and nongranulomatous iridocyclitis (Fig. 4). In these inflammatory conditions macular edema has been thought to be due to prostaglandins (PGs) or PG-like substances released from the inflamed tissue. It has been shown that PG-like substances are released in substantial amounts in acute anterior uveitis in both rabbits and man (50). PGs increase permeability of the iris vessels (49). Similarly, PGs could be the causative factor in the breakdown of the blood-retinal barrier in the macula.

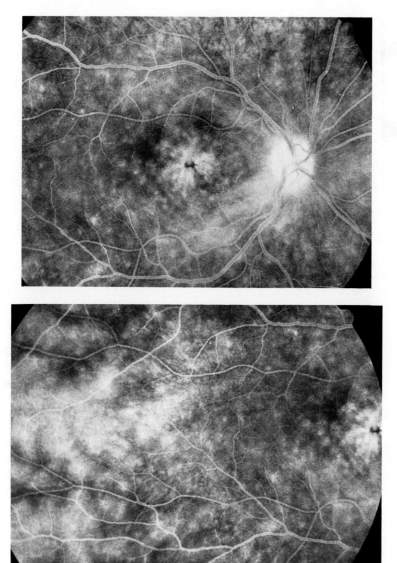

FIG. 4. Cystoid macular edema and mild leakage of peripapillary **(top)** and peripheral **(bottom)** retinal vessels in nongranulomatous iridocyclitis.

Archer (1) studied the effect of PGE on the blood-retinal barrier experimentally by perfusing the retinal vasculature via the carotid artery with varying concentrations of PGE_1. He found that the healthy retinal vascular endothelium remained intact even to large concentrations of PG, but following short periods of ischemia, the administration of relatively small quantities of PGE_1 produced rapid and marked breakdown of the blood-retinal barrier and extensive edema.

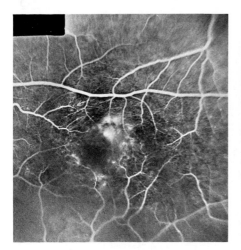 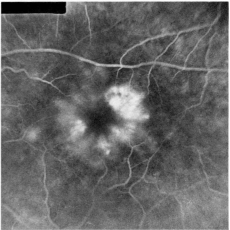

FIG. 5. Aphakic cystoid macular edema. Dilated capillaries **(left)** with late petaloid accumulation of fluorescein in the cystoid spaces **(right)**. Clear view of the fundus partly obscured by vitreous opacities.

CME in Toxic Conditions

Topical administration of epinephrine may result in CME, particularly in aphakic eyes. In 1968, Kolker and Becker (25) reported a reversible macular edema in 22 eyes of 15 patients under epinephrine therapy for chronic open-angle glaucoma. Fourteen patients were aphakic and one had dislocated lens. After epinephrine therapy, the time required for visual improvement varied from 1 week to several months, and 6 or more months were usually needed for complete return of vision and disappearance of macular edema. In 4 cases cystoid maculopathy reappeared when the drug was used again. These findings were confirmed by Thomas and co-workers (45), who found CME in 28% of aphakic eyes under epinephrine therapy, whereas for aphakic glaucomatous eyes not being treated with epinephrine this percentage was 13%. In 6 of 7 eyes, edema resolved within 6 months to 1 year after cessation of topical epinephrine.

Being an adrenergic vasoconstrictor, epinephrine may have a direct effect on the ocular vasculature. Experimental studies on rabbits and cats have shown that the retinal uptake of radioactively labeled, topically administered epinephrine was significantly higher in an aphakic eye than an eye that retains the lens as a barrier to anterior-to-posterior drug migration (28).

Recently the role of ultraviolet light as a cause of CME has been suggested. Tennant (44) reported that by using a 400-nm light filter on the operating microscope and similar protective lenses for the correction of aphakia the incidence of macular edema, demonstrated by fluorescein angiography 5 to 6 weeks postoperatively, decreased from 36% in the unfiltered group to 20% in the filtered group, and the incidence of clinical CME with reduced visual

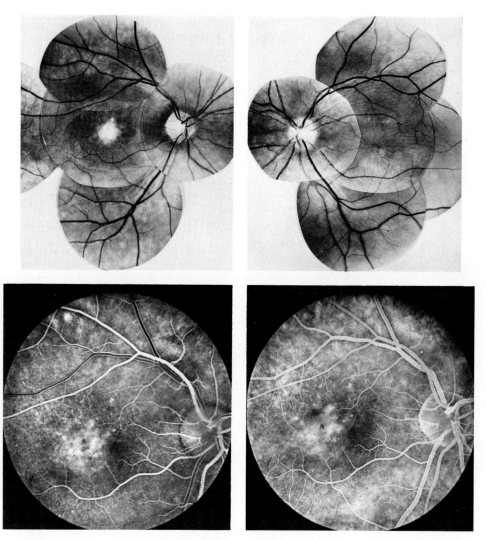

FIG. 6. Cystoid macular edema in vitelliform macular dystrophy. **Top left:** Right eye; **top right:** left eye. **Bottom left and right:** Accumulation of fluorescein in the right macula due to pigment epithelial changes. (**Top** figures are reprinted from ref. 30 with permission of the author and *International Ophthalmology*.)

acuity of less than 20/40 decreased from 3% in the control group to 0.76% in the filtered group.

Aphakic CME

CME has been supposed to be the most common complication following cataract surgery (19) (Fig. 5). In 1953, S. R. Irvine (21) described a "vitreous syndrome" consisting of delayed rupture of the vitreous face followed by adherence of the herniated vitreous to the cataract wound and subsequent decrease in visual acuity associated with reversible macular changes. In 1966, Gass and Norton (12) demonstrated in their fluorescein angiographic studies that cystoid edema in the macula after cataract extraction was secondary to alteration in the capillary permeability of the macula.

After routine intracapsular cataract surgery the incidence of clinically significant CME is about 2% (21,22), and after intra- or extracapsular cataract extraction with various types of intraocular lenses the incidence varies from 0% to 20% (22,41,42). By fluorescein angiography, increased permeability of the macular capillaries at some time after cataract surgery has been found in a much higher percentage of eyes. Between the 4th and 16th weeks the incidence of angiographic CME may be 40% to 60% (14,19,20,33,37).

The prognosis of aphakic CME is usually good. The time of onset of edema varies from a few weeks to several years. In most cases edema subsides within 6 to 12 months with good recovery of vision. Gass and Norton (13) found clear correlation between prognosis and vitreous adherence to the cataract wound. In eyes without vitreous incarceration, macular edema resolved in 79%, and the average time required was 25 weeks; whereas in eyes with vitreous incarceration, edema resolved in 60%, and the average time required was 65 weeks.

The pathomechanism of postoperative cystoid edema has been the subject of a great controversy. In aphakic eyes, the two possible mechanisms suggested by Irvine (21) were vitreous traction on the macula or secondary iritis produced by vitreous traction on the iris and ciliary body, both secondary to delayed rupture of the vitreous face. Support to the theory of vitreous traction on the macula was presented by Tolentino and Schepens (46), who found vitreoretinal adhesion and traction in all but 1 eye in a series of 25 eyes with CME following cataract extraction. They suggested that after removal of the lens the vitreous body was able to move forward, which resulted in posterior vitreous detachment. At the macula and optic disc, where the adhesion between retina and vitreous was firm, vitreoretinal adhesion remained and caused traction and edema of the retina. In a recent report Ho and Tolentino (16) again emphasized the role of vitreomacular traction in the development of aphakic CME. Gass and Norton (12,13), however, were unable to demonstrate vitreous adherence to the macula in CME. In postmortem studies on aphakic eyes Foos (9) found that 77% of 62 eyes had complete and 16% had partial posterior vitreous detachment, but he too was unable to find any vitreomacular adhesions with the exception of eyes that had paramacular preretinal neovascularization.

A theory of microconcussions of the retina caused by oscillations of the liquid vitreous during saccadic movement of the aphakic eye (endophthalmodonesis) was presented by Binkhorst (2). The studies that compare the occurrence of CME after extracapsular cataract extraction with or without posterior capsulotomy give some support to the role of the vitreous movements as a cause of macular damage. Chambless (5) reported that in a group of 1,055 extracapsular cataract extractions the incidence of CME was 7.3% in cases with open capsules but only 0.9% when the capsules were left intact. By preventing a forward displacement of the vitreous body, an intact posterior capsule could both prevent endophthalmodonesis and rupture of the vitreous face and diminish vitreous traction on the retina. On the other hand, Chambless (5) could not find any significant difference in the incidence of CME between capsulotomy without vitreous disturbance and capsulotomy with vitreous prolapse or loss, and the occurrence of CME was independent of the size or timing of the opening of the posterior capsule. The low incidence of CME in eyes with an intact posterior capsule could also be due to prevention of continued mechanical irritation of the iris and ciliary body caused by vitreous touch. After extracapsular surgery with an intraocular lens implant, the implant may have a similar protective effect, because in these eyes Jaffe and co-workers (23) found no significant difference in the incidence of CME in their two series with an intact capsule or with primary posterior capsulotomy.

The role of intraocular inflammation as a cause of aphakic CME has been widely accepted (12–14,20,37,42,51). The clinical and fluorescein angiographic picture of aphakic CME is identical to that seen in chronic cyclitis and other inflammatory diseases. Most eyes with CME show mild irritability and some inflammatory reaction in the vitreous. Fluorescein angiographic studies of the iris have shown that vascular changes in aphakic CME are not restricted to the macula and the disc, but iris vessels may also be congested and leak fluorescein (4,26). It has been suggested that increased permeability of the macular capillaries could be due to breakdown of the blood-aqueous barrier and release of PGs and other inflammatory mediators initiated by surgical trauma as well as continued mechanical irritation by vitreous or an intraocular lens implant (37,51). Significant reduction in the immediate postoperative incidence of CME after intracapsular surgery was obtained by topical (37,51) or oral (24) administration of a PG inhibitor, indomethacin.

The incidence of CME and its severity seem to be highest after intracapsular cataract extraction with vitreous incarceration to the cataract wound and following intracapsular cataract extraction with an iris-fixated intraocular lens. Stern et al. (42) reported that an overall incidence of clinical CME following implantation of an iris-fixated lens was 6.1%. In most of their cases CME was recurrent, and in 44% of them the vision did not recover better than 20/40. Correspondingly, Stark et al. (41) found the highest incidence of persistent CME (7%) in eyes with contaminated iris-fixated lenses, which also had severest postoperative inflammation.

Eyes with iridocapsular or posterior chamber lenses following extracapsular cataract extraction seem to have less CME than eyes operated on by intracapsular cataract extraction with or without intraocular lenses (22,41). In the Food and Drug Administration report, the incidences of persistent (at 1 year)

CME following the various types of intraocular lens implants were 2.2% with an anterior chamber lens, 2.4% with an iris-fixated lens, 0.3% with an iridocapsular lens, and 0.8% with a posterior chamber lens.

The 40% to 60% incidence of angiographic edema following cataract surgery (15,19,20,33,37) indicates that some vasoactive factor may be released in every operation, but the susceptibility of the vasculature varies. This susceptibility could depend on general systemic factors like age or vascular disease (13,15,20,33). A recent report on cataract surgery in infants showed, however, that aphakic CME may also develop in children. Following transpupillary lensectomy and anterior vitrectomy CME developed in 10 of 27 eyes (17). Postoperative hypotension or hypertension (15) or the use of α-chymotrypsin (44) or retrobulbar hyaluronidase (27) seem to have no effect on the development of CME. In experimental studies, Tso (47) found that leakage of the retinal vasculature alone did not cause CME. He suggested that ischemia resulting in microinfarction could be one of the important factors in the production of CME.

In phakic eyes postoperative CME is only infrequently seen. Among their patients, Hitchings and co-workers (15) found no cases of CME following elective glaucoma surgery. Susceptibility of the aphakic eyes to CME could be due to disruption of the barrier between the anterior part of the eye and the vitreous. The possible role of ultraviolet light as a cause of aphakic CME is discussed earlier in this text. It has been shown experimentally that the retinal uptake of radioactively labeled, topically administered epinephrine was significantly higher in aphakic than phakic eyes when an intracapsular technique of cataract surgery was used (28). In aphakic eyes, particularly following intracapsular cataract extraction or posterior capsulotomy and rupture of the vitreous face, vasoactive substances released from the iris or the ciliary body could readily get into the vitreous body, accumulate there, and gradually penetrate into the retina.

The predilection of macula for cystoid edema has been explained by various theories. Gass and Norton (12) stated that the macular region by virtue of its structure is the site of predilection for the accumulation of interstitial fluid. The internal limiting lamina is thinner over the central macula and the disc than over the rest of the postequatorial retina (10). This would allow vasoactive factors to penetrate into the retina. In addition, the high metabolic activity of the macula and the lack of capillaries in the center of the macula may increase its susceptibility to edema.

CME may also develop following other surgical procedures, particularly in aphakic eyes. Following aphakic penetrating keratoplasty, West and co-workers (48) found macular edema on fluorescein angiography in 27 (64%) of 42 eyes, in 14 eyes after a combined keratoplasty and lens extraction, and in 28 eyes after keratoplasty following previous lens extraction. CME has also been demonstrated following vitrectomy (35) and detachment surgery (39); as well as following prophylactic procedures for the treatment of retinal holes (40). There seem to be no reports in the literature on CME after laser trabeculoplasty in aphakia. Nonetheless, about a year ago I had a patient who had had chronic open-angle glaucoma and aphakia for 3 years. Since cataract surgery the vision had been normal, and no signs of maculopathy had been detected. Three months after trabeculoplasty with argon laser, the vision dropped to 20/200 due to significant CME. In this eye macular edema seems to be persistent with permanent loss of central vision. No other obvious cause than the laser treatment could be found for the CME.

CME in Retinal Detachment

CME is a common complication in eyes with retinal detachment and may be one of the causes of poor visual recovery after detachment surgery (6,31,39). Postdetachment CME is more common in aphakic than in phakic eyes. Using fluorescein angiography and color stereophotography, Meredith and co-workers (34) found CME in 25% of 67 phakic eyes and in 40% of 33 aphakic eyes studied 6 weeks after successful scleral buckling surgery. Correspondingly, Lobes and Grand (31) found 28% incidence of CME in phakic eyes and 64% incidence in aphakic eyes after retinal detachment surgery.

Because of the similarities between postcataract and postdetachment CME, the same causative factors could be suspected. Inflammatory cause is indicated by the findings of Miyake and co-workers (36), who found that topical indomethacin decreased the incidence of CME after detachment surgery from 33% in the placebo group to 13% in the indomethacin-treated group. Further, they found more clinically severe cases of CME in the placebo group than in the indomethacin-treated group. In both groups, aphakic eyes had a higher incidence of CME than eyes with intact lenses. Meredith and co-workers (34) stated, however, that although inflammation may be a necessary factor, it is insufficient in creating postsurgical macular edema, because all their eyes showed signs of inflammation but only the older eyes developed CME.

In experimental rhegmatogenous detachment in owl monkey, Machemer (32) found that cyst formation started in the inner retinal layers and later larger cysts formed in the outer layers. Machemer suggested that retinal edema in these eyes must be due to a metabolic change in the retina secondary to detachment of the sensory retina from the pigment epithelium. The clinical fluorescein angiographic studies on eyes with CME following detachment surgery have shown that in some of these eyes macular capillaries do not leak fluorescein (6,31). In these eyes cystoid spaces may be the result of loss of retinal tissue following metabolic changes that occur after separation of the neuroretina from the pigment epithelium and failure of the pigment epithelial pump to remove fluid from the retina.

CME in Choroidal Tumors

Reduced visual acuity due to CME may be the first clinical sign of choroidal melanoma (3,38). CME may develop even in eyes in which the tumor does not extend near the macula. Usually, however, inflammatory cells are found in the vitreous. Brownstein and co-workers (3) reported a case of spindle-β melanoma of the choroid in which they found lymphocytic cell infiltrate around some of the retinal vessels and mononuclear cells in the vitreous adjacent to the retina. Thus, inflammatory cells in the vitreous and cystoid edema of the macula may represent immunologic reactions to tumor antigens or tumor necrosis.

CME in Hereditary Macular Dystrophies

Leakage of macular capillaries and CME may also occur in some hereditary dystrophies. In dominant CME, described by Deutman and co-workers (7), leaking perimacular capillaries are the predominant finding, although other capillaries at the posterior pole may leak as well. In addition to vascular changes, these patients have moderate to high hyperopia, a subnormal electro-oculogram together with a normal electroretinogram, and some patients show whitish punctate opacities in the vitreous body. CME has also been described in some cases of retinitis pigmentosa (8,18). It is possible that the vascular changes in these conditions are secondary to hypoxia or toxic products produced by the dystrophic process. In retinitis pigmentosa and in the advanced forms of vitelliform dystrophy (30) CME may also occur without retinal vascular leakage (Fig. 6). In these eyes cystoid edema could be secondary to the defective pigment epithelium.

CME in Degenerative Macular Diseases

In degenerative macular diseases such as senile maculopathy, CME seems to be secondary to alterations in the retinal pigment epithelium or development of subretinal neovascular membranes with exudates and hemorrhages that disturb the normal metabolic interaction between the sensory retina and retinal pigment epithelium.

REFERENCES

1. Archer, D. B. (1975): The overall mechanism of macular edema. Macular Workshop, Bath.
2. Binkhorst, C. D. (1980): Corneal and retinal complications after cataract extraction. The mechanical aspect of endophthalmodonesis. *Ophthalmology,* 87:609–617.
3. Brownstein, S., Orton, R., and Jackson, W. B. (1978): Cystoid macular edema with equatorial choroidal melanoma. *Arch. Ophthalmol.,* 96:2105–2107.
4. Burnett, J., Tessler, H., Isenberg, S., and Tso, M. O. M. (1979): Clinical trial of fenoprofen in the treatment of aphakic cystoid macular edema. *Invest. Ophthalmol. Vis. Sci.,* 18(ARVO Suppl.):255.
5. Chambless, W. S. (1979): Phacoemulsification and the retina: Cystoid macular edema. *Ophthalmology,* 86:2019–2022.
6. Cleary, P. E., and Leaver, P. K. (1978): Macular abnormalities in the reattached retina. *Br. J. Ophthalmol.,* 62:595–603.
7. Deutman, A. F., Pinckers, A. J. L. G., and Aan de Kerk, A. L. (1976): Dominantly inherited cystoid macular edema. *Am. J. Ophthalmol.,* 82:540–548.

8. Fishman, G. A., Fishman, M., and Maggiano, J. (1977): Macular lesions associated with retinitis pigmentosa. *Arch. Ophthalmol.,* 95:798–803.
9. Foos, R. Y. (1972): Posterior vitreous detachment. *Trans. Am. Acad. Ophthalmol. Otolaryngol.,* 76:480–497.
10. Foos, R. Y. (1972): Vitreoretinal juncture; topographical variations. *Invest. Ophthalmol. Vis. Sci.,* 11:801–808.
11. Gass, J. D. M. (1976): Lamellar macular hole. A complication of cystoid macular edema after cataract extraction. *Arch. Ophthalmol.,* 94:793–800.
12. Gass, J. D. M., and Norton, E. W. D. (1966): Cystoid macular edema and papilledema following cataract extraction. A fluorescein fundoscopic and angiographic study. *Arch. Ophthalmol.,* 76:646–661.
13. Gass, J. D. M., and Norton, E. W. D. (1969): Follow-up study of cystoid macular edema following cataract extraction. *Trans. Am. Acad. Ophthalmol. Otolaryngol.,* 73:665–682.
14. Hitchings, R. A., and Chisholm, I. H. (1975): Incidence of aphakic macular oedema. A prospective study. *Br. J. Ophthalmol.,* 59:444–450.
15. Hitchings, R. A., Chisholm, I. H., and Bird, A. C. (1975): Aphakic macular edema: Incidence and pathogenesis. *Invest. Ophthalmol. Vis. Sci.,* 14:68–72.
16. Ho, P. C., and Tolentino, F. I. (1982): The role of vitreous in aphakic cystoid macular edema: A review. *Am. Intra-ocular. Implant Soc. J.,* 8:258–264.
17. Hoyt, C. S., and Nickel, B. (1982): Aphakic cystoid macular edema. Occurrence in infants and children after transpupillary lensectomy and anterior vitrectomy. *Arch. Ophthalmol.,* 100:746–749.
18. Hyvärinen, L., Maumenee, A. E., Kelley, J., and Cantollino, S. (1971): Fluorescein angiographic findings in retinitis pigmentosa. *Am. J. Ophthalmol.,* 71:17–26.
19. Irvine, A. R. (1976): Cystoid maculopathy. *Surv. Ophthalmol.,* 21:1–17.
20. Irvine, A. R., Bresky, R., Crowder, B. M., Forster, R. K., Hunter, D. M., and Kulvin, S. M. (1971): Macular edema after cataract extraction. *Ann. Ophthalmol.,* 3:1234–1240.
21. Irvine, S. R. (1953): A newly defined vitreous syndrome following cataract surgery. *Am. J. Ophthalmol.,* 36:599–619.
22. Jaffe, N. S., Clayman, H. M., and Jaffe, M. S. (1982): Cystoid macular edema after intracapsular and extracapsular cataract extraction with and without an intraocular lens. *Ophthalmology,* 89:25–29.
23. Jaffe, N. S., Luscombe, S. M., Clayman, H. M., and Gass, J. D. M. (1981): A fluorescein angiographic study of cystoid macular edema. *Am. J. Ophthalmol.,* 92:775–777.
24. Klein, R. M., Katzin, H. M., and Yannuzzi, L. A. (1979): The effect of indomethacin pretreatment on aphakic cystoid macular edema. *Am. J. Ophthalmol.,* 87:487–489.
25. Kolker, A. E., and Becker, B. (1968): Epinephrine maculopathy. *Arch. Ophthalmol.,* 79:552–562.
26. Kottow, M., and Hendrickson, P. (1975): Iris angiography in cystoid macular edema after cataract extraction. *Arch. Ophthalmol.,* 93:487–493.
27. Kraff, M. C., Sanders, D. R., Jampol, L. M., and Lieberman, H. L. (1983): Effect of retrobulbar hyaluronidase on pseudophakic cystoid macular edema. *Am. Intra-ocular Implant. Soc. J.,* 9:184–185.
28. Kramer, S. G. (1976): Retinal uptake of topical epinephrine in aphakia. In: *Symposium on Ocular Therapy,* vol. 9, edited by I. H. Leopold and R. P. Burns, pp. 73–83. John Wiley, New York.
29. Laatikainen, L. (1976): Vascular changes after central retinal vein occlusion. *Trans. Ophthalmol. Soc. U.K.,* 96:190–192.
30. Laatikainen, L. (1979): Presumed vitelliform dystrophy with perimacular flecks and retinal detachment. *Int. Ophthalmol.,* 1:163–170.
31. Lobes, L. A., Jr., and Grand, M. G. (1980): Incidence of cystoid macular edema following scleral buckling procedure. *Arch. Ophthalmol.,* 98:1230–1232.
32. Machemer, R. (1968): Experimental retinal detachment in the owl monkey. II. Histology of retina and pigment epithelium. *Am. J. Ophthalmol.,* 66:396–410.
33. Meredith, T. A., Kenyon, K. R., Singerman, L. J., and Fine, S. L. (1976): Perifoveal vascular leakage and macular oedema after intracapsular cataract extraction. *Br. J. Ophthalmol.,* 60:765–769.
34. Meredith, T. A., Reeser, F. H., Topping, T. M., and Aaberg, T. M. (1980): Cystoid macular edema after retinal detachment surgery. *Ophthalmology,* 87:1090–1095.

35. Michels, R. G. (1981): *Vitreous Surgery*, pp. 423–425. C. V. Mosby, St. Louis.
36. Miyake, K., Miyake, Y., Maekubo, K., Asakura, M., and Manabe, R. (1983): Incidence of cystoid macular edema after retinal detachment surgery and the use of topical indomethacin. *Am. J. Ophthalmol.*, 95:451–456.
37. Miyake, K., Sakamura, S., and Miura, H. (1980): Long-term follow-up study on prevention of aphakic cystoid macular oedema by topical indomethacin. *Br. J. Ophthalmol.*, 64:324–328.
38. Newsom, W. A., Hood, C. I., Horwitz, J. A., Fine, S. L., and Sewell, J. H. (1972): Cystoid macular edema: Histopathologic and angiographic correlations. A clinicopathologic case report. *Trans. Am. Acad. Ophthalmol. Otolaryngol.*, 76:1005–1009.
39. Reese, A. B. (1937): Defective central vision following successful operations for detachment of the retina. *Am. J. Ophthalmol.*, 20:591–598.
40. Ryan, S. J., Jr. (1973): Cystoid maculopathy in phakic retinal detachment procedures. *Am. J. Ophthalmol.*, 76:519–522.
41. Stark, W. J., Maumenee, A. E., Dangel, M. E., Martin, N. F., and Hirst, L. W. (1982): Intraocular lenses. Experience at the Wilmer Institute. *Ophthalmology*, 89:104–108.
42. Stern, A. L., Taylor, D. M., Dalburg, L. A., and Cosentino, R. T. (1981): Pseudophakic cystoid maculopathy. *Ophthalmology*, 88:942–946.
43. Tarkkanen, A., and Laatikainen, L. (1983): Coats's disease: Clinical, angiographic, histopathological findings and clinical management. *Br. J. Ophthalmol.*, 67:766–776.
44. Tennant, J. L. (1983): *Cystoid Macular Edema*. Audio-Digest Foundation. Ophthalmology, vol. 21, no. 15.
45. Thomas, J. V., Gragoudas, E. S., Blair, N. P., and Lapus, J. V. (1978): Correlation of epinephrine use and macular edema in aphakic glaucomatous eyes. *Arch. Ophthalmol.*, 96:625–628.
46. Tolentino, F. I., and Schepens, C. L. (1965): Edema of posterior pole after cataract extraction. A biomicroscopic study. *Arch. Ophthalmol.*, 74:781–786.
47. Tso, M. O. M. (1981): Pathology and pathogenesis of cystoid macular edema. *Ophthalmologica*, 183:46–54.
48. West, C. E., Fitzgerald, C. R., and Sewell, J. H. (1973): Cystoid macular edema following aphakic keratoplasty. *Am. J. Ophthalmol.*, 75:77–81.
49. Whitelocke, R. A. F., and Eakins, K. E. (1973): Vascular changes in the anterior uvea of the rabbit produced by prostaglandins. *Arch. Ophthalmol.*, 89:495–499.
50. Whitelocke, R. A. F., Eakins, K. E., and Bennett, A. (1973): Prostaglandins and the eye. *Proc. R. Soc. Med.*, 66:429–434.
51. Yannuzzi, L. A., Landau, A. N., and Turtz, A. I. (1981): Incidence of aphakic cystoid macular edema with the use of topical indomethacin. *Ophthalmology*, 88:947–954.

Commentary

Therapy of Cystoid Macular Edema

The first descriptions of cystoid macular edema (CME) are referenced in Duke-Elder's 1941 volume, *Diseases of the Inner Eye* (2). CME was studied by Bangerter in 1945 (1), and, in 1950, Hruby (4) described the appearance of CME in eyes from which cataract was removed. In 1953, Irvine (5) produced a well-defined clinical description of aphakic CME. In 1966 Gass and Norton (3) firmly fixed the syndrome in the minds of ophthalmologists with their wonderful angiographic study of the lesion.

Gass and Norton (3) pointed out the high incidence of postoperative CME and its relative benignity. In this regard it is important in any consideration of CME occurring after cataract surgery to distinguish between CME that affects visual acuity and CME demonstrable only by fluorescein angiography. The low incidence of the former and the high incidence of the latter suggests that not enough consideration has been given to how the defect is repaired. In other words, the angiographic defect occurs in many, many of whom repair the lesion, and some few of whom do not. Why? Further, it is important to distinguish between the various kinds of "trauma" that occur intraoperatively, and, those events occurring postoperatively that may initiate, aggravate or prolong either visually important CME, e.g., perhaps chronic inflammation, retained lens cortex, leaky barrier, or (?) ultraviolet light.

Once the barrier has been disrupted, the inflammatory cascade begins. Thus it is simpler to prevent than to cure CME. Hence, the emphasis on prophylaxis. Among the many ophthalmologists who have contributed to increased knowledge about this intriguing lesion and its occurrence, Jampol (6), Kraff and coworkers (9) stand high. Others have contributed consistently to pharmacotherapy of this modality, among whom are Yannuzi (13), Miyake (12), KeulendeVos (8), to mention a few. A few words about adverse effects of prolonged use of oral nonsteroidal agents are in order. Topical use is definitely better, from a prophylactic point of view. The nonsalicylate nonsteroidal anti-inflammatory agents given orally all cause gastrointestinal toxicity. They can cause hepatic dysfunction and decrease in renal blood flow. They have the potential to cause blood dyscrasias. They all produce CNS toxicity. Prolonged systemic use of these compounds must not be taken lightly. On the other hand, to use these compounds preoperatively and even postoperatively for a short time may have certain advantages.

With regard to potency ratios for the nonsteroidal agents, a recent experimental publication dealing with the ocular tissues of the rabbit indicates that aspirin is more potent than flurbiprofen which is more potent than indomethacin in suppressing the degree of inflammation. As the authors point out, the discrepancies among these several drugs may be due to their differential effects on the two important pathways implicated in inflammatory responses, the cyclooxygenase and lipoxygenase mediated routes. It should be mentioned that the drugs were equipotent after topical administration (10).

There is controversy (that may be difficult to resolve) concerning the role of ultraviolet light as a contributing factor to visual loss, either by a separate lesion on its own or by contribution to CME. There is no doubt that one can produce a lesion with ultraviolet light in a "trapped" eye (11), but whether this actually takes place in an efficient operative situation is a question that has supporters of both negative (7) and positive answers (see M. Tso, *this volume*). Recently, Jampol et al. (7) have indicated that the incorporation of an ultraviolet filter in the illumination system of the surgical microscope made no difference in the immediate postoperative incidence of CME, but that postoperative CME *was* reduced by the use of an ultraviolet absorbing IOL (9). The latter paper may speak not so much to the cause of CME as to its rate of repair, i.e. inactivation of certain enzymes such as prostaglandin dehydrogenase or the persistence of oxygen derived free radicals, as these factors relate to the rate of repair of the lesion, may be more important.

Another point on a closely related subject: to say that postoperative posterior capsulotomy increases the incidence of CME is to begin from a biased base. Those may be the very eyes that are inflamed enough to require posterior capsulotomy for a good visual result; i.e. in some of these instances, whatever created the need for capsulotomy also created the setting for the development of CME.

For reasons stressed elsewhere (see Commentary to Dr. Leopold's chapter), it may be important to incorporate preoperative steroids in any regimen calculated to reduce the organism's reaction to surgical trauma. Finally, it should be remembered that in evaluating the surgical results of some authors (see W. Stark et al., *this volume*), it is clear that the best prophylaxis is efficient, excellent surgery with maximal preservation of the blood-aqueous barrier. The *repair* of angiographically defective perifoveal capillary leakage is a question that has not as yet been fully addressed.

The Editors

REFERENCES

1. Bangerter, A. (1945): Zur Diagnose, Differentialdiagnose und Therapie des cystoiden Maculaödems (Maculacysten). *Ophthalmologica,* 109:102–122.

2. Duke-Elder, W. S. (1941): *Text-Book of Ophthalmology,* Vol. 3, *Diseases of the Inner Eye,* p. 2592. CV Mosby, St. Louis.
3. Gass, J. D. M., and Norton, E. W. D. (1966): Cystoid macular edema and papilledema following cataract extraction. A fluorescein fundoscopic and angiographic study. *Arch. Ophthalmol.,* 76:646–661.
4. Hruby, K. (1950): Spaltlampenmikroskopie des hinteren Augenabschnittes. Urban und Schwarzenberg, Wien-Innsbruck.
5. Irvine, S. R. (1953): A newly defined vitreous syndrome following cataract surgery. *Am. J. Ophthalmol.,* 36:599–619.
6. Jampol, L. M. (1982): Pharmacologic therapy of aphakic cystoid macular edema. *Ophthalmology,* 89:891–897.
7. Jampol, L. M., Kraff, M. C., Sanders, D. R., et al (1985): Near-UV radiation from the operating microscope and pseudophakic cystoid macular edema. *Arch. Ophthalmol.,* 103:28–30.
8. Keulen-deVos, H. C. J., Van Rij, G., Renardel de LaValette, J. C. G., and Jansen, J. T. G. (1983): Effect of indomethacin in preventing surgically induced miosis. *Br. J. Ophthalmol.,* 67:94–96.
9. Kraff, M. C., Sanders, D. R., Jampol, L. M., Lieberman, H. L. (1985): Effect of an ultraviolet-filtering intraocular lens on cystoid macular edema. *Ophthalmology,* 92:366–369.
10. Kulkarni, P. S., and Srinivasan, D. (1985): Comparative *in vivo* inhibitory effects of nonsteroidal anti-inflammatory agents on prostaglandin synthesis in rabbit ocular tissues. *Arch. Ophthalmol.,* 103:103–106.
11. McDonald, H. R., and Irvine, A. R. (1983): Light-induced maculopathy from the operating microscope in extracapsular cataract extraction and intraocular lens implantation. *Ophthalmology,* 90:945–951.
12. Miyake, K. (1978): Prevention of cystoid macular edema after lens extraction by topical indomethacin. II: A control study in bilateral extractions. *Jpn. J. Ophthalmol.,* 22:80–94.
13. Yannuzzi, L. A., Klein, R. M., Wallyn, R. M., Cohen, N., and Katz, I. (1977): Ineffectiveness of indomethacin in the treatment of chronic cystoid macular edema. *Am. J. Ophthalmol.,* 84:517–519.

Surgical Pharmacology of the Eye,
edited by M. Sears and A. Tarkkanen.
Raven Press, New York © 1985.

Therapy of Cystoid Macular Edema

Lee M. Jampol

*Department of Ophthalmology, Northwestern University School
of Medicine, Chicago, Illinois 60611*

SUMMARY: Cystoid macular edema may be seen in a wide variety of postoperative situations and with vascular, hereditary, inflammatory, and other diseases. In patients with aphakic CME (ACME), prophylaxis and therapy has concentrated on anti-inflammatory drugs, including the prostaglandin synthesis inhibitors and corticosteroids. Prostaglandin synthesis inhibitors appear to be of some value in the prophylaxis of ACME. Corticosteroids appear to be of some therapeutic benefit. Unfortunately, cases that are refractory to these therapies can occur, and permanent visual loss is still seen. The development of surgical techniques and intraocular lenses that minimize the occurrence of cystoid macular edema is desirable. Patients with retinal vasculopathies, including diabetes mellitus and retinal venous obstruction, develop macular edema as well. The exact role of photocoagulation, either of focal or grid type, for these patients is uncertain. It is hoped that ongoing trials of photocoagulation will reveal the value of these therapies. In patients with uveitis syndromes, anti-inflammatory drugs, especially corticosteroids, appear to be of value in the therapy of cystoid macular edema. In patients with hereditary diseases, no known therapy for the cystoid macular edema exists.

The occurrence of macular edema with a cystoid anatomic configuration can be seen in a wide variety of clinical situations (L. Laatikainen, *this volume*). It is seen as a postoperative complication, particularly following cataract surgery, retinal detachment repair, vitrectomy, or keratoplasty. It is also a common finding in patients with retinal vascular diseases including diabetes mellitus, retinal venous obstruction, Coats' disease, von Hippel's disease, parafoveal telangiectasia, and macroaneurysm. Macular edema can be seen in patients with epiretinal membranes, uveitis, hereditary diseases (especially retinitis pigmentosa), following the use of topical epinephrine in the aphakic eye, and also in patients with choroidal diseases (e.g., melanoma) and pigment epithelial disease (e.g., subretinal neovascularization). It is unclear if all of these diverse diseases have common final pathways (e.g., synthesis of prostaglandins) accounting for the similarities of the clinical findings. On scrutiny of these entities it is apparent that in some situations the leakage is from the retinal vasculature; the inner blood-retinal barrier is deficient (e.g., aphakic cystoid macular edema). In other situations the leakage is at the outer blood-retinal barrier, at the level of the pigment epithelium, (e.g., choroidal tumors and subretinal neovascularization). The therapies available for cystoid macular edema will be reviewed.

POSTOPERATIVE CYSTOID MACULAR EDEMA

Angiographic aphakic cystoid macular edema (ACME) is a common finding, being seen, for example, in up to 60% to 77% of patients undergoing intracapsular cataract extraction (32,33). Many of these cases of ACME do not affect visual acuity. Perhaps 2% to 10% of aphakic eyes will have visually significant ACME. In the vast majority of these cases, the macular edema clears and the final visual acuity is unaffected. A small percentage (perhaps 1% to 3%) of patients will show chronic macular edema with visual loss.

Many clinicians believe that extracapsular cataract extraction with an intact posterior capsule has a lower incidence of angiographic and clinical cystoid macular edema (21). The performance of posterior capsulotomy, however, definitely increases the incidence of angiographic cystoid macular edema (Kraff, Sanders, and Jampol, *to be published*), although it is unclear if this raises the incidence of visually significant cystoid macular edema. Complications during cataract surgery, especially vitreous loss, result in an increased incidence and increased persistence of cystoid macular edema. The manner in which the vitreous loss is handled (e.g., automated vitrectomy versus cellulose sponge vitrectomy) does not seem crucial (3), but vitreous incarceration should be avoided. In addition, the placement of some types of intraocular lenses, especially some iris-supported lenses, (metal loop lenses or Copeland lenses) is associated with increased incidence of cystoid macular edema (21). Loose anterior chamber lenses also frequently cause cystoid macular edema (5). In our experience the performance of extracapsular surgery with a posterior chamber implant has a very low incidence of visually significant ACME.

Medical Therapy—ACME

Many eyes with ACME (the Irvine-Gass syndrome) have evidence of inflammation, including discomfort, circumlimbal injection, mild anterior chamber reaction, and vitreal cells. Histopathologic studies have shown inflammation with retinal vasculitis (30). As a result, therapy has concentrated on the use of anti-inflammatory agents (19). There is strong evidence that the *prophylactic* use of topical indomethacin and perhaps other prostaglandin synthesis inhibitors (20) is associated with a reduced incidence of angiographic cystoid macular edema (19). This has been shown by studies by Miyake (33), Yannuzzi and colleagues (49), and Kraff and co-workers (26) (for a detailed review see ref. 19). In the last study, for example, the incidence of angiographic ACME 2½ to 5 months postoperatively in eyes undergoing extracapsular surgery with a posterior chamber implant was 18% in control eyes versus 10% in eyes treated with topical indomethacin (26). In none of these studies has this effect been demonstrated to be sustained beyond 1 year. In addition, since such a small percentage of eyes have clinically significant cystoid macular edema, no study to date has been able to demonstrate the value of prophylactic topical prostaglandin synthesis inhibitors on the incidence of *visually significant* cystoid macular edema (19). In fact, the number of patients to demonstrate this is so large that this study will most likely never be performed.

Use of systemic prostaglandin synthesis inhibitors such as indomethacin has also been demonstrated to be of value in the prophylaxis of ACME (24). However, systemic side effects were common in this study. The value of either topical or systemic corticosteroids in the prophylaxis of ACME remains uncertain. In view of the marked anti-inflammatory effect of corticosteroids and their value in reducing the breakdown of the blood-aqueous barrier following cataract surgery (37), it seems logical that they may be of value in the prevention of ACME. To date, however, no randomized studies have addressed this issue.

Once clinically significant aphakic or pseudophakic cystoid macular edema has occurred, therapy has again primarily utilized anti-inflammatory agents. Stern and co-workers (42) have presented evidence that systemic corticosteroids are of some value in treating pseudophakic (iris-supported lenses) cystoid macular edema. Forty of 49 cases treated with systemic steroids responded at least once. In many cases, the authors used 60 mg of prednisone daily with subsequent tapering. Sub-Tenon's injections were also utilized. These investigators noted recurrences on discontinuation of therapy.

The value of topical corticosteroids in the therapy of ACME is uncertain (19). McEntyre (31) noted he could often produce in patients a rise in intraocular pressure with topical corticosteroids. He reported clearing of cystoid macular edema in many of these patients. He suggested that the cystoid macular edema cleared because of a hydrostatic effect from the increased intraocular pressure. This study had no controls and has not been confirmed; thus, the value of topical corticosteroids remains uncertain.

Topical and systemic prostaglandin synthesis inhibitors are also of possible benefit in the therapy of ACME (19). A study by Burnett and colleagues (7) with topical fenoprofen did not demonstrate an effect on established ACME. However, the number of treated eyes was very small. Yannuzzi and co-workers (48) found that systemic indomethacin given to patients with well-established ACME had no effect. I have seen patients treated with topical or systemic indomethacin in whom the clearing of ACME seemed to correspond to the institution of therapy. However, the value of this therapy has yet to be demonstrated by a controlled prospective study.

Surgical Intervention—ACME

Although Zweng (50) has suggested that photocoagulation might be of benefit for patients with ACME, this has not been confirmed and at present there is no demonstrated efficacy. In patients in whom vitreous incarceration is present in association with ACME, several studies have suggested that surgical intervention with removal of the vitreous has a beneficial effect (9,15). In fact, Fung (16) is currently supervising a prospective randomized study attempting to demonstrate the value of vitrectomy for ACME in patients with vitreous incarceration. Preliminary results have suggested a beneficial effect of treatment. The advent of the neodymium-YAG laser has provided another method of transecting vitreous strands going to the cataract incision. Cutting the vitreous bands is easily performed with minimal risk or complications in most patients. Katzen and co-workers have suggested that cutting the vitreous bands results in clearing of the cystoid macular edema and visual improvement (22,23). There are many problems with these studies as pointed out by Weingeist (46), especially the absence of a control group. It is imperative that a prospective controlled study comparing YAG laser therapy with a control group be performed.

Retinal Detachment, Keratoplasty and Cystoid Macular Edema

Patients undergoing retinal detachment surgery including scleral buckling can also develop cystoid macular edema (28,34). Recently Miyake and co-workers (34) have demonstrated that prophylactic topical prostaglandin synthesis inhibitors are of value in reducing the incidence of cystoid macular edema in these patients. These data showed that topical indomethacin decreased the incidence of the cystoid macular edema after retinal detachment from 33% in the control group to 13% in the treated group. In addition, the severity of the cystoid macular edema was decreased. The value of other anti-inflammatory therapy, such as corticosteroids, in preventing or treating cystoid macular edema associated with retinal detachment or vitreous surgery remains uncertain. Patients undergoing keratoplasty, especially aphakic patients have a very high incidence of cystoid macular edema (47). Again, anti-inflammatory drugs such as prostaglandin synthesis inhibitors and corticosteroids may be of value, but this has not been proved.

RETINAL VASCULOPATHIES

Diabetes Mellitus

Macular edema is a major problem in patients with diabetic retinopathy (10,36,39). As recently reviewed by Bresnick (6), this edema can be subdivided into focal or diffuse leakage. Patients with focal leakage may demonstrate local edema and circinate rings of lipid surrounding leaking microaneurysms. In this situation, photocoagulation of the microaneurysms is often a benefit in reducing the leakage and the lipid exudation (40). Visual improvement may be observed. In patients with multiple focal leaking spots, focal photocoagulation has been used, and some believe that this is of value in reducing leakage

(4,29,36). A few clinical trials have suggested that focal photocoagulation for macular edema may delay or prevent further deterioration of vision but often does not restore the visual acuity to normal (4,36). Both xenon arc and argon laser photocoagulation have been used. It is hoped the Early Treatment Diabetic Retinopathy Study (ETDRS) will clarify the value of focal photocoagulation.

In patients with diffuse macular edema, a common finding, the appropriate interventions are not as clear. If hypertension is present, it has been suggested that reduction of the blood pressure may be of value in reducing macular edema (6). Similarly, improvement in renal and cardiac function, fluid balance, and perhaps better diabetic control may be of value, but this has certainly not been proved. In patients with diffuse macular edema, the relative roles of retinal vascular versus retinal pigment epithelial leakage remains uncertain. Tso and co-workers (45) have emphasized the possible importance of retinal pigment epithelium abnormalities and leakage in the pathogenesis of diabetic retinopathy. Recent therapies have included an attempt to utilize a grid type of macular photocoagulation (almost a scatter type of pattern) in hopes of reducing the edema (6). Some preliminary observations have suggested that this may be of value in reducing macular edema. The protocol for the ETDRS is to investigate the value of placement of 200-μm argon laser burns in the macula. Whether these burns will open up pathways for the egress of fluid from the retina or rather will affect pigment epithelial function is unclear. The ETDRS should establish the value of this therapy in reducing macular edema in diabetes.

Retinal Vein Occlusion

Vision in patients with central retinal vein occlusion may be reduced by macular edema, often taking a cystoid pattern. In young patients, without ischemia, this may be the major cause of visual loss. In some patients resolution of the venous obstruction, with a return of the vasculature toward normal, is associated with reduced macular edema and improvement in the central visual acuity. Unfortunately, other patients do not show clearing, and permanent cystoid macular changes may remain. In addition, scarring of the macula may occur, with permanent visual loss, even if the edema clears. To date, no therapy has been proved of value for patients with this macular edema. Hayreh (18) has suggested that corticosteroids (systemic or retrobulbar) may be of some value in patients with central retinal vein occlusion and macular edema. It has also been suggested that a grid type of photocoagulation might be of value in clearing the edema. Both therapies remain unproved.

Patients with branch retinal vein occlusions may have macular edema with a decrease in visual acuity. In cases where retinal ischemia is absent or does not involve the fovea, clearing of the macular edema is often associated with improvement in the visual acuity. The Branch Retinal Vein Occlusion Study, a multicenter study supported by the National Eye Institute, is investigating the value of scatter photocoagulation in the distribution of the obstructed vein in clearing the macular edema. Some investigations, based on anecdotal cases and nonrandomized series, have suggested that scatter photocoagulation is of value in hastening the clearing of the macular edema (38). Preliminary results of the Branch of Retinal Vein Occlusion Study have confirmed some benefit of scatter photocoagulation in patients with persistent macular edema.

Coats' Disease, von Hippel's Disease, and Parafoveal Telangiectasis

Many patients with Coats' disease (41) (retinal microaneurysms and telangiectasis) or von Hippel's disease (1) may show macular exudation and edema. It has been shown that photocoagulation or cryotherapy of the peripheral vascular abnormalities can result in a decrease in the exudation and fluid in the macular area. Dramatic visual improvement can occur if permanent foveal damage is not present. Some patients show localized parafoveal telangiectasis with secondary macular edema. Gass and Oyakawa (17) have recently classified several varieties of this disorder. The origin of these changes remains uncertain although it is possible that some patients have pigment epithelial disease that precedes the occurrence of the retinal telangiectasis. No therapy has been demonstrated to be of value for this focal leakage. I have utilized indomethacin in several cases without benefit. Since the telangiectasis is often in the macula, it usually cannot be treated with focal photocoagulation.

Macroaneurysm and Epiretinal Membrane

Patients with retinal arterial macroaneurysms also may show macular edema and exudation (2). Focal photocoagulation can be of benefit in treating these patients. Partial or complete closure of the macroaneurysm (either spontaneous or from photocoagulation) usually results in decreased macular edema. Patients with epiretinal membranes also frequently show macular edema. Surgical stripping of these membranes can be associated with a dramatic improvement in the appearance of the retina and a decrease in retinal vascular leakage. Visual improvement may be seen, although a return to normal vision is unusual. These membranes may also peel spontaneously or after photocoagulation of the retina (43).

UVEITIS

Cystoid macular edema is seen in association with uveitis, including pars planitis, nonspecific iridocyclitis, and Behçet's disease. The edema is usually associated with anterior chamber reaction and vitreal cells. It has been widely accepted that anti-inflammatory therapies, especially periocular and systemic corticosteroids, are of value in treating these uveitis syndromes. In more severe cases cytotoxic immunosuppressive drugs may be required. Recently cyclosporin, an immunosuppressive drug that acts on the T-lymphocyte, has been used in patients with uveitis that is refractory to standard therapy (35). Patients may show a resolution of the cystoid macular edema as the uveitis responds. The response to anti-inflammatory therapy, however, may be transient, and recurrences are common as the drugs are tapered.

HEREDITARY DISEASES

Patients with retinitis pigmentosa (11,12) may demonstrate cystoid macular edema, and this may in fact be the cause of the central visual loss in these patients. In addition, patients with Favre-Goldmann retinoschisis show dramatic retinal vascular leakage, leading to macular edema (14). Deutman (8) and others (13) have described an autosomal-dominant disorder characterized by leaking retinal vessels and cystoid macular edema. The origin of the retinal vascular changes in all of these hereditary diseases remains uncertain. No therapies are currently available.

EPINEPHRINE MACULOPATHY

Aphakic patients treated with topical dipivalyl epinephrine or epinephrine may demonstrate cystoid macular edema (25,44). There is good evidence that epinephrine can penetrate to the posterior segment of the eye (27) and affect the vasculature, resulting in cystoid macular edema. Fortunately, this macular edema is usually reversible on discontinuation of these medications.

CHOROIDAL TUMORS AND RETINAL PIGMENT EPITHELIAL DISEASES

The occurrence of choroidal tumors, such as malignant melanoma and hemangioma, can result in overlying degeneration of the pigment epithelium and the occurrence of cystoid changes in the macula area. In addition, pigment epithelial diseases can disrupt the outer blood-retinal barrier and cause cystoid macular edema. Patients with subretinal neovascularization, especially those with senile macular degeneration, may demonstrate, in addition to subretinal neovascularization or retinal pigment epithelial detachment, the occurrence of overlying cystoid macular edema. In these situations the leakage appears to be through the pigment epithelium into the retina. Treatment of the underlying disease, such as the choroidal tumor or the subretinal neovascularization, may result in clearing of the cystoid macular edema.

REFERENCES

1. Annesley, W. H., Jr., Leonard, B. C., Shields, J. A., and Tasman, W. S. (1977): Fifteen year review of treated cases of retinal angiomatosis. *Trans. Am. Acad. Ophthal. Otolaryngol.* 83:446–453.

2. Asdourian, G. K., Goldberg, M. F., Jampol, L. M., and Rabb, M. (1977): Retinal macroaneurysms. *Arch. Ophthalmol.,* 95:624–629.
3. Berger, B. B., Zweig, K. C., and Peyman, G. A. (1980): Vitreous loss managed by anterior vitrectomy. Long term follow-up of 59 cases. *Arch. Ophthalmol.,* 98:1245–1247.
4. Blankenship, G. W. (1979): Diabetic macular edema and argon laser photocoagulation: A prospective randomized study. *Ophthalmology,* 86:69–78.
5. Braude, L. S., Feigelman, M. J., Sugar, J., and Jampol, L. M. (1984): Management of loose Choyce-style anterior chamber lenses. *Ophthalmic Surg.,* 15:502–507.
6. Bresnick, G. H. (1983): Diabetic maculopathy. A critical review highlighting diffuse macular edema. *Ophthalmology,* 90:1301–1317.
7. Burnett, J., Tessler, H., Isenberg, S., et al. (1983): Double-masked trial of fenoprofen sodium: Treatment of chronic aphakic cystoid macular edema. *Ophthalmic Surg.,* 17:150–152.
8. Deutman, A. F., Pinckers, A. J. L. G., and Aan de Kerk, A. L. (1976): Dominantly inherited cystoid macular edema. *Am. J. Ophthalmol.,* 82:540–548.
9. Federman, J. L., Annesley, W. H., Jr., Sarin, L. K., and Remer, P. (1980): Vitrectomy and cystoid macular edema. *Ophthalmology,* 87:622–628.
10. Ferris, F. L., and Patz, A. (1983): Macular edema—a major complication of diabetic retinopathy. Symposium on medical and surgical diseases of the retina and vitreous. *Trans. New Orleans Acad. Ophthalmol.,* pp. 307–316.
11. Fetkenhour, C. L., Choromokos, E., Weinstein, G., Jr., and Shoch, D. (1977): Cystoid macular edema in retinitis pigmentosa. *Trans. Am. Acad. Ophthalmol. Otolaryngol.,* 83:515–521.
12. Fishman, G. A., Fishman, M., and Maggiano, J. M. (1977): Macular lesions associated with retinitis pigmentosa. *Arch. Ophthalmol.,* 95:798–803.
13. Fishman, G. A., Goldberg, M. F., and Trautmann, J. C. (1979): Dominantly inherited cystoid macular edema. *Ann. Ophthalmol.,* 11:21–27.
14. Fishman, G. A., Jampol, L. M., and Goldberg, M. F. (1976): Diagnostic feature of the Favre-Goldmann syndrome. *Br. J. Ophthalmol.,* 60:345–353.
15. Fung, W. E. (1980): Anterior vitrectomy for chronic aphakic cystoid macular edema. *Ophthalmology,* 87:189–193.
16. Fung, W. E. (1982): Surgical therapy for chronic aphakic cystoid macular edema. *Ophthalmology,* 89:898–901.
17. Gass, J. D., and Oyakawa, R. T. (1982): Idiopathic juxtafoveal retinal telangiectasis. *Arch. Ophthalmol.,* 100:769–780.
18. Hayreh, S. S. (1977): Central retinal vein occlusion. Differential diagnosis and management. *Trans. Am. Acad. Ophthalmol. Otolaryngol.,* 83:379–391.
19. Jampol, L. M. (1982): Pharmacologic therapy of aphakic cystoid macular edema. A review. *Ophthalmology,* 80:891–897.
20. Jampol, L. M. (1984): Nonsteroidal antiinflammatory drugs in ophthalmology. American Academy of Ophthalmology Module 3. *Focal Points 1984:1–7.*
21. Jampol, L. M., Sanders, D. R., and Kraff, M. C. (1984): Prophylaxis and therapy of aphakic cystoid macular edema. *Surv. Ophthalmol.,* 28(Suppl.):535–539.
22. Katzen, L. E., Fleischman, J. A., and Trokel, S. (1983): YAG laser treatment of cystoid macular edema. *Am. J. Ophthalmol.,* 95:589–592.
23. Katzen, L. E., Lapinsky, P. T., Fleischman, J. A., and Trokel, S. (1984): YAG laser treatment of cystoid macular edema—clinical update. *Cataract,* 1:27–29.
24. Klein, R. M., Katzin, H. M., and Yannuzzi, L. A. (1979): The effect of indomethacin pretreatment on aphakic cystoid macular edema. *Am. J. Ophthalmol.,* 87:487–489.
25. Kolker, A. E., and Becker, B. (1968): Epinephrine maculopathy. *Arch. Ophthalmol.,* 79:552–562.
26. Kraff, M. C., Sanders, D. R., Jampol, L. M., et al. (1982): Prophylaxis of pseudophakic cystoid macular edema with topical indomethacin. *Ophthalmology,* 89:885–890.
27. Kramer, S. G. (1976): Retinal uptake of topical epinephrine in aphakia. *Symposium on Ocular Therapy,* edited by I. H. Leopold and R. P. Burns, pp. 73–83. John Wiley, New York.
28. Lobes, L. A., Jr., and Grand, M. G. (1980): Incidence of cystoid macular edema following scleral buckling procedures. *Arch. Ophthalmol.,* 98:1230–1232.
29. Marous, D. F., and Aaberg, T. M. (1977): Argon laser photocoagulation of diabetic cystoid maculopathy. *Ann. Ophthalmol.,* 9:365–372.
30. Martin, N. F., Green, W. R., and Martin, L. W. (1983): Retinal phlebitis in the Irvine-Gass Syndrome. *Am. J. Ophthalmol.,* 83:377–386.

31. McEntyre, J. M. (1978): A successful treatment for aphakic cystoid macular edema. *Ann. Ophthalmol.,* 10:1219–1224.
32. Meredith, T. A., Kenyon, K. R., Singerman, L. J., et al. (1976): Perifoveal vascular leakage and macular edema after intracapsular cataract extraction. *Br. J. Ophthalmol.,* 60:765–769.
33. Miyake, K. (1977): Prevention of cystoid macular edema after lens extraction by topical indomethacin. 1. A preliminary report. *Albrecht von Graefes Arch. Klin. Exp. Ophthalmol.,* 203:81–88.
34. Miyake, K., Miyake, Y., Maekubo, K., Asakura, M., and Manabe, R. (1983): Incidence of cystoid macular edema after retinal detachment surgery and the use of topical indomethacin. *Am. J. Ophthalmol.,* 95:451–456.
35. Nussenblatt, R. B., Palestine, A. G., Rook, A. H., Scher, I., Wacker, W. B., and Gery, I. (1983): Treatment of intraocular inflammatory diseases with cyclosporin A. *Lancet,* 2:235–238.
36. Patz, A., Schatz, H., Berkow, J. W., Gittelsohn, A. M., and Ticho, U. (1973): Macular edema—an overlooked complication of diabetic retinopathy. *Trans. Am. Acad. Ophthalmol. Otolaryngol.,* 77:34–42.
37. Sanders, D. R., Kraff, M. C., Lieberman, H. L., et al. (1982): Breakdown and reestablishment of blood-aqueous barrier with implant surgery. *Arch. Ophthalmol.,* 100:588–590.
38. Schatz, H. (1981): Treatment of foveal cystic edema caused by branch vein occlusion. *Ophthalmology,* 88(Suppl):49.
39. Schatz, H., and Patz, A. (1976): Cystoid maculopathy in diabetics. *Arch. Ophthalmol.,* 94:761–768.
40. Spalter, H. F. (1971): Photocoagulation of circinate maculopathy in diabetic retinopathy. *Am. J. Ophthalmol.,* 71:242–250.
41. Spitznas, M., Joussen, F., and Wessing, A. (1976): Treatment of Coats' disease with photocoagulation. *Albrecht v. Graefes Arch. Klin. Exp. Ophthalmol.,* 199:31–37.
42. Stern, A. L., Taylor, D. M., Dalburg, L. A., and Cosentino, R. T. (1981): Pseudophakic cystoid maculopathy, a study of 50 cases. *Ophthalmology,* 88:942–946.
43. Sumers, K. D., Jampol, L. M., Goldberg, M. F., and Huamonte, F. U. (1980): Spontaneous separation of epiretinal membranes. *Arch. Ophthalmol.,* 98:318–320.
44. Thomas, J. V., Gragoudas, E. S., Blair, N. P., et al. (1978): Correlation of epinephrine use and macular edema in aphakic glaucomatous eyes. *Arch. Ophthalmol.,* 96:625–628.
45. Tso, M. O. M., Cunha-Vaz, J. G. F., Shih, C. Y., and Jones, C. W. (1979): A clinicopathologic study of the blood-retinal barrier in experimental diabetes. *Invest. Ophthalmol. Vis. Sci.,* 18(Suppl):169.
46. Weingeist, T. (1983): YAG laser treatment of cystoid macular edema. *Am. J. Ophthalmol.,* 96:407–408.
47. West, C. E., Fitzgerald, C. R., and Sewell, J. H. (1973): Cystoid macular edema following aphakic keratoplasty. *Am. J. Ophthalmol.,* 75:77–81.
48. Yannuzzi, L. A., Klein, R. M., Wallyn, R. H., Cohen, N., and Katz, I. (1977): Ineffectiveness of indomethacin in the treatment of chronic cystoid macular edema. *Am. J. Ophthalmol.,* 84:517–519.
49. Yannuzzi, L. A., Landau, A. N., and Turtz, A. I. (1981): Incidence of aphakic cystoid macular edema with the use of topical indomethacin. *Ophthalmology,* 88:947–954.
50. Zweng, H. C., Little, H. L., and Peabody, R. R. (1968): Laser photocoagulation of macular lesions. *Trans. Am. Acad. Ophthalmol. Otolaryngol.,* 72:377–388.

Subject Index